CONNECTIVE TISSUE DISEASES

CONNECTIVE TISSUE DISEASES

Edited by

Jill J. F. Belch MB, FRCP, MD

Reader, Consultant Physician and Head of Section of Vascular and Inflammatory Medicine, Ninewells Hospital and Medical School, Dundee, UK

and

Robert B. Zurier MD

Professor of Medicine, Director, Division of Rheumatology, University of Massachusetts Medical Center, Worcester, Massachusetts, USA

CHAPMAN & HALL MEDICAL

London · Glasgow · Weinheim · New York · Tokyo · Melbourne · Madras

Published by
Chapman & Hall, 2–6 Boundary Row, London SE1 8HN, UK

Chapman & Hall, 2–6 Boundary Row, London SE1 8HN, UK

Blackie Academic & Professional, Wester Cleddens Road, Bishopbriggs, Glasgow G64 2NZ, UK

Chapman & Hall GmbH, Pappelallee 3, 69469 Weinheim, Germany

Chapman & Hall USA, 115 Fifth Avenue, New York, NY 10003, USA

Chapman & Hall Japan, ITP-Japan, Kyowa Building, 3F, 2-2-1 Hirakawacho, Chiyoda-ku, Tokyo 102, Japan

Chapman & Hall Australia, 102 Dodds Street, South Melbourne, Victoria 3205, Australia

Chapman & Hall India, R. Seshadri, 32 Second Main Road, CIT East, Madras 600 035, India

First edition 1995

© 1995 Chapman & Hall

Typeset in 10/12pt Palatino by Type Study, Scarborough
Printed in Great Britain at the University Press, Cambridge

ISBN 0 412 48620 2

A catalogue record for this book is available from the British Library

Library of Congress Catalog Card Number: 94-74689

CONTENTS

CONTRIBUTORS

S. B. ABRAMSON
Chairman
Department of Rheumatology
Hospital for Joint Diseases
301E 17th Street
New York
NY 10003
USA

K. F. AL-JARALLAH
Department of Medicine
McMaster University
Hamilton
Ontario
Canada L8N 325

N. B. ALLEN
Associate Professor
Division of Rheumatology and Immunology
Duke University Medical Center
Durham
North Carolina 27710
USA

B. M. ANSELL
Retired Head of Division of Rheumatology
Clinical Research Centre
Northwick Park Hospital
Harrow
UK

J. J. F. BELCH
Consultant Physician and Reader
Head of Section of Vascular and
    Inflammatory Medicine
University Department of Medicine
Ninewells Hospital and Medical School
Dundee DD1 9S7
UK

H. BIRD
Reader in Rheumatology
University of Leeds
Clinical Pharmacology Unit
Chapel Allerton Hospital
Chapeltown Road
Leeds LS7 4SA
UK

W. W. BUCHANAN
Department of Medicine
McMaster University
Hamilton
Ontario
Canada L8N 325

E. H. S. CHOY
Lecturer and Senior Registrar
Rheumatology Unit
Guy's Hospital
St Thomas' Street
London SE1 9RT
UK

D. M. FAGUNDUS
Senior Fellow in Rheumatology
Division of Rheumatology and Immunology
Department of Medicine
Medical University of South Carolina
171 Ashley Avenue
Charleston
SC 29425–2229
USA

K. A. HAINES
The Hospital for Joint Diseases
301E 17th Street
New York
NY 10003
USA

R. W. HOFFMAN
Associate Professor of Internal Medicine and
    Pathology
Division of Immunology and Rheumatology
University of Missouri-Columbia
Columbia
MO 65212
USA

C. A. LANGFORD
Fellow
Division of Rheumatology and Immunology
Duke University Arthritis Center
Duke University Medical Center
Durham
North Carolina
USA

E. C. LeROY
Professor of Medicine (Rheumatology)
Director
Division of Rheumatology and Immunology
Department of Medicine
Medical University of South Carolina
171 Ashley Avenue
Charleston
SC 29425-2229
USA

R. M. McCALLUM
Assistant Professor of Medicine
Division of Rheumatology and Immunology
Duke University Arthritis Center
Duke University Medical Center
Durham
North Carolina
USA

C. MAPLE
ARC Research Fellow
University Department of Medicine
Ninewells Hospital and Medical School
Dundee DD1 9SY
UK

T. A. MEDSGER, JR.
Professor of Medicine
Chief of Division of Rheumatology and
    Clinical Immunology
Department of Medicine
University of Pittsburgh School of Medicine
Pittsburgh
PA 15261
USA

A. MORGAN
Research Fellow in Rheumatology
University of Leeds
Clinical Pharmacology Unit
Chapel Allerton Hospital
Chapeltown Road
Leeds LS7 4SA
UK

H. M. MOUTSOPOULOS
Professor of Medicine and Director
Department of Pathophysiology
School of Medicine
National University of Athens
Athens
Greece

C. V. ODDIS
Associate Professor of Medicine
Division of Rheumatology and Clinical
    Immunology
Department of Medicine
University of Pittsburgh School of Medicine
Pittsburgh
PA 15261
USA

G. S. PANAYI
ARC Professor of Rheumatology
Rheumatology Unit
Guy's Hospital
St Thomas' Street
London SE1 9RT
UK

J. K. RAO
Fellow
Division of Rheumatology and Immunology
Duke University Medical Center and
    Center for Health Services Research in
    Primary Care
Durham Veterans Affairs Medical Center
Durham
North Carolina 27710
USA

D. G. I. SCOTT
Consultant in Rheumatology
Department of Rheumatology
Norfolk and Norwich Hospital
Brunswick Road
Norwich
Norfolk NR1 3SR
UK

G. C. SHARP
Curators' Professor of Internal Medicine and
    Pathology
Director
Division of Immunology and Rheumatology
University of Missouri-Columbia
Columbia
MO 65212
USA

C. B. TALLMAN
University of Massachusetts
Medical Center
55 Lake Avenue
Worcester
MA 01655
USA

A. G. TZIOUFAS
Rheumatologist
Department of Pathophysiology
School of Medicine
National University of Athens
Athens
Greece

A. K. VAISHNAW
Research Registrar
Rheumatology Unit
Department of Medicine
Hammersmith Hospital
Du Cane Road
London W12 0NN
UK

M. J. WALPORT
Professor of Medicine
Head
Rheumatology Unit
Department of Medicine
Royal Postgraduate Medical School
Hammersmith Hospital
Du Cane Road
London W12 0NN
UK

R. A. WATTS
Senior Registrar in Rheumatology
Norfolk and Norwich Hospital
Brunswick Road
Norfolk
Norwich NR1 3SR
UK

R. B. ZURIER
Professor of Medicine
Director
Division of Rheumatology
University of Massachusetts
Medical Center
55 Lake Avenue
Worcester
MA 01655
USA

PREFACE

Connective Tissue Diseases represents an attempt to gather under one cover information about the connective tissue disorders. Many book chapters and journals address this area but only a few books are devoted solely to this subject. The term '**Connective Tissue Diseases**' describes a group of conditions characterized by multisystem involvement, and abnormal immunological features such as auto-antibodies and immune complex deposition. They have a world-wide distribution and usually affect the middle-aged population who are the main work force of the community.

Because of the systemic nature of these diseases, medical practitioners of all disciplines will be involved in the management of these conditions at some stage of their career. For the same reason, connective tissue diseases often appear in lists of differential diagnoses for other conditions. Considerable overlap exists in the presenting features amongst these conditions. Fortunately, recent advances in immunology have contributed a great deal to the understanding of these disorders leading to new classification systems. Improved knowledge of the immunogenesis of connective tissue disease has also allowed earlier cases to be identified thus improving the overall prognosis of these conditions. On the other hand, discovery of new auto-antibodies make study of this disorder more difficult for the non-specialist. Despite our much improved knowledge of the immunological basis and classification of these diseases the initial diagnosis and management of these serious conditions remain difficult tasks for the physician. Nonetheless, not many textbooks are devoted to discussion of connective tissue diseases alone. This book is intended for the physician who may be involved in management of patients with connective tissue disease.

This book gives a detailed and comprehensive account of the major connective tissue diseases. In addition, two chapters are devoted to Sjögren's syndrome and Raynaud's Phenomenon which may exist on their own as distinct entities, or as initial presenting problems of connective tissue disease. A full chapter is also devoted to Rheumatoid Arthritis, a disorder which some consider to be a true connective tissue disease. Each chapter includes a historical background of the condition followed by a summary of the epidemiology, pathophysiology, clinical manifestations, investigation procedures and treatment strategies. All the chapters are authored by leaders in their field based either in Europe or the USA. We hope the reader will find the text clear, informative and up-to-date.

Jill J. F. Belch
Robert B. Zurier

INFLAMMATORY MEDIATORS IN CONNECTIVE TISSUE DISORDERS

1

K. A. Haines and S. B. Abramson

INTRODUCTION

Inflammation, both acute and chronic, is mediated by a complex interaction of the cellular and humoral components of the immune system. In conditions of bacterial infection or tissue injury, the sequence of events begins with a known inflammatory trigger and a discussion of the process of inflammation can proceed in a logical order. However, etiologies of the various connective tissue diseases remain undefined. One must, therefore, arbitrarily dissect the inflammation of autoimmune disorders into its component parts while keeping in mind the complex interaction of these components. This chapter will review both inflammatory mediators released from cells – neutrophils, monocytes and platelets – as well as humoral activators of these cells with particular emphasis upon chemoattractants, complement components and immune complexes. The pathogenic mechanisms by which inflammatory mediators provoke vascular injury in systemic lupus erythematosus will also be discussed.

CELLULAR MEDIATORS OF INFLAMMATION

Three types of myeloid-derived cells – neutrophils, macrophages and platelets – play a central role in the development of acute, subacute and chronic immunologically-mediated tissue injury. The activation of these cells in response to chemoattractants, immune complexes and other stimuli provokes the release of inflammatory mediators which account for the diverse manifestations of autoimmune disease.

NEUTROPHILS

Release of toxic proteolytic enzymes

While the chief function of polymorphonuclear leukocytes is phagocytosis and destruction of microorganisms, these cells also mediate tissue injury in necrotizing vasculitis and contribute to the synovitis in the inflammatory arthritides, such as rheumatoid arthritis[1]. Neutrophil responses following activation include adherence, chemotaxis and the release of toxic mediators. In autoimmune diseases, immune complexes and activated complement components engage specific cell surface receptors, and thereby induce the secretion of inflammatory mediators (e.g. proteolytic enzymes and superoxide anion) with resultant tissue injury. Neutrophils contain two morphologically distinct granules (specific and azurophilic) that contain proteases, which under normal circumstances are

Connective Tissue Diseases. Edited by Jill J. F. Belch and Robert B. Zurier. Published in 1995 by Chapman & Hall, London. ISBN 0 412 48620 2

sequestered within the granule and the phagosome, presenting no threat to the host. However, the extracellular release of granule contents may promote inflammation and damage at tissue sites. Phagocytosis is not necessary for neutrophil degranulation, which may be provoked by soluble stimuli (e.g. C5a, interleukin-8 (IL-8)). Degranulation is augmented when neutrophils encounter stimuli deposited on a surface: lysosomal release unfolds by a process of reverse endocytosis, or what has been called 'frustrated phagocytosis'. This exuberant release of lysosomal enzymes from neutrophils may be relevant to the pathogenesis of tissue injury in diseases characterized by the deposition of immune complexes on cell surfaces or on such extracellular surfaces as vascular basement membranes or articular cartilage[2].

Table 1.1 Potential effects of oxygen-free radicals*

On cells
Killing of microbes (e.g. viruses, bacteria, fungi, protozoa)
Injury of tumor cells
Stimulation of secretion by platelets, mast cells, endothelial cells, glomerular cells
Mutagenesis of bacteria and mammalian cells
Tumor promotion and carcinogenesis

On extracellular products
Generation of chemotactic lipids from arachidonate
Activation of leukocyte collagenase, gelatinase
Inactivation of chemotactic leukotrienes, chemotactic peptides, α-1-antiprotease, met-enkephalin, leukocyte hydrolases, bacterial toxins

* Adapted from [3]

Production of toxic oxygen radicals

When phagocytic leukocytes are activated, molecular oxygen consumption by the leukocyte is increased. The majority of this oxygen is transformed directly into superoxide anion radicals. This toxic free radical is produced by the addition of an extra electron to molecular oxygen by an assembled multiprotein complex which requires membrane-bound cytochrome b_{558} and key cytosolic proteins (including a *ras*-related low molecular weight GTP-binding protein). Stimulated neutrophils also produce hydrogen peroxide, hydroxyl radicals and, possibly, singlet oxygen. Oxygen-derived free radicals are significant mediators of inflammation causing tissue injury and irreversible modification of macromolecules[3] (Table 1.1).

Complement receptors and neutrophil adhesion

Phagocytic cells also express receptors for the complement fragment C3b (designated CR1) and its inactivated cleavage product iC3b (designated CR3, or CD11b/CD18)[4]. On the surface of phagocytes, both CR1 and CR3 play important roles in the clearance of particles, such as opsonized bacteria, to which C3b or iC3b are bound. This clearance mechanism is essential for the removal of immune complexes containing C3b and iC3b[5]. In addition to its role as a receptor for iC3b, CR3 is the major neutrophil adhesion molecule responsible for the capacity of the neutrophil to adhere to vascular endothelium and to other neutrophils[6]. This adhesion of activated neutrophils to vascular endothelium is one of the initial events in the inflammatory process. Adhesion depends in part upon the activation of surface glycoproteins known as β_2 integrins which are heterodimers consisting of a common beta subunit (CD18) and distinct alpha subunits (CD11a, CD11b, CD11c). In the neutrophil the most important β_2 integrin appears to be CD11b/CD18 (CR3), required for normal phagocytosis, aggregation, adhesion and chemotaxis. Intercellular adhesion molecule-1 (ICAM-1), expressed on resting and activated endothelial cells, has been identified as a ligand for the CD18 integrins[7]. Interaction between CD18 and ICAM-1 modulates both the adhesion of neutrophils to vascular endothelium and their egress to the extravascular space. The initial rolling of activated neutrophils on endothelium, a prerequisite for CD18-dependent adhesion under conditions of flow, is mediated by a separate molecular interaction: that between the selectins, E-selectin and P-selectin, on the endothelial cell and a carbohydrate ligand, sialyl-Le^x, on the neutrophil[7–9]. In addition, the neutrophil expresses L-selectin on its surface, which also promotes rolling, and is shed from the plasma membrane upon cell activation. The redundancy with regard to selectin function may in part be explained by the different kinetics of their participation in the events of intracellular adhesion: L-selectin is shed within **seconds** of neutrophil activation; P-selectin is stored in the Weibel–Palade bodies in endothelial cells and expressed on the surface within **minutes** following exposure of the cells to acute stimuli, such as thrombin; and E-selectin is upregulated over several **hours** following cytokine exposure in a process which requires transcription and translation of new protein.

Important therapeutic strategies have evolved from the recent recognition that the ability of toxic mediators released by activated neutrophils to injure vascular endothelium is dependent upon their capacity to adhere to the target cell. Experimental models of immune-complex mediated lung injury, ischemia-reperfusion injury, and adjuvant arthritis can each be ameliorated by strategies which utilize blocking antibodies to CD18, ICAM-1 or selectins in order to prevent neutrophil-endothelial cell attachment. It is likely that these antiadhesion strategies will lead to novel clinical interventions.

MACROPHAGES AS SECRETORY CELLS IN INFLAMMATION

Release of proteases

Macrophages express the three major classes of Fc receptors as well as B_1, B_2 and B_3

Table 1.2 Secretory products of mononuclear phagocytes*

Polypeptide hormones
Interleukin 1-α and 1-β (collectively IL-1)
Tumor necrosis factor-α (cachectin)
Interferon-α
Interferon-γ (confirmation needed)
Platelet-derived growth factor(s)
Transforming growth factor-β
β-Endorphin
Neutrophil-activating factor/interleukin-8

Complement (C) components
Classical path: C1, C4, C2, C3, C5
Alternative path: factor B, factor D, properdin
Inhibitors: C3b inactivator, β-1H

Coagulation factors
Intrinsic path: IX, X, V, prothrombin
Extrinsic path: VII
Surface activities: tissue factor, prothrombinase
Prothrombolytic activity: plasminogen activator
    inhibitors, plasmin inhibitors

Bioactive lipids
Cyclooxygenase products: prostaglandin E_2,
    prostaglandin $F_{2\alpha}$, prostacyclin, thromboxane
Lipoxygenase products:
    monohydroxyeicosatetraenoic acids,
    dihydroxyeicosatetraenoic acids, leukotrienes B,
    C, D, E
Platelet-activating factors (1 O-alkyl-2-acetyl-*sn*-
    glyceryl-3-phosphorylcholine)

Reactive oxygen intermediates (e.g. superoxide anion)

Reactive nitrogen intermediates (e.g. nitric oxide)

* Adapted from [3]

integrins. These surface receptors facilitate phagocytosis of opsonized particles, intercellular adhesion and adhesion to extracellular matrix proteins. Macrophages secrete up to 100 substances, ranging from free radicals, such as superoxide anion, to large macromolecules, such as fibronectin[3]. Some products are secreted in response to inflammatory stimuli while others are constitutively released (Table 1.2). For example, plasminogen activator, which converts plasminogen to plasmin, is secreted at low levels by mono-cytes or non-stimulated macrophages, and is augmented by inflammatory stimuli. Plasmin not only degrades fibrin, but also activates complement components, C1 and C3. Acti-vated macrophages produce plasminogen ac-tivator in two forms: a soluble form released into the extracellular medium and a cell-associated form. Collagenase is another neutral protease constitutively secreted at low levels by non-activated macrophages; stimu-lation with interleukin-1 (IL-1) and toxin augments secretion. In such chronic inflam-matory sites as the rheumatoid synovium, collagen may be partially degraded by macro-phage-secreted collagenases. Lysozyme, a cationic protein which hydrolyses the glucose linkages in bacterial cell walls, is also a macro-phage secretory product. It has also been detected in human osteoarthritic cartilage where it is believed to be secreted by activated chondrocytes.

When stimulated by exposure to immune complexes, endotoxin, IL-1, or C3b-coated particles, macrophages and monocytes ex-hibit a procoagulant activity[10]. The pro-coagulant products include tissue factor (identified as a receptor for factor VII), factor X activator, prothrombin activator, and vitamin K-dependent clotting factors II, VII, IX and X. Monocytes in rheumatic disease patients dis-play a higher procoagulant-producing activity than normal – likely a result of exposure to cytokines and cleavage products of comp-lement. Increased procoagulant activity may contribute to fibrin deposition at sites of in-flammation. Whether such increased procoa-gulant activity observed in these conditions also promotes a 'hypercoagulable' state (e.g. as observed in SLE) remains unknown.

Production of cytokines

As shown in Table 1.2, macrophages also secrete a variety of polypeptide hormones which regulate immune function and in-flammation as well as wound healing and repair[11]. Macrophages, for example, pro-duce three cytokines, interleukin-1α(IL-1α), IL-1β and tumor necrosis factor-α (TNF-α), which not only have overlapping functions, but are also capable of inducing each others release by macrophages themselves[3]. Macrophages also produce the cytokine neutrophil-activating peptide-1/IL-8 which is a potent neutrophil chemoattractant. The pro-duction of IL-8, induced by IL-1α, IL-1β and TNF-α has been described in a variety of IL-1β tissues, including alveolar macrophages, renal mesangial cells and psoriatic skin lesions[12].

Arachidonate-derived mediators of inflammation

In addition to the capacity to secrete diverse biologically active proteins, monocytes and macrophages are significant sources of lipid mediators of inflammation which are derived from arachidonic acid. Arachidonic acid is stored in the cell membrane as a component of its constituent phospholipids, primarily phos-phatidylcholine and phosphatidylinositol. Arachidonate is cleaved from the glycerol backbone (R_2 position) of these phospholipids after stimulation of inflammatory cells and activation of phospholipase A_2. Arachidonate may be a second messenger in its own right[13]. However, it is also metabolized via two distinct enzymatic pathways, the cyclo-oxygenase pathway and the lipoxygenase pathway, generating prostaglandins and leukotrienes, respectively.

Prostaglandin G/H synthase is the initial enzyme in the prostaglandin pathway, and is the target enzyme for inactivation by non-steroidal anti-inflammatory drugs. There are two isoforms of this enzyme which, although products of two distinct genes, are highly homologous. Despite the structural hom-ology, these genes are under separate control. The first gene identified, PGH-1, appears to be constituitively expressed in a variety of cells. Expression of PGH synthase-2 may be re-stricted to inflammatory cells, is induced by a variety of cytokines and growth factors and is inhibited by dexamethosone (reviewed in[14]). Of interest, neutrophils make little, if any, prostaglandins whereas monocyte/ macrophages, platelets, endothelial cells and tissue mast cells (among others) actively secrete prostaglandins in response to inflammatory stimuli. Activation of PGH synthase(s) results in the generation of the unstable endoperoxides, PGG and PGH. These products are metabolized to PGD_2, PGE_2 and $PGF_{2\alpha}$ by distinct isomerases or by spontaneous hydrolysis of the peroxide ring. Thromboxane (TXA_2) and prostacyclin (PGI_2) are synthesized by specific isomerases from PGG and PGH.

The stable prostaglandins are at least in part pro-inflammatory compounds. They cause fever, vasodilatation, potentiate the activity of the kinins and augment neutrophil chemotaxis. However, prostaglandins also have significant anti-inflammatory effects. As early as 1973, Zurier and Ballas demonstrated that high doses of PGE inhibit the development of adjuvant arthritis[15], most likely due to their ability to provoke increments in cyclic AMP. In parallel, it has been demonstrated that treatment of neutrophils with PGE_1 inhibits activation of these cells to a large degree: aggregation, superoxide anion generation and lysosomal enzyme release provoked by N-formyl-methionyl-phenylalanine (FMLP) are all inhibited[16]. Moreover, treatment of neutrophils with the cyclooxygenase inhibitors, NSAIDS, **potentiates**, rather than inhibits the prostaglandin effect[17]. Thus, not only can prostaglandins be anti-inflammatory, NSAIDs are unlikely to be exerting their anti-inflammatory effects via inhibition of prostaglandin synthases. It is more likely that non-steroidal anti-inflammatory agents, at the relatively high dose required to inhibit inflammation, inhibit neutrophil responses via their capacity to uncouple membrane receptors for chemoattractants, immune complexes, etc. from cellular activation systems[18].

Arachidonic acid is also metabolized by the lipoxygenase pathway of enzyme activation which generates such mediators of acute inflammation as leukotriene B_4, the sulfidopeptide leukotrienes, LTC_4, D_4 and E_4 and the lipoxins, LXA_4 and LXB_4. These compounds all bind to specific receptors on a variety of cell types. They provoke chemotactic activity and stimulate secretion from their various leukocyte targets. (Lipoxins have also been described as competitive inhibitors of leukotrienes.) The leukotrienes and lipoxins trigger other functions involved in acute inflammation, e.g. vasodilatation and smooth muscle contraction, upon binding to other cell types. There are several lipoxygenases, each with its own cell distribution. Myeloid cells (neutrophils, eosinophils, monocytes/macrophages, basophils, mast cells) contain the 5-lipoxygenase enzyme[19]; platelets and neural cells contain the 12-lipoxygenase enzyme [20,21]; neutrophils, eosinophils, reticulocytes and airway epithelium contain the 15-lipoxygenase enzyme[22]. 5-lipoxygenase activity is critical in the formation of leukotrines. In resting cells the 5-lipoxygenase is in the cytosol as a ferrous (Fe^{2+}) enzyme. Upon activation of the cell, the lipoxygenase is converted to the ferric (Fe^{3+}) state and translocates to the cell membrane. There it complexes with the 'five lipoxygenase activating protein' known as FLAP and converts arachidonic acid to 5-hydroperoxyeicosatetraenoic acid and subsequently to leukotriene A_4 (LTA_4). LTA_4 can be metabolized to LTB_4 (neutrophils and macrophages) or to LTC_4, D_4 and E_4 (eosinophils, mast cells, basophils, macrophages) or secreted. This secreted form takes on critical importance as few cells other than myeloid cells contain the 5-lipoxygenase; however, most cells contain an LTA_4 hydrolase and may be able to convert this product to leukotrienes. Indeed, the lipoxins are generated by a second lipoxygenation step – coincubation of activated neutrophils and platelets results in the generation of lipoxin A_4, B_4 and their isomers [23,24].

Nitric oxide as a modulator of inflammation

Macrophages are also among the cellular sources of reactive nitrogen intermediates, such as nitric oxide. Nitric oxide, although originally identified as a product of endothelial cells which accounts for 'endothelium derived relaxation factor' activity, is now appreciated to be a highly reactive molecule with diverse biological functions. The exposure of macrophages to cytokines (e.g. IL-1β, interferon-γ) markedly increases nitric oxide production. Activities of nitric oxide, which may be important in the inflammatory response, include vasodilation and its capacity to react with superoxide anion to form toxic perioxynitrite compounds. Consistent with a pro-inflammatory role, the inhibition of nitric oxide synthesis has recently been demonstrated to reduce the severity of disease in streptococcal cell wall-induced arthritis in Lewis rats[25]. However, like stable prostaglandins, nitric oxide may exert anti-inflammatory properties particularly with regard to the protection of endothelial cells from activated neutrophils and platelets. For example, nitric oxide inhibits neutrophil and platelet aggregation, inhibits the adhesion of neutrophils to endothelial cells and inhibits neutrophil oxidant production, and thereby may provide a 'teflon coat' for the blood vessel walls[26].

PLATELETS

Platelets, derived from marrow megakaryocytes, are involved in hemostasis, wound healing and cellular responses to injury [27,28]. In primitive organisms, a single cell type served both leukocyte and platelet functions. In higher organisms, platelets have retained some properties of inflammatory cells. For example, platelets:

- release inflammatory mediators upon activation and aggregation;
- are activated by phlogistic agents (such as complement activation products);
- play a role in animal models of inflammatory disease; and
- have been identified in localization and activation at tissue injury sites in human inflammatory diseases.

Platelet activation at sites of tissue injury is achieved by such hemostatic factors as thrombin, adenosine diphosphate, arachidonate derivates and exposed subendothelial collagen. There is evidence for platelet activation in some immunologically mediated diseases, such as asthma, cold urticaria, scleroderma and systemic lupus erythematosus[29–31].

At sites of inflammation activated platelets release a variety of both protein and lipid-derived mediators with inflammatory potential. Stimuli that activate platelet adhesion and degranulation also trigger the release of arachidonic acid from the membrane. This initiates the synthesis of thromboxane A_2 (TxA$_2$) and 12-hydroxytetraenoic acid (12-HETE). TxA$_2$ promotes platelet aggregation and vasoconstriction; 12-HETE activates neutrophils and macrophages.

Products released from platelets, which may promote local inflammation, are classified according to their intracellular granule of origin. Dense granules release ADP, which activates platelet fibrinogen binding sites of the β3 integrin gpIIb/IIIa, and serotonin, a potent vasoconstrictor. Alpha granule components, platelet factor 4 and β-thromboglobulin have been reported to activate both mononuclear and polymorphonuclear leukocytes. Alpha granules are also the source of platelet-derived growth factor (PDGF) which stimulates proliferation of smooth muscle cells and fibroblasts; thrombospondin, which promotes neutrophil adherence to blood vessel walls; factor VIII: von Willebrand factor antigen (VWF); factor V; fibrinogen and fibronectin.

Platelets express two surface adhesion promoting molecules; gpIIb/IIIa (activated by ADP) which binds fibrinogen, fibronectin, vitronection, and VWF[32]. Second, P-selectin

Table 1.3 Classification of the major Fcγ receptors

Characteristics	FcRγI	FcRγII	FcRγIII (types IIIA and B)
Genetic polymorphism	No	Yes	Yes
Affinity for IgG	High	Low	Low
CD classification	CD64	CD32	CD16
Membrane linkage	Transmembrane	Transmembrane	Transmembrane (IIIA) Phosphatidylinositol-glycan linked (IIIB)
Cell distribution	Monocytes Neutrophils (activated)	Monocytes Neutrophils Eosinophils Platelets B cells	NK cells (IIIA) Neutrophils (IIIB) Eosinophils (activated, IIIB) Monocytes (activated, IIIA)

(GMP-140, PADGEM), a member of the selectin family of adhesion molecules, is a membrane glycoprotein located in the alpha granules of platelets and Weibel–Palade bodies of endothelium. When these cells are activated by agents such as thrombin, P-selectin is rapidly translocated to the plasma membrane where it functions as a receptor for neutrophils and monocytes. Expression of P-selectin on activated platelets may therefore facilitate recruitment of neutrophils and monocytes to sites of thrombosis or inflammation[8].

HUMORAL MEDIATORS

COMPLEMENT AND OTHER CHEMOATTRACTANTS

The complement system

The complement system is comprised of at least 20 plasma proteins which participate in a variety of host defense and immunological reactions. Each complement component is cleaved via a limited proteolytic reaction which proceeds by either the **classical** or **alternative** pathway. The alternative pathway is more primitive and may be activated by contact with a variety of substances including polysaccharides (such as endotoxin) found in the cell walls of microorganisms. The activation of the classical pathway by immune complexes requires binding of the first complement component, C1, to sites on the Fc portions of immunoglobulins, particularly of the IgG-1, IgG-3 and IgM isotypes.

Activation of C3

Activation of the third component of complement is central to both the classical and alternative pathways. C3 is cleaved by convertases to two active products, C3a and C3b. C3a, released into the fluid phase, provokes the release of histamine from mast cells and basophils, causes smooth muscle contraction and induces platelet aggregation. C3b has two functions: C3b is part of the C5 convertase which continues the complement cascade; C3b is also the major opsonin of the complement system. It binds to immune complexes and to a variety of activators such as microbial organisms. The binding of C3b to these particles facilitates the attachment of the particle to the C3b receptor on cells, CR1 which is present on erythrocytes, neutrophils, monocytes, B-lymphocytes and glomerular podocytes. CR1 on phagocytes potentiates phagocytosis. CR1 on erythrocytes, which accounts for approximately 90% of CR1 in blood, facilitates the clearance of immune

Table 1.4   Chemoattractants and hematopoietic cells

Chemoattractant	Class (structure)	Target cell	Stimulates
FMLP	Bacterial product (tripeptide)	Neutrophils, monocytes	Chemotaxis secretion
C5a	Complement split product (11 kDa peptide)	Neutrophils, monocytes, mast cells, eosinophils	Chemotaxis secretion
Leukotriene B$_4$	Arachidonic acid metabolite (hydroxy fatty acid)	Neutrophils, monocytes, eosinophils	Chemotaxis secretion
Interleukin-8	Cytokine (12 kDa peptide)	Neutrophils, monocytes, eosinophils, basophils, memory T-cells	Chemotaxis secretion
TGF-β1	Growth factor (25 kDa polypeptide)	Neutrophils, monocytes, lymphocytes	Chemotaxis
Substance P	Tachykinin (12 kDa peptide)	Neutrophils, monocytes, basophils	Chemotaxis

complexes from the circulation by transporting erythrocyte-bound complexes to the liver and spleen for removal.

Activation of C5

In addition to its role as an opsonin, C3b also forms part of the C5 convertase which leads to the generation of C5a and C5b. C5a, like C3a, is an anaphylotoxin, capable of activating basophils and mast cells. C5a is also among the most potent biological chemoattractants for neutrophils, as will be discussed below. C5b, which will attach to the surface of cells and microrganisms, is the first component in the assembly of the membrane attack complex, C5b–9.

Membrane attack complex

The membrane attack complex (MAC), or the terminal complement assembly of C5b–9, has long been known as lytic bacteria. However, assembly of MAC on homologous leukocytes is not a cytotoxic event. After insertion of MAC into a leukocyte membrane, the cell sheds a small membrane vesicle containing the MAC complex. What is less appreciated is that insertion of MAC into the cell membrane

triggers cell activation before it is shed[33,34]. MAC acts as an ionophore, provoking increases in cytosolic calcium and consequently triggering cell functions (reviewed in[35]). These include generation of toxic oxygen products as well as activation of both the cyclooxygenase (platelets, monocyte/macrophages, synoviocytes) and lipoxygenase pathways of arachidonate metabolism. Furthermore, the deposition of MAC increases the surface expression of P-selectin on the endothelial cell surface, promoting adhesion to circulating neutrophils[36]. *In vivo* evidence that vascular endothelium represents a site of C5b–9 deposition has been demonstrated in immune vasculitis[37–39] and infarcted myocardium[40].

Activation of phagocytic cells by C5a and other chemoattractants

Chemoattractants are defined as soluble molecules which provoke the directed migration of leukocytes towards increasing concentration of that molecule. They are of diverse biological types: peptides, polypeptides and lipids (Table 1.4). C5a, the complement-derived chemoattractant, activates cells via a specific cell surface receptor which shares many characteristics with the well-studied bacterial chemoattractant FMLP. Receptors for these chemoattractants are members of a family of seven transmembrane spanning glycoproteins that are coupled to hetero-trimeric GTP-binding proteins or G-proteins. In the inactive state G-proteins remain as heterotrimers, consisting of α, β and γ sub-units. GDP is bound to the α subunit. Engage-ment of chemoattractant receptors by their respective ligands activates these GTP-binding proteins to release the GDP and bind GTP. The β–γ subunit dissociates and the GTP-bound α subunit becomes coupled to, and activates, a phosphatidylinositol specific phospholipase C. This enzyme cleaves the membrane phospholipid, phosphatidylino-sitol 4,5 *bis*phosphate (PIP$_2$) into two intra-cellular messengers: inositol 1,4,5 *tris*phosphate (IP$_3$) and diacylgylcerol (DAG)[41]. These two compounds respect-ively trigger release of calcium from intracellu-lar stores and activation of the isoforms of a serine-threonine protein kinase, protein ki-nase C (PKC). PKC has many intracellular substrates; among them is a second phospho-lipase, phosphatidylcholine-specific phos-pholipase D[42]. Activation of this enzyme results in the generation of phosphatidic acid, a second messenger closely correlated with production of toxic oxygen metabol-ites[43,44]. Ligation of chemoattractant recep-tors also triggers activation of a phosphatidylcholine-specific phospholipase C[45] directly producing DAG. How this li-pase is activated by receptor-chemoattractant interaction is unclear; however, generation of DAG is closely correlated with leukocyte de-granulation. Activation of other signal trans-duction systems in leukocytes is provoked by engagement of chemoattractant receptors. Among them are tyrosine kinases, adenylate and guanylate cyclases and *ras*-related pro-teins; how these are coupled to receptor ligation remains to be defined.

Perhaps most interestingly, the signal transduction pathways involved in the function of chemotaxis, *per se*, are, as yet, undefined. Substance P, a neurotransmitter, transforming growth factor β1 an inhibitory growth factor, and fibrinopeptide B, a product of the clotting cascade are unique chemo-attractants in that they all provoke neutrophil chemotaxis without stimulating secret-ion[46,47]. We have therefore proposed that the chemoattractant class of inflammatory molecules be divided into two families, 'classi-cal chemoattractants', those that can also trigger secretion, and 'pure chemoattrac-tants', those that cannot. None of the pure chemoattractants trigger release of calcium, inositol phosphates or the lipid second mess-engers discussed above, although they weakly activate membrane-associated GTPases. Their effect on microtubules, tyro-sine phosphorylation or *ras*-related proteins remains to be determined.

IMMUNE COMPLEXES

Autoimmune disorders are characterized by the production of autoantibodies of a wide range of specificities. IgM and multimeric IgG can trigger complement-mediated end-organ damage by binding to tissue-specific antigens via their antigen binding sites. Insoluble im-mune complexes, however, precipitate in tis-sues and provoke significant destruction by direct activation of inflammatory cells. By activating cells at the site of deposition, these immune aggregates can provoke release of proteolytic enzymes and toxic oxygen metabolites along endothelial basement mem-branes. Neutrophils, monocytes/macro-phages, platelets and B-lymphocytes and natural killer cells all express receptors for immune complexes[48]. These receptors pri-marily bind aggregated IgG although recep-tors for IgE, most commonly expressed on mast cells, are found at a low level on these cells. There are three types of receptors for multimeric IgG which bind these complexes via their Fc fragments; hence, these receptors are termed FcγRI, II and III. Immune complex receptors differ widely both in cell distribution, and primary structure as reflected by affinity, antigenicity and mechanisms of membrane attachment (Table 1.3). FcγRII is the most widely expressed of these receptors, found on essentially all cells of the immune system.

Immune complexes trigger neutrophil activation by the generation of similar intracellular messengers to those provoked by treatment with chemoattractants. Engagement of FcR provokes rises in inositol phosphates, cytosolic Ca^{2+}[49], diacylglycerol[50,51] and phosphatidic acid. In addition, immune complexes activate membrane-bound GTPases as well as cytosolic tyrosine kinases in inflammatory cells[52–54]. However, immune complex activation of inflammatory cells utilize enzymatic pathways of signal transduction that are distinct from those triggered by chemoattractants. The generation of these second messengers by immune complexes differ kinetically and in sensitivity to inhibitors (pertussis toxin, gonococcal *Por* protein) from those triggered by chemoattractants[50,51,55–57].

Because of the multiple classes of FcR expressed on individual cell types, it has been difficult to dissect the role of the various receptors in cell activation (although platelets, posessing only FcγRII are an exception). By means of monoclonal antibodies generated against FcγRII (MAb IV.3) or FcγRIII (MAb 3G8) which block binding of immune complexes to the respective receptor on neutrophils[50,55], it has been demonstrated that ligation of the unblocked FcγR can still provoke lysosomal enzyme release from neutrophils. Similar effects have been shown for other neutrophil functions, such as actin polymerization[58], phagocytosis[59] and superoxide anion generation[60]. However, the maximal cellular response to immune complexes is a synergistic one, requiring engagement of both FcγRII and III. One would infer from these data that the engagement of either receptor activates a distinct signal transduction mechanism, sufficient in itself for cell activation but capable of 'priming' the other. Clear evidence for this has been demonstrated with regard to calcium fluxes; engagement of FcγRII can provoke early and sustained increments in Ca^{2+} whereas FcγRIII activation triggers a more transient release of Ca^{2+}[37,61]. Whether either receptor can provoke influx of extracellular Ca^{2+} is not yet clear[37,62].

INFLAMMATORY MEDIATORS IN THE PATHOGENESIS OF TISSUE INJURY IN SLE

Systemic lupus erythematosus is the connective tissue disease which best exemplifies the consequences of the systemic generation of humoral inflammatory mediators and the activation of the cellular constituents of inflammation as outlined above. Immune complex formation, the episodic bursts of complement activation and the recruitment of stimulated leukocytes into a variety of tissues, makes SLE a disease which has attracted great interest in the attempt to understand immune-mediated injury.

COMPLEMENT COMPONENTS AND SLE DISEASE ACTIVITY

The activation of complement via proteolytic cascade plays a central role in the pathogenesis of SLE[63,64] (Figure 1.1). The consumption of complement components and their deposition in tissue is reflected by a decrease in serum levels of C3 and C4 in most patients with active disease[65,66]. However, since the synthesis of both C3 and C4 increases during periods of disease activity, the serum levels of these proteins may be normal despite accelerated consumption[67,68]. Conversely, chronically depressed levels of individual complement components due to decreased synthesis, hereditary deficiencies or increased extravascular distribution of complement proteins has been reported in SLE[69,70]. The

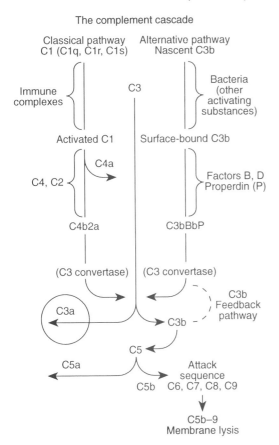

Fig. 1.1 Complement cascade. Classical and alternative pathways of complement activation.

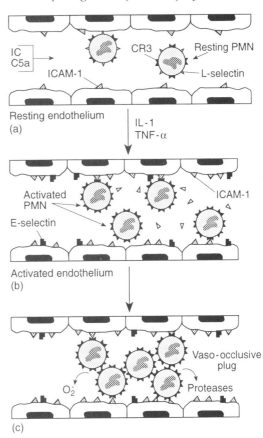

Fig. 1.2 Intravascular activation of neutrophils in SLE. Resting neutrophils (PMN) are either free in circulation or 'rolling', by means of L-selectin's adhesion to carbohydrates on the endothelial cell lining of vessel walls (A). Intravascular activation of neutrophils by immune complexes or complement split products provoke shedding of L-selectin and increased expression of CR3. IL-1 or TNF-α increase the constitutive expression of ICAM-1 and induce the synthesis and expression of E-selectin on the surface of endothelial cells (B). Finally, activated neutrophils adhere to endothelium, release inflammatory mediators and, in some settings, aggregate causing occlusion of small blood vessels (C).

decreased serum complement levels in these patients may lead to the mistaken conclusion that excessive complement activation is ongoing. To define more precisely the role of complement activation with respect to clinical disease activity of SLE, we[71–74] and others[75,76] have measured circulating levels of complement degradation products during periods of active and inactive disease. Levels of plasma C3a, Ba and the serum complement attack complex, SC5b–9, were each shown to be more sensitive indicators of disease activity than either total C3 level or C4. Elevations of plasma C3a levels may precede other serologic or clinical evidence of an impending disease flare[72].

COMPLEMENT ACTIVATION AND TISSUE INJURY

It is well appreciated that serological abnormalities of the complement system serve not

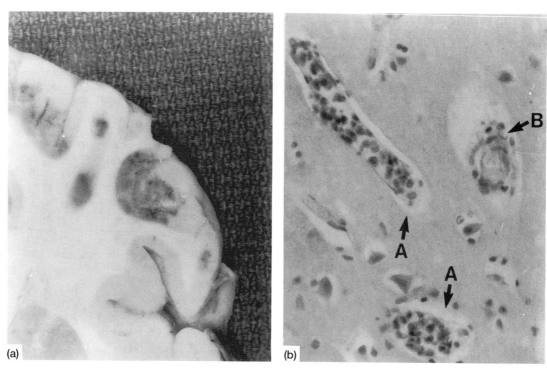

Fig. 1.3 Pathology of CNS lupus. In a patient who died with CNS lupus, cerebral infarcts were subtended by vessels occluded by leukocyte aggregates (A), or fibrin thrombi (B), similar to those observed in a Shwartzman reaction. (Photographs courtesy of Dr Nelson Torre, Buffalo, NY.)

only as biological markers of active disease, but are also reflective of the generation of complement-derived inflammatory mediators (e.g. C5a) in tissues which mediate end-organ damage. The capacity of activated complement components to promote the release of inflammatory mediators from mast cells (C3a, C5a), neutrophils (C5a) and platelets (C3a) accounts for their central role in the pathogenesis of immune-mediated injury. Activated complement derived proteins may act locally at sites of immune complex deposition or be generated in the circulation, creating the potential for widespread vascular injury as discussed below[6,77–79].

In patients with SLE the mechanisms of tissue injury are complex and reflect the diversity of autoantibody production. First, injury can result directly from the action of autoantibodies cytotoxic for certain cell types, including red cells and platelets with resulting hemolytic anemia or thrombocytopenia. Secondly, circulating complexes (such as DNA/anti-DNA) are deposited in the subendothelial layers of the vascular basement membrane in multiple organs, such as skin, kidney and serosal surfaces. The deposited immune complexes can initiate a localized inflammatory response characterized by the activation of complement, the infiltration of neutrophils and later of mononuclear cells. Nuclear debris resulting from necrosis reacts with antinuclear antibodies forming basophilic-staining hematoxylin bodies. A third mechanism of tissue damage in SLE, which can occur in the absence of local immune complex deposition, results from the intravascular activation of the complement system. As noted above, in patients with active disease there are marked elevations in plasma of biologically active complement split products such as C3a and C5a. These split products activate inflammatory cells, such as neutrophils and platelets, causing them to aggregate and to adhere to vascular endothelium (Figure 1.2). Evidence that circulating neutrophils have been exposed to secretagogues is provided by the upregulation of CD11b/CD18 on their surface during periods of active, but not inactive disease[80]. During flares of disease the vascular endothelium is also activated to express abnormal amounts of surface adhesion molecules (such as E-selectin and ICAM-1) which promote leukocyte-endothelial attachment [81]. The exposure of circulating neutrophils to elevated plasma levels of complement split products, in association with endothelial cell activation, can lead to widespread tissue injury (Figure 1.3). This mechanism is similar to that described in the Schwartzman reaction[82] and may account for organ injury in endotoxic shock, ischemia-reperfusion injury and the adult respiratory distress syndrome [78]. We have provided evidence that a similar pathogenic mechanism contributes to the syndromes of cerebritis[72,77] and reversible hypoxemia in SLE[83].

REFERENCES

1. Kitsis, E. A. and Weissmann, G. (1991) The role of the neutrophil in rheumatoid arthritis. *Clin. Orthopaed. Rel. Res.*, **265**, 63–72.
2. Weissmann, G., Korchak, H. M., Perez, H. D. *et al.* (1981) *Neutrophils as Secretory Organs*, PSG Publishing Co., Boston, pp. 175–91.
3. Nathan, C. F. (1987) Secretory products of macrophages. *J. Clin. Invest.*, **79**, 319–26.
4. Ross, G. D. and Medof, M. E. (1985) Membrane complement receptors specific for bound fragments of C3. *Adv. Immunol.*, **37**, 217–67.
5. Schifferli, J. A., Ng, Y. C. and Peters, D. K. (1986) The role of complement and its receptor in the elimination of immune complexes. *N. Eng. J. Med.*, **315**, 488–95.
6. Philips, M. R., Abramson, S. B. and Wiessmann, G. (1989) Neutrophil adhesion and autoimmune vascular injury. *Clin. Aspects Autoimmun.*, **3**, 6–15.
7. Yong, K. and Khwaja, A. (1990) Leucocyte cellular adhesion molecules. *Blood Rev.*, **4**, 211–25.
8. McEver, R. B. (1991) Selectins: novel receptors that mediate leukocyte adhesion during inflammation, *Thromb. and Haemostasis*, **65**, 233–8.
9. Lawrence, M. B. and Springer, T. A. (1991) Leukocytes roll on a selection of physiologic flow rates: distinction from and prerequisite for adhesion through integrins. *Cell*, **65**, 859–73.
10. Wharram, B. L., Fitting, K., Kunkel, S. L. *et al.* (1991) Tissue factors expression in endothelial cell/monocyte co-cultures stimulated by lipopolysaccharide and/or aggregated IgG. Mechanisms of cell-cell communication. *J. Immunol.*, **146**, 1437–45.
11. Schultz, G. and Rotater, D. S. (1991) EGF and TGF-alpha in wound healing and repair. *J. Cell: Biol.*, **45**, 346–52.
12. Kusner, D. J., Luebbers, E. L., Nowinski, R. J. *et al.* (1991) Cytokine- and LPS-induced synthesis of interleukin-8 from human mesangial cells. *Kidney Int.*, **39**, 1240–8.
13. Abramson, S. B., Leszczynska-Piziak, J. and Weissmann, G. (1991) Arachidonic acid as a second messenger. Interactions with a GTP-binding protein of human neutrophils. *J. Immunol.*, **147**, 231–6.
14. Baird, N. R. and Morrison, A. R. (1993) Amplification of the arachidonic acid cascade: implications for pharmacologic intervention. *Am. J. Kidney Dis.*, **21**, 557–64.
15. Zurier, R. B. and Ballas, M. (1973) Prostaglandin E: suppression of adjuvant arthritis: histopathology. *Arth. Rheum.*, **16**, 251–8.
16. Abramson, S. B., Cherksey, B., Gude, D. *et al.* (1990) Nonsteroidal antiinflammatory drugs exert differential effects on neutrophil function and plasma membrane viscosity: studies in human neutrophils and liposomes. *Inflammation*, **14**, 11–30.
17. Kitsis, E. A., Weissmann, G. and Abramson, S. B. (1991) The prostaglandin paradox: additive inhibition of neutrophil function by aspirin-like drugs and the prostaglandin E1 analog misoprostol. *J. Rheum.*, **18**, 1461–5.
18. Abramson, S., Korchak, H., Ludewig, R. *et al.* (1985) Modes of action of aspirin-like drugs. *Proc. Nat. Acad. Sci. USA*, **82**, 7227–31.
19. Musser, J. H. and Kreft, A. F. (1992) 5-lipoxygenase: properties, pharmacology and the quinolinyl(bridged)aryl class of inhibitors. *J. Medic. Chem.*, **35**, 2501–24.

20. Hamberg, M. and Samuelsson, B. (1974) Prostaglandin endoperoxides. Novel transformations of arachidonic acid in human platelets. *Proc. Nat. Acad. Sci. USA*, **71**, 3400–4.

21. Adesuyi, S. A., Cockrell, C. S., Gamache, D. A. *et al.* (1985) Lipoxygenase metabolism of arachidonic acid in brain. *J. Neurochem.*, **45**, 770–6.

22. Izumi, T., Radmark, O. and Samuelsson, B. (1991) Purification of 15-lipoxygenase for human leukocytes, evidence for the presence of isozymes. *Adv. Prost. Thromb. Leuk. Res.*, **21**, 101–4.

23. Fiore, S., Romano, M. and Serhan, C. N. (1991) Lipoxin and leukotriene production during receptor-activated interactions between human platelets and cytokine-primed neutrophils. *Adv. Prost. Thromb. Leuk. Res.*, **21**, 93–6.

24. Edenius, C., Forsberg, I., Stenke, L. *et al.* (1991) Lipoxin formation in human platelets. *Adv. Prost. Thromb. Leuk. Res.*, **21**, 97–100.

25. McCartney-Francis, N., Allen, J. B., Mizel, D. E. *et al.* (1993) Suppression of arthritis by an inhibitor of nitric oxide synthase. *J. Exp. Med.*, **178**, 749–54.

26. Clancy, R. M., Leszczynska-Piziak, J. and Abramson, S. B. (1992) Nitric oxide, an endothelial cell relaxation factor, inhibits neutrophil superoxide anion production via a direct action on the NADPH oxidase. *J. Clin. Invest.*, **90**, 1116–21.

27. Weksler, B. B. (1988) Platelets, in *Inflammation Basic Principles and Clinical Correlates*, (eds J. I. Gallin, M. Goldstein and R. N. Y. Snyderman), Raven Press, pp. 543–57.

28. Skaer, R. J. (1981) Platelet degranulation, in *Platelets in Biology and Pathology*, vol. 2, (ed. J. L. Gordon) Elsevier/North-Holland, Amsterdam, pp. 321–48.

29. Krauer, K. A. (1981) Platelet activation during antigen-induced airway reactions in asthmatic subjects. *N. Engl J. Med.*, **304**, 1404–6.

30. Grandel, K. E., Farr, R. S. and Wanderer, A. A. (1985) Association of platelet activating factor with primary acquired cold urticaria. *N. Engl J. Med.*, **313**, 405–9.

31. Ginsberg, M. H. (1986) Role of platelets in inflammation and rheumatic disease. *Adv. Inflamm. Res.*, **2**, 53–71.

32. Pytela, R., Pierschbacher, M., Ginsberg, M. *et al.* (1986) Platelet membrane glycoprotein IIb/IIIa: a member of a family of Arg-Gly-Asp-specific adhesion receptors. *Science*, **231**, 1559–62.

33. Stein, J. M. and Luzio, J. P. (1989) Membrane sorting during vesicle shedding from neutrophils during sublytic complement attack. *Biochem. Soc. Trans.*, **16**, 1082–3.

34. Morgan, B. P., Dankert, J. R. and Esser, A. F. (1987) Recovery of human neutrophils from complement attack: removal of the membrane attack complex by endocytosis and exocytosis. *J. Immunol.*, **138**, 246–53.

35. Morgan, B. P. (1989) Complement membrane attack on nucleated cells: resistance, recovery and non-lethal effects. *Biochem. J.*, **264**, 1–14.

36. Hattori, R., Hamilton, K. K., McEver, R. P. *et al.* (1989) Complement proteins C5b–9 induce secretion of high molecular weight multimers of endothelial von Willebrand Factor and translocation of granule membrane. *J. Biol. Chem.*, **264**, 9053–60.

37. Biesecker, G., Katz, S. and Koffler, D. (1981) Renal localization of the membrane attack complex in systemic lupus erythematosus nephritis. *J. Exp.Med.*, **154**, 1779–94.

38. Biesecker, G., Lavin, L., Zisking, M. *et al.* (1982) Cutaneous localization of the membrane attack complex in discoid and systemic lupus erythematosus. *N. Eng. J. Med.*, **306**, 264–70.

39. Kissel, J. T., Mendell, J. R. and Rammohan, K. W. (1986) Microvascular deposition of complement membrane attack complex in dermatomyositis. *N. Engl. J. Med.*, **314**, 329–334.

40. Schafer, H., Mathey, D., Hugo, F. *et al.* (1986) Deposition of the terminal C5b–9 complement complex in infarcted areas of human myocardium. *J. Immunol.*, **137**, 1945–9.

41. Berridge, M. J. and Irvine, R. F. (1989) Inositol phosphates and cell signalling. *Nature*, **341**, 197–204.

42. Exton, J. H. (1990) Signaling through phosphatidylcholine breakdown. *J. Biol. Chem.*, **265**, 1–4.

43. Korchak, H. M., Vosshall, L. B., Haines, K. A. *et al.* (1988) Activation of the human neutrophil by calcium-mobilizing ligands II. Correlation of calcium, diacyl glycerol and phosphatidic acid generation with superoxide anion generation. *J. Biol. Chem.*, **263**, 11098–105.

44. Bauldry, S. A., Bass, D. A.,Cousart, S. L. *et al.* (1991) Tumour necrosis factor α priming of phospholipase D in human neutrophils. Correlation between phosphatidic acid production and superoxide generation. *J. Biol. Chem.*, **266**, 4173–9.

45. Haines, K. A., Reibman, J., Tang, X. *et al.* (1991) Effects of protein I of *N. gonorrhoeae* on

neutrophil activation: I. Generation of diacylglycerol from phosphatidylcholine via a specific phospholipase C is associated with exocytosis. *J. Cell Biol.*, **114**, 433–42.

46. Mulder, K. M. and Morris, S. L. (1992) Activation of p21ras by transforming growth factor in epithelial cells. *J. Biol. Chem.*, **267**, 5029–31.

47. Haines, K. A., Kolasinski, S. L., Cronstein, B. N. *et al.* (1993) Chemoattraction of neutrophils by Substance P and Transforming Growth Factor-1 is inadequately explained by current models of lipid remodeling. *J. Immunol.*, **151**, 1491–9.

48. Ravetch, J. V. and Kinet, J.-P. (1991) Fc receptors. *Annu Rev. Immunol.*, **9**, 457–92.

49. Kimberly, R. P., Ahlstrom, J. W., Click, M. E. *et al.* (1990) The glycosyl phosphatidylinositol-linked FcγRIIIPMN mediates transmembrane signaling events distinct from FcγRII. *J. Exp. Med.*, **171**, 1239–55.

50. Reibman, J., Haines, K. A., Gude, D. *et al.* (1991) Differences in signal transduction between two Fcγ receptors for the chemoattractant fMLP in neutrophils: effects of colchicine on pertussis toxin sensitivity and diacylglycerol formation. *J. Immunol.*, **146**, 988–96.

51. Haines, K. A. and Weissmann, G. (1990) Protein I of *N.gonorrhoeae* shows that phosphatidate from phosphatidylcholine via phospholipase C is an intracellular messenger in neutrophil activation by chemoattractants, in *Advances in Prostaglandin, Thromboxane and Leukotriene Research*, (eds B. Samuelsson, R. Paoletti, P. W. Ramwell *et al.*), Raven Press, E. New York, pp. 545–52.

52. Blackburn Jr. W. D., and Heck, L. W. (1989) Neutrophil activation by surface bound IgG is via a pertussis insensitive G protein. *Biochem. Biophys. Res. Commun.*, **164**, 983–9.

53. Huang, M. M., Indik, Z., Brass, L.F. *et al.* (1992) Activation of Fc (gamma) RII induces tyrosine phosphorylation of multiple proteins including Fc (gamma) RII. *J. Biol. Chem.*, **267**, 5467–73.

54. Rubinstein, E., Urso, I., Boucheix, C. *et al.* (1992) Platelet activation by cross-linking HLA class I molecules and Fc receptor. *Blood*, **79**, 2901–8.

55. Walker, B. A. M., Hagenlocker, B. E., Stubbs Jr. E. B. *et al.* (1991) Signal transduction events and FcγR engagement in human neutrophils stimulated with immune complexes. *J. Immunol.*, **146**, 735–41.

56. Feister, A. J., Browder, B., Willis, H. E. *et al.* (1988) Pertussis toxin inhibits human neutrophil responses mediated by the 42-kilodalton IgG Fc receptor. *J. Immunol.*, **141**, 228–33.

57. Brennan, P. J., Zigmond, S. H., Schreiber, A. D. *et al.* (1991) Binding of IgG containing immune complexes to a human neutrophil Fc(gamma)RII and Fc(gamma)RIII induces actin polymerization by a pertussis toxin-insensitive transduction pathway. *J. Immunol.*, **146**, 4282–8.

58. Salmon, J. E., Brogle, N. L., Edberg, J. C. *et al.* (1991) Fcγ Receptor III induces actin polymerizarion in human neutrophils and primes phagocytosis mediated by Fcγ receptor II. *J. Immunol.*, **146**, 997–1004.

59. Rosales, C. and Brown, E. J. (1991) Two mechanisms for IgG Fc-receptor-mediated phagocytosis by human neutrophils. *J. Immunol.*, **146**, 3937–44.

60. Brunkhorst, B.A., Strohmeier, G., Lazzari, K. *et al.* (1992) Differential roles of Fc(gamma)RII and Fc(gamma)RIII in immune complex stimulation of human neutrophils. *J. Biol. Chem.*, **267**, 20659–66.

61. Stadler, J., Harbrecht, B. G., DiSilvio, M. *et al.* (1993) Endogenous nitric oxide inhibits the synthesis of cyclooxygenase products and interleukin-6 by rat kupffer cells. *J. Leukocyte Bio.* **53**, 165–72.

62. Bulkley, B. H. and Roberts, W. C. (1975) The heart in systemic lupus erythematosus and the changes induced in it by corticosteroid therapy. *Am. J. Med.*, **58**, 243–64.

63. Schur, P. H. and Sandson, J. (1968) Immunologic factors and clinical activity in systemic lupus erythematosus. *N. Eng. J. Med.*, **278**, 533–8.

64. Lange, K., Wasserman, E. and Slobody, L. B. (1960) Significance of serum complement levels for diagnosis and prognosis of acute and subacute glomerulonephritis and lupus erythematosus disseminatus. *Ann. Intern. Med.*, **53**, 636–46.

65. Ruddy, S., Carpenter, C. B., Chin, K. W. *et al.* (1975) Human complement metabolism: an analysis of 144 studies. *Medicine (Baltimore)*, **54**, 165–78.

66. Alper, C. A. and Rosen, F. (1967) Studies of the *in vitro* behavior of human C3 in normal subjects and patients. *J. Clin. Invest.*, **46**, 2021–34.

67. Sliwinski, A. J. and Zvaifler, N. J. (1972) Decreased synthesis of the third component (C3) in hypocomplementemic systemic lupus erythematosus. *Clin. Exp. Immunol.*, **11**, 21–9.

68. Charlesworth, J.A., Williams, D. G., Sherington, E. *et al.* (1974) Metabolic studies of the third component of complement and the glycine rich glycoprotein in patients with hypocomplementemia. *J. Clin. Invest.*, **53**, 1578–87.

69. Prentice, R. L., Shimizu, Y., Lin, C. H. *et al.* (1982) Serial blood pressure measurements and cardiovascular disease in a Japanese cohort. *Am. J. Epid.*, **116**, 1–28.

70. Shimizu, Y., Kato, H., Lin, C. H. *et al.* (1986) Relationship between longitudinal changes in blood pressure and stroke incidence. *Radiation Effects Res. Fndn.*, **TR 5–84**, 1–18.

71. Belmont, H. M., Hopkins, P., Edelson, H. S. *et al.* (1986) Complement activation during systemic lupus erythematosus. C3a and C5a anaphylatoxins circulate during exacerbations of disease. *Arth. Rheum.*, **29**, 1085–9.

72. Hopkins, P. T., Belmont, H. M., Buyon, J. *et al.* (1988) Increased levels of plasma anaphylatoxins in systemic lupus erythematosus predict flares of the disease and may elicit vascular injury in lupus cerebritis. *Arth. Rheum.*, **31**, 632–41.

73. Buyon, J., Tamerius, J., Belmont, H. M. *et al.* (1992) Assessment of disease activity and impending flare in patients with systemic lupus erythematosus: comparison of the use of complement split products and conventional measurements of complement. *Arth. Rheum.*, **35**, 1028–37.

74. Buyon, J., Tamerius, J., Ordica, S. *et al.* (1992) Activation of the alternative complement pathway accompanies disease flares in systemic lupus erythematosus during pregnancy. *Arth. Rheum.*, **35**, 55–61.

75. Falk, R. J., Dalmasso, A. P., Kim, Y. *et al.* (1985) Radioimmunoassay of the attack complex of complement in serum from patients with systemic lupus erythematosus. *N. Eng. J. Med.*, **312**, 1594–9.

76. Kerr, L., Adelsberg, B. R., Schulman, P. *et al.* (1989) Factor B activation products in patients with systemic lupus erythematosus: a marker of severe disease activity. *Arth. Rheum.*, **32**, 1406–13.

77. Abramson, S. B. and Weissmann, G. (1988) Complement split products and the pathogenesis of SLE. *Hosp. Prac.*, **23**(12), 45–55.

78. Jacob, H. S., Craddock, P. R., Hammerschmidt, D. E. *et al.* (1980) Complement-induced granulocyte aggregation: an unsuspected mechanism of disease. *N. Eng. J. Med.*, **302**, 789–94.

79. Shwartzman, G. (1937) *Phenomenon of Local Tissue Reactivity*, Paul Hoeber, New York.

80. Buyon, J. P., Shadick, N., Berkman, R. *et al.* (1988) Surface expression of gp165/95, the complement receptor CR3, as a marker of disease activity in systemic lupus erythematosus. *Clin. Immunol. Immunopath.*, **46**, 141–9.

81. Belmont, H. M., Buyon, J., Giorno, R. *et al.* (1994) Upregulation of endothelial cell adhesion molecules characterizes disease activity in systemic lupus erythematosus: the Shwartzman Phenomenon revised. *Arth. Rheum.* **37**, 376–83.

82. Argenbright, L. and Barton, R. (1992) Interactions of leukocyte integrins with intercellular adhesion molecule 1 in the production of inflammatory vascular injury in vivo. The Shwartzman phenomenon revisited. *J. Clin. Invest.*, **89**, 259–73.

83. Abramson, S. B., Dobro, J., Eberle, M. A. *et al.* (1991) Acute reversible hypoxemia in systemic lupus erythematosus. *Ann. Int. Med.*, **114**, 941–7.

A. K. Vaishnaw and M. J. Walport

INTRODUCTION

Systemic lupus erythematosus (SLE) is a multisystem disease which predominantly affects women. It is a heterogeneous disorder and is defined according to a set of disease classification criteria devised by the American Rheumatism Association[1]. The unifying feature is the presence of autoantibodies against a wide array of highly conserved intracellular autoantigens including nucleic acids, molecules involved in the transcription and translation of nucleic acids and constituents of cell membranes. Immune complexes, comprising autoantibodies bound to their respective autoantigens, may be the major stimulus to inflammation in SLE (Chapter 1). However, the presence of autoantibodies alone is not sufficient to cause disease and cell-mediated immunity and other factors play an important role.

Loss of tolerance to self-antigens is central to the induction of all autoimmune syndromes. In SLE there are multiple qualitative and quantitative abnormalities of T- and B-cells and their regulatory cytokines. Animal models of lupus have shown that genetic factors have an important role in permitting the breakdown of tolerance and the generation of autoantibodies. Disease susceptibility genes have been identified in human lupus but environmental triggers, such as ultraviolet radiation and drugs, are also strongly implicated. The etiology of SLE appears to be multifactorial with disease expression initiated by a variety of environmental insults acting in genetically susceptible individuals.

EPIDEMIOLOGY

Lupus is an uncommon disease associated with significant morbidity and mortality. The incidence is estimated between 1–8/100 000 per year and appears to be rising. This is probably partly due to the improved diagnosis of mild cases secondary to improvements in serological analysis. Prevalence varies from 12–50/100 000 and is influenced dramatically by age, sex and race. The female to male ratio is 9:1 in the age range 20–40 years and 2:1 thereafter. Lupus is up to four times commoner in blacks than whites, particularly in the USA and Jamaica, although it is rare in rural Africa.

AUTOANTIBODIES IN SLE

Autoantibodies are the most consistent manifestation of autoimmunity in lupus. They are implicated in the pathogenesis and are important markers of disease. The earliest description of an autoantibody-mediated phenomenon in lupus was the demonstration of LE cells by Hargraves *et al.* in 1948[2]. This was followed in 1957 by the description of antinuclear factor, subsequently characterized as antinuclear antibodies (ANA). ANA comprise a series of autoantibodies against

Connective Tissue Diseases. Edited by Jill J. F. Belch and Robert B. Zurier. Published in 1995 by Chapman & Hall, London. ISBN 0 412 48620 2

Table 2.1   Autoantibody specificities in SLE

Antibody	Antigen	Prevalence	Association/comment	Ref
native DNA	dsDNA	40–65%	Peripheral nuclear staining, lupus nephritis	[3]
denat. DNA	ssDNA	>70%	–	
Histones	H1, H2A, H2B	50–70%	Homogeneous nuclear staining Drug-induced LE	(4, 5)
Sm	Peptides B, B', D, E complexed with uridine rich RNAs	up to 25%	Membranous nephritis.	[6, 7]
U1 RNP	Peptides '70 kDa', A, C complexed with uridine rich RNAs	30%	High titer+ MCTD	[7, 8]
Ro	60 and 52 kDa peptides complexed with Y1-Y5 RNAs	30%	SCLE, neonatal lupus, Sjögen's syndrome	[9–12]
La	48 kDa peptide associated with Y series and other RNA	15%	Similar to anti-Ro	[7, 13]
rRNP	15, 16, 38 kDa phosphoproteins ass. with ribosomal RNA	10%	?Cerebral lupus	[14, 15]
Ku	DNA binding protein	10%	Sclerodactyly	[16]
PCNA	36 kDa auxiliary protein for DNA pol. delta	10%	Severe disease	[17]
Hsp 90	Part of heat shock protein family	50%	?	[18]
Phospholipid	Cardiolipin/B2 glycoprotein I	30–40%	Thrombosis, abortion	[19, 20]
Lymphocytoxins	?	>50%	Lymphopenia Bone marrow toxicity	[21, 31, 33]

nuclear antigens including double-standed DNA (dsDNA), histones and the 'extractable nuclear antigens' which are a series of ribonucleoproteins.

Indirect immunofluorescence shows that the vast majority of lupus sera have ANA activity, which is most commonly directed against dsDNA or histones. The presences of high titers of anti-dsDNA antibodies is virtually pathognomonic of SLE, present in up to 65% of patients. Autoantibodies against one of the extractable nuclear antigens, 'Sm', are also disease-specific but occur in fewer patients. A wide spectrum of other auto antibodies are detected with variable frequency and these have proved important in defining subsets of disease (Table 2.1). Detailed analysis of autoantibody specifities, by techniques such as immunoprecipitation and Western blotting, has shown that there are two groups of target antigens[22]: intracellular and membrane associated.

ANTIBODIES TO INTRACELLULAR ANTIGENS

Study of autoantibodies against intracellular antigens has led to several fundamental observations:

1. Three highly conserved 'particles' serve as the major autoantigenic stimuli in SLE. These are nucleoprotein complexes comprising nucleic acid bound to protein:
   (a) the nucleosome, which is associated with anti-ds DNA and anti-histone antibodies;
   (b) small nuclear ribonucleoproteins (snRNP), associated with anti-Sm and anti-U1 RNP antibodies; and
   (c) small cytoplasmic ribonucleoproteins (scRNP), associated with anti-Ro and anti-La antibodies.
2. Autoimmunity to each of these subcellular particles usually takes the form of autoantibody production against more than one component of the complex. Thus the occurrence of anti-dsDNA antibodies is paralleled by that of anti-histone antibodies[23]. Similarly, anti-Sm often coexists with anti-U1RNP as does anti-Ro with anti-La.
3. The autoantibody response to individual autoantigens is polyclonal[24] and multiple, non-cross-reactive epitopes are recognized[25–27].

These observations imply that the relevant immunogen in SLE is the intact subcellular complex of nucleic acid and protein[28]. This has proved extremely difficult to demonstrate in the case of native DNA. However, autoantibodies to the extractable nuclear antigens have been easier to generate upon immunization of mice with purified heterologous antigens[29,30].

ANTIBODIES TO MEMBRANE-ASSOCIATED ANTIGENS

Autoantibodies to cell surface constituents are common. They form an ill-defined group of specificities which often have complex cross-reactivities and are associated with some of the hematological manifestations of lupus. They are typically low affinity and IgM class. In many cases the autoantigen has not yet been identified. Three groups of these autoantibodies have been described:

1. Cross reacting anti-nuclear antibodies. There is evidence that subpopulations of anti-dsDNA and anti-histone antibodies cross-react with lymphocyte, neutrophil and neuronal cell surfaces[31]. Similarly anti-P ribosomal antibodies have been shown to cross-react with the cell surface of a neuroblastoma cell line[32].
2. Antibodies reacting primarily with cell surface antigens[33]. A variety of surface antigens have been identified. These include B2 microglobulin, MHC class II molecules and a range of T-cell markers.
3. Receptor-mediated binding of autoantibodies to cells. Autoantibodies within immune complexes may localize to a variety of cell types via surface Fc and complement receptors. In the case of erythrocytes, opsonized immune complexes bind the surface complement receptor, CR1, but are not internalized (see Chapter 1). DNA can bind to the surface of monocytes, T- and B-lymphocytes and neutrophils via a 30 kDa 'DNA receptor'[34]. This may play a role in the binding of anti-DNA antibodies to these cell surfaces.

ANTIBODIES TO PHOSPHOLIPIDS

Phospholipids are the major structural component of cell membranes. In the last decade it has been demonstrated that antibodies to anionic phospholipids are strongly correlated with thrombotic events in SLE[19]. These anti-phospholipid (APL) antibodies are detected in 30–40% of lupus patients, depending on the assay used. There are currently three main assays: the lupus anticoagulant test, cardiolipin-based immunoassay and the Venereal Disease Research Laboratory (VDRL) test. *In vitro*, APL antibodies may prolong clotting time in a phospholipid-based assay such as the kaolin cephalin clotting time (KCCT) – this is termed lupus anticoagulant

(LA) activity, in practice. Many patients with LA activity will also produce a positive reaction in immunoassays using cardiolipin as the antigen – hence anti-cardiolipin antibodies. The third assay which detects APL antibodies, the VDRL test, is a flocculation assay utilizing carbon particles coated with several phospholipids, including cardiolipin.

Each of these assays identifies a slightly different range of specificities and individual patients may show positive reactivity in one or more assay. APL antibodies are a heterogeneous group of immunoglobulins with complex and partially over-lapping cross-reactivities. This has made characterization of the relevant autoantigen(s) difficult.

PATHOGENICITY OF AUTOANTIBODIES

Evidence is accumulating for the pathogenicity of autoantibodies and their direct role in tissue damage. Their presence alone, however, is not sufficient to cause disease. In 1958, in an experiment which would now be considered unethical, a group of patients with advanced malignancy were transfused with lupus sera. Fortunately, this did not result in any overt manifestations of SLE. Similarly, the transplacental passage of IgG autoantibodies has been well documented but is only rarely associated with neonatal lupus (see below).

ANTI-DNA ANTIBODIES

There is compelling circumstantial evidence to implicate anti-dsDNA antibodies in the pathogenesis of lupus nephritis[35]. In both murine and human lupus, DNA, anti-dsDNA antibodies and complement can be eluted from inflamed kidneys[36]. In contrast to other autoantibodies, there is a longitudinal correlation in many patients between levels of anti-dsDNA, disease activity and treatment[35,37,38]. Experimentally, the infusion of anti-DNA antibodies into normal mice has resulted in a variety of renal immune deposits and even proliferative nephritis[39,40].

Despite these data, the exact mechanism whereby autoantibodies may cause nephritis is not known. Immune complexes containing DNA and anti-DNA antibodies have been detected in the circulation, albeit rarely, and could be deposited in the kidneys[41]. Alternatively, antibodies may bind *in situ*, either to DNA or cross-reacting glomerular antigens, such as heparan sulphate.

From the entire range of anti-DNA antibodies, the subpopulations which are associated with nephritis have certain properties[42]. They are usually anti-dsDNA, IgG class, high affinity, cationic and fix complement. This may explain why only a proportion of patients with anti-DNA antibodies develop renal disease.

ANTI-RO ANTIBODIES

Anti-Ro antibodies almost certainly mediate the neonatal lupus syndrome and the photosensitive rash of subacute cutaneous lupus erythematosus (SCLE). Ro antigen is known to have a low level of cell surface expression. This has been shown to upregulate when keratinocytes are exposed to ultraviolet radiation[43] and may explain the sensitivity of SCLE patients to sunlight. Furthermore, when anti-Ro sera were infused into immunodeficient mice with engrafted human skin, the antibodies preferentially bound to the human keratinocytes and gave a pattern of IgG deposition identical to that seen in neonatal lupus and SCLE[44]. Recent data have also demonstrated that exposure of neonatal rabbit cardiomyocytes to anti-Ro caused a delay in the action potential, which was not the case for adult tissue[45]. This has given insight into the potential pathogenicity of anti-Ro antibodies in the congenital complete heart block seen in some cases of neonatal lupus.

ANTI-PHOSPHOLIPID ANTIBODIES

The risk of thrombosis in lupus is three to four times higher in the presence of APL antibodies which implies that they have pathogenic capability. APL antibodies may also be detected during the course of chronic infections (e.g. syphilis, leprosy and malaria) and drug-induced LE. The origin of these antibodies is probably different to that in SLE; they are typically IgM isotype, cross-react with neutral phospholipids and are not associated with thrombosis. In lupus, thrombotic complications have been most frequently associated with high titer IgG anti-cardiolipin antibodies, which cross-react with negatively charged phospholipids, such as phosphotidyl serine[46,47].

The exact mechanism of pathogenicity remains unknown. In contrast to the majority of lesions seen in SLE, those associated with APL antibodies are thrombotic rather than inflammatory. One attractive hypothesis is that the autoantibodies bind to cell membrane phospholipids and activate platelets or interfere with endothelial prostacyclin release. However, there is no direct evidence to support this and it has been alternatively proposed that APL antibodies bind to coagulation factors. In this regard, it has been demonstrated that anti-cardiolipin antibodies require the co-factor B2 glycoprotein I in order to bind anionic phospholipid[48]. B2 glycoprotein I is known to have anti-thrombotic properties and furthermore, immunization with this glycoprotein has been shown to induce APL antibodies in experimental animals[49].

OTHER AUTOANTIBODIES

The relevance of other autoantibodies is as yet unknown. Antibodies to cell surface constituents appear to play a role in hemolysis, leucopenia and thrombocytopenia. They may also have subtle effects on various T-cell subsets including depression of $CD4^+$ and/or $CD8^+$ T-lymphocytes. *In vivo*, the level of these lymphocytotoxic antibodies correlates with T-lymphopenia and other parameters of active lupus and their potential role in pathogenesis has been recently reviewed[33].

ORIGINS OF AUTOANTIBODIES

The autoantibody response in lupus appears to be specific and driven by antigen. The magnitude of the response can be great and individual autoantibodies may constitute a large fraction of the total circulating immunoglobulin, e.g. up to 15 g/l anti-Sm[24] and 30 g/l anti-Ro[50]. Iso-electric focusing has shown that autoantibodies to DNA, Sm, Ro, La and RNP are typically polyclonal[24]. Their immunoglobulin class and subclass distributions are similar to those observed following immunization and, importantly, they also show class switching.

Some genes that encode autoantibodies have been sequenced in order to delineate the exact mechanisms that underlie their production. There is controversy regarding germ-line polymorphisms in the immunoglobulin constant domains and whether any of these correlate with disease. Study of the variable region sequences in a variety of autoantibodies, however, has generally shown somatic mutation in their variable regions – as exemplified by anti-DNA antibodies[51]. This is powerful data supporting the hypothesis that the generation of autoantibody to autoantigen involves conventional maturation of the immune response. This in turn implies a breakdown of tolerance to self and raises questions regarding B- and T-cell function.

B-CELLS

No specific B-cell phenotype has been implicated in the pathogenesis of human lupus although $CD5^+$ B-lymphocytes, which synthesize low affinity IgM autoantibodies, may play a role in the New Zealand mouse model[52]. A predominant feature of both murine and human SLE is B-cell hyperactivity and hypergammaglobulinemia[53,54]. In animal models, the induction of polyclonal B-cell activation is associated with autoantibody synthesis[55] and this was originally taken as evidence for non-specific autoantibody production in lupus. It is now acknowledged that the normal B-cell repertoire has a large number of precursors for anti-DNA production which can be induced by a variety of non-specific means. However, these so-called 'natural autoantibodies' are generally polyspecific, IgM and of doubtful pathogenicity. The current postulate is that an early phase of non-specific B-cell activation is followed by more selective autoantibody synthesis with class switching and skewing of the repertoire secondary to antigen drive. In murine lupus, longitudinal analysis of the B-cell and autoantibody response supports this[56,57].

B-cells also show enhanced response to T-cell derived cytokine signals, e.g. I1–2, and combinations of I1–4, 5 and 6[58]. Indeed, much of the B-cell hyperactivity observed in SLE appears to be T-cell driven.

T-CELLS

Lymphopenia and abnormalities of specific T-cell subsets are typical of lupus (see above). Whether these disturbances underlie the autoimmune process or merely reflect disease activity is unknown. Current understanding does implicate T-cells in the pathogenesis of SLE. The bulk of the autoantibody response is IgG_1 and IgG_3; the generation of which is thought to be dependent on T-cell help. Despite the lymphopenia, surface markers demonstrate T-cell activation during exacerbations of lupus[33,59]. Follow-up studies also show a correlation between the T-cell activating cytokine I1–2 and disease activity[58]. More specifically, T-cells derived from lupus patients have been shown to augment anti-DNA production *in vitro*[60]. In murine SLE, the depletion of T-cells using anti-$CD4^+$ monoclonal antibodies has been associated with an improvement in nephritis and increased life span[61,62].

However, crucial evidence for specificity of the T-cell response at the level of the T-cell receptor is lacking. Nor are there any data as yet demonstrating T-cell proliferative responses to processed native antigen. An expansion in this area of understanding will be important in deciphering the events that lead to autoreactivity in SLE.

IMMUNE COMPLEXES AND COMPLEMENT

There is good evidence of a pathogenic role for immune complexes in SLE (Chapter 1). First, immune complexes and complement are deposited in various organs, including skin, kidney, brain, joints and lungs. Secondly, the binding of autoantibodies to circulating autoantigen, or to antigen *in situ*, leads to activation of the classical pathway of the complement system. Indeed, hypocomplementemia is a useful test of active lupus.

IMMUNE COMPLEXES

Circulating immune complexes (CIC) were first detected in lupus sera as cryoglobulins; containing IgG, IgM and complement proteins[63]. There have been subsequent attempts to correlate CIC with disease activity. However, the interpretation of data from these longitudinal studies has been problematic because of autoantibodies in lupus sera reacting against assay components, e.g. anti-C1q antibodies (see below). The practical impact of these difficulties has been that the measurement of CIC is no longer routinely performed by most clinical laboratories.

Specialized assays using monoclonal antibodies against neoantigens only expressed during complement activation[64] gave positive results with lupus sera, which in general correlated with disease activity. Despite this, identifying the antigen and antibody specificities within CIC has been difficult, and the presence[65] or absence of DNA[66] is controversial.

COMPLEMENT

Complement activity in lupus sera is reduced, relates to disease activity and improves with treatment. Complement deposition, and in particular the membrane attack complex, may be detected in inflamed skin and glomeruli. Levels of the classical pathway proteins, C1q, C2, and C4 are often markedly reduced in lupus[38]. C3 levels are less frequently abnormal and reduced levels are often an indication of severe disease[67,68]. However, studies of cohorts of patients with SLE show weak (albeit highly significant) correlation in the levels of individual complement proteins with disease activity[37,69].

DISEASE SUSCEPTIBILITY GENES

The contribution of genetic factors to disease is studied by comparing the concordance rates for identical and dizygotic twins. For human lupus, these values are 24% for monozygotic and 5% for dizygotic twins[70]. The rate for dizygotic twins is similar to that for first degree relatives[71]. These figures confirm the role of genetic factors in susceptibility to SLE although the observation that the concordance rate for monozygotic twins is 24%, rather than 100%, also implicates environmental factors.

COMPLEMENT GENES AND SLE

The strongest disease susceptibility genes to be identified in humans are those encoding deficiencies of classical pathway complement components, especially C1q, C2, and C4[72]. Although individuals who are homozygous for such deficiencies are rare, the vast majority have SLE. There is a gradation of disease severity in these patients. C1q deficiency is associated with a full array of autoantibodies, rashes, glomerulonephritis, cerebral lupus and often early death. C4 or C2 deficiency are complicated by SLE of lesser severity.

C4 has two isotypic variants, C4A and C4B. Studies of large lupus populations have identified null alleles (which are associated with no expressed protein) of C4A as a putative susceptibility gene in > 50% of caucasoid patients and similar data exists for other racial groups[73,74]. The key role of classical pathway components in the solubilization and removal of CIC makes deficiency of any of these proteins a strong predisposing factor to the development of SLE (see below).

MHC ASSOCIATIONS

It is still not certain which MHC gene(s) confer increased susceptibility to the development of SLE. The two groups of genes encoded within the MHC that have attracted greatest interest are the class II genes and the class III complement genes, particularly those encoding C4 and C2. Tumor necrosis factors α and β are also encoded in the class III locus and in murine SLE there have been data suggesting that low expression of TNF may be associated with severe disease[75].

Initial studies of class II antigens showed a raised prevalence of HLA-DR2 and HLA-DR3 among caucasoid SLE patients, though the relative risk of disease associated with possession of these antigens was only 2–3 fold[76]. Subsequent studies confirmed a significant association between B8 and DR3 and SLE[77,78]. Family studies demonstrated that in fact the haplotype HLA-A1, B8, DR3 was increased in prevalence in SLE[73]. Importantly, this haplotype also encodes a C4A null allele, located in the intervening region between the class I and II genes. The occurrence of linkage disequilibrium over large fragments of DNA has led to difficulty in attributing susceptibility to any one locus on such an extended haplotype. However, the detection of an excess of C4 null alleles in all lupus populations studied, including those which rarely express DR3 e.g. Japanese, has strengthened the candidacy of the C4 null allele as the relevant disease susceptibility gene in the extended haplotype, HLA A1, B8, C4AQ*0, DR3.

Recently, there has been evidence cited that B8-DR3 is in linkage with alleles at the DQ locus (DQw2.1) and that these are prevalent in patients expressing anti-Ro antibodies[79]. However, the frequent presence of anti-Ro in patients with any inherited classical pathway complement deficiency (and therefore not necessarily DR3 positive), argues against a prime role for the DQ locus on the induction of these antibodies.

HORMONES

Steroid hormones are known to exert profound effects on the immune system. The predominance of SLE in females of reproductive age has therefore focused attention on the role of sex hormones in lupus. In the New Zealand mouse model of SLE, prepubertal orchidectomy or the administration of estrogens accelerated disease in male mice, whereas oophorectomy or testosterone injections appeared to be protective and reduced mortality in females[80]. With respect to human lupus, Lahita and co-workers have demonstrated an excess of estrogenic activity in both sexes and reduced levels of testosterone in females[81,82]. There is some evidence that lupus flares are more frequent during the hyperestrogenic state of pregnancy, although this area is extremely controversial. The use of exogenous estrogens, e.g. 17-ethinyl estradiol, in the oral contraceptive pill, has been more clearly associated with worsening of the disease in females[83]. In view of these data, suggesting a role for female sex hormones in promoting disease, androgenic hormone therapy has been tried in both males and females[84]. However, this approach has been unsuccessful, raising questions as to whether the observed sex steroid abnormalities are cause or effect.

ENVIRONMENTAL FACTORS IN SLE

Although environmental factors are important in the expression of autoimmune disease, our understanding of their role in SLE is rudimentary. Many drugs are capable of inducing a lupus-like illness or exacerbating existing disease (see below). In addition, it is now recognized that certain drugs are commonly associated with allergic reactions in lupus patients, e.g. sulfonamides. Exposure to ultraviolet radiation is related to many of the acute rashes of lupus and may even cause a systemic flare of disease. The clinical nature of lupus – a febrile, remitting and relapsing illness with chronic immune perturbation – has led to the hypothesis that a persistent viral infection may be important etiologically. A number of viral illnesses are associated with autoimmune phenomena including HIV, Epstein–Barr, hepatitis B or cytomegalovirus infections. The mechanisms by which viruses may lead to autoimmunity are discussed below, but as yet there are no convincing data documenting an infectious agent as a cause for SLE. Interestingly, however, there have been recent anecdotal reports of parvovirus infection preceding the onset of lupus in some patients[85,86].

ANIMAL MODELS

Lupus-prone mice have given important insights into the pathogenesis of SLE. There are three strains of mice that are especially susceptible to the development of an SLE-like illness[80]: the New Zealand mice (NZB, NZW and their F1 hybrid), the BXSB mouse and the MRL mouse.

The NZB strain spontaneously develops hemolytic anemia whilst the NZW strain is essentially normal. However, the F1 offspring of a NZB × NZW cross develop an autoimmune syndrome of autoantibodies, hemolytic anemia and glomerulonephritis leading to premature death. This model further resembles human disease in that females have a more severe phenotype and die before males. In contrast, the BXSB model shows accelerated disease in males and a milder, delayed onset in females. The MRL/*lpr* model exhibits marked lymphoproliferation, splenomegaly and systemic autoimmunity. Two congenic strains have been produced; MRL-*lpr/lpr*, which has accelerated disease, and MRL-+/+ which expresses milder, late-onset disease.

There is considerable clinical variation between these three models but significantly they are all characterized by hypergammaglobulinemia, anti-DNA and other antinuclear antibodies, circulating immune complexes, glomerulonephritis and a degree of vasculitis. Experiments with these three models have confirmed the heterogeneity of SLE and shown that, as in humans, murine SLE is a polygenic and multifactorial process. Several conclusions regarding the etiopathogenesis of disease in lupus mice have been drawn:

1. Disease may be transmitted by transplantation of bone marrow from lupus-prone strains of mice to their normal, irradiated counterparts. This shows that expression of the disease susceptibility gene(s) within cells arising from hematopoietic stem cells is sufficient to induce disease.
2. There is marked genetic heterogeneity among the several strains of mice that develop lupus. Four types of genes controlling disease in mice have been recognized:
   (a) Disease susceptibility genes. The introduction of these genes in isolation into normal mice leads to the development of autoimmune phenomena, although not necessarily SLE. Apoptosis, or programed cell death, is a crucial mechanism whereby autoreactive lymphocytes of the immune system are eliminated. The *lpr* gene encodes for a mutant of a T-lymphocyte cell surface antigen termed Fas. The *lpr* mutation leads to defective Fas function and failure of apoptosis[87]. This mechanism is thought to account for the phenotype of the MRL-*lpr/lpr* model which is homozygous with respect to the *lpr* mutation. There is another gene involved in apoptosis termed *gld*, which may encode a ligand to the Fas antigen[88]. Mutations at the *gld* locus are also associated with autoimmunity in other mice models [89].
   (b) Disease accelerating genes. The presence of these genes in isolation in a normal mouse is not sufficient to cause SLE, but their introduction into a lupus-prone strain hastens disease. Examples of this are:
      (i) those determining sex-hormone production in NZB/W mice;
      (ii) a Y chromosome gene in the BXSB mouse; and
      (iii) the *lpr* gene in MRL mice.
   (c) Genes controlling individual manifestations of disease. The most dramatic of several examples of this is the H-2 bm12 polymorphism in the mouse MHC locus. The introduction of bm12 into the NZB model leads to intense production of anti-dsDNA antibodies [90].
   (d) Protective genes which inhibit the development of disease: e.g. *xid*. The *xid* mutation is normally associated with an X-linked immunodeficiency syndrome, but in lupus-prone strains it appears to suppress disease[91].
3. The single abnormality of immune cellular function common to all strains is excessive activation of B-lymphocytes. It is not yet clear whether this is due to their excessive sensitivity to normally-derived signals from cytokines or whether they are stimulated excessively by abnormal production of cytokines from other activated cells, e.g.

helper CD4$^+$ T-cells. In the case of the MRL strain, the *lpr* gene is associated with massive lymphadenopathy secondary to accumulation of CD4 CD8 double negative T-lymphocytes. It is tempting to speculate that these accelerate disease by the secretion of B-cell stimulatory cytokines.

4. The various lupus-prone strains of mice do not share a particular MHC haplotype at the H-2 locus. A gene in, or linked to, the H-2^z haplotype of NZW mice, appears to be the dominant disease susceptibility gene in promoting high levels of anti-DNA antibodies and early nephritis in (NZB = NZW)F1 hybrids[92]. There is little evidence that inherited complement deficiency plays an important role in disease susceptibility to spontaneous murine lupus, in contrast to the situation in humans.

5. There are environmental as well as genetic accelerating factors that hasten or delay the onset of disease in lupus-prone animals. Viral (e.g. Gross virus or lymphocytic choriomeningitis virus) and bacterial infection accelerate the onset of disease.

ETIOLOGICAL HYPOTHESES

A message from all of these studies in animals is that SLE is a syndrome with similar final pathways of disease expression, but may have diverse causes. The processes which initiate disease may well be different from those that perpetuate it. Four groups of hypotheses proposing explanations for the etiology of SLE in humans will be considered:

1. failure of the mononuclear phagocytic system to clear immune complexes leading to stimulation of autoimmunity by auto-antigens;
2. aberrant polyclonal activation of B-lymphocytes resulting in autoantibody production;
3. abnormality of 'idiotypic networks';
4. viruses as a cause of disease.

Is SLE due to failure of the physiological clearance mechanisms of immune complexes?

One hypothesis for the etiology of SLE is that there is failure of the physiological mechanisms of immune complex (IC) clearance. In the normal situation, generation of IC in the circulation or at sites of tissue deposition, leads to activation of complement and opsonization of the complexes. Opsonized IC can then bind via C3b to the complement receptor CR1 on red blood cells and are transported to the fixed mononuclear phagocyte system in the liver and spleen for further processing. Abnormal clearance has been demonstrated in primates which had been either depleted of complement[93] or infused with poorly complement-fixing IC[94].

The strongest disease susceptibility genes characterized for the development of SLE are null alleles for the complement proteins C1q, C2, and C4 (above). These proteins are encoded at distinct genetic loci which implies a pathophysiological link between complement deficiency and lupus. This is further supported by the observation that acquired complement deficiency states, such as those associated with inherited C1 inhibitor deficiency and C3 nephritic factor, are also associated with a raised prevalence of autoimmunity.

A possible pathophysiological mechanism for the association of complement deficiency with SLE is shown in Figure 2.1. The interaction of IC with complement inhibits their precipitation from solution and solubilizes complexes deposited in tissues[95]. C3b, iC3b and C4b bound to complexes are ligands for complement receptors on a variety of cells leading to:

1. opsonization for phagocytosis by neutrophils;
2. binding to CR1 on erythrocytes and transport to the liver and spleen; and
3. binding of immune complexes to antigen-presenting and to B-cells.

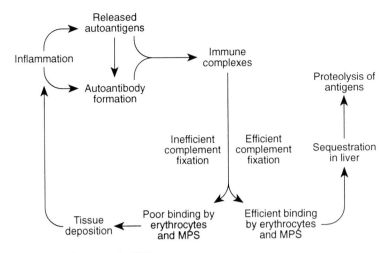

Fig. 2.1 Immune complex clearance in SLE.

It follows that complement deficiency will result in defective binding of C4 and C3 to IC and thus impair each of these activities. The persistence of IC may stimulate autoimmunity through antigen associated with the IC or as a consequence of antigens released after IC-mediated tissue injury[96]. Recently, a patient with C2 deficiency and SLE has been described[97]. Splenic uptake of IC was entirely absent in this patient but could be restored by the infusion of fresh frozen plasma containing C2. Interestingly, regular fresh frozen plasma treatment was also associated with clinical remission.

However, only a very small minority of SLE patients have total, inherited deficiency of a complement protein and it is harder to explain a physiological link between heterozygous deficiency of C4A, apparently the commonest disease susceptibility gene to SLE, and impaired immune complex handling *in vivo*. It has been shown that as little as 1% of C4A is sufficient to inhibit immune precipitation of immune complexes *in vitro* and normal adherence of immune complexes to erythrocytes[98]. However, complement functions as an extravascular, as well as an intravascular, enzyme cascade and it is therefore possible that C4A levels are lower in the extravascular

space in heterozygote subjects, which may allow the triggering of SLE.

Once the process of immune complex formation is started, activation of the classical and alternative pathways of complement leads to increased turnover and reduced levels of complement proteins. This may be a factor which perpetuates disease, by further impairing the mechanisms of disposal of immune complexes. It is possible that the reduction of CR1 on erythrocytes, which is seen in patients with active SLE, may also contribute to disease persistence in a similar manner to reduced C4 levels[99]. Indeed, *in vivo* IC clearance studies in patients with active disease, hypocomplementemia and reduced CR1 levels, have shown reduced splenic clearance of complexes and an abnormal localization pattern in the liver[100]. These data give insight into the failure of IC clearance mechanisms, even in patients who do not have homozygous deficiencies of complement proteins.

Is SLE due to polyclonal activation of lymphocytes?

One hypothesis for the development of SLE is that polyclonal activation of B-lymphocytes leads to unregulated proliferation of all antibody-producing cells, including those producing autoantibodies. This could follow from extrinsic activation of lymphocytes, e.g. stimulated by viral infection, or from breakdown of immunoregulatory mechanisms. Experimental evidence in mice demonstrated that the immune response to autoantigens (such as DNA), and external antigens (such as ovalbumin) is qualitatively the same in autoimmune strains of mice and normal mice, but quantitatively different[101]. However, other studies of human and murine lupus (reviewed above) have provided strong evidence that the autoantibody response is selective, driven by antigen, and that there is not polyclonal activation of all B-cells. These latter data do not exclude the possibility that the early phase of SLE is initiated by polyclonal B-cell activation, with a secondary antigen-specific phase in which disease is expressed.

Disturbances of idiotypic networks

Antibodies bear their own antigenic determinants, termed idiotypes, that may induce production of anti-idiotype antibodies. The finding of cross-reactive idiotypes on autoantibodies, some of which are represented on several of the characteristic lupus autoantibodies has led to the hypothesis that a disturbance in the putative network of idiotypes and anti-idiotypes may stimulate autoantibody production[102,103]. The evidence for the existence *in vivo* of networks of autoantibodies and anti-idiotypes is very limited, although a number of groups have found anti-idiotypic antibodies to anti-DNA antibodies in sera from patients, particularly those with inactive disease[104,105].

The hypothesis that antibody production may be regulated by anti-idiotypes has therapeutic implications. It has been tested by Hahn and Ebling[106] who attempted to suppress expression of a cross-reactive idiotype on murine anti-dsDNA antibodies using a monoclonal anti-idiotypic antibody.

Although the idiotype could be suppressed, with transient therapeutic benefit, this was soon overcome by the development of large quantities of anti-dsDNA antibodies bearing other idiotypes. This result is strongly in favor of the hypothesis of an antigen-driven immune response. An augmentation of idiotype production was found when MRL mice were administered polyclonal anti-idiotypic antibodies[107]. Much of the evidence against the hypothesis that polyclonal activation is the cause of autoantibody production, can also be used to counter the hypothesis that a disturbance of idiotypic networks is responsible. In particular, the spectrum of SLE autoantigens and the multiple epitopes which are recognized by autoantibodies would be difficult to reconcile simply with a disturbed idiotypic network.

Viruses as a cause of SLE

Viruses could, in theory, cause SLE by:

1. infecting lymphoid cells and perturbing their function;
2. interacting with host machinery for the replication of nucleic acids and creating neoantigens which could break immunological tolerance;
3. stimulating the production of anti-idiotypic antibodies which could interact with receptors for viruses on cells;
4. cross-reactive epitopes between viral and host antigens, termed molecular mimicry; or
5. infection of non-lymphoid cells causing prolonged release of autoantigens.

There is a virtually total lack of evidence in strong support of any of these hypotheses.

There has been great interest in possible roles of retroviruses in SLE. Retroviral gene sequences are integrated into the host genome and are transmissible vertically from generation to generation. The discovery of antibodies to C-type retroviruses in NZB mice raised the possibility that such viruses play an

Table 2.2 The 1982 ARA criteria for the classification of SLE [1]

1. Malar rash
2. Discoid rash
3. Photosensitivity
4. Oral ulcers
5. Non-erosive arthritis of two or more joints
6. Serositis (pleurisy or pericarditis)
7. Renal disorder (proteinuria >0.5 g/day, or cellular casts)
8. Neurological disorder (seizure or psychosis)
9. Hematological disorder (hemolytic anemia, leucopenia $<4 \times 10^9/l$ on two or more occasions, lymphopenia $<1.5 \times 10^9/l$ on two or more occasions or thrombocytopenia $<100 \times 10^9/l$)
10. Immunological disorder (positive LE cell, anti-dsDNA, anti-Sm or false-positive syphilis serology)
11. Positive ANA

A diagnosis of SLE can be made if four or more of these criteria are detected over any period of time.

etiological role in murine lupus[108]. Antibodies to the viral *env* gene product, Gp70, are produced in large amounts in these animals and immune complexes comprising Gp70-anti-Gp70 have been shown to participate in the lesions of glomerulonephritis. However, it has been shown that expression of retroviral antigens is not essential for the development of lupus in NZB mice[109]. Recently, a study has shown expression of a novel 8.4 kilobase retroviral transcript in the thymus and spleen of several lupus-prone mouse strains but not in controls. Retroviral expression was shown to precede development of lupus and could be mapped to a bone-marrow stem cell[110]. It is interesting that murine lupus is transmissible by bone marrow transplantation from a lupus-prone strain to normal mice. However, as yet there is very little evidence for the participation of retroviruses in human SLE.

CLINICAL FEATURES

The clinical manifestations of lupus are diverse and vary greatly from patient to patient. Milder disease with fever and polyarthalgia may be confused with early rheumatoid arthritis. The initial manifestation of lupus may predominantly involve a single organ system – nephritis, thrombocytopenia, rash or psychosis – and it is not unusual for lupus patients to present to the rheumatologist via another clinic. Another common scenario is the thrombotic pattern of disease seen in association with APL antibodies. There is no single classical presentation and the diagnosis of SLE is based on a set of disease classification criteria (Table 2.2).

GENERAL

Fever, malaise, anorexia and weight loss are common features of lupus. Lymphadenopathy with small 'rubbery' nodes is seen in up to 30% of patients. The ESR is typically elevated in active lupus although a corresponding rise in the CRP titer is rare and, when present, is suggestive of infection[111].

MUSCULOSKELETAL

Polyarthralgia is the commonest manifestation of SLE, occurring in over 90% of patients. The arthropathy is typically episodic, symmetrical and involves small joints of the hands and feet, wrists, ankles and knees. It is non-erosive and generally non-deforming with involvement of peri-articular tissues rather than cartilage or juxta-articular bone. These are important distinguishing features from rheumatoid arthritis. Rarely (< 10%), tenosynovitis is severe and causes tendon contractures in the hands. This gives rise to a deforming pseudo-rheumatoid picture termed Jaccoud's arthritis (Figure 2.2).

Avascular necrosis of bone is increasingly recognized as a complication of SLE (Figure 2.3). It often occurs in the context of high-dose corticosteroids, and should be considered when pain occurs in large joints, e.g. hip. Similarly, myopathy is more likely to be the result of steroid usage rather than a true

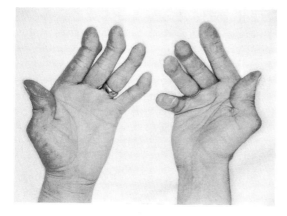

Fig. 2.2 Jaccoud's arthropathy occurs in up to 10% of patients, with swan-neck changes, Z-shaped thumbs and ulnar drift of the digits. Radiograph did not show any erosive changes.

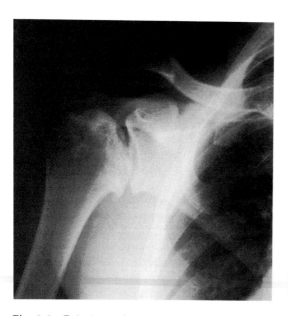

Fig. 2.3 Pain in a solitary large joint should raise the possibility of sepsis or, as in this case, avascular necrosis of bone. The shoulder joint of this patient who had received corticosteroids, shows irregular bone texture with sclerosis and peri-articular cystic changes. There are also early osteoarthritic changes.

inflammatory myositis, which is seen in less than 5% of patients. Very rarely myasthenia

gravis or the Eaton–Lambert syndrome have been described co-existing with SLE.

SKIN AND MUCOUS MEMBRANES

The skin is affected in the majority of SLE patients. Skin involvement is characterized histologically by the deposition of IgG, IgM and/or complement at the dermoepidermal junction. Paradoxically, these immune deposits may also be detected in areas of unaffected skin in lupus; and this forms the basis of the 'lupus band test'. However, deposition of complement membrane attack complex components is predominantly seen in areas of active inflammation.

Acute rashes in lupus are often associated with photosensitivity (Plate 1). The characteristic lesion is the erythematous butterfly/malar rash. Generalized erythema and localized photosensitive eruptions may also occur; these are occasionally bullous. Subacute cutaneous lupus erythematosus (SCLE) is characterized by annular or psoriaform photosensitive eruptions. Chronic rashes occur in 15% of cases of SLE. In contrast to the other rashes, these are typically scarring and associated with skin atrophy. The most frequently described chronic lesions are discoid lupus with erythema, scaling, follicular plugging, telangiectasia and atrophy. Like SCLE, discoid lupus erythematosus may also occur as a distinct syndrome (see below). Lupus panniculitis is one of the rare forms of skin involvement and causes inflammation and hyaline necrosis of subcutaneous adipocytes.

A number of other rashes occur in SLE. These comprise the network-like rash of livedo reticularis (often in association with APL antibodies), urticaria, nail fold capillaritis and vasculitis (Figure 2.4). Raynaud's phenomenon is an extremely common symptom. Mucosal ulceration can occur at any site but is most prevalent in the oral cavity. Perhaps the most distressing skin manifestation is alopecia. It can be generalized or local and, as in discoid LE, may result in scarring.

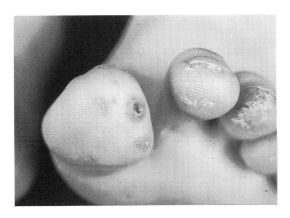

Fig. 2.4 Vasculitis affecting skin usually occurs in the context of active systemic disease. In this patient, tender purpuric lesions with areas of central ulceration were noted. Often there are associated nail-fold changes with splinter hemorrhages and peri-ungual erythema.

Hair loss is seen in up to 60% of patients and often requires cosmetic treatment as response to drugs is poor.

HEART

Fibrinoid pericarditis and small pericardial effusions are common in SLE, although tamponade is rare. Minor ECG abnormalities including non-specific T-wave changes are frequently seen. Cardiomyopathy, verrucous (Libman–Sachs) endocarditis and conduction defects (PR interval prolongation, atrioventricular block) have been reported but are unusual. Most of these cardiac complications have been found to be more prevalent in post-mortem as compared with ante-mortem series.

Systolic murmurs are audible in over 30% of patients and were previously attributed to a hyperdynamic circulation or anemia. However, more recent echocardiographic surveys have detected valvular thickening in 27–47% of patients and this complication may be associated with APL antibodies[112,113]. Valvular pathology does not generally lead to hemodynamic compromise.

Coronary artery disease is increasingly recognized as a late cardiac complication (see below). Duration of disease and steroid therapy appear to play a role, in addition to the usual risk factors for atherosclerosis[114].

LUNGS

Dyspnea, cough and chest pain are frequent symptoms in SLE. Clinically, 60% of patients will experience pleurisy with or without an inflammatory exudate at some stage of disease. Pulmonary function tests are abnormal in 80% with minor changes in the transfer factor and lung volumes. Pleuropericardial disease generally responds to a combination of non-steroidal anti-inflammatory drugs, steroids and aspiration as indicated.

There are several more insidious complications which affect the lung parenchyma and are much harder to manage. These comprise chronic interstitial lung disease, pulmonary hemorrhage, pulmonary hypertension (possibly secondary to APL antibodies) and a shrinking lung syndrome secondary to diaphragmatic involvement. Pulmonary function tests are sensitive in demonstrating parenchymal disease and sequential follow-up of the transfer factor may be particularly useful. Radiographic screening is less sensitive but will reveal pulmonary infiltrates. When present these are rarely due to a 'lupus pneumonitis' and vigilance has to be maintained for an infectious cause which is the more likely explanation, especially when a patient is on steroids/immunosuppressants.

KIDNEYS

Renal involvement will occur in the majority of patients. In up to 30–40% of patients there will be readily detectable manifestations of renal disease. Severe lupus nephritis is a serious adverse prognostic feature and currently 5-year renal survival from diagnosis is estimated between 74–87%[115,116]. SLE is responsible for approximately 3% of all end-stage renal failure patients. These data emphasize the need for a high index of suspicion for renal disease in all patients, especially given the success of cytotoxic drugs in retarding renal deterioration[117,118].

The presentation of renal disease is variable. Rarely, SLE may present as a rapidly progressive glomerulonephritis (GN) with advanced renal failure. More frequently, renal involvement is insidious, and urinalysis and blood pressure monitoring should be performed assiduously. In established nephritis the two most serious patterns are, a nephritic syndrome with focal/diffuse proliferative nephropathy or a nephrotic syndrome with membranous nephropathy (Plate 2). There is considerable clinical and histological overlap between the various patterns of lupus nephritis.

A causal role for autoantibodies and complement in renal inflammation is likely and many groups have found correlations between the severity of nephritis, systemic complement activation and levels of anti-dsDNA antibodies (reviewed earlier). However, renal involvement in SLE is complex and it results from several pathological processes:

1. Lupus nephritis. Glomerular injury is determined by the site of the deposition of antibody and complement. In membranous nephropathy this is the subepithelial space of the glomerular capillaries resulting in proteinuria, while in proliferative GN deposition is widespread and leads to both glomerular and tubular injury. A role for cell-mediated damage is supported by the intense mononuclear infiltrate leading to glomerular crescents and tubular inflammation in diffuse proliferative GN.
2. Hypertension and its effects on the kidney.
3. Glomerular thrombosis. This is commonly found in patients with focal and diffuse proliferative GN and is associated with deposition of complement and immune complexes, and with thrombocytopenia [119]. It is also found in patients with APL antibodies and in this circumstance is associated with little glomerular inflammation[119].

The assessment of lupus nephritis has been aided by a WHO classification of lupus renal histology[120] summarized in Table 2.3. This classification is useful both diagnostically and in the assessment of renal prognosis. 'Chronicity' and 'activity' indices of renal biopsy appearances have proved disappointing in predicting outcome[121]. Progressive renal failure is largely predicted by three factors: WHO grade IV biopsy (in particular tubulointerstitial damage), the presence of hypertension and a raised serum creatinine level at time of diagnosis[115,116]. In view of the high morbidity and mortality of renal disease in SLE and the value of therapeutic interventions, the need for regular screening (urinalysis, BP measurements, creatinine) and early use of renal biopsy cannot be overstated.

CENTRAL NERVOUS SYSTEM (CNS)

Primary CNS pathology in SLE is poorly understood. Almost a half of patients have some degree of cerebral involvement which is usually non-focal, manifesting as cognitive impairment, major psychosis, affective disorder or neurosis. Recurrent headaches and migraine are common. Epilepsy, like psychosis, may be the presenting feature of disease. Focal CNS involvement occurs in 10–35% of cases typically causing stroke, transverse myelitis or cranial neuropathy. Retinal involvement is relatively common and results in soft exudates termed 'cytoid bodies'. Basal ganglia syndromes and peripheral neuropathy are rare but demonstrate how SLE can affect any part of the CNS.

The pathological basis of these various clinical disorders is unclear. In post-mortem series microthrombi and infarction have been reported far more frequently (40%) than

Table 2.3 WHO classification of renal histology in SLE

Group	Major histological features	Site of immune deposit	Clinical features
I Minimal	Minimal or no change	None	Mild hematuria/proteinuria
II Mesangial GN	Mesangial hypercellularity	Mesangial	Hematuria/proteinuria
III Focal proliferative GN	Segmental glomerular involvement with hypercellularity and necrosis	Largely mesangial	Hematuria/proteinuria (sometimes heavy), nephritic syndrome possible
IV Diffuse proliferative GN	Diffuse glomerular hypercellularity with crescents, segmental glomerular necrosis, thrombosis, and tubulointerstitial inflammation	Mesangial, subendothelial extra glomerular	Nephritic syndrome, possibly nephrotic syndrome
V Membranous nephropathy	Thickening of glomerular capillaries	Capillary subepithelial	Nephrotic syndrome

immune complexes and vasculitis (10%) [122,123]. The choroid plexus, which is similar in structure to glomeruli, is a common site for the deposition of antibodies and complement, but there is no evidence that this has a pathological role. Cerebrospinal fluid protein levels suggest that there is no significant breach of the blood-brain barrier, however, oligoclonal IgG bands provide evidence of intrathecal immunoglobulin synthesis in some patients[124].

A variety of autoantibodies are prevalent in patients with CNS disease and include:

1. cross-reacting lymphocytotoxic antibodies [125,126];
2. anti-neuronal antibodies[127];
3. anti-cardiolipin antibodies, associated with cerebral vascular disease, chorea and migraine;
4. anti-ribosomal P antibodies, associated with lupus psychosis[15]; and
5. anti-neurofilament antibodies[128].

Whether these antibodies gain access to the CNS is unknown and their pathological significance is therefore uncertain.

The assessment of CNS disease is notoriously difficult given its protean manifestations and poor understanding of its pathology. Further difficulty may arise because of CNS effects secondary to metabolic disturbance, severe hypertension, sepsis or steroid therapy. The diagnosis of focal CNS lupus and of organic brain syndromes with cerebral atrophy has been considerably improved by advances in magnetic resonance imaging[129]. Where this is not available, CT scanning is still of value, especially in the context of acute cerebrovascular disease.

Other investigations, such as angiography, EEG and the analysis of cerebrospinal fluid and serum, have limited sensitivity and specificity but are sometimes useful.

LIVER AND GUT

Anorexia and abdominal pain occur in up to 30% of patients but more severe manifestations are unusual. Liver involvement is recognized, although rare. Hepatic steatosis is the most common finding but this is often the result of steroids. SLE may have a direct effect on the liver, occasionally causing arteritis with infarction. Vasculitis of the gut may cause intestinal angina and infarction.

RETICULOENDOTHELIAL SYSTEM

It is rare for patients to present with massive lymphadenopathy. Interestingly, two patients have been described with unexplained massive lymphadenopathy and a lupus-like disorder[130]. Accumulation of CD4 CD8 double negative T-cells in the lymph nodes was noted. The immunological and clinical features were similar to the *lpr* mouse model.

The role of T-cells has already been discussed and the extent of T-cell dysfunction is reflected in the reduction of cell-mediated responses to DTH antigens in active SLE. Antibody responses to foreign antigens are normal or slightly reduced. Splenomegaly occurs in less than 15% of cases although 'functional hyposplenism' has been described.

BLOOD

There is widespread hematological involvement affecting all cell types in both peripheral blood and bone marrow. Normochromic, normocytic anemia is seen in up to 75% of patients. In addition to the anemia of chronic disease, there is often some degree of hemolytic anemia. This may be Coombs' positive or negative, acute or chronic. When anti-red cell antibodies are detected, they are often 'warm-type' and fix complement.

Lymphocytotoxic antibodies are found in the majority of lupus sera. Both cold- and warm-reactive, they correlate with the lymphopenia, a cardinal feature of active disease. In contrast, other vasculitic illnesses are usually associated with a normal or raised white cell count. Thrombocytopenia is common, but in 5% of cases it may be severe and ultimately require splenectomy. Thrombocytopenia occurring in isolation and antedating other signs of lupus is well recognized. The possibility of SLE should therefore be considered before making a diagnosis of idiopathic thrombocytopenic purpura.

SUBSETS OF DISEASE

The heterogeneity of lupus is reflected in the number of autoimmune syndromes which are similar to SLE and often do not fulfil the ARA classification criteria. These have been classified as disease subsets of SLE. Figure 2.5 illustrates how they constitute a group of disorders with overlapping features with classical SLE. It is not known whether they are due to genetically encoded variation in host responsiveness to a single etiological stimulus, or whether different patterns of disease are responses to different etiological agents. Evidence for the former hypothesis comes

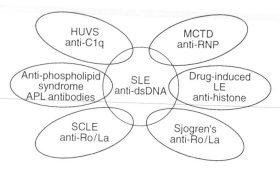

Fig. 2.5 SLE and its disease subsets showing autoantibody overlap.

from studies of families in whom one member may suffer from discoid lupus, while another has SLE which is fully expressed. Subclassification of disease has led to the realization that certain autoantibodies appear to be associated with particular patterns of illness, e.g. anti-Ro with cutaneous disease, antiphospholipid antibodies with thrombosis. It has also allowed the designation of variants of SLE with a favorable prognosis.

SUBACUTE CUTANEOUS LUPUS ERYTHEMATOSUS (SCLE)

SCLE may exist as a separate syndrome with mild systemic features and a number of important associations. It may overlap with primary Sjögren's syndrome with which it shares serological characteristics which include antibodies to Ro and La, rheumatoid factor and hyperglobulinemia. There is a strong association between this subtype of disease and HLA-B8,-DR3. Previously, up to 5% of SLE patients were thought to be negative for ANA and typically suffer from an SCLE-like illness. Use of the modern and more sensitive Hep-2 cell line, as a substrate for ANA detection, has revealed that most of these patients are ANA positive.

DISCOID LUPUS ERYTHEMATOSUS (DLE)

DLE most commonly occurs as a distinct syndrome with little systemic involvement and a good prognosis with only 5% progressing to generalized disease. DLE has important epidemiological differences from SLE. Onset is generally later in DLE and the female-to-male ratio is lower at 2:1. However, these patients show many of the immunological features of lupus[131] and DLE patients often have a family history of SLE.

NEONATAL LUPUS

The neonatal lupus syndrome comprises complete congenital heart block, photosensitive rash, hepatitis and thrombocytopenia (Chapter 12). One of the surprising features of SLE, apparently mediated by IgG autoantibodies, is the rarity of neonatal disease[132,133]. The cutaneous manifestations of neonatal lupus closely resemble those of SCLE and both show extremely strong associations with autoantibodies to Ro and La[132]. There are equally strong associations between antibodies to Ro and La and congenital cardiac disease[134], although the prevalence of congenital cardiac disease in children born of mothers with anti-Ro antibodies is less than 5%[132,133]. The role of these antibodies in the causation of fetal myocarditis progressing to congenital heart block and, occasionally, generalized cardiac fibrosis has not been established, though immunoglobulin deposits have been described in cardiac tissue[135].

PRIMARY SJÖGREN'S SYNDROME

This disease is considered in Chapter 5. The characteristic autoantibodies of primary Sjögren's syndrome are anti-Ro, anti-La and rheumatoid factor. The clinical features of SLE and primary Sjögren's syndrome overlap considerably[136] and the MHC haplotype, HLA-A1, B8, DR3, C4AQ 0, C4B1, BfS, C2-1, has a raised prevalence among patients with both diseases. It is unknown whether SLE and primary Sjögren's syndrome are part of the spectrum of a single disease or have different etiologies.

MCTD

Antibodies to RNP have been associated with an overlap disorder between SLE, myositis and scleroderma – 'mixed connective tissue disease' (MCTD)[8]. In low titer, anti-RNP antibodies are found in up to 30% of SLE patients. In high titer, and in the absence of antibodies to dsDNA or Sm, they are associated with MCTD, in which the most consistent clinical feature is severe Raynaud's phenomenon. An erosive polyarthritis with prominent swelling of fingers is another common clinical feature of MCTD, distinguishing patients from those with classical SLE. Patients with MCTD seem to have a slightly different spectrum of reactivity to the proteins of U1RNP than patients with SLE. Antibodies to the 68 kDa protein are much commoner in MCTD than in SLE[137]. Antibodies to RNP certainly do not define a unique subset of disease. The clinical features of the original series of patients described as having MCTD evolved into those found in a variety of diseases including SLE, scleroderma, and rheumatoid arthritis[138].

HYPOCOMPLEMENTEMIC URTICARIAL VASCULITIS SYNDROME [HUVS)

Recurrent lower limb urticaria is common in SLE and on biopsy there may be changes of a leukocytoclastic vasculitis. A syndrome comprising urticarial vasculitis and hypocomplementemia (HUVS) without the features of classical SLE is recognized[139]. There is a close relationship between HUVS and SLE since urticarial vasculitis is associated both with reduced serum complement, specifically very low C1q, low C4 and C2, and normal to low C3. Arthritis and glomerulonephritis are also seen in HUVS which may occasionally progress to SLE. It is now appreciated that the common denominator between the two syndromes is the presence of autoantibodies to the complement protein C1q[140].

DRUG-INDUCED LE

The multifactorial etiology of SLE and the interplay of genes and environmental agents is exemplified by the lupus-like illness that may follow the ingestion of certain drugs. Drug-induced LE is generally seen in an older group of patients and affects males and females equally. A growing list of agents are implicated including hydralazine, procainamide, phenytoin, isoniazid, chlorpromazine, estrogens and more recently drugs used in the treatment of rheumatic disease, such as D-penicillamine and sulfasalazine[141]. The pattern of disease resembles idiopathic SLE but there is a preponderance of pulmonary involvement and less CNS and renal disease. The outcome is generally favorable on cessation of the offending drug although a short course of steroids may be required.

Certain drugs, e.g. hydralazine, induce ANA in a dose-dependent fashion but only a minority develop signs of lupus. There is an inherited polymorphism of the drug-metabolizing acetyltransferase enzyme and hydralazine-induced lupus is much more prevalent among slow acetylators than fast[142]. The autoantibody response associated with drug-induced disease is qualitatively different from idiopathic SLE, and this may give insight into the origins of the autoantibodies in the two conditions. Anti-histone antibodies are common but anti-dsDNA antibodies are rarely detected. In addition, the specificity of the antibodies seems to vary according to the agent inciting disease. Hydralazine and procainamide are associated with antibodies to trypsin-resistant epitopes on histones H2A-H2B, whereas chlorpromazine and, to a lesser extent, procainamide[143] are associated with the development of lupus anticoagulant activity. The histone specificity contrasts with idiopathic SLE where the trypsin-sensitive epitopes on H1 and H2B are targeted. The genetic predisposition to hydralazine-induced lupus appears to differ from that of 'idiopathic' SLE. A raised prevalence of HLA-DR4 has been found in two groups of patients with hydralazine-induced lupus[144].

The mechanism of induction of disease by drugs is unknown and a number of hypotheses have been explored which include:

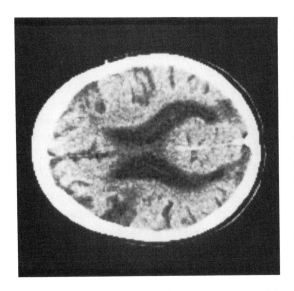

Fig. 2.6 Multiple cerebral infarcts in a patient with high titre anti-cardiolipin antibodies on CT scanning.

1. direct interaction of drug with DNA resulting in modified antigenicity.[145];
2. inhibition of DNA-methylation altering T-cell reactivity[146]; and
3. nucleophilic inactivation of complement C4, causing acquired C4 deficiency[147].

ANTI-PHOSPHOLIPID SYNDROME

The clinical features of this variant of SLE are venous and arterial thrombosis, hemolytic anemia, thrombocytopenia, livedo reticularis and cardiac valvular lesions. APL antibodies are probably responsible for much of the CNS pathology in lupus (Figure 2.6). There also appears to be an association with recurrent spontaneous abortion in the second or third trimester. This complication may be secondary to a placental vasculopathy. The nature of anti-phospholipid antibodies and the associated immunopathology have been explored above. Despite strong epidemiological evidence, a causal role for APL antibodies in the etiology of these lesions has not yet been established[47]. The prevalence of anti-phospholipid antibodies among patients who fulfil the ARA classification criteria for SLE is almost 40% using cardiolipin immunoassay. A subgroup of patients have been identified who have the clinical features associated with APL antibodies, but who do not have other features of SLE. These patients have been designated by some authors as suffering from the 'primary anti-phospholipid syndrome'.

There have been no controlled trials of treatment for the complications of the anti-phospholipid syndrome and there is considerable uncertainty regarding management. Following a significant venous thrombosis, anti-coagulation with warfarin is recommended. The ideal duration of anti-coagulation is unclear but there have been several reports of recurrent thrombosis after withdrawal. Consequently, long-term anti-coagulation is generally preferred. Low-dose aspirin may inhibit those components of the thrombotic tendency associated with platelet activation but the role of full anti-coagulation in arterial thrombosis is uncertain.

The management of recurrent pregnancy loss has fluctuated from a conservative approach to high-dose steroids and/or plasma exchange. Early reports showed benefit from high-dose prednisolone and aspirin[148] although adverse outcome, with an increased risk of pre-eclampsia, has been reported subsequently[149]. The rationale for steroids is debatable:

1. The pathogenesis of this syndrome is thrombotic rather than inflammatory.
2. Levels of APL antibodies do not seem to be influenced by immunosuppression.

   The use of low-dose aspirin, known to be beneficial in pre-eclampsia, and careful fetal monitoring seems prudent. Women who are already anticoagulated for prior thrombotic complications, should be switched to subcutaneous heparin to avoid the teratogenic effects of warfarin. In pregnancy, the use of steroid should mainly be reserved to treat the inflammatory complications of disease.

MANAGEMENT OF SLE

The reported survival of patients with SLE has progressively improved during the past 40 years. There is increasing evidence from controlled studies that the use of disease modifying therapies has led to genuinely improved survival in SLE. Specific combinations of prednisolone with cytotoxic drugs have improved outcome in patients with severe nephritis, both in terms of survival and prevention of renal failure.

GENERAL MEASURES

1. It is essential to establish good patient rapport, especially in view of the natural history of lupus and the complicated treatment regimens used during severe episodes. This also ensures ease of access to clinics and allows early detection of change in status.
2. Patients should be made aware of potential disease triggers, which have been outlined above.
3. Counselling and careful attention to family planning are required because of the possible interactions between estrogens and lupus.
4. The assistance of other medical specialities at an early stage is crucial when there is serious involvement of major organs.
5. Rigorous monitoring of disease activity and for side-effects of treatment is essential.

SPECIFIC MEASURES

The enormous clinical variation in the manifestations of SLE determines that the organ(s) involved should be identified for each patient.

Whenever possible, objective measures of disease activity and reversibility should then be defined for each affected organ, e.g. for renal disease: urinary sediment, 24-hour proteinuria, creatinine clearance, blood pressure. These should be recorded sequentially on flow charts. Most patients learn subjective criteria to assess their own disease activity, such as increased hair loss, arthralgia and malaise. Although the pattern of organ involvement in any given patient often becomes established early in the course of disease, it is essential to remain alert to the onset of new organ involvement, particularly the development of renal disease.

Having defined the extent of target organ involvement, the next step is to form an overall assessment of disease activity. There are three broad categories of disease, each of which has different treatment implications, considered below:

1. mild: cutaneous or joint involvement in the absence of significant constitutional symptoms;
2. moderate: inflammatory involvement of other organs, e.g. heart and/or lungs plus or minus constitutional symptoms – this category would include patients with mesangial nephritis (WHO grade II);
3. severe: severe inflammatory involvement of vital organs, e.g. patients with neuropsychiatric disease, cardiac, severe pulmonary or severe renal involvement (focal or diffuse proliferative nephritis, WHO grades III and IV).

Treatment of mild disease and cutaneous disease

Patients with malaise and arthralgia may be adequately managed by rest and non-steroidal anti-inflammatory drugs alone. Antimalarial drugs, particularly hydroxychloroquine, may be helpful for the treatment of mild to moderate manifestations of SLE, including rash, arthralgia and mild constitutional symptoms. Objective evidence of the effectiveness of anti-malarials has now been provided by a placebo-controlled trial of withdrawal of hydroxychloroquine in a group of 47 patients with stable mild SLE who had been using the drug for a mean of 3 years[150]. Over 6 months there were 9 flares of disease in the treatment group compared with 16 flares in the placebo group.

By consensus the hydroxychloroquine dosage should be less than 6.5 mg/kg ideal body weight per day (in practical terms up to 400 mg/day) to minimize the risks of ocular toxicity. However, 6-monthly ocular monitoring should still be performed by:

1. counselling patients to report development of scotomata, loss of color vision or dark adaptation; and
2. regular screening for scotomata using an Amsler grid, as a small risk of toxicity remains[151].

It may be possible to discontinue hydroxychloroquine therapy during the winter months in patients in whom photosensitivity is a major feature in the exacerbation of rash.

Treatment of the more severe manifestations of cutaneous disease

Photosensitivity may provide an important contribution to the rash of SLE and may even cause a systemic disease flare. Patients should therefore be counselled about ultraviolet light (UV) avoidance and the use of broad spectrum UVA and UVB-blocking creams and ointments. Judicious use of topical steroids and intralesional steroids may also prove effective. A range of drugs have been used in patients with severe cutaneous LE, unresponsive to topical therapy, without evidence of severe systemic disease, in whom there is a need to avoid the toxicity of high-dose prednisolone and cytotoxic drugs. These include other anti-malarial drugs, such as mepacrine, which causes skin yellowing and may cause mood disturbance, and chloroquine, which probably

carries a greater risk than hydroxychloroquine of retinal toxicity. Combinations of hydroxychloroquine and mepacrine may be useful in severe cutaneous LE.

Dapsone and thalidomide are also used but formal trial data are lacking. Dapsone is usually given in a dose of 50–100 mg daily, and is thought to be of particular value in urticarial vasculitis[152,153]. The major side-effect of dapsone is microangiopathic hemolytic anemia, which is common and dose-related and needs to be monitored by regular measurement of hemoglobin, inspection of blood film, and bilirubin levels. It is contraindicated in glucose-6-phosphate dehydrogenase deficiency. There are several reports of the use of thalidomide in small series of patients with discoid lupus[154], lupus panniculitis[155] and subacute cutaneous lupus erythematosus[156]. Thalidomide carries the risk of fetal malformation, sedation and peripheral neuropathy. Patients need to be carefully counselled before prescription of this drug. The neuropathy associated with thalidomide appears to be related to the cumulative dosage. The maintenance dose should therefore be minimized to delay the onset of this side-effect which should be monitored by regular electrophysiological testing[157].

Treatment of moderate disease

Steroids

Although no controlled trials exist for the use of steroids in SLE, a number of empirically derived principles have emerged. The starting dose should be chosen according to the disease severity and is usually given once daily. Mild to moderate inflammatory disease is treated initially with doses of 0.5 mg/kg/day, severe with 1–1.5 mg/kg. Whenever possible, escalating doses of steroids should be avoided.

Once commenced, the aim should be to control disease activity before reducing prednisolone and most clinicians would maintain the starting dose for approximately 4 weeks. Treatment should then be tapered to a maintenance regime but here clinical practice is diverse. Some use alternate day steroid therapy, others maintain a daily dose. One approach is to reduce treatment to prednisolone 10 mg daily over 2–3 months with further reduction of not more than 1 mg/month. More rapid withdrawal of treatment may be associated with a flare of disease leading to rebound prescription of high doses of prednisolone. Therefore, it is prudent to maintain patients on doses of 5–7 mg of prednisolone for many months – until there is clinical and serological evidence of remission – before attempting to tail off the prednisolone completely.

Azathiorpine

Azathioprine, at a dose of approximately 2.5 mg/kg, has an important role as a steroid-sparing agent in patients with moderate to severe SLE. Approximately 0.3% of the population show virtually absent activity of the enzyme thiopurine methyltransferase which metabolizes azathioprine[158]. These individuals develop profound marrow suppression after taking azathioprine and obsessive hematological monitoring is essential, especially over the first 6 weeks. Long-term monitoring of the blood count is essential in all patients receiving cytotoxic drugs.

Treatment of severe disease

Cytotoxic agents

These drugs are used in addition to high-dose corticosteroid treatment when there is life-threatening vital organ involvement in lupus. A variety of cytotoxic drugs have been used in the rheumatic diseases, including azathioprine, cyclophosphamide, methotrexate and cylosporin. Methotrexate has not been properly evaluated in lupus and the use of cyclosporin is limited by its potential renal toxicity, which makes monitoring difficult in lupus nephritis. Therefore, in SLE, azathioprine and cyclophosphamide are the agents that have been most widely used. The two commonest indications for this treatment are active cerebral disease and severe nephritis with impaired renal function. Histologically, the latter correlates with focal and diffuse proliferative nephritis (WHO grades III and IV) accompanied by crescents, sclerosis and tubulointerstitial changes (above).

Prolonged studies using pulse cyclophosphamide have been conducted by workers at NIH[117,118]. Entry criteria were the presence of SLE with severe nephritis (grades III and IV). Five different treatments were compared:

1. prednisolone alone;
2. azathioprine plus prednisolone;
3. oral cyclophosphamide plus prednisolone;
4. oral azathioprine plus oral cyclophosphamide plus prednisolone;
5. IV pulse cyclophosphamide plus prednisolone.

Numbers of patients in each group varied from 18–30 patients and the follow-up on 19 of the patients now extends to 15 years or more. The end-points measured were progression to end stage renal failure and death. The three treatment regimens that included cyclophosphamide were significantly better in retarding progression to renal failure.

Pulsed cyclophosphamide has been used in other settings in SLE. The NIH group have published[159] an uncontrolled study using pulsed intravenous cyclophosphamide in 9 patients with severe neuropsychiatric lupus, most of whom were refractory to high-dose prednisolone. In 8 of these patients, recovery was graded as good or excellent. A similar regime for children with diffuse proliferative nephritis is also in use[160].

There are limited data regarding duration of treatment with pulse cyclophosphamide. Investigators at NIH randomized 65 patients with severe lupus nephritis to three groups:

1. 6 pulses of methylprednisolone at monthly intervals;
2. 6 pulses of cyclophosphamide at monthly intervals; and
3. 6 pulses of cyclophosphamide at monthly intervals followed by 8 pulses at intervals of 3 months[161].

During 5-year follow up the number of patients doubling their serum creatinine was significantly lower in the long-course cyclophosphamide group than the methylprednisolone group. The probability of developing an exacerbation after the first 6 months of treatment was also significantly lower in the group receiving long-course cyclophosphamide compared with that receiving short-course cyclophosphamide.

The optimal dose, route of administration and interval between pulses of cyclophosphamide is unknown. The NIH group titrate the dose from 500 mg to 1 gm/m^2 of body surface area, aiming to maintain the leucocyte count between 1.5×109 and $3.0 \times 109/l$ at the nadir of the leucopenia which occurs between 10 and 14 days after drug administration[161]. The Ann Arbor group titrate to higher doses if necessary, with the aim of achieving a nadir of $2.0–3.0 \times 109$ leucocytes/l at 7 or 14 days after treatment (the lymphocyte nadir is at 7 days, the neutrophil at approximately 14 days) – a detailed protocol is given in[162]. The administration of cyclophosphamide should be accompanied by a high fluid intake to minimize bladder toxicity. Some also co-administer mesna to inactivate acrolein, a toxic metabolite of cyclophosphamide which causes the bladder-urothelial injury. It has recently been appreciated that allergic reactions to mesna are common[163].

It is important to obtain informed consent from patients before prescription of cytotoxic agents. For cyclophosphamide it is necessary to warn patients of the risks of acute hematological and bladder toxicity and of the possibilities of long-term induction of infertility (up to 50%), bladder and lymphoid neoplasia.

The success of treatments for the severe inflammatory manifestations of SLE mean that late complications of treatment are now much commoner. In summary, there are two important caveats about the use of cytotoxic agents in SLE:

1. patients need to be counselled in detail regarding the risk/benefits of treatments; and
2. the attending physician must be obsessive in monitoring of the treatment.

Plasma exchange

The role of plasmapheresis in SLE is uncertain. The results of a large controlled study of plasma exchange in patients with severe lupus nephritis are not encouraging[164]. Eighty-six patients with WHO grade III, IV or V lupus nephritis were randomized to receive oral cyclophosphamide and high-dose prednisolone plus or minus 4 weeks of plasma exchange carried out 3 times each week. There were no significant differences between the two groups in any of the outcome measures, including death and renal failure despite significant early reduction in IgG, anti-dsDNA antibody and cryoglobulin levels in the plasmapheresis group. However, it may be premature to reject plasmapheresis in lupus and currently trials are being conducted to assess the combined effect of plasma exchange with synchronized administration of cytotoxic drugs to counteract the rebound B-cell activity that occurs after plasmapheresis.

Treatment of hypertension

Elevated systolic blood pressure has been identified as the most significant correlate of early mortality in SLE[165]. This may be explained by hypertension acting as a surrogate marker for the presence of nephritis, although this is not always the case[166] and hypertension may precede overt nephritis.

The adverse effect of hypertension on renal prognosis has been demonstrated in a variety of nephropathies. This appears to be the case in lupus nephritis[167] and aggressive management of hypertension may therefore be as important as immunosuppressive treatment itself.

OUTCOME IN SLE

The reported survival of patients with SLE has progressively improved over the past 40 years. The 5-year survival rate was less than 50% in 1955 and by 1990 had risen to over 90%. The explanation for this change is likely to be complex and not just simply improved management protocols. The increase in the number and availability of serological tests has undoubtedly led to the earlier recognition of milder cases. Inclusion of such cases in large studies may have contributed to the improved survival data.

Mortality is influenced by a number of factors not directly related to disease[168]. Some evidence suggests age at onset is important and that childhood SLE is associated with the worst prognosis. There is controversy regarding the relative severity of disease in males and females and reports differ. Black patients are considered to have a poorer outcome as compared to caucasians. In part this has been attributed to socioeconomic factors but an underlying genetic predisposition may also be at play. Prevalence of anti-Sm antibodies is much higher in black patients (>25%) than caucasians (10%)[169], and it has been proposed that blacks have a tendency to more severe complications, such as nephritis.

What are the causes of death in patients with SLE? Two studies by Urowitz and colleagues some years ago showed a bimodal pattern of deaths[170,171]. Those occurring in the first two years of disease were caused in approximately equal numbers by infection and the direct effects of the SLE, usually cerebral or renal disease. The second cluster of deaths, occurring after more than 5 years of disease, was found to be due to either active SLE or cardiovascular complications, particularly coronary artery disease.

These findings have stimulated several studies into the factors which may predispose to death from infection or coronary artery disease.

INFECTIONS IN SLE

A retrospective study by Ginzler and colleagues[172] attempted to identify risk factors for sepsis in SLE. Significant factors which emerged were increasing steroid dosage, active lupus nephritis, uremia and bone marrow toxicity secondary to azathioprine therapy. Azathioprine treatment was associated with an increased incidence of herpes zoster infection. Other factors which may contribute to sepsis in SLE are:

1. severe hypocomplementemia, a well-characterized risk factor for the development of pyogenic sepsis, particularly meningococcal disease; and
2. hyposplenism, either surgical as treatment of ITP or occurring as part of the disease process[173].

ACCELERATED CARDIOVASCULAR DISEASE

There are many factors which may play a role in accelerating cardiovascular disease in patients with SLE. These include:

1. damage to the coronary arteries by vasculitis;
2. hyperlipidemia secondary to the nephrotic syndrome and/or corticosteroid therapy;
3. hypertension secondary to nephritis and/or corticosteroids; and
4. coronary artery thrombosis associated with the presence of anticardiolipin antibodies.

A number of recent studies have examined risk factors for cardiovascular disease in SLE patients[114,174]. Important risk factors were hypertension, hypercholesterolemia and obesity, coupled with age and duration of prednisolone usage.

THE FUTURE

Controlled studies of agents already in clinical practice will refine treatment of lupus patients in maximizing benefit and reducing side-effects. As more is understood about the autoimmune basis of SLE at a molecular level, it may be possible to design more specifically targeted therapy. Current knowledge of how the immune response is generated together with developments in monoclonal antibody technology enable targeting of the immune system at several levels. The relative importance of some class II and III MHC associations, involvement of various T-cell subsets and specific clones of T-cells as well as the role of cytokines has been discussed above and is covered in greater detail in Chapter 14. This knowledge is still rudimentary, however, and the exact molecular events that cause autoimmunity are not understood. Preliminary studies in lupus mice have successfully used $CD4^+$ T-cells as targets for antibody therapy leading to remission[61,62]. Similar experimental therapies in human rheumatic diseases have been directed against lymphocytes and there are reports of treatment with anti-CD4 antibodies[175] (Chapter 14).

Evidence gathered from studies of humans and mice with SLE supports the hypothesis that SLE is a syndrome in which disease is caused by a final common pathway of inflammation initiated by many different stimuli. Both genetic susceptibility to disease and provocative environmental stimuli appear to be heterogeneous. High titers of autoantibodies accompanied by evidence of complement activation are the most striking abnormalities detected in patients with SLE. While the presence of autoantibodies is not sufficient for the development of inflammation, it is probable that they are necessary. A role for cell-mediated mechanisms of disease has been suggested by some studies and more work is needed to define these. In this regard, the use of animal models and the ability to conduct transgenic experiments will enable a more careful dissection of the autoimmune process and facilitate our understanding of the pathogenesis of SLE.

REFERENCES

1. Tan, E. M., Cohen, A. S., Fries, J. F. *et al.* (1982) The 1982 revised criteria for the classification of systemic lupus erythematosus. *Arth. Rheum.*, **25**, 1271–7.
2. Hargraves, M. M., Richmond, H. and Morton, R. (1948) Presentation of two bone marrow elements: The 'tart' cell and the 'LE' cell. *Proc. of the Staff Meetings at Mayo Clinic*, **23**, 25–8.
3. Tan, E. M., Schur, P. H., Carr, R. I. *et al.* (1966) Deoxyribonucleic acid (DNA) and antibodies to DNA in the serum of patients with systemic lupus erythematosus. *J. Clin. Invest.*, **45**, 1732–40.
4. Fritzler, M. J. and Tan, E. M. (1978) Antibodies to histones in drug-induced and idiopathic lupus erythematosus. *J. Clin. Invest.*, **62**, 560–7.
5. Rubin, R. L., Joslin, F. G. and Tan, E. M. (1982) Specificity of anti-histone antibodies in systemic lupus erythematosus. *Arth. Rheum.*, **25**, 779–82.
6. Tan, E. M. and Kunkel, H. G. (1966) Characteristics of a soluble nuclear antigen precipitating with sera of patients with systemic lupus erythematosus. *J. Immunol.*, **96**, 464–71.
7. Lerner, M. R. and Steitz, J. A. (1979) Antibodies to small nuclear RNAs complexed with proteins are produced by patients with systemic lupus erythematosus. *Proc. Nat. Acad. Sci. USA*, **76**, 5495–7.
8. Sharp, G. C., Irvin, W. S., Tan, E. M. *et al.* (1972) Mixed connective tissue disease – an apparently distinct rheumatic disease syndrome associated with a specific antibody to an extractable nuclear antigen (ENA). *Am. J. Med.*, **52**, 148–59.
9. Mattioli, M. and Reichlin, M. (1974) Heterogeneity of RNA-protein antigens reactive with sera of patients with systemic lupus erythematosus. *Arth. Rheum.*, **17**, 421–9.
10. Wolin, S. L. and Steitz, J. A. (1984) The Ro

small cytoplasmic ribonucleoproteins: identification of the antigenic protein and its binding site on the Ro RNAs. *Proc. Nat. Acad. Sci. USA*, **81**, 1996–2000.

11. Yang, V. W., Lerner, M. R., Steitz, J. A. *et al.* (1981) A small nuclear ribonucleoprotein is required for splicing of adenoviral early RNA sequences. *Proc. Nat. Acad. Sci. USA*, **78**, 1371–5.

12. Connor, G. E., Nelson, G., Wiesnieweloski, R. *et al.* (1982) Protein antigens of the RNA-protein complexes detected by anti-Sm and anti-RNP antibodies found in the serum of patients with systemic lupus erythematosus and related disorders. *J. Exp. Med.*, **156**, 1475–86.

13. Lerner, M. R., Boyle, J. A., Hardin, J. A. *et al.* (1981) Two novel classes of ribonucleoproteins detected by antibodies associated with lupus erythematosus. *Science*, **211**, 400–2.

14. Francoeur, A. M., Peebles, C. L., Heckman, K. J. *et al.* (1985) Identification of ribosomal protein autoantigens. *J. Immunol.*, **135**, 2378–84.

15. Bonfa, E., Golombek, S. J., Kaufman, L. D. *et al.* (1987) Association between lupus psychosis and anti-ribosomal P protein antibodies. *N. Eng. J. Med.*, **317**, 265–71.

16. Mimori, T., Akizuki, M., Yamagata, H. *et al.* (1981) Characterization of a high molecular weight acidic nuclear protein recognized by autoantibodies in sera from patients with polymyositis-scleroderma overlap. *J. Clin. Invest.*, **68**, 611–20.

17. Miyachi, K., Fritzler, M. J. and Tan, E. M. (1978) Autoantibody to a nuclear antigen in proliferating cells. *J. Immunol.*, **121**, 2228–34.

18. Minota, S., Koyasu, S., Yahara, I. *et al.* (1988) Autoantibodies to the heat-shock protein hsp90 in systemic lupus erythematosus. *J. Clin. Invest.*, **81**, 106–9.

19. Harris, E. N., Asherson, R. A. and Hughes, G. R. (1988) Antiphospholipid antibodies – autoantibodies with a difference. *Ann. Rev. Med.*, **39**, 261–71.

20. McNeil, H. P., Simpson, R. J., Chesterman, C. N. *et al.* (1990) Anti-phospholipid antibodies are directed against a complex antigen that includes a lipid-binding inhibitor of coagulation: beta 2-glycoprotein I (apolipoprotein H). *Proc. Nat. Acad. Sci. USA*, **87**, 4120–4.

21. Terasaki, P. I., Mottironi, V. D. and Barnett, E. V. (1970) Cytotoxins in disease. Autocytotoxins in lupus. *N. Eng. J. Med.*, **283**, 724–7.

22. Tan, E. M. (1989) Antinuclear antibodies: diagnostic markers for autoimmune diseases and probes for cell biology. *Advan. Immunol.*, **44**, 93–151.

23. Rubin, R. L. and Waga, S. (1987) Antihistone antibodies in systemic lupus erythematosus. *J. Rheum.*, **14**, 118–26.

24. Eisenberg, R. A., Dyer, K., Craven, S. Y. *et al.* (1985) Subclass restriction and polyclonality of the systemic lupus erythematosus marker antibody anti-Sm. *J. Clin. Invest.*, **75**, 1270–7.

25. Chan, E. K. L. and Tan E. M. (1986) Epitopes and structural domains of a RNA-binding nuclear protein, SS-B/La: similarities with adenovirus DNA-binding protein. *Scan. J. Rheum.*, **61**, 102–5.

26. Ogata, K., Ogata, Y., Takasaki, T. *et al.* (1987) Epitopes on proliferating cell nuclear antigen recognized by human lupus autoantibody and murine monoclonal antibody. *J. Immunol.*, **139**, 2942–6.

27. James, J. A. and Harley, J. B. (1992) Linear epitope mapping of an Sm B/B' polypeptide. *J. Immunol.*, **148**, 2074–9.

28. Hardin, J. A. and Thomas, J. O. (1983) Antibodies to histones in systemic lupus erythematosus: localization of prominant autoantigens in H1 and H2B. *Proc. Nat. Acad. Sci. USA*, **80**, 7410–14.

29. Reuter, R. and Luhrmann, R. (1986) Immunization of mice with purified U1 small nuclear ribonucleoprotein (RNP) induces a pattern of antibody specificities characteristic of the anti-Sm and anti-RNP autoimmune response of patients with lupus erythematosus, as measured by monoclonal antibodies. *Proc. Nat. Acad. Sci. USA*, **83**, 8689–93.

30. Shores, E. W., Eisenberg, R. A. and Cohen, P. L. (1986) Role of the Sm antigen in the generation of anti-Sm autoantibodies in the SLE-prone MRL mouse. *J. Immunol.*, **136**, 3662–7.

31. Rekvig, O. P. and Hannestad, K. (1980) Human autoantibodies that react with both cell nuclei and plasma membranes display specificity for the octamer of histones H2A, H2B, H3, and H4 in high salt. *J. Exp. Med.*, **152**, 1720–33.

32. Cameron, J. S., Turner, D. R., Heaton, J. *et al.* (1983) Idiopathic mesangiocapillary glomerulonephritis. Comparison of types I

and II in children and adults and long-term prognosis. *Am. J. Med.*, **74**, 175–92.

33. Winfield, J. B. and Mimura, T. (1992) Pathogenetic significance of anti-lymphocyte autoantibodies in systemic lupus erythematosus. *Clin. Immunol. Immunopath.*, **63**, 13–16.

34. Bennett, R. M., Kotzin, B. L. and Merritt, M. J. (1987) DNA receptor dysfunction in systemic lupus erythematosus and kindred disorders. Induction by anti-DNA antibodies, antihistone antibodies, and antireceptor antibodies. *J. Exp. Med.*, **166**, 850–63.

35. Fournie, G. J. (1988) Circulating DNA and lupus nephritis. *Kid. Int.*, **33**, 487–97.

36. Krishnan, C. and Kaplan, M. H. (1967) Immunopathologic studies of systemic lupus erythematosus. II. Anti-nuclear reaction of gamma-globulin eluted from homogenates and isolated glomeruli of kidneys from patients with lupus nephritis. *J. Clin. Invest.*, **46**, 569.

37. Cameron, J. S., Lessof, M. H., Ogg, C. S. *et al.* (1976) Disease activity in the nephritis of systemic lupus erythematosus in relation to serum complement concentrations. DNA-binding capacity and precipitating anti-DNA antibody. *Clin. Exp. Immunol.*, **25**, 418–27.

38. Schur, P. H. and Sandson, J. (1968) Immunologic factors and clinical activity in systemic lupus erythematosus. *N. Eng. J. Med.*, **278**, 533–7.

39. Koren, E., Reichlin, M. W., Koscec, M. *et al.* (1992) Autoantibodies to ribosomal P proteins react with a plasma membrane-related target on human cells. *J. Clin. Invest.*, **89**, 1236–41.

40. Katz, M. S., Foster, M. H. and Madaio, M. P. (1993) Independently derived murine glomerular immune deposit-forming anti-DNA are encoded by near identical Vh gene sequences. *J. Clin. Invest.*, **91**, 402–8.

41. Tan, E. M., Schur, P. H., Carr, R. I. *et al.* (1966) Deoxyribonucleic acid (DNA) and antibodies to DNA in the serum of patients with systemic lupus erythematosus. *J. Clin. Invest.*, **45**, 1732–40.

42. Pisetsky, D. S. (1992) Anti-DNA antibodies in systemic lupus erythematosus. *Rheum. Dis. Clin. N. Am.*, **18**, 437–54.

43. LeFeber, W. P., Norris, D. A., Ryan, S. R. *et al.* (1984) Ultraviolet light induces binding of antibodies to selected nuclear antigens on cultured human keratinocytes. *J. Clin. Invest.*, **74**, 1545–51.

44. Lee, L. A., Gaither, K. K., Coulter, S. N. *et al.*

(1989) Pattern of cutaneous immunoglobulin G deposition in subacute cutaneous lupus erythematosus is reproduced by infusing purified anti-Ro (SSA) autoantibodies into human skin-grafted mice. *J. Clin. Invest.*, **83**, 1556–62.

45. Alexander, E., Buyon, J. P., Provost, T. T. *et al.* (1992) Anti-Ro/SS-A antibodies in the pathophysiology of congenital heart block in neonatal lupus syndrome, an experimental approach. *In vitro* electrophysiologic and immunocytochemical studies. *Arth. Rheum.*, **35**,176–89.

46. Loizou, S., Byron, M. A., Englert, H. J. *et al.* (1988) Association of quantitative anti-cardiolipin antibody levels with fetal loss and time of loss in systemic lupus erythematosus. *Q. J. Med.*, **68**, 525–31.

47. McNeil, H. P., Chesterman, C. N. and Krilis, S. A. (1991) Immunology and clinical importance of anti-phospholipid antibodies. *Advan. Immunol.*, **49**, 193–280.

48. McNeil, H. P., Simpson, R. J., Chesterman, C. N. *et al.* (1990) Anti-phospholipid antibodies are directed against a complex antigen that includes a lipid-binding inhibitor of co-agulation: beta-2 glycoprotein I (apolipoprotein H). *Proc. Nat. Acad. Sci. USA*, **87**, 4120–4.

49. Gharavi, A. E., Sammaritano, L. R., Wen, J. *et al.* (1992) Induction of anti-phospholipid autoantibodies by immunisation with beta 2-glycoprotein I (apolipoprotein H). *J. Clin. Invest.*, **90**, 1105–9.

50. Harley, J. B., Alexander, E. M., Bias, W. B. *et al.* (1986) Anti-Ro (SS-A) and anti-La (SS-B) in patients with Sjögren's syndrome. *Arth. Rheum.*, **29**, 196–9.

51. Diamond, B., Katz, J. B., Paul, E. *et al.* (1992) The role of somatic mutation in the pathogenic anti-DNA response. *Ann. Rev. Immunol.*, **10**, 731–57.

52. Hayakawa, K. and Hardy, R. R. (1988) Normal, autoimmune and malignant CD5 + B cells: the Ly-1 lineage. *Ann. Rev. Immunol.*, **6**, 197–218.

53. Budman, D. R., Merchant, E. B., Steinberg, A. D. *et al.* (1977) Increased spontaneous activity of antibody-forming cells in the peripheral blood of patients with active SLE. *Arth. Rheum.*, **20**, 829–33.

54. Blaese, R. M., Grayson, J. and Steinberg, A. D. (1980) Increased immunoglobulin-secreting cells in the blood of patients with active

systemic lupus erythematosus. *Am. J. Med.*, **69**, 345–50.

55. Izui, S., Kobayakawa, T., Zryd, M. J. *et al.* (1977) Mechanism for induction of anti-DNA antibodies by bacterial lipopolysaccharides in mice; II. Correlation between anti-DNA induction and polyclonal antibody formation by various polyclonal B lymphocyte activators. *J. Immunol.*, **119**, 2157–62.

56. Klinman, D. M., Eisenberg, R. A. and Steinberg, A. D. (1990) Development of the autoimmune B cell repertoire in MRL-lpr/lpr mice. *J. Immunol.*, **144**, 506–11.

57. Burlingame, R. W., Rubin, R. L., Balderas, R. S. *et al.* (1993) Genesis and evolution of antichromatin autoantibodies in murine lupus implicates T-dependent immunisation with self antigen. *J. Clin. Invest.*, **91**, 1687–96.

58. Linker-Israeli, M. (1992) Cytokine abnormalities in human lupus. *Clin. Immunol. Immunopath.*, **63**, 10–12.

59. Yu, D. T., Winchester, R. J., Fu, S. M. *et al.* (1980) Peripheral blood Ia-positive T cells increases in certain diseases and after immunisation. *J. Exp. Med.*, **151**, 91–100.

60. Rajagopalan, S., Zordan, T., Tsokos, G. C. *et al.* (1990) Pathogenic anti-DNA autoantibody-inducing T helper cell lines from patients with active lupus nephritis: isolation CD4-8-T helper cell lines that express the gamma delta T-cell antigen receptor. *Proc. Nat. Acad. Sci. USA*, **87**, 7020–4.

61. Wofsy, D. and Seaman, W. E. (1986) Successful treatment of autoimmunity in NZB/NZW F1 mice with monoclonal antibody to L3T4. *J. Exp. Med.*, **161**, 378–91.

62. Seaman, W. E. and Wofsy, D. (1989) Selective manipulation of the immune response *in vivo* by monoclonal antibodies. *Ann. Rev. Med.*, **39**, 231–41.

63. Christian, C. L., Hatfield, W. B. and Chase, P. H. (1963) Systemic lupus erythematosus: cryoprecipitation of sera. *J. Clin. Invest.*, **42**, 823–6.

64. Aguado, M. T., Lambria, J. D., Tsokos, G. C. *et al.* (1985) Monoclonal antibodies against complement 3 neoantigens for detection of immune complexes and complement activation. *J. Clin. Invest.*, **76**, 1418–26.

65. Davis IV, J. S., Godfrey, S. M. and Winfield, J. B. (1978) Direct evidence for circulating DNA-anti-DNA complexes in systemic lupus erythematosus. *Arth. Rheum.*, **21**, 17–22.

66. Izui, S., Lambert, P. H. and Miescher, P. A. (1977) Failure to detect circulating DNA-anti-DNA complexes by four radioimmunological methods in patients with systemic lupus erythematosus. *Clin. Exp. Immunol.*, **30**, 384.

67. Lloyd, W. and Schur, P. H. (1981) Immune complexes, complement, and anti-DNA in exacerbations of systemic lupus erythematosus (SLE). *Med. (Baltimore)*, **1**, 208–17.

68. Weinstein, A., Bordwell, B., Stone, B. *et al.* (1983) Antibodies to native DNA and serum complement (C3) levels. *Am. J. Med.*, **74**, 206–16.

69. Valentijn, R. M., van Overhagen, H., Hazevoet, H. M. *et al.* (1985) The value of complement and immune complex determinations in monitoring disease activity in patients with systemic lupus erythematosus. *Arth. Rheum.*, **28**, 904–13.

70. Deapen, D., Escalante, A., Weinrib, L. *et al.* (1992) A revised estimate of twin concordance in systemic lupus erythematosus. *Arth. Rheum.*, **35**, 311–8.

71. Estes, D. and Christian, C. L. (1971) The natural history of systemic lupus erythematosus by prospective analysis. *Med. (Baltimore)*, **50**, 85–95.

72. Morgan, B. P. and Walport, M. J. (1991) Complement deficiency and disease. *Immunol. Today*, **12**, 301–6.

73. Fielder, A. H. L., Walport, M. J., Batchelor, J. R. *et al.* (1983) Family study of the major histocompatibility complex in patients with systemic lupus erythematosus: importance of null alleles of C4A and C4B in determining disease susceptibility. *Br. Med. J.*, **286**, 425–8.

74. Dunckley, H., Gatenby, P. A., Hawkins, B. *et al.* (1987) Deficiency of C4A is a genetic determinant of systemic lupus erythematosus in three ethnic groups. *J. Immunol.*, **14**, 209–18.

75. Jacob C. O. and McDevitt, H. O. (1988) Tumour necrosis factor-alpha production in murine autoimmune 'lupus' nephritis. *Nature*, **331**(6154), 356–8.

76. Walport, M. J., Black, C. M. and Batchelor, J. R. (1982) The immunogenetics of SLE. *Clin. Rheum. Dis. (London)*, **8**, 3–21.

77. Bell, D. A., Rigby, R., Stiller, C. R. *et al.* (1984) HLA antigens in systemic lupus erythematosus: relationship to disease severity, age at onset, and sex. *J. Rheum.*, **11**, 475–9.

78. Reveille, J. D., Bias, W. B., Winkelstein, J. A. *et al.* (1983) Familial systemic lupus erythematosus: immunogenetic studies in eight families. *Med. (Baltimore)*, **62**, 21–35.

79. Reveille, J. D., Macleod, M. J., Whittington, K. *et al.* (1991) Specific amino acid residues in the second hypervariable region of HLA-DQA1 and DQB1 chain genes promote the Ro (SS-A)/La (SS-B) autoantibody responses. *J. Immunol.*, **146**, 3871–6.

80. Theofilopoulos, A. N. and Dixon, F. J. (1985) Murine models of systemic lupus erythematosus. *Advan. Immunol.*, **37**, 269–389.

81. Lahita, R. G., Bradlow, H. L., Kunkel, H. G. *et al.* (1981) Increased 16alpha-hydroxylation of estradiol in systemic lupus erythematosus. *J. Clin. Endocrin. Metabol.*, **53**, 174–8.

82. Lahita, R. G., Kunkel, H. G. and Bradlow, H. L. (1983) Increased oxidation of testosterone in systemic lupus erythematosus. *Arth. Rheum.*, **26**, 1517–21.

83. Jungers, P., Dougados, M., Pelissier, C. *et al.* (1982) Influence of oral contraceptive therapy on the activity of systemic lupus erythematosus. *Arth. Rheum.*, **25**, 618–23.

84. Asherson, R. A. and Lahita, R. G. (1991) Sex hormone modulation in systemic lupus erythematosus: still a therapeutic option? *Ann. Rheum. Dis.*, **50**, 897–8.

85. Chassagne, P., Mejjad, O., Gourmelen, O. *et al.* (1993) Exacerbation of systemic lupus erythematosus during human parvovirus B19 infection. *Br. J. Rheum.*, **32**, 158–9.

86. Sasaki, T., Takahashi, Y., Yoshinaga, K. *et al.* (1989) An association between human parvovirus B19 infection and autoantibody production. *J. Rheum.*, **16**, 708–9.

87. Watanabe-Fukunaga, R., Brannan, C. I., Copeland, N. G. *et al.* (1992) Lymphoproliferation disorder in mice explained by defects in Fas antigen that mediates apoptosis. *Nature*, **356**(6367), 314–7.

88. Allen, R. D., Marshall, J. D., Roths, J. B. *et al.* (1990) Differences defined by bone marrow transplantation suggest that *lpr* and *gld* are mutations of genes encoding an interacting pair of molecules. *J. Exp. Med.*, **172**, 1367–75.

89. Ishigatsubo, Y., Steinberg, A. D. and Klinman, D. M. (1988) Autoantibody production is associated with polyclonal B cell activation in autoimmune mice which express the *lpr* or *gld* genes. *Eur. J. Immunol.*, **18**, 1809–94.

90. Chiang, B-L., Bearer, E., Ansari, A. *et al.* (1990) The BM12 mutation and autoantibodies to dsDNA in NZB.H-2 bm12 mice. *J. Immunol.*, **145**, 94–101.

91. Fieser, T. M., Gershwin, M. E., Steinberg, A. D. *et al.* (1984) Abrogation of murine lupus by

the xid gene is associated with reduced responsiveness of B cells to C-cell-helper signals. *Cell. Immunol.*, **87**, 708–13.

92. Kotzin, B. L. and Palmer, E. (1987) The contribution of NZW genes to lupus-like disease in (NZB × NZW)F1 mice. *J. Exp. Med.*, **165**, 1237–51.

93. Waxman, F. J., Hebert, L. A., Comacoff, J. B. *et al.* (1984) Complement depletion accelerates the clearance of immune-complexes from the circulation of primates. *J. Clin. Invest.*, **74**, 1329–40.

94. Waxman, F. J., Hebert, L. A., Cosio, F. G. *et al.* (1986) Differential binding of immunoglobulin A and immunoglobulin G1 immune complexes to primate erythrocytes *in vivo*. *J. Clin. Invest.*, **77**, 82–9.

95. Schifferli, J. A., Ng, Y. C. and Peters, D. K. (1986) The role of complement and its receptor in the elimination of immune complexes. *N. Eng. J. Med.*, **315**, 488–95.

96. Lachmann, P. J. and Walport, M. J. (1987) Deficiency of the effector mechanisms of the immune response and autoimmunity, in *Autoimmunity and Autoimmune Disease, Ciba Foundation Symposium*, **no 129** (ed. J. Whelan), Wiley, Chichester, pp. 149–71.

97. Davies, K. A., Erlendsson, K., Beynon, H. L. C. *et al.* (1993) Splenic uptake of immune complexes in man is complement-dependent. *J. Immunol.*, **151**, 3866–73.

98. Schifferli, J. A., Hauptmann, G. and Paccaud, J-P. (1987) Complement-mediated adherence of immune complexes to human erythrocytes. *FEBS Letters*, **213**, 415–18.

99. Walport, M. J. and Lachmann, P. J. (1988) Erythrocyte complement receptor type 1, immune complexes and the rheumatic diseases. *Arth. Rheum.*, **31**, 153–8.

100. Davies, K. A., Peters, A. M., Beynon, H. L. C. *et al.* (1992) Immune complex processing in patients with systemic lupus erythematosus – *in vivo* imaging and clearance studies. *J. Clin. Invest.*, **90**, 2075–83.

101. Fauci, A. S. (1980) Immunoregulation in autoimmunity. *J. Aller. Clin. Immunol.*, **66**, 5–17.

102. Schwartz, R. S. and Stollar, B. D. (1985) Origins of anti-DNA autoantibodies. *J. Clin. Invest.*, **75**, 321–7.

103. Zouali, M., Stollar, B. D. and Schwartz, R. S. (1988) Origin and diversification of anti-DNA antibodies. *Immunol. Rev.*, **105**, 137–59.

104. Abdou, N. I., Wall, H., Lindsley, H. B. *et al.* (1981) Network theory in autoimmunity. *In*

vitro suppression of serum anti-DNA anti-body binding to DNA by anti-idiotypic antibody in systemic lupus erythematosus. *J. Clin. Invest.*, **67**, 1297–304.

105. Muryoi, T., Sasaki, T., Harata, N. *et al.* (1988) Heterogeneity of anti-idiotypic antibodies to anti-DNA antibodies in humans. *Clin. Exp. Immunol.*, **71**, 67–72.

106. Hahn, B. H. and Ebling, F. M. (1984) Suppression of murine lupus nephritis by administration of an anti-idiotypic antibody to anti-DNA. *J. Immunol.*, **132**, 187–90.

107. Teitelbaum, D., Rauch, J., Stollar, B. D. *et al.* (1984) *In vivo* effects of antibodies against a high frequency idiotype of anti-DNA antibodies in MRL mice. *J. Immunol.*, **132**, 1282.

108. Mellors, R. C. and Huang, C. Y. (1967) Immunopathology of NZB/BL mice. VI. Virus separable from spleen and pathogenic for Swiss mice. *J. Exp. Med.*, **126**, 53–62.

109. Datta, S. K., Manny, N., Andrzejewski, C. *et al.* (1978) Genetic studies of autoimmunity and retrovirus expression in crosses of New Zealand black mice I. Xenotropic virus. *J. Exp. Med.*, **147**, 854–71.

110. Krieg, A. M., Gourley, M. F. and Steinberg, A. D. (1991) Association of murine lupus and thymic full-length endogenous retroviral expression maps to a bone marrow stem cell. *J. Immunol.*, **146**, 3002–5.

111. Becker, G. J., Waldburger, M., Hughes, G. R. *et al.* (1980) Value of serum C-reactive protein measurement in the investigation of fever in systemic lupus erythematosus. *Ann. Rheum. Dis.*, **39**, 50–2.

112. Wener, M. H., Uwatoko, S. and Mannik, M. (1989) Antibodies to the collagen-like region of C1q in sera of patients with autoimmune rheumatic diseases. *Arth. Rheum.*, **32**, 544–51.

113. Roldan, C. A., Shively, B. K., Lau, C. C. *et al.* (1992) Systemic lupus erythematosus valve disease by transesophageal echocardiography and the role of anti-phospholipid antibodies. *J. Am. Coll. Card.*, **20**, 1127–34.

114. Petri, M., Perez-Gutthann, S., Spence, D. *et al.* (1992) Risk factors for coronary artery disease in patients with systemic lupus erythematosus. *Am. J. Med.*, **93**, 513–19.

115. Gruppo Italiano per lo Studio della Nefrite lupica (GISNEL), (1992) Lupus nephritis: prognostic factors and probability of maintaining life-supporting renal function 10 years after the diagnosis. *Am. J. Kid. Dis.*, **19**, 473–9.

116. Ward, M. M. and Studenski, S. (1992) Clinical prognostic factors in lupus nephritis. The importance of hypertension and smoking. *Arch. Int. Med.*, **152**, 2082–8.

117. Austin, H. A., Klippel, J. H., Balow, J. E. *et al.* (1986) Therapy of lupus nephritis. Controlled trial of prednisone and cytotoxic drugs. *N. Eng. J. Med.*, **314**, 614–19.

118. Steinberg, A. D. and Steinberg, S. C. (1991) Long-term preservation of renal function in patients with lupus nephritis receiving treatment that includes cyclophoshamide versus those treated with prednisone only. *Arth. Rheum.*, **34**, 945–50.

119. Kant, K. S., Pollak, V. E., Weiss, M. A. *et al.* (1981) Glomerular thrombosis in systemic lupus erythematosus: prevalence and significance. *Med. (Baltimore)*, **60**, 71–86.

120. Balow, J. E. and Austin, H. A. (1988) Renal disease in systemic lupus erythematosus. *Rheum. Dis. Clin. N. Am.*, **14**, 117–33.

121. Schwartz, M. M., Lan, S. P., Bernstein, J. *et al.* (1992) Role of pathology indices in the management of severe lupus glomerulonephritis. Lupus Nephritis Collaborative Study Group. *Kid. Int.*, **42**, 743–8.

122. Johnson, R. T. and Richardson, E. P. (1968) The neurological manifestations of systemic lupus erythematosus. A clinical-pathologic study of 24 cases and review of the literature. *Med. (Baltimore)*, **47**, 337–65.

123. Hanly, J. G., Walsh, N. M. and Sangalang, V. (1992) Brain pathology in systemic lupus erythematosus. *J. Rheum.*, **19**, 732–41.

124. Winfield, J. B., Shaw, M., Silverman, L. M. *et al.* (1983) Intrathecal IgG synthesis and blood-brain barrier impairment in patients with systemic lupus erythematosus and central nervous system dysfunction. *Am. J. Med.*, **74**, 837–44.

125. Bluestein, H. G. and Zvaifler, N. J. (1976) Brain-reactive lymphocytotoxic antibodies in the serum of patients with systemic lupus erythematosus. *J. Clin. Invest.*, **57**, 509–16.

126. Bresnihan, B., Hohmeister, R., Cutting, J. *et al.* (1979) The neuropsychiatric disorder in systemic lupus erythematosus: evidence for both vascular and immune mechanisms. *Ann. Rheum. Dis.*, **38**, 301–6.

127. Zvaifler, N. J. and Bluestein, H. G. (1982) The pathogenesis of central nervous system manifestations of systemic lupus erythematosus. *Arth. Rheum.*, **25**, 862–6.

128. Robbins, M. L., Kornguth, S. E., Bell, C. L.

et al. (1988) Antineurofilament antibody evaluation in neuropsychiatric systemic lupus erythematosus. Combination with anticardiolipin antibody assay and magnetic resonance imaging. *Arth. Rheum.*, **31**, 623–31.

129. Bell, C. L., Partington, C., Robbins, M. *et al.* (1991) Magnetic resonance imaging of central nervous system lesions in patients with lupus erythematosus. Correlation with clinical remission and antineurofilament and anticardiolipin antibody titers. *Arth. Rheum.*, **34**, 432–41.

130. Sneller, M. C., Straus, S. E., Jaffe, E. S. *et al.* (1992) A novel lymphoproliferative/autoimmune syndrome resembling murine *lpr/gld* disease. *J. Clin. Invest.*, **90**, 334–41.

131. Wallace, D. J., Pistiner, M., Nessim, S. *et al.* (1992) Cutaneous lupus erythematosus without systemic lupus erythematosus: clinical and laboratory features. *Sem. Arth. Rheum.*, **21**, 221–6.

132. Watson, R. M., Lane, A. T., Barnett, N. K. *et al.* (1984) Neonatal lupus erythematosus. *Med. (Baltimore)*, **63**, 362–78.

133. Lockshin, M. D., Bonfa, E., Elkon, K. *et al.* (1988) Neonatal risk to newborns of mothers with systemic lupus erythematosus. *Arth. Rheum.*, **31**, 697–701.

134. Scott, J. S., Maddison, P. J., Taylor, P. V. *et al.* (1983) Connective-tissue disease, antibodies to ribonucleoprotein, and congenital heart block. *N. Eng. J. Med.*, **309**, 209–12.

135. Litsey, S. E., Noonan, J. A., O'Connor, W. N. *et al.* (1985) Maternal connective tissue disease and congenital heart block. *N. Eng. J. Med.*, **312**, 98–100.

136. Provost, T. T., Talal, N., Harley, J. B. *et al.* (1988) The relationship between anti-Ro (SS-A) antibody-positive Sjögren's syndrome and anti-Ro (SS-A) antibody-positive lupus erythematosus. *Arch. Dermatol.*, **124**, 63–71.

137. Pettersson, I., Wang, G., Smith, E. I. *et al.* (1986) The use of immunoblotting and immunoprecipitation of (U) small nuclear ribonucleoproteins in the analysis of sera of patients with mixed connective tissue disease and systemic lupus erythematosus. A cross-sectional, longitudinal study. *Arth. Rheum.*, **29**, 986–96.

138. Nimelstein, S. H., Brody, S., McShane, D. *et al.* (1980) Mixed connective tissue disease: a subsequent evaluation of the original 25 patients. *Med. (Baltimore)*, **59**, 239–48.

139. Agnello, V., Koffler, D., Eisenberg, J. W. *et al.* (1971) C1q precipitins in the sera of patients with systemic lupus erythematosus and other hypocomplementemic states: characterisation of high and low molecular weight types. *J. Exp. Med.*, **134**, 228–41.

140. Uwatoko, S. and Mannik, M. (1988) Low-molecular weight C1q-binding immunoglobulin G in patients with systemic lupus erythematosus consists of autoantibodies to the collagen-like region of C1q. *J. Clin. Invest.*, **82**, 816–24.

141. Vyse, T. and So, A. K. (1992) Sulphasalazine induced autoimmune syndrome. *B. J. Rheum.*, **31**, 115–6.

142. Woolsey, R. L., Drayer, D. E., Reidenberg, M. M. *et al.* (1978) Effect of acetylator phenotype on the rate at which procainamide induces antinuclear antibodies and the lupus syndrome. *N. Eng. J. Med.*, **298**, 1157–9.

143. Davis, S., Furie, B. C., Griffin, J. H. *et al.* (1978) Circulating inhibitors of blood coagulation associated with procainamide-induced lupus erythematosus. *Am. J. Hematol.*, **4**, 401–7.

144. Batchelor, J. R., Welsh, K. I. and Tinoco, R. M. (1980) Hydralazine-induced systemic lupus erythematosus: influence of HLA-DR and sex on susceptibility. *Lancet*, **1**, 1107–9.

145. Thomas, T. J. and Messner, R. P. (1986) Effects of lupus-inducing drugs on the B to Z transition of synthetic DNA. *Arth. Rheum.*, **29**, 638–45.

146. Cornacchia, E., Golbus, J., Maybaum, J. *et al.* (1988) Hydralazine and procainamide inhibit T cell DNA methylation and induce autoreactivity. *J. Immunol.*, **140**, 2197–200.

147. Sim, E., Gill, E. W. and Sim, R. B. (1984) Drugs that induce systemic lupus erythematosus inhibit complement component C4. *Lancet*, **2**, 422–4.

148. Lubbe, W. F., Palmer, S. J., Butler, W. S. *et al.* (1983) Fetal survival after prednisone suppression of maternal lupus-anticoagulant. *Lancet*, **1**, 1361–3.

149. Lockshin, M. D., Druzin, M. L. and Qamar, T. (1989) Prednisolone does not prevent recurrent fetal death in women with anti-phospholipid antibody. *Am. J. Obstet. Gynecol.*, **160**, 439–43.

150. The Canadian Hydroxychloroquine Study Group. (1991) A randomised study of the effect of withdrawing hydroxychloroquine sulphate in systemic lupus erythematosus. *N. Eng. J. Med.*, **324**, 150–4.

151. Easterbrook, M. (1988) Ocular effects and safety of antimalarial agents. *Am. J. Med.*, **85**, 23–9.

152. Ruzicka, T. and Goerz, G. (1981) Dapsone in the treatment of lupus erythematosus. *Br. J. Dermatol.*, **104**, 53–6.

153. Fredenberg, M. F. and Malkinson, F. D. (1987) Sulfone therapy in the treatment of leukocytoclastic vasculitis. Report of three cases. *J. Am. Acad. Dermatol.*, **16**, 772–8.

154. Knop, J., Bonsmann, G., Happle, R. *et al.* (1983) Thalidomide in the treatment of sixty cases of chronic discoid lupus erythematosus. *Br. J. Dermatol.*, **108**, 461–6.

155. Burrows, N. P., Walport, M. J., Hammond, A. H. *et al.* (1991) Lupus erythematosus profundus with partial C4 deficiency responding to thalidomide. *Br. J. Dermatol.*, **125**, 62–7.

156. Naafs, B., Bakkers, E. J., Flinterman, J. *et al.* (1982) Thalidomide treatment of subacute cutaneous lupus erythematosus. *Br. J. Dermatol.*, **107**, 83–6.

157. Wulff, C. H., Hoyer, H., Asboe Hansen, G. *et al.* (1985) Development of polyneuropathy during thalidomide therapy. *B. J. Dermatol.*, **112**, 475–80.

158. Lennard, L., Loon, J. A. van and Weinshilboum, R. M. (1989) Pharmacogenetics of acute azathioprine toxicity: relationship to thiopurine methyltransferase genetic polymorphism. *Clin. Pharmacol. Ther.*, **46**, 149–54.

159. Boumpas, D. T., Yamada, H., Patronas, N. J. *et al.* (1991) Pulse cyclophosphamide for severe neuropsychiatric lupus. *Q. J. Med.*, **81**, 975–84.

160. Lehman, T. J. (1992) Current concepts in immunosuppressive drug therapy of systemic lupus erythematosus. *J. Rheum.* Suppl., **33**, 20–2.

161. Boumpas, D. T., Austin, H. A., Vaughn, E. M. *et al.* (1992) Controlled trial of pulse methylprednisolone versus two regimens of pulse cyclophosphamide in severe lupus nephritis. *Lancet*, **340**, 741–5.

162. McCune, W. J., Golbus, J., Zeldes, W. *et al.* (1988) Clinical and immunologic effects of monthly administration of intravenous cyclophosphamide in severe systemic lupus erythematosus. *N. Eng. J. Med.*, **318**, 1423–31.

163. Zonzits, E., Aberer, W. and Tappeiner, G. (1992) Drug eruptions from mesna. After cyclophosphamide treatment of patients with systemic lupus erythematosus and dermatomyositis. *Arch. Dermatol.*, **128**, 80–2.

164. Lewis, E. J., Hunsicker, L. G., Lan, S. P. *et al.* (1992) A controlled trial of plasmapheresis therapy in severe lupus nephritis. The Lupus Nephritis Collaborative Study Group [see comments]. *N. Eng. J. Med.*, **326**, 1373–9.

165. Seleznick, M. J. and Fries, J. F. (1991) Variables associated with decreased survival in systemic lupus erythematosus. *Sem. Arth. Rheum.*, **21**, 73–80.

166. Budman, D. R. and Steinberg, A. D. (1976) Hypertension and renal disease in systemic lupus erythematosus. *Arch. Int. Med.*, **136**, 1003–7.

167. Dinant, H. J., Decker, J. L., Klippel, J. H. *et al.* (1982) Alternative modes of cyclophosphamide and azathioprine therapy in lupus nephritis. *Ann. Int. Med.*, **96**, 728–36.

168. Ginzler, E. M. and Schorn, K. (1988) Outcome and prognosis in systemic lupus erythematosus. *Rheum. Dis. Clin. N. Am.*, **14**, 67–78.

169. Arnett, F. C., Hamilton, R. G., Roebber, M. G. *et al.* (1988) Increased frequencies of Sm and nRNP autoantibodies in American blacks compared to whites with systemic lupus erythematosus. *J. Rheum.*, **15**, 1773–6.

170. Urowitz, M. B., Bookman, A. A. M., Koehler, B. E. *et al.* (1976) The bimodal mortality of systemic lupus erythematosus. *Am. J. Med.*, **60**, 221–5.

171. Rubin, L. A., Urowitz, M. B. and Gladman, D. D. (1985) Mortality in systemic lupus erythematosus: the bimodal pattern revisited. *Q. J. Med.*, **216**, 87–98.

172. Ginzler, E., Diamond, H., Kaplan, D. *et al.* (1978) Computer analysis of factors influencing frequency of infection in systemic lupus erythematosus. *Arth. Rheum.*, **21**, 37–44.

173. Dillon, A. M., Stein, H. B. and English, R. A. (1982) Splenic atrophy in systemic lupus erythematosus. *Ann. Int. Med.*, **96**, 40–3.

174. Petri, M., Spence, D., Bone, L. R. *et al.* (1992) Coronary artery disease risk factors in the Johns Hopkins Lupus Cohort: prevalence, recognition by patients, and preventive practices. *Med. (Baltimore)*, **71**, 291–302.

175. Hiepe, F., Volk, H. D., Apostoloff, E. *et al.* (1991) Treatment of severe systemic lupus erythematosus with anti-CD4 monoclonal antibody [letter]. *Lancet*, **338**, 1529–30.

D. M. Fagundus and E. C. LeRoy

INTRODUCTION

The disease systemic sclerosis (SSc) is a broad-based challenge to the physician, which includes the clinical aspects of diagnosis, evaluation and treatment; the demographic variables (which groups develop particular manifestations) and the fundamental questions which explore cell-cell and cell-matrix interactions resulting in perivascular mononuclear infiltrates and increased deposition of extracellular matrix, the pathologic lesions characteristic of scleroderma. The spectrum of clinical manifestations ranges from subtle thickening of an isolated discrete patch of skin usually of largely cosmetic importance, to rapidly progressive involvement of both skin and internal organs resulting in significant mortality.

Localized scleroderma, or morphea, usually has an insidious onset in the first two decades of life, being first noticed as dry or discolored skin (Chapter 12). These changes may stabilize or may proceed to more obvious thickened skin by either increases in existing patches or the appearance of new patches. Localized scleroderma is quite variable and can be described by its pattern, including guttate, linear or isolated. The common link between these different patterns is a nearly universal lack of internal organ involvement. Another important distinguishing feature from systemic sclerosis is the absence of Raynaud's phenomenon (RP) and the presence of normal nailfold capillaries. Tests for antinuclear antibodies are positive in about one-half of patients and peripheral eosinophilia is present in about one-third. Involvement may include only the dermis or may penetrate through subcutaneous tissue to fascia, periostium and muscle, resulting in a contracture when such involvement crosses a joint or significant hemiatrophy of an extremity when onset occurs prior to puberty and restricts epiphyseal long bone growth. Localized scleroderma is histologically indistinguishable from systemic sclerosis with perivascular inflammation and matrix deposition. Treatment is largely observational and supportive. *En coup de sabre* describes a cosmetically devastating linear pattern of scleroderma affecting the face and scalp, usually of young patients which may result in facial hemiatrophy, a distribution which can be associated with seizures and ocular malalignment. An abnormal embryonic neural crest migration has been proposed to explain the pathogenesis of localized scleroderma; nonetheless, the full etiology remains unknown[1].

Systemic sclerosis, or generalized scleroderma, can be classified as either limited (lSSc) or diffuse (dSSc). Other nomenclature, such as progressive systemic sclerosis, is discouraged since it can confuse diagnosis and possible therapy and it imposes unnecessary and often inaccurate emotional burdens on the patient (v.i. for CREST syndrome). Epidemiologic studies have yielded an incidence of 10

Connective Tissue Diseases. Edited by Jill J. F. Belch and Robert B. Zurier. Published in 1995 by Chapman & Hall, London.
ISBN 0 412 48620 2

Table 3.1   Subsets of systemic sclerosis (SSc)

Diffuse cutaneous SSc (dSSc)*

Onset of Raynaud's phenomenon within 1 year of onset of skin changes (puffy or hidebound)

Truncal and acral skin involvement

Presence of tendon friction rubs

Early and significant incidence of interstitial lung disease, oliguric renal failure, diffuse gastrointestinal disease, and myocardial involvement

Absence of anticentromere antibodies (ACA)

Nailfold capillary dilatation and capillary destruction[†]

Antitopoisomerase antibodies (30% of patients)

Limited cutaneous SSc (lSSc)

Raynaud's phenomenon for years (occasionally decades)

Skin involvement limited to hands, face, feet and forearms (acral) or absent

A significant late incidence of pulmonary hypertension, with or without interstitial lung disease, trigeminal neuralgia, skin calcifications, telangiectasia

A high incidence of ACA (70–80%)

Dilated nailfold capillary loops, usually without capillary dropout

---

* Experienced observers note some patients with dSSc who do not develop organ insufficiency and suggest the term chronic dSSc for these patients.

[†] Nailford capillary dilatation and destruction may also be seen in patients with dermatomyositis, overlap syndromes and undifferentiated connective tissue disease. These syndromes may be considered as part of the spectrum of scleroderma-associated disorders.

From *J. Rheum.* **15**, 202–5, 1988.

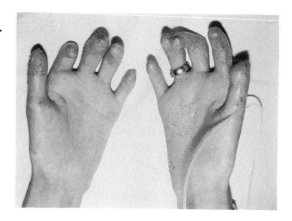

Fig. 3.1   Severe scleroderma affecting the hands.

cases per million with a female prevalence which is especially apparent in young adults (7:1) compared to subjects over 50 years of age (2:1). Attempts have been made to unify the broad clinical spectrum of systemic sclerosis with diagnostic criteria having both high sensitivity and specificity[2] (Table 3.1). These criteria do not fare well when applied to patients with lSSc, because they require taut skin proximal to the metacarpophalangeal joints excluding 3–4 fold more subjects (versus those fulfilling criteria) with combinations of RP, sclerodactaly and scleroderma-like nailfold capillary abnormalities. The true defining

cutaneous difference between patients with limited and diffuse SSc is that the latter require skin changes proximal to the elbow (excluding the face and neck, which are characteristic of lSSc) at some time during the disease. Generally, dSSc patients are more apt to have both proximal cutaneous and significant internal organ involvement earlier in their course (e.g. in the first decade of symptoms).

Patients with dSSc usually present complaining of recent onset RP (over the last several weeks to months) associated with edematous ('puffy') fingers, hands and face. They often have proximal skin thickening within one year of symptoms (Figure 3.1). Initial complaints are most likely related to the skin with excessive pain, burning, puritis and swelling. Examination may reveal elevated blood pressure, tendon friction rubs and pulmonary bibasilar crackles in addition to skin thickening of the extremities and trunk. These patients should undergo immediate and regularly repeated evaluation for end-organ involvement as detailed below.

Limited (lSSc) patients may be older and may experience less severe RP for decades, often not requiring medical attention. In addition to an acral distribution of skin involvement, attention should be given to possible symptoms and signs of pulmonary hypertension, since lSSc patients are susceptible to this often lethal involvement. These patients, usually more stable and often non-progressive, are those to which the previously used CREST syndrome (Calcinosis, Raynaud's phenomenon, Esopageal dysmotility, Sclerodactaly and Telangectasias) was applied. The frequent failure of these patients to have these features simultaneously or at all, as well as the anatomic constraints of sclerodactyly coupled with the fact that dSSc patients often have several CREST features permits the conclusion that CREST is neither precise nor a preferred term.

Occasionally, patients will have features of two or more connective tissue diseases including SSc, systemic lupus erythematosus, Sjögrens syndrome, rheumatoid arthritis and polymyositis/dermatomyositis, constituting an overlap syndrome. Uncommonly, a patient will have RP, positive confirmatory tests for SSc and characteristic internal organ involvement without skin thickening. This presentation defines SSc sine scleroderma. A number of these patients probably remain undiagnosed while receiving treatment for gastrointestinal dysmotility, pulmonary hypertension or interstitial pulmonary fibrosis. Altman *et al.* determined that risk factors including age greater than 64 years, anemia (hemoglobin less than 11 gm/dl) and impaired renal function (blood urea nitrogen greater than 16 mg/dl) were early predictors of increased mortality for all SSc patients[3].

There are several conflicting reports linking SSc and cancer. Those from tertiary care centers and involving post-mortem examinations did not establish an increased incidence of malignancy in scleroderma patients[4]. This contrasted with anecdotal case reports associating alveolar cell carcinoma with SSc[5]. More recently, several investigators have noted a coexistence of cancer and SSc ranging from 3–7%[6]. Malignancies were either primarily non-alveolar cell lung cancer occurring in patients (many non-smokers) with established chronic interstitial lung disease or breast cancer detected at or near the time of diagnosis. Medsger has recommended close surveillance with serial chest X-rays and mammography, respectively[7]. Also, the increasing use of immunosuppressive medications in rheumatologic disorders has been associated with hematologic malignancies (3 out of 26 patients in one cohort)[7]. These patients should make informed decisions regarding therapy with their physician and have routine hematologic monitoring.

ENVIRONMENTAL TRIGGERS OF SCLERODERMA-LIKE SYNDROMES

The first environmental association of scleroderma was made by Bramwell in stone masons exposed to silica[8]. Since then, many geographic, occupational and chemical associations linking SSc with environmental exposures have been reported. Offenders include bleomycin, vinyl chloride monomer, epoxy resin compounds and organic solvents including toluene, benzene, xylene and trichloroethylene. The degree and pattern of skin involvement, internal organ involvement, Raynaud's phenomenon, and epidemiology vary greatly.

The association with exposure to silica and its derivatives first made by Bramwell has been confirmed in miners from different geographic locations. More recently, claims of connective tissue diseases including SSc linked to silicone gel-filled breast implants have been made and are being explored in both the scientific and judicial communities. Several case reports are countered by a larger case-control study not demonstrating an increased incidence of connective tissue diseases in subjects with breast implants[9].

Toxic oil syndrome (TOS) was a scleroderma-like disease which appeared in Spain in 1981 as an epidemic affecting 20 000 users of adulterated rapeseed oil used for cooking[10]. The denaturing contaminant, aniline, was implicated as the causative agent. The cause of over 800 deaths, long-term sequelae of TOS include scleroderma-like skin changes,

Sjögren's-like signs and symptoms, periph-eral neuropathy and also pulmonary hyper-tension which continues to cause mortality now a decade after exposure[11].

Eosinophilia-myalgia syndrome (EMS) was first described in 1989[12]. Commonly used for insomnia and depression, L-tryptophan was available in over-the-counter preparations and has probably caused EMS in over 4000 individuals. Initial symptoms included arthralgia, dyspnea and debilitating myalgia. Examination revealed erythe-matosus macules on the trunk and ex-tremities, significant subcutaneous edema and thickening of the skin in a central distribution. Laboratory findings included a peripheral eosinophilia (1×10^9/l), and an elevated serum aldolase with a normal crea-tine kinase. Skin lesion histology revealed inflammation and fibrosis extending from the dermis to the perimysium with a peri-vascular mononuclear infiltrate most promi-nent in the fascia (fasciitis). Peripheral neuropathy and neurocognitive dysfunction were common. A definite association has been made with contamination by at least one chemical, 1,1-ethylidene bis (L-tryptophan) (EBT), detected by high-performance liquid chromatography (hence, peak E) in batches of contaminated L-tryptophan. Optimal treatment has not been determined although patients had partial amelioration of EMS symptoms with gluco-corticoids. Chronic problems include a per-sistent skin rash, myalgia, muscle cramps and neurocognitive dysfunction. The skin lesions are indistinguishable from those of idiopathic fasciitis.

The pathogenesis of EMS was probably in part due to induction of an alternate path-way of L-tryptophan metabolism resulting in accumation of kynurenine metabolites[13]. Several cytokines, including transforming growth factor-β (TGF-β), interferon-γ and interleukin-4 (IL-4), show increased ex-pression in EMS and may have been respon-sible for generating fibrotic manifestations.

PATHOGENESIS

For any hypothesis of the pathogenesis of sclerderma to be tenable, it must explain events leading to the perivascular mononu-clear inflammation and increased deposition of extracellular matrix, both well recognized as the terminus in a series of still largely unknown individual susceptibilities, environ-mental triggers and cellular events. Further-more, this hypothesis regarding scleroderma must include vascular endothelial injury and activation, cell-mediated immune system acti-vation and fibrosis of both vascular and inter-stitial compartments. Certainly, the primary clinical benefits for understanding fibrosis in scleroderma would be to develop specific management strategies to include detecting an individual's susceptibility to fibrosis and stopping or reversing these processes at a prefibrotic stage. This optimism is tempered by the low probability of only one element interacting solely with another when there is already assembled a complicated network of cytokines triggering both paracrine and auto-crine effects involving fibroblasts and endo-thelial cells as both effector and target cells in seemingly unrelated exchanges whose key events remain elusive. In short, our under-standing of the pathogenesis of SSc remains distinctly limited.

FIBROBLAST

An abnormal scleroderma fibroblast pheno-type was established over 20 years ago when these cells were shown to produce increased amounts of collagen[14]. Increased produc-tion of collagens I, III, V, VI, VII, fibronectin and proteoglycan by SSc fibroblasts has been demonstrated to occur at a pretranslational level by detection of increased amounts of corresponding mRNA. Furthermore, the scleroderma fibroblast demonstrates altered responses to growth factors and insensitivity to acquisition of quiescence *in vitro*, instead continuing to express matrix products and the c-myc proto-oncogene, one of the immediate response competence genes. TGF-β, a strong fibrogenic cytokine, does not have the same stimulatory effect on SSc fibroblasts cultures that it does on normal fibroblasts. A postulated autocrine effect of TGF-β *in vivo* is thought to result in persistent SSc fibroblast activation *in vitro*[15]. This altered growth regulation seems to be due in part to TGF-β and increased levels of platelet derived growth factor (PDGF), in particular upregulation of the PDGF-AA ligand PDGF-αα receptor complex system on SSc fibroblasts detected after TFG-β exposure. Identification of the mechanism responsible for upregulation of certain matrix genes would provide a target for therapeutic intervention. One example currently under study utilizes promoter-reporter constructs to probe the increased COLIA2 gene expression (the alpha 2(I) collagen gene)[16]. The upregulation of this gene in SSc maps identically to the TGF-β dependent responsive nucleotide element. Alternatively, therapy aimed to block assembly of matrix proteins utilizing analogues of collagen-specific amino acids preventing secondary and tertiary collagen conformation might allow further degradation by collagenase (which is produced normally by SSc fibroblasts), preventing clinically evident fibrosis. There are multiple potential pathways to interrupt collagen deposition as a strategy to block fibrosis. None has been successful in humans.

VASCULAR

A re-evaluation of the endothelium from functioning as a passive barrier to an active organ capable of autocrine and paracrine effects permeating the entire vascular system has paralleled the description of its role in SSc pathogenesis[17]. A deranged endothelium was postulated to be present following the description of localized perivascular infiltrates occurring early in the course of SSc prior to excessive matrix deposition. A protease released from activated T-cell granules in increased quantities in SSc, granzyme one, is cytotoxic to endothelium and can be blocked by antigranzyme antibodies. This damaged endothelium not only results in increased permeability, but also is capable of participating in both humoral and cell-mediated events. T-cell activation and adherence to endothelium, possibly triggered by exposure and antigenicity of basement membrane components type IV collagen and laminin, may result in a self-perpetuating cycle of IL-2 dependent, CD4+, T-cell activation, followed by endothelial damage, cytokine release, increased permeability, decreased blood flow, increased thrombogenicity and fibroblast activation resulting in matrix proliferation and release of T-cell activating cytokines. Markers of endothelial dysfunction include plasma factor VIII – von Willibrand factor and serum angiotensin converting enzyme levels which may aid in quantitating future therapy targeting endothelial cytotoxic factors.

IMMUNE

The presence of several autoantibodies in the serum of SSc patients lends support to an immune-mediated, autoimmune component in SSc[17]. Also, the localization of primarily CD4+, T-helper, IL-2 dependent lymphocytes in the perivascular lesions of SSc colocalized with cytokines detected by immunohistochemical techniques lends further credence to T-cell dependent, pathogenetically important events. Serum levels of IL-2 and IL-2 receptors are elevated in SSc. A relative increase of CD4+, T-helper, IL-2 secreting lymphocytes, which could be fibrogenic if they secrete the profibrogenic IL-4 but could also be 'protective' if they secrete the potent collagen inhibitor gamma interferon compared with a relative decrease of CD8+, T-cytolytic, lymphocytes could partially explain fibrosis in SSc. Mechanisms of T-cell activation remain elusive. From the perspective of an immunogenetic predisposition for a specific immune response, the strongest HLA major histo-compatibility complex associations are with the class II antigens DR-1 and DR-5 being associated with anticentromere and anti-topoisomerase antibodies, respectively. Exposure of vascular extracellular matrix epitopes contained in the basal lamina, namely laminin and collagen type IV, may promote lymphocyte adherence via a mechanism of costimulation involving beta one integrins (also called very late antigens, VLA) present on T-cell membranes. Likewise, an antigen specific T-cell receptor ($CD3^+$) or a superantigen independent of MHC presentation may be responsible for T-cell activation. Defining the precise mechanism(s) of T-cell activation may lead to therapeutic interventions.

EARLY DETECTION OF THE SUBJECT AT RISK

A unifying feature of all patients with SSc is Raynaud's phenomenon (RP). Its specificity and use as a diagnostic criteria for SSc by itself is poor. However, RP is very sensitive for SSc and present in nearly all patients prior to diagnosis of SSc (Chapter 6). The prognostic significance of evaluating RP falls into predicting which individuals are at risk of developing a connective tissue disease. Secondary RP may be associated with connective tissue diseases including SSc. Recently, the traditional prognostic gold standard of time (i.e. waiting for 2 years to see if connective tissue disease occurs) has been essentially replaced by the development of a sensitive HEp-2 substrate for detecting antinuclear antibodies (ANA) and a reliable microscopic evaluation of nailfold capillaries which, together with a rheumatologists' history and physical examination, constitute a powerful mechanism for distinguishing primary and secondary RP during the initial evaluation.

Antinuclear antibodies in SSc are of prognostic importance since their recognized specificity for SSc subsets does not change

Table 3.2 Autoimmune serology in systemic sclerosis (SSc)

Anti-centromere antibodies
Anti-nuclear antibodies (speckled, nucleolar, other)
Anti-nucleolar antibodies
RNA polymerase I, II and III
Fibrillarin (U3 RNA protein complex)
Nucleolar 4-65 RNA
U2 RNA protein complex
Polymyositis/SSc overlap (Pm/Scl)
Anti-topoisomerase I (formerly Scl-70)
Anti-collagen type I
(interstitial collagen, ubiquitous)
Anti-collagen type IV
(basement membrane structure)
Anti-laminin
(basement membrane adhesion protein)
Anti-ribonucleoprotein (RNP)
Jo-1 (Anti-histidyl-transfer RNA [tRNA] synthetase) SS-A (Ro), SS-B (La) Ku

From *J. Dermatol.*, **19**, 509–23, 1992.

with time. Kallenberg *et al.* completed ANA studies on RP patients followed for 6 years using both indirect immunofluorescence and more sensitive immunoblotting techniques[18]. The latter technique supported the prediction that patients with an anti-centromere antibody (ACA) pattern would develop lSSc (sensitivity 60%, specificity 98%) and that those with antitopoisomerase I antibodies would develop dSSc (sensitivity 38%, specificity 100%). These predictions confirm known autoantibody associations for SSc subsets.

Antitopoisomerase I antibody, associated with dSSc and originally called anti-Scl-70 antibody, was discovered by detection of an apparent 70 kDa protein using SDS gel electrophoresis. Subsequently, anti-Scl-70 antibodies were found to react with a 100 kDa molecular weight DNA topoisomerase I protein. This enzyme is also localized to the nucleolus, as are other enzymes associated with SSc, including RNA polymerase, I, II and III, fibrillarin and others.

Patients with lSSc may exhibit ACA. Described as a speckled pattern using indirect immunofluorescence, this antigen is a highly conserved protein localized to the kinetochore structure of metaphase chromosomes. ACA are quite specific for lSSc. Other autoantibodies (Table 3.2) are recognized in SSc but not widely utilized clinically. Because of the frequency of speckled ANA positivity in SSc patients, one wit labeled sclerodermologists as 'The Speckled Band'.

Patients with SSc and dermatomyositis have a microangiopathy visible at the nailfold capillary bed by low magnitude widefield microscopy. These vascular abnormalities, analagous to abnormalities in internal organs in SSc, are detectable because of the longitudinal, easily visible (via widefield microscopy) arrangement of capillaries in the nailfold. PRP patients have normal capillaries; however, lSSc and dSSc have distinct patterns of dilatation only and of dilatation, disorganization and dropout, respectively[19]. This test is both sensitive and extremely specific for SSc.

ORGAN SPECIFIC INVOLVEMENT AND TREATMENT

SKIN

Thickening of the skin is a defining feature of scleroderma. Universally, patients with SSc skin thickening will have cutaneous involvement of the fingers. Skin sclerosis is best examined by visual inspection, light palpation and gentle pinching. A skilled examiner may differentiate skin changes due to scleroderma from other diseases, such as eosinophillic fasciitis (which spares the fingers, presents normal nailfold capillaries and is negative for RP). Digital pits and scars may be present. Digital ulcers secondary to RP are at increased risk of infection. Prophylactic measures should include early topical wound care with regular cleaning combined with calcium channel blockers and, possibly, light applications of topical nitrates at the base of the digital

arteries to selectively increase regional blood flow. Intravenous antibiotics and careful debridment may be indicated for chronic ulcers. Carpal tunnel syndrome is often an early finding and may predate skin thickening. Calcinosis is frequently a late finding often located on the palmer aspects of the fingers, extensor surface of the arms and, in the bedridden, on the ischial tuberosities. Telangectasia, if present, are typically in an acral distribution.

Quantitative measurements of skin sclerosis, or skin scores, aid in diagnosis, classification and accurate assessment of progression of disease[20]. There is acceptable reproducibility between skilled examiners in quantitating both the distribution and degree of skin thickness from normal to hidebound. Following the course of skin involvement is worthwhile since three distinct phases have been recognized. First, patients may experience a puffy, edematous, pruritic, aching phase later followed by variable degrees of skin thickening. After many years, an atrophic phase may occur during which patients experience significant dermal softening but retain epidermal atrophy; however, the sclerodactaly and associated finger flexion contractures usually remain a constant reminder of the diagnosis.

LUNG

Pulmonary involvement ranks second only to esophageal hypomotility and its sequelae in frequency of internal organ involvement in SSc. Mortality from the pulmonary manifestations of SSc, including interstitial lung disease and pulmonary hypertension, has displaced renal crisis as the most common end stage organ involvement since 1980, when the common use of angiotension converting enzyme (ACE) inhibitors dramatically decreased the incidence of scleroderma renal crisis.

Interstitial lung disease (ILD) is a common finding on SSc post-mortem examinations, occurring in nearly three-quarters of examinations. Roughly one-half of patients will have

ILD symptoms of cough and, more likely, dyspnea on exertion. Rarely, hemopstysis may be present, which should prompt a search for pulmonary malignancy. Physical examination may be entirely normal or reveal bibasilar crackles ('velcro rales'). Right-sided heart strain secondary to cor pulmonale may be revealed by the presence of a right ventricular lift, an increased fixed and split second heart sound, an S_3 or murmurs of tricuspid or pulmonary insufficiency.

Chest roentenograms are not early indicators of pulmonary disease. Abnormalities in different series vary widely. Changes cannot be correlated with ILD but may include linear and nodular fibrosis resembling honeycombing in the lower lobes in more advanced patients. Gallium scans are also not reliable for evaluating SSc lung disease.

Pulmonary function testing (PFT) is a noninvasive, easily administered, readily available, sensitive method of detecting early lung involvement. The earliest abnormality, also the most sensitive, is a fall of the diffusing capacity (DLco). This reflects decreased lung compliance and ventilatory volumes. In dSSc, this may be followed by a decrease in total lung capacity (TLC), vital capacity (VC) and forced vital capacity (FVC). A small number (15%) of patients will have an obstructive pattern. Less than 10% of patients with an isolated DLco below 40% will be alive after 5 years compared with a 75% 5-year survival of patients with a DLco greater than 40%.

Thin-section computerized tomography (CT) of the chest in the prone position is another reliable non-invasive means to evaluate pulmonary disease. Peripheral crescents of high attenuation in the lower lobes are an early radiographic finding of ILD. Other abnormalities may include thickened septal and subpleural lines, parenchymal bands, subpleural cysts, mediastinal lymphadenopathy and, later, honeycombing. In one series, 44% of SSC patients with a normal X-ray had abnormalities on CT scan[21].

Bronchoalveolar lavage (BAL) provides a reproducible, sensitive method to evaluate active inflammation of the lower respiratory tract in dSSC which may precede clinical symptoms[22]. BAL abnormalities in SSc associated with a decreased DLco, dyspnea and an abnormal open lung biopsy include increased total cellularity comprised of alveolar macrophages, eosinophils and granulocytes. Normal BAL findings (the absence of alveolitis) predict no significant morbidity secondary to ILD, while an abnormal BAL portends worsening pulmonary disease confirmed longitudinally by abnormal chest film and PFTs. *In vitro* studies of the cellular lavage of pulmonary fibroblasts and of cytokines obtained by BAL have implicated all of these elements in the pathogenesis of SSc ILD which closely resembles idiopathic pulmonary fibrosis.

Pathologic studies of patients with SSc ILD often reveal pleural effusions along with fibrosis of the interstitium, alveolar septae and bronchial walls. This is accompanied by congestion of capillaries and edema near alveolar septae. Other vessels may exhibit concentric intimal proliferation, medial hypertrophy and perivascular fibrosis resulting in luminal narrowing and obliteration of vessels. The vasculopathy may be evident when isolated pulmonary hypertension is present.

Hopefully, the correlation of BAL with ILD severity will provide a yardstick to evaluate clinical treatment. D-penicillamine has been associated with a stable or improved DLco but no change in FVC. Cyclophosphamide and low-dose prednisone have been associated with stabilization of clinical symptoms, pulmonary volumes and diffusing capacity[23]. Long-term controlled multicenter studies are needed to determine optimal treatment.

Pulmonary hypertension (PH) in SSc is frequently associated with limited disease. Pulmonary hypertension secondary to interstitial lung disease is usually seen in dSSc patients. Once again, the most common symptom is dyspnea often of rather sudden onset. Physical examination may reveal a pulmonic lift, an increased pulmonic component of the second heart sound, an S_4, an attenuated a wave in the jugular venous pulsation and bibasilar crackles over the lungs if ILD is present. A decreased DLco is the most common objective abnormality in isolated pulmonary hypertension and has been detected in up to 40% of patients tested. A significant isolated reduction in DLco ($<50\%$ predicted) has been associated with development of isolated PH, exclusive to lSSc. Steen *et al.* detected isolated pulmonary hypertension in 11% of patients followed for 7 years with an initially decreased DLco[24]. All had lSSc and died within two years of detection of PH. Further evaluation may include doppler 2-D echocardiography revealing elevated resting and exercise pulmonary artery pressures, right-side chamber enlargements, asymmetric septal hypertrophy and paradoxical motion. Sensitivity of echocardiography may be decreased for patients with mild or reversible PH. Cardiac catherization, which can confirm suspected PH, is usually avoided secondary to invasiveness, costs and risks of acute induction of further pulmonary vasoconstriction which can be lethal in some cases. A vasospastic component is supported by an exercise induced component to PH and the nearly universal finding of RP in these patients. Overall, a non-invasive gold standard for detecting PH has not been devised. Rather, in patients with lSSc, an isolated decrease of the DLco and an abnormal echocardiogram should prompt immediate treatment with calcium channel blockers. Controlled clinical trials are lacking (and would probably be unethical) and extrapolation from studies of primary pulmonary hypertension may not be completely valid. Recently, ACE inhibitors have also been used in treating pulmonary hypertension. Monitoring by echo doppler has improved management but has not as yet had a measurable effect on outcome.

HEART

Cardiac involvement in SSc is not often initially apparent clinically; however, it is common in dSSc and will be more evident as patients with SSc survive for longer periods of time. Case reports and pathologic studies by Weiss *et al.* in 1943 noted random patchy areas of myocardial fibrosis with normal epicardial arteries consistent with contraction band necrosis[25]. This scarring is probably the result of a vasospastic RP of the small myocardial vessels resulting in repeated ischemic episodes with reperfusion, a hypothesis supported by the association of cold induced regional perfusion defects and left ventricular dysfunction, as well as by pathologic studies demonstrating increased myofibrosis in SSc hearts with primary ventricular dysfunction compared to those with secondary dysfunction (i.e. cor pulmonale)[26–28]. Post-mortem examinations report myocardial fibrosis in 70% of SSc compared to 37% in a control group[28]. Evaluation with echocardiography may reveal regional wall motion abnormalities that correlate variably with thallium perfusion defects. These patients do not have an increased incidence of atherosclerotic coronary artery disease (ASCAD), implicating small vessel disease as the basis for the observed functional abnormalities. Further support for a cardiac microvascular etiology comes from successful treatment of these patients with calcium channel blockers. Generally, SSc patients with ASCAD are poor candidates for bypass revascularization, often not surviving the perioperative period secondary to pulmonary or myocardial complications, at least in part due to the microvascular disease.

Pericardial effusion represents the most common cardiac abnormality of SSc. Rarely does an effusion present as cardiac tamponade; rather, it is usually discovered during the evaluation of a SSc patient with peripheral edema that is in excess of puffy skin attributable to active cutaneous SSc. In the first several years after the onset of SSc symptoms, effusions will be more frequent in dSSc patients; lSSc patients also have effusions and cardiac involvement, usually in the second to fourth decades of their illness. Treatment with diuretics should be avoided, so as to reduce the likelihood of impaired renal function. A pericardial window may be indicated for progressive effusions not responsive to medical treatment. These patients are also at risk for scleroderma renal crisis within 6 months of the onset of cardiac symptoms, a part of the dSSc constellation.

Conduction abnormalities determined by electrocardiography, Holter monitoring and electrophysiology include sinus node dysfunction, supraventricular tachycardia, atrial fibrillation, premature atrial and junctional contractions and ventricular premature contractions and fibrillation. Pathologic studies cannot always correlate anatomic myofibrosis with conduction abnormalities. Correlation does exist between significant ventricular ectopy and sudden death. Unfortunately, the majority of these arthythmias often occur in patients without symptoms of palpitation or syncope. Predictors of decreased survival from SSc heart disease include left axis deviation, a moderate to large pericardial effusion and significant thallium perfusion abnormalities[29,30].

GUT

Gastrointestinal (GI) manifestations account for the most frequent internal organ involvement in SSc. The most common complaints, present in over 85% of patients, are referable to esophageal hypomotility and reflux. Common symptoms include progressive dysphagia to solids and nocturnal or recumbent heartburn secondary to esophageal dysmotility and gastroesophageal reflux, respectively. Smooth muscle hypomotility of the distal two-thirds of the esophagous and decreased lower esophageal sphincter pressure may be screened for with quantitative esophageal scintigraphy (determining eso-

phageal transit time) and barium swallow esophagram (in the prone position using low-density barium). Esophageal manometry remains the standard for evaluation of esophageal hypomotility. A complaint of emesis of ingested food shortly after a meal should be evaluated expeditiously with esophagogastroduodenoscopy to rule out obstruction resulting from an esophageal stricture. Although strictures and Barrett's metaplasia are not uncommon in SSc, transformation to malignancy is no higher than the general population and routine screening is not indicated. This may change if the control of renal and pulmonary SSc permit longer life spans.

Motility defects may be found in all sections of the GI tract. An abnormal response to the neurogenic signal triggered by an intraluminal fluid load has been noted in both the small and large intestine in SSc[31,32]. More severe gastroesophageal reflux has been linked to significant duodenal dysmotility supporting a possible role for prokinetic drugs in treatment. Clinical manifestations range from a constipation-diarrhea-obstipation cycle reminiscent of irritable bowel syndrome to abdominal distention, postprandial bloating and diffuse pain with or without steatorrhea constituting the pseudobstruction syndrome. This latter entity, resulting from hypomotility, dilatation, distention, bacterial overgrowth and malabsorption may be evaluated with an upper GI barium swallow with small bowel follow through (Figure 3.2). Universal involvement of the esophagus will be present in SSc patients with intestinal disease. Histologic changes of the bowel in SSc include muscularis mucosae atrophy and increased collagen deposition in the submucosa and lamina propria (which is also rich in immunomodulatory cells). Perivascular fibrosis may be present. A fibrotic serosal surface may be present on the atonic segments of bowel.

Pancreatic insufficiency as a source of steatorrhea in SSc is rare. Other manifestations of GI involvement may include

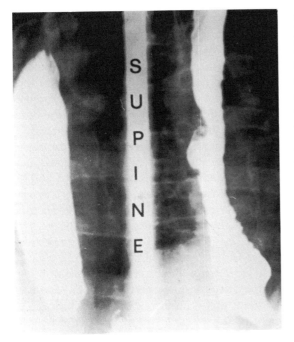

Fig. 3.2 Barium swallow showing poor esophageal mobility in SSc patient (left) compared to control (right).

primary biliary cirrhosis, primarily associated with lSSc, wide mouth diverticula in the large intestine, gastric antral vascular ectasia (the watermelon stomach) and telangectasias throughout the GI tract rarely resulting in symptomatic blood loss.

Treatment of GI disease is routinely dictated by symptoms; therefore, universal radiographic evaluation is not warranted. Symptomatic treatment of reflux with smaller, more frequent and agreeable meals along with a 4 in elevation of the head of the bed should accompany any pharmacologic interventions with antacids, H_2-blockers, sulcrafate and more recently omeprazole for reflux esophagitis. Promotility drugs (such as metaclopramide) have not been fully endorsed because their effects on not only hypokinetic but also dyskinetic SSc GI smooth muscle may be erratic. Also, these compounds may be associated with depression, dopaminergic extrapyramidal symptoms and tardive dyskinesia. A newer non-dopaminergic prokinetic agent lacking extrapyramidal effects, cisapride, awaits a thorough clinical evaluation in SSc. Avoidance of constipating narcotics and judicious use of fiber and stool softeners may ameliorate intestinal symptoms. Suspected intestinal bacterial overgrowth in pseudobstruction may respond to alternating courses of antibiotics. Resection or ostomies are rarely indicated. As an artificial and expensive last resort only, SSc patients with established non-functional bowel may achieve adequate nutrition with a well coordinated nocturnal total parenteral nutrition program resulting in improved activities of daily living and self-worth.

KIDNEY

Early indicators of renal involvement in SSc include proteinuria, hypertension and impaired glomerular filtration rate. Renal involvement usually occurs in dSSc patients within 5 years of diagnosis and may be associated with anemia, pericardial effusion, congestive heart failure and rapid progression of skin involvement. The incidence approaches 50% in clinical evaluations with higher involvement on autopsy. Previously associated with near universal mortality despite employing polypharmacy antihypertensive regimens and even nephectomy, recognition of SSc renal crisis as an alteration of the renin-angiotensin-aldosterone axis and treatment with converting enzymes inhibitors (CEI) has decreased the severity to such a degree that it is no longer the leading cause of mortality in SSc.

Patients should be screened with frequent home blood pressure measurements and renal function. Proteinuria greater than 0.5 g/24 hours or creatinure clearance of less than 60 cc/min should prompt further intervention. Lack of early treatment with CEIs may result in a triad of malignant hypertension, thrombotic microangiopathy and renal failure constituting SSc renal crisis. A subset of these patients may not have hypertension; also an association with recent steroid use has been made[33]. Renal histopathologic changes reflect the vascular etiology with intimal thickening of the small- and medium-size arteries accompanied by medial atrophy and luminal occlusion. Fibrinoid necrosis and periadventitial fibrosis also contribute to the characteristic of advanced SSc renal disease. Progressive glomerulonecrosis with basement membrane thickening may be present, immunofluorescence staining is usually unremarkable.

Treatment with CEIs has decreased mortality significantly; however, a significant number of patients are refractory to treatment. CEIs may actually reverse scleroderma renal crisis acutely and prevent or reverse the need for dialysis chronically. Achieving satisfactory vascular access for hemodialysis may be difficult; however, the ability of patients to use this as a bridge for treatment while receiving CEIs justifies its utilization. Peritoneal dialysis is complicated by fibrosis of the peritoneal membrane and decreased clearance secondary to a physiologic peritoneal RP. A final caveat is to avoid the simultaneous use of D-penicillamine and captopril, since the presence of sulfhydryl groups in each compound may increase side-effects caused by this moiety; numerous CEI alternatives are available.

TREATMENT

The treatment of scleroderma, although studied widely, is limited in altering the natural history of the disease. Significant advances have been made treating organ involvement (e.g. CEIs in renal disease) but reproducible studies of disease modifying agents that withstand scientific review are lacking. The reasons for this have been editorialized[34,35]. SSc is a sufficiently rare disease to make generating significant numbers of patients difficult, resulting in a sparse number of multicenter trials. The lack of controls, placebo responses and the natural history of regressive skin involvement complicate outcome measurement. Other outcomes including internal organ involvement, mortality and quality of life need to be included in prolonged trials in which subjects are entered at the time of clinical disease onset. Analyses comparing the effects of a therapeutic agent during a non-responsive fibrotic phase or a regressing atrophic phase cannot be applied to earlier 'active' phases of disease. As more is learned about the pathogenesis of SSc, therapeutic trials with biologic response modifiers (so called 'magic bullets') aimed at specific triggers can be developed and hopefully evaluated in a scientific manner. In uncontrolled studies, numerous agents have been reported to have therapeutic responses including D-penicillamine, cyclosporin-A, methotrexate, colchicine and recombinant interferon-γ. Many of the studies were limited by toxic side effects outweighing modest beneficial responses. Controlled long-term studies of therapy targeting fibrogenic mechanisms with easily quantifiable outcomes is a goal that can be accomplished with developing technologies.

REFERENCES

1. David, J., Wilson J. and Woo, P. (1991) Scleroderma 'en coup de sabre'. *Ann. Rheum. Dis.*, **50**, 260–62.
2. LeRoy, E. C., Black, C., Fleischmajer, R. *et al.* (1988) Scleroderma (systemic sclerosis): classification, subsets and pathogenesis. *J. Rheumatol.*, **15**(2), 202–5.
3. Altman, R. D., Medsger Jr., T. A., Bloch, D. A. *et al.* (1991) Predictors of survival in systemic sclerosis (scleroderma). *Arth. Rheum.*, **34**(4), 403–13.
4. Black, K. A., Zilko, P. J., Dawkin, R. L. *et al.* (1982) Cancer in connective tissue disease. *Arth. Rheum.*, **25**(9), 1130–33.
5. Zatuchni, J., Campbell, W. N. and Zarofonetis, C. J. D. (1953) Pulmonary fibrosis and terminal bronchiolar carcinoma in scleroderma, *Cancer*, **6**, 1147–58.

6. Duncan, S. C., Winkelmann, R. K. (1979) Cancer and scleroderma. *Arch. Dermatol.*, **115**, 950–5.

7. Medsger Jr., T. A. (1985) Systemic sclerosis and malignancy – are they related? *J. Rheum.*, **12**(6), 1041–3.

8. Bramwell, B. (1914) Diffuse scleroderma: its frequency; its occurence in stone-masons: its treatment by fibrolysin – elevations of temperature due to fibrolysin injections. *Edin. Med. J.*, **12**, 387–401.

9. Wigley, F. M., Miller, R., Hochberg, M. C. *et al.* (1992) Augmentation mammoplasty in patients with systemic sclerosis: data from the Baltimore scleroderma research center and Pittsburgh scleroderma data bank. *Arth. Rheum.*, **35**: S46, (abstr).

10. Kilbourne, E. M., Posada de la Paz, M. and Abaitua Borda, I. (1992) *Epidemiologic Studies in Toxic Oil Syndrome. Current knowledge and future perspectives*, World Health Organization Regional Publications, European Series, No. 42, pp. 5–26.

11. Abaitua Borda, I. and Posada de la Paz, M. (1992) *Clinical findings, in Toxic Oil Syndrome. Current knowledge and future perspectives*, World Health Organization Regional Publications, European Series, No. 42, pp. 5–26.

12. Silver, R. M. (1991) Unraveling the eosinophilia-myalgia syndrome. *Arch. Dermatol.*, **127**, 1214–16.

13. Silver, R. M., McKinley, K., Smith, E. A. *et al.* (1992) Tryptophan metabolism via the kynurenine pathway in patients with the eosinophilia-myalgia syndrome. *Arth.Rheum.*, **35**(9), 1097–105.

14. LeRoy, E. C. (1972) Connective tissue synthesis by scleroderma skin fibroblasts in cell culture. *J. Exp. Med.*, **135**, 1351–62.

15. LeRoy, E. C., Smith, E. A., Kahaleh, M. B. *et al.* (1989) A strategy for determining the pathogenesis of systemic sclerosis. Is transforming growth factor β the answer? *Arth. Rheum.*, **32**(7), 817–25.

16. Kikuchi, K., Hartl, C. W., Smith, E. A. *et al.* (1992) Direct demonstration of transcriptional activation of collagen gene expression in systemic sclerosis fibroblasts: insensitivity to TGFβ1 stimulation. *Biochem. Biophys. Res. Commun.*, **187**(1), 45–50.

17. LeRoy, E. C. (1992) A brief overview of the pathogenesis of scleroderma (systemic sclerosis). *Ann. Rheum. Dis.*, **51**, 286–8.

18. Kallenberg, C. G. M., Wouda, A. A., Hoet, M. H. *et al.* (1988) Development of connective tissue disease in patients presenting with Raynaud's phenomenon: a six year follow up with emphasis on the predictive value of antinuclear antibodies as detected by immunoblotting. *Ann. Rheum. Dis.*, **47**, 634–41.

19. Carpentier, P. H. and Maricq, H. R. (1990) Microvasculature in systemic sclerosis, in *Rheumatic Disease Clinics of North America*, (ed. E. C. LeRoy), W. B. Saunders Co., Philadelphia, **16**, pp. 75–92.

20. Kahaleh, M. B., Sultany, G. L., Smith, E. A. *et al.* (1986) A modified scleroderma skin scoring method. *Clin. Exper. Rheum.*, **4**, 367–9.

21. Harrison, N. K., Glanville, A. R., Strickland, B. *et al.* (1989) Pulmonary involvement in systemic sclerosis: the detection of early changes by thin section CT scan, bronchoalveolar lavage and 99mTc-DTPA clearance. *Respir. Med.*, **83**, 403–14.

22. Wallert, B. K., Hatron, P., Grosbois, J. *et al.* (1986) Subclinical pulmonary involvement in collagen vascular disease assessed by bronchoalveolar lavage: relationship between alveolitis and subsequent changes in lung function. *Am. Rev. Respir. Dis.*, **133**, 574–80.

23. Silver, R. M., Warrick, J. H., Kinsella, M. B. *et al.* (1993) Cyclophosphamide and low-dose prednisone therapy in patients with systemic sclerosis (scleroderma) with interstitial lung disease. *J. Rheum.*, **20**(5), 838–44.

24. Steen, V. D., Graham, G., Conte, C. *et al.* (1992) Isolated diffusing capacity reduction in systemic sclerosis. *Arth. Rheum.*, **35**(7), 765–70.

25. Weiss, S., Stead, Jr., E. A., Warren, J V. *et al.* (1943) Scleroderma heart disease with a consideration of certain other visceral manifestations of scleroderma. *Arch. Inter. Med.*, **71**, 749–76.

26. Alexander, E. L., Firestein, G. S., Weiss, J. L. *et al.* (1986) Reversible cold-induced abnormalities in myocardial perfusion and function in systemic sclerosis. *Ann. Intern. Med.*, **105**, 661–8.

27. Ellis, W. W., Baer, A. N., Robertson, R. M. *et al.* (1986) Left ventricular dysfunction induced by cold exposure in patients with systemic sclerosis. *Am. J. Med.*, **80**, 385–92.

28. Follansbee, W. P., Miller, T. R., Curtiss, E. I. *et al.* (1990) A controlled clinicopathologic study of myocardial fibrosis in systemic sclerosis (scleroderma). *J Rheum.*, **17**(5), 656–62.

29. Clements, P. J., Lachenbruch, P. A., Furst, D.

E. *et al.* (1991) Cardiac score – a semiquantitative measure of cardiac involvement that improves prediction of prognosis in systemic sclerosis. *Arth. Rheum.*, **34**(11), 1371–80.

30. Follansbee, W. P., Curtiss, E. I., Medsger, Jr., T. A. *et al.* (1984) Physiologic abnormalities of cardiac function in progressive systemic sclerosis with diffuse scleroderma. *N. Engl. J. Med.*, **310**, 142–5.

31. DiMarino, A. J., Carlson, G., Myers, A. *et al.* (1973) Duodenal myoelectric activity in scleroderma. Abnormal responses to mechanical and hormonal stimuli. *N. Engl. J. Med.*, **289**, 1220–3.

32. Battle, W. M., Snape Jr., W. J., Wright, *et al.* (1981) Abnormal colonic motility in progressive systemic sclerosis. *Ann. Intern. Med.*, **94**, 749–52.

33. Helfrich, D. J., Banner, B., Steen, V. D. *et al.* (1989) Normotensive renal failure in systemic sclerosis. *Arth. Rheum.*, **32**(9), 1128–34.

34. Seibold, J. R., Furst, D. E., Clements, P. J. (1992) Why everything (or nothing) seems to work in the treatment of scleroderma. *J. Rheum.*, **19**(5), 673–6.

35. Wigley, F. M. (1992) Treatment of systemic sclerosis, in *Current Opin Rheumatol*, (ed. E. C. LeRoy), **4**(6), 878–6.

POLYMYOSITIS AND DERMATOMYOSITIS

T. A. Medsger, Jr. and C. V. Oddis

INTRODUCTION

Polymyositis (PM) and dermatomyositis (DM) are acquired chronic inflammatory disorders which primarily affect skeletal muscle, leading to proximal muscle weakness. When a characteristic rash is present, the term dermatomyositis is used. These conditions belong to a single spectrum of disease, but many distinctive syndromes exist within this rubric. The heterogeneity of clinical manifestations suggests multiple etiologies. However, certain common features, such as the presence of lymphocytes in muscle biopsy specimens, the frequent occurrence of serum autoantibodies and responsiveness to corticosteroids and immunosuppressive drugs, favor autoimmune mechanisms participating in pathogenesis.

EPIDEMIOLOGY

The epidemiology of the inflammatory myopathies has been a topic of considerable interest, resulting in a number of important publications and reviews[1–7].

CLASSIFICATION

Disease classification in PM/DM serves to identify clinically homogeneous subsets of patients, with the ultimate goals of facilitating studies of natural history and response to treatment as well as laboratory investigations of pathogenesis and etiology. Currently employed classification systems separate DM from PM, and childhood from adult onset disease, as well as distinguish myositis associated with malignancy or with other connective tissue diseases ('overlap' syndromes) [8–10]. Evidence has been presented recently that a three-way classification system best explains the observed demographic, histologic, immunopathologic and therapeutic features of these diseases; the major distinct patient groups proposed are PM, DM and inclusion body myositis (IBM)[11]. It is uncertain if separate categories should be used for myositis associated with malignancy or with other connective tissue diseases, but clinical features and outcome are clearly different in these patient subsets. For the purposes of this chapter, we will use the classification system listed in Table 4.1, recognizing that new knowledge will lead to appropriate revision in the future.

Table 4.1 Classification

1. Polymyositis
2. Dermatomyositis
3. Myositis associated with another connective tissue disease
4. Myositis associated with malignancy
5. Inclusion body myositis

Connective Tissue Diseases. Edited by Jill J. F. Belch and Robert B. Zurier. Published in 1995 by Chapman & Hall, London. ISBN 0 412 48620 2

Table 4.2   Reported incidence of PM/DM in different populations

First author (year)	Geographic area	Inclusive dates of study	Incidence (per million)	Comments
Rose (1966)[4]	Northeast England	1954–64	2.25	Patients classified using Walton and Adams criteria
Kurland (1969)[2]	Rochester, Minn.	1957–67	6.0	Population almost exclusively white
Findlay (1969)[6]	Transvaal, South Africa	1960–7	7.5	Includes DM cases only
Medsger (1970)[1]	Memphis and Shelby County, Tenn.	1947–68	5.0	Population 40% black
Benbassat (1980)[3]	Israel	1960–76	2.2	Includes hospital diagnosed cases; Bohan and Peter criteria for diagnosis
Oddis (1990)[5]	Allegheny County, Penna.	1963–82	5.5	Population 90% white; incidence 8.9/million during 1973–82
Koh (1993)[7]	Singapore	1986–91	7.7	EMG laboratories and primary medical center; Bohan and Peter criteria for diagnosis

Myositis-specific serum antibodies (MSA) are found in approximately 40% of patients with inflammatory myopathy. As with disease-specific autoantibodies in other connective tissue diseases, notably systemic lupus erythematosus and systemic sclerosis, MSA define homogeneous patient subsets, and several MSA have strong immunogenetic associations (section on 'Serum autoantibodies', below). These antibodies have been suggested as useful contributors to classification[12]. It is likely that, in the future, both clinical and serologic features will be combined to best classify inflammatory myopathy patients.

DIAGNOSTIC CRITERIA

For purposes of defining patient groups in population studies, clinical research and aiding in the diagnosis of the individual patient, the 1975 diagnostic criteria of Bohan and Peter[8] have served well for two decades. These criteria include proximal muscle weakness, three types of laboratory confirmation of muscle inflammation (serum enzymes,

electromyogram and biopsy) and the rash of DM. Definite, probable and possible disease can be defined using these criteria. The sensitivity of the Bohan and Peter criteria in seven published series has been summarized and averages 70% definite and 20% probable, with most probable and possible cases downgraded not because of uncertainty about diagnosis, but rather because one or more of the laboratory tests of muscle inflammation were not performed[13]. Their specificity against 436 lupus and scleroderma patients combined was 93%[14].

INCIDENCE

The annual incidence of PM/DM reported in community studies has ranged from 2–10 new cases per million persons at risk[1–7] (Table 4.2). Published rates would appear to be underestimates since most often limited searches (i.e. hospitals only) were performed and patients with potential misdiagnoses (e.g. muscular dystrophy) were not examined. Although there are increasing incidence rates over time in several communities, these trends are more likely due to increased physician awareness than to a true increase in disease occurrence.

In a northeast section of England, 89 new cases of PM/DM were detected in a population of 3.2 million over a 12-year time period for an annual incidence of 2.25 per million[4]. In the small, almost exclusively white population of northern European origin from Rochester and Olmstead County, Minnesota, incidence was determined to be 6.0 per million per year[2]. We have performed two hospital-based studies using similar methodology[1,5]. In Memphis and Shelby County, Tennessee, a large and racially mixed population with 40% African Americans, the annual incidence was 5.0 per million overall, rising to 8.4 per million during the last six years (1963–8) of the 22-year survey. Similarly, our results in Pittsburgh and Allegheny County, Pennsylvania, showed a PM/DM incidence of 5.5 per million persons which was highest (10.0 per million) in the last decade of the study (1973–82).

The pattern of incidence by age suggests childhood and adulthood peaks with a paucity of patients diagnosed during the adolescent and young adult years of 15–24. This finding supports the separation of childhood from adult disease. The mean age at myositis onset is increased when there is an accompanying malignancy.

The overall female-to-male ratio in reported epidemiologic studies is 2.5:1, but subset differences are evident. The sex ratio is nearly equal in childhood onset and malignancy-associated disease, yet females dominate (10:1) when there are features of another connective tissue disease (overlap).

PM/DM has a 3–4:1 African American to white incidence ratio with a distinct peak among young adult African Americans. The tendency for the latter group to be affected by PM/DM at earlier ages is a feature shared with systemic lupus erythematosus and systemic sclerosis (Chapters 2 and 3). Polymyositis is more frequent than dermatomyositis in African Americans.

PREVALENCE

Based on only three living cases in Olmstead County, Minnesota, the estimated prevalence of polymyositis in 1968 was 63 per million population[2]. A similar figure of 50 per million was reported in Kumamoto, Japan in 1982–3[15]. Considering more recent improved survival, a more reasonable estimate would be 150 per million calculated as incidence (10/million/year) times average disease duration (15 years).

ENVIRONMENTAL FACTORS

No convincing associations of inflammatory myopathies with environmental factors have been recognized. Antecedent heavy muscular exertion and emotional stress during the 12 months preceding disease onset were found significantly more frequently in PM/DM than in sex-matched unaffected sibling controls[16]. Disease onset was more frequent in the winter and spring months in two studies[1,17], especially in childhood cases[1]. Suspicious geographic and spring month onset 'clustering' of patients with anti-Jo-1 antibody have been observed, but not further analyzed[18]. These findings are consistent with precipitation by viral and/or bacterial infections, but in the above sibling study, upper respiratory infection and pharyngitis occurred in similar frequencies in cases and controls[16]. When the spectrum of muscle disease is enlarged to also include non-inflammatory myopathies, a variety of drugs, chemicals, dietary supplements and occupational and toxic exposures are implicated[19].

GENETIC FACTORS

PM/DM has been reported in monozygotic twins[20] and in first degree relatives of index cases[21]. First-degree relatives and other family members frequently suffer from another closely related connective tissue disease[22].

When the accepted clinical classification subsets were examined, HLA associations were weak. White children with DM and adults with PM had an increased frequency of HLA-B8, DR3[23,24], while African Americans with PM more often had HLA-B7, DRw6[24]. Adults with DM in overlap with another connective tissue disease more commonly had HLA B14 and B40[25]. Children with DM had an increased frequency of C4A null alleles, which are in linkage disequilibrium with B8 and DR3[26].

When serum autoantibody status is used to define patient subsets, immunogenetic associations are much more striking. Anti-Jo1 antibody positive patients, who have polymyositis and several other distinctive clinical manifestations (below), have a significantly increased frequency of HLA-DRw52 compared with controls[27]. Those myositis patients with anti-PM-Sc1, who also typically have scleroderma features, nearly all possess HLA-DR3 or DRw52[28,29]. It is thus likely that certain persons are immunogenetically predisposed to acquire clinically and serologically linked myositis syndromes.

CLINICAL PRESENTATIONS

The clinical features and syndromes at the time of presentation vary considerably from patient to patient[30,31] (Table 4.3). The most frequent and hallmark complaint is insidious, progressive, painless proximal muscle weakness during the prior 3–6 months. In children and young adults with DM, the onset is often more acute, with constitutional features (fever, fatigue) and muscle pain and weakness developing rapidly over several weeks. In contrast, a recently recognized subset of patients has very slowly evolving weakness over 5–10 years. Patients are typically men with both pelvic girdle and distal extremity muscle weakness who have inclusion body myositis on muscle biopsy. If this characteristic histologic finding is absent, differentiation from adult onset muscular dystrophy may be difficult. Finally, a few patients have

Table 4.3 Types and frequencies of presenting clinical syndromes in PM/DM

Syndrome	Estimated frequency
1. Painless proximal weakness (over 3–6 months)	55%
2. Acute or subacute proximal pain and weakness (over weeks to 2 months)	30%
3. Insidious proximal and distal weakness (over 1–10 years)	10%
4. Proximal myalgia alone	5%
5. Dermatomyositis rash alone	<1%

Revised from *Rheumatology* (eds J. Klippel and P. Dieppe), Gower Medical Publishing, London, 1994, with permission.

myalgia in proximal muscles without evident weakness or the pathognomonic rash of DM. Distal extremity and neck muscle weakness is most often absent in patients with malignancy.

Other striated muscles may be weak besides the shoulder and pelvic girdle. On occasion, weakness in these muscle groups may result in the most prominent symptoms of the illness. Examples are hoarseness and dysphonia due to bulbar muscle weakness, regurgitation of liquids through the nose and aspiration pneumonia secondary to pharyngeal dysphagia, and dyspnea resulting from respiratory muscle weakness with or without interstitial lung disease. Ocular and facial muscle involvement should not occur, even in severe cases of inflammatory myopathy.

The rash of DM can precede myositis[32]. Patients with anti-synthetase antibodies may first note Raynaud's phenomenon, polyarthralgias and/or polyarthritis, or dyspnea due to interstitial lung disease. In overlap syndromes, one may encounter early scleroderma features including puffy fingers, sclerodactyly and distal dysphagia or heartburn, or lupus findings, such as photosensitive and/or malar skin rash, alopecia, pleurisy or oral ulceration.

DIFFERENTIAL DIAGNOSIS

HISTORY AND PHYSICAL EXAMINATION

In patients with impaired proximal skeletal muscle function, half complain about 'weakness' and the remainder tend to use the terms 'tiredness' and 'fatigue'. It is thus important to differentiate between difficulty in performing a motor task (weakness) or its repetitive performance (muscle fatigue) and difficulty doing activities of daily living that require more endurance than muscle strength. Weakness and muscle fatigue with activity imply primary disease of muscle or the neuromuscular unit, while lack of endurance may be associated with, or be solely due to, cardiovascular, metabolic, endocrine or psychiatric disorders. The more non-specific term 'fatigue' describes a variety of patient complaints that have the common feature of loss of sense of well-being. It may include indifference to tasks at hand, preoccupation with unimportant activities or difficulty initiating or sustaining an activity. The patient often does not separate physical from mental activity. For example, disinclination to interact with one's family members and friends during leisure hours may be termed 'fatigue' by the patient, but be interpreted as a symptom of depression by the discerning physician.

If muscle weakness is suspected based on careful evaluation of the history, then exploration of other dimensions of this complaint are useful. Was the onset insidious or abrupt? Is the weakness episodic or persistent; global or localized; symmetrical or asymmetrical; proximal, distal, truncal or facial? Is it affected by prolonged muscle use; time of day; diet; environmental factors such as temperature; or medications? Is there associated muscle pain or tenderness; cramps or fasciculations; sensory symptoms; arthritis; skin rash; or a family history of myopathy?

NON-INFLAMMATORY MYOPATHIES

The differential diagnosis of adult PM (Table 4.4) is broad and includes numerous conditions capable of causing skeletal muscle weakness[30]. History, physical examination, laboratory test result differences and muscle biopsy serve as the primary differentiating features between these conditions.

Primary diseases of nerve include the spinal muscular atrophies, autosomal recessive disorders leading to slowly progressive degeneration of spinal anterior horn cells (weakness, wasting) and amyotrophic lateral sclerosis, resulting in more rapid degeneration of both lower and upper motor neurons (bulbar or pseudobulbar palsy).

Myasthenia gravis is the prototype disorder of the neuromuscular junction, in which weakness often affects the extraocular and bulbar muscles and becomes worse with repetitive contraction. A similar pattern of activity-increased weakness is found in Eaton–Lambert syndrome. Both of these diseases can cause proximal muscle weakness, but are distinguished from PM/DM by their characteristic electromyographic patterns as well as absence of serum muscle enzyme elevation.

The muscular dystrophies are predominantly heritable conditions with onset of symptoms either in childhood or adulthood and slow but steady progression. Their primary genetic and clinical features are well-described. Glycogen storage diseases result from enzyme deficiencies involving the glycolytic pathway. McArdle's disease, or myophosphorylase deficiency, is caused by failure to degrade glycogen for energy under anaerobic conditions. It is characterized by acute episodes of pain, weakness and swelling in muscles after frequent voluntary movements or prolonged contraction. On occasion, a late proximal myopathy occurs that can simulate PM. Ischemic exercise testing results in failure to produce lactate and muscle biopsy shows glycogen accumulation and absence of myophosphorylase. Adult maltase deficiency results in excessive accumulation of glycogen in membrane-bound lysozymes. Progressive proximal weakness, a myotonic electromyogram and glycogen deposition on muscle biopsy are observed.

Table 4.4   Differential diagnosis of inflammatory myopathy

Endocrine-metabolic
Thyroid (hyper-, hypo-)
Adrenal (hyper-, hypo-)
Parathyroid (hyper-, hypo-)
Acromegaly
Calcium (hyper-, hypo-)
Magnesium (hypo-)
Potassium (hypo-)
Carbohydrate, lipid, purine metabolic disorders
Nutritional (vitamin D, E deficiencies; malabsorption)
Organ failure (renal, hepatic)

Drug-induced
Ethanol
D-penicillamine
Chloroquine
Emetine
Ipecac
Zidovudine (AZT)
Colchicine
Cholesterol lowering agents
Corticosteroids
Pentazocine

Other autoimmune and connective tissue diseases
Rheumatoid arthritis
Systemic lupus erythematosus
Vasculitis
Sjörgen's syndrome
Polymyalgia rheumatica
Systemic sclerosis
Eosinophilia-myalgia syndrome

Neuromuscular
Denervation (spinal muscular atrophies; amyotrophic lateral sclerosis)
Neuromuscular junction (Eaton–Lambert syndrome; myasthenia gravis)
Paraneoplastic (carcinomatous neuromyopathy)
Proximal neuropathies (Guillain–Barré syndrome; acute intermittent porphyria; diabetic amyotrophy)

Genetic and congenital
Muscular dystrophies (Duchenne's fascioscapulohumeral; limb girdle; Becker's; others)
Myotonic dystrophy; myotonia congenita
Congenital myopathies (nemaline; mitochondrial; centronuclear; central core)

Infectious
Bacterial (*Staphylococcus*; *Streptococcus*; *Clostridium welchii*; *Salmonella*; leprosy)
Viral (influenza; Coxsackie; echovirus; Epstein–Barr, rubella/rubella vaccination; human immunodeficiency; *Rickettsia*)
Parasitic (*Trichinella*; *Toxoplasma*; *Schistosoma*; *Sarcosporidia*; cysticerci)

Other
Rhabdomyolysis
Myositis ossificans
Microembolization (atheroma, carcinoma)

Disorders of muscle lipid metabolism may also mimic PM. Carnitine deficiency results in the inability to transport long-chain fatty acids into mitochondria for oxidation, leading to lipid accumulation in muscle fibers and a chronic proximal myopathy. The enzyme carnitine palmityl transferase may also be lacking, resulting in a syndrome resembling McArdle's disease, with exertional pain and weakness due to inadequate ATP production from lipids. A similar symptom complex can occur with myoadenylate deaminase deficiency.

Other causes of proximal myopathy include hypokalemia, vitamin D deficiency, adrenal insufficiency, hypophosphatemia, hyperthyroidism, carcinomatous neuromyopathy and exposures to various toxic substances. A variety of drugs are capable of producing non-inflammatory myopathy.

OTHER INFLAMMATORY MYOPATHIES

Infectious agents are capable of producing myositis. Myositis secondary to influenza[33], Coxsackie virus[34], echovirus[35] and human immunodeficiency virus[36] are well-documented. Echovirus has been associated with myositis in patients with x-linked hypo-gammaglobulinemia. In contrast to PM, the duration of myositis in these cases is self-limited and no patients have been reported to evolve to chronic PM. Complement-fixing IgG and neutralizing antibodies to Coxsackie B viruses are found two-fold more frequently in juvenile DM compared with juvenile rheumatoid arthritis and hospital controls[34] and viral protein sequences have been detected in affected muscle[37]. Other infectious agents capable of causing myositis are trichinosis, toxoplasma[38], *Borrelia burgdorferi* (Lyme disease)[39] and staphylococci (pyomyositis)[40].

Drug-induced PM may occur with D-penicillamine therapy[41]. 'Contaminated' L-tryptophan in the recent eosinophilia-myalgia syndrome epidemic mentioned in Chapter 3 led to interstitial and perivascular eosinophilic infiltration of muscle and neuromyopathy with prominent muscle pain and cramps but no myofibril degeneration and normal creatine kinase levels[42]. Focal or nodular myositis with eosinophilic inflammatory infiltration may also be part of the spectrum of the hypereosinophilic syndrome.

Focal nodular myositis, presenting with tumor-like masses and curiously limited to one or several extremities, has been reported. Giant cell myositis is rare but can be encountered in sarcoidosis. Regenerating muscle in other conditions may have a multinucleate appearance that must be distinguished from true giant cells in a typical granuloma.

CLINICAL AND LABORATORY MANIFESTATIONS

CONSTITUTIONAL

Patients with myositis may present with a variety of constitutional symptoms. Fatigue is present in most patients and appears distinct from muscular complaints. Fever, sometimes found in childhood DM and younger adults, is also commonly seen during flares of myositis in patients with autoantibodies directed against the amino-acyl-tRNA synthetases (below). Weight loss is uncommon except in patients with an associated malignancy, severe depression or significant pharyngeal involvement that interferes with swallowing.

SKELETAL MUSCLE

The hallmark clinical feature of inflammatory myopathy, and typically the dominant symptom, is muscle weakness, which affects nearly every patient at some time during the illness. The shoulder and hip girdle muscles are equally involved and weakness is bilateral and symmetrical. Weakness usually develops over a period of weeks to months. Patients with inclusion body myositis (IBM) have a more insidious onset of weakness characterized by both proximal and distal involvement. Patients with PM and DM complain of difficulty rising from a chair, walking up steps, lifting their heads off a pillow and raising their arms above head level for activities such as combing their hair. Their gait becomes clumsy and sometimes waddling. Falling episodes are common in IBM owing to marked quadriceps atrophy. Fine motor movements that depend on distal muscle strength are also compromised in IBM, but distal weakness is rare in early PM and DM. Muscle pain and tenderness are occasionally reported, most frequently in DM patients.

Involvement of pharyngeal striated muscles leads to dysphonia, proximal dysphagia, difficulty in initiating swallowing and regurgitation of liquids through the nose. Tracheobronchial aspiration may result, leading to chemical or infectious pneumonitis. Respiratory muscle involvement with ventilatory insufficiency is seen with acute or advanced cases of myositis.

A combination of neuropathic and myopathic features is characteristic of IBM patients. Weakness and atrophy are more asymmetric compared to PM and DM with selective involvement of the quadriceps, biceps and triceps muscles. Distal muscle involvement with foot extensor (foot drop) and finger flexor weakness is common. Weakness of the deep finger flexors of the third, fourth and fifth digits in association with atrophy of the flexor digitorum muscle of the forearm is felt to be pathognomonic for IBM[11].

Swelling of muscle is unusual in idiopathic myositis. Firmness to palpitation with incomplete passive stretching suggests fibrous replacement of muscle with contracture. Muscle hypertrophy is not observed in PM or DM; this finding favors one or another form of muscular dystrophy.

The laboratory evaluation of myositis includes a number of studies. In active inflammation, muscle enzymes leak from injured muscle fibers, leading to increased serum levels. Creatine kinase (CK) is the most sensitive enzyme indicator of muscle injury, but aldolase, aspartate aminotransaminase (AST or SGOT), alanine aminotransaminase (ALT or SGPT) and lactate dehydrogenase (LDH) may also be elevated. Raised transaminases and LDH in a patient with fatigue and nonspecific weakness has led to the inaccurate diagnosis of hepatitis and to an unnecessary liver biopsy. The CK is elevated at some time in the course of myositis in 95% of patients. However, there are many reported instances of normal CK at the time of biopsy-proved active myositis, especially in DM (including childhood DM) and malignancy[43]. In some cases, a serum inhibitor of creatine kinase present in patients with muscle disease or injury, but not in normal individuals, interferes with the detection of CK activity[44].

Release of myoglobin from muscle is a more sensitive indicator of injury than the serum CK. When large amounts of myoglobin are filtered by the kidney, tubular necrosis with acute renal failure may ensue[45]. The measurement of blood and urine myoglobin is tedious and expensive, but a rapid, more convenient immunoturbidimetric assay may become available[46]. Unfortunately, this advance will not solve the problem of specificity,

as myoglobin is also found in cardiac muscle. New markers are being evaluated that are specific for only myocardium (troponin) or skeletal muscle (carbonic anhydrase III)[47].

Electromyography (EMG) is a sensitive but non-specific diagnostic tool in the evaluation of inflammatory myopathy. Affected proximal muscles demonstrate myopathic motor unit potentials that, on voluntary contraction, are polyphasic in type and of short duration and low amplitude. Increased spontaneous activity is evidenced by fibrillation potentials, complex repetitive discharges and positive sharp waves. A normal EMG is rarely found in myositis; over 90% of patients with active disease demonstrate changes when weak, but not atrophic, muscles are studied. The EMG may be helpful in selecting an appropriate site for a muscle biopsy and also may be used clinically to assess puzzling patients, such as those with normal serum enzyme levels and a physical examination that is difficult to interpret. The electromyographic changes of steroid myopathy are not nearly as severe as those seen with active inflammation.

Muscle biopsy is recommended in all cases of suspected myositis to confirm the diagnosis. Unfortunately, sampling errors limits the sensitivity of the procedure, as up to 20% of biopsies in typical myositis cases are normal. This supports the concept that histologic changes are patchy and emphasizes the need for other criteria in the diagnosis of myositis. The pathognomonic finding is the presence of chronic inflammatory cells in the perivascular and interstitial areas (Figure 4.1). The infiltrate is predominantly lymphocytic, but may also include histiocytes, plasma cells, eosinophils and even polymorphonuclear cells. Other findings include degeneration and necrosis of myofibrils as well as regeneration. More chronic changes consist of an increase in fibrous connective tissue between fascicles and fatty replacement of damaged myofibrils. DM is associated with perifascicular atrophy, capillary damage and depletion, and even overt vasculitis (especially in children),

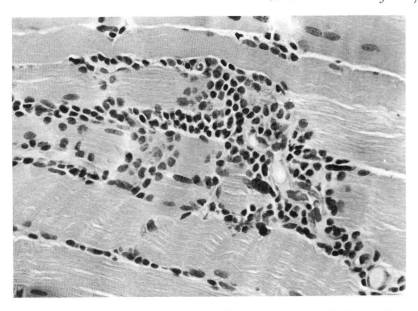

Fig. 4.1 Hematoxylin and eosin stain of a paraffin section of muscle biopsy from a patient with polymyositis demonstrating perivascular and endomysial mononuclear (predominantly lymphocytic) inflammatory infiltrate; total magnification 190× (Photograph courtesy of Dr David Lacomis).

changes that are not found in PM (Figure 4.2). The muscle chosen for biopsy should demonstrate classic electromyographic changes and be weak but not atrophic or endstage. The opposite side of the body from the EMG should be biopsied to avoid the focal myositis artefact that can result from needle insertion into muscle. Although open surgical biopsy is preferred, the diagnosis can also be made with needle biopsy (personal observation).

Magnetic resonance imaging (MRI) is a non-invasive diagnostic tool used only recently in the diagnosis and management of inflammatory myopathies. Recognition of muscle pathology has been enhanced with newer MRI techniques that selectively suppress the signal from fat, thus accentuating the increase in signal intensity from the inflammatory process in muscle[48] (Figure 4.3). This fat-suppressed (STIR) image signal intensity has been shown to correlate with both clinical disease activity and inflammatory changes on muscle biopsy in several studies of adult and childhood myositis patients[48–50]. In 40 patients with inflammatory myopathy, the muscle STIR signal intensity was higher in patients with active versus inactive disease and was more sensitive in detecting active disease than the muscle biopsy[49]. Three patients were followed longitudinally with MRI, and the signal intensity changes correlated well with clinical disease activity scores. The investigators also found that IBM patients had significantly more anterior than posterior compartment thigh involvement, as well as a more focal pattern of increased signal compared to PM or DM patients. In a prospective study of 24 children (19 CDM), all patients with clinically active disease had abnormal MRI findings, whereas those with inactive disease had a normal MRI[50]. Although markedly abnormal signal intensities were associated with high CK levels, MRI changes were also seen in children with normal muscle enzymes. Considering the invasiveness and limitations of the muscle

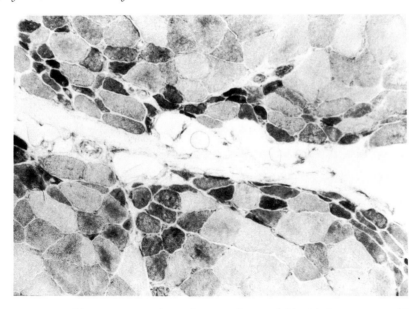

Fig. 4.2   NADH stain of frozen section of muscle tissue from a child with dermatomyositis demonstrating marked perifascicular atrophy, total magnification 100× (Photograph courtesy of Dr David Lacomis).

biopsy, MRI may be a reasonable alternative for diagnosis, confirmation of disease flare (particularly in patients with normal muscle enzymes), directing the selection of a site for biopsy, and allowing non-invasive assessment of disease activity (deterioration or improvement) over time[50]. Its current considerable expense will be a limiting factor.

CUTANEOUS

The cutaneous lesions of DM are virtually pathognomonic and they may precede, accompany or follow the onset of muscle weakness. Gottron's papules, found in nearly three-quarters of DM patients, are erythematosus, scaly, slightly raised plaques over the finger joints or other extensor surfaces such as the elbows, knees and hands (Plate 3). The heliotrope rash is less common (50% patients) and is an erythematous or violaceous rash affecting the upper eyelids with or without edema. Photosensitivity is common and periungual changes with cuticular hypertrophy, telangiectasias and dilated, enlarged capillary loops may be seen[51]. Chronically, the skin lesions become shiny, atrophic and often hypopigmented. 'Mechanics hands' (Plate 4) are characterized by painful lateral and palmar digital fissuring and are found in PM as well as DM patients in association with anti-synthetase or anti-PM-Scl antibodies[29,31]. Other cutaneous findings reported in myositis patients include panniculitis[52], cutaneous mucinosis, vitiligo[53] and multifocal lipoatrophy[54].

The term 'amyopathic dermatomyositis' or 'DM sine myositis' refers to the unusual patient who demonstrates the classic skin lesions of DM without clinical or laboratory evidence of muscle disease. Recent studies have described nine adult DM patients followed for a mean of 6.1 years after the diagnosis of DM sine myositis was made [55,56].

The skin histology in early DM is similar to that seen in systemic lupus and reveals epidermal atrophy, liquefaction degeneration of the basal cell layer and perivascular infiltration of lymphocytes in the upper dermis.

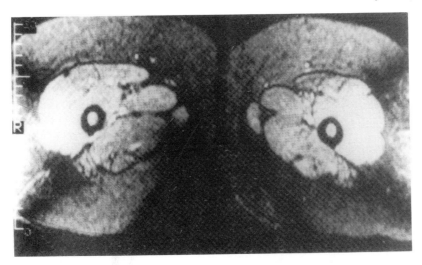

Fig. 4.3   Magnetic resonance imaging of the thigh of a patient with acute dermatomyositis. This fat suppressed image demonstrates an increased STIR signal intensity (white appearance) in the vastus lateralis secondary to muscle inflammation. (Reprinted from Fraser, D. D. *et al.* (1991) Magnetic resonance imaging in idiopathic inflammatory myopathy, *J. Rheum.*, with permission.)

Unlike lupus, immunofluorescence does not show immunoglobulin or complement at the dermal-epidermal junction.

ARTICULAR

Inflammatory polyarthralgias and/or polyarthritis may occur as an initial manifestation of myositis or during the course of the disease. Articular symptoms are more common in patients with myositis in overlap with another connective tissue disease, but are also frequently found in the subset of patients with the anti-Jo-1 antibody. The distribution of articular involvement is rheumatoid-like with the wrists, knees and small joints of the hands most frequently affected[57]. The arthritis is generally mild and very responsive to the dose of corticosteroid used to treat the myositis. However, an erosive arthritis of the hands with periosteal calcifications and interphalangeal thumb joint instability ('floppy thumb sign'), and a predominantly subluxing, deforming non-erosive arthropathy in association with the anti-Jo1 antibody have been described[58,59] (Figures 4.4, 4.5).

PULMONARY

Lung involvement in myositis may be secondary to respiratory muscle weakness, interstitial lung disease, a complication of treatment or other organ (e.g. heart, esophagus) involvement. When muscle weakness is severe, inspiratory and expiratory muscles (diaphragm, intercostal muscles) may be affected, leading to respiratory compromise. In a study of 53 patients with proximal myopathies, hypercapnia was likely when respiratory muscle strength was less than 30% of normal, and when vital capacity was less than 55% predicted[60]. Patients with severe weakness and, in particular, marked pharyngeal involvement should be aggressively treated, as respiratory failure requiring ventilatory assistance may ensue[61]. Individuals with proximal dysphagia are at high risk of aspiration pneumonia. Swallowing function should be evaluated and followed by barium swallow in these patients, with appropriate aspiration prophylaxis.

The clinical characteristics of interstitial lung disease (ILD) are similar to findings in

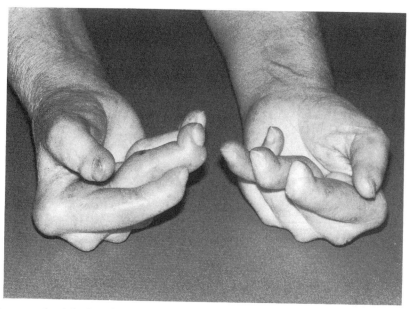

Fig. 4.4 Photograph of the hands of a 45-year-old female with polymyositis and the anti-Jo-1 antibody. Note the symmetric, rheumatoid-like deformities with subluxation. The interphalangeal joints of the thumb have been surgically fused.

primary ILD or that seen with other connective tissue diseases. A severe fatal form of rapidly progressive, diffuse alveolitis may occur, but most patients have a mild, slowly progressive form of ILD, or only radiographic (bibasilar fibrosis) or physiologic (abnormal pulmonary function test) abnormalities. One unique feature of ILD in myositis is its strong association with the anti-aminoacyl-tRNA synthetases autoantibodies[62]. Three patients with the anti-Jo1 antibody and ILD developed rapidly progressive and fatal adult respiratory distress syndrome[63].

Infectious pneumonitis from common bacterial or opportunistic organisms can complicate corticosteroid or cytotoxic therapy, and drug-induced pneumonitis may result from methotrexate or cyclophosphamide. Isolated pleurisy and/or pleural effusions are infrequent in myositis. Congestive heart failure due to myocarditis or cardiac arrhythmias secondary to conduction system disease may lead to pulmonary edema.

As described above, the typical chest radiograph in ILD demonstrates bibasilar fibrotic changes. However, some patients with a normal chest film have evidence of interstitial fibrosis on thin section computerized axial tomography[64]. A restrictive pattern with a reduced forced vital capacity and reduced diffusing capacity for carbon monoxide are characteristic pulmonary function test abnormalities. With active alveolitis, the gallium scan is often abnormal, and bronchoalveolar lavage fluid contains increased numbers of macrophages, lymphocytes and neutrophils. Lung biopsy shows an interstitial infiltrate of chronic inflammatory cells along with fibrosis and vascular thickening[65].

CARDIAC

Due to reporting biases and probable under-ascertainment, the true prevalence of cardiac involvement is difficult to determine. It may be asymptomatic until very advanced[66]. The most frequent findings are electrocardiographic abnormalities, such as ectopic beats or conduction defects[67]. Congestive heart failure is less common and may be due to either

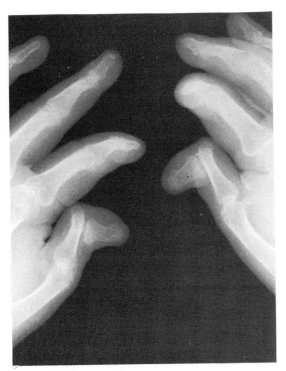

Fig. 4.5. Radiograph of the hands of the same patient depicted in Figure 4.4 prior to thumb surgery. Note the bilateral complete subluxation (dislocation) of the distal phalanges of the thumb (the 'floppy thumb sign'). There are no obvious bony erosive changes.

inflammation (myocarditis) or fibrous replacement of the myocardium. Pericarditis is uncommon, but pericardial tamponade has been reported in childhood DM[68]. Endomyocardial fibrosis was seen in one adult patient[69]. Some investigators believe that a persistent CK-MB fraction over 3% indicates underlying cardiac disease from myositis[70]. However, the MB fraction may be elevated in patients without cardiac disease, presumably due to release of this enzyme fraction from regenerating skeletal muscle[71].

GASTROINTESTINAL

Proximal dysphagia in myositis patients is secondary to involvement of the pharyngeal musculature and, as discussed earlier, may lead to tracheobronchial aspiration and chemical or infectious pneumonitis. Dysphagia may also result from cricopharyngeal muscle dysfunction which often leads to obstruction[72]. Surgery in the form of a cricopharyngeal myotomy may be required to alleviate the symptoms of cricopharyngeal dysfunction. Distal dysphagia and heartburn secondary to the dysmotility associated with esophageal smooth muscle dysfunction may develop in pure PM or DM as well as in myositis in overlap syndromes[73]. Duodenal and small intestinal hypomotility are unusual but, if present, can result in malabsorption syndrome causing post-prandial abdominal bloating, pain, frequent diarrhea and significant weight loss. A life-threatening manifestation of childhood DM is gastrointestinal mucosal ulceration with hemorrhage secondary to vasculitis. Gastrointestinal evaluation of 14 adult patients with PM revealed celiac disease in 5[74]. The inflammatory myopathy in these 5 patients is clearly different from the myopathy often seen in celiac disease patients that is due to osteomalacia and secondary vitamin D deficiency.

OTHER

Soft-tissue calcification is an occasionally disabling complication of childhood DM but is uncommon in adults[75]. Various deep and superficial patterns of soft-tissue calcification were identified in 16 out of 40 (40%) pediatric patients in one series[76]. Calcification was generally associated with severe unremitting myositis in these children. Interfascial calcification interferes with muscle function and often limits the effectiveness of physical therapy (Figure 4.6). Adjacent skin and soft tissue may become inflamed and eventually ulcerate with drainage of calcareous material.

Raynaud's phenomenon is a frequent accompanying complaint in myositis patients, particularly in individuals with DM, connective tissue disease overlap syndromes and the anti-Jo1 antibody. Digital tip ulcerations and

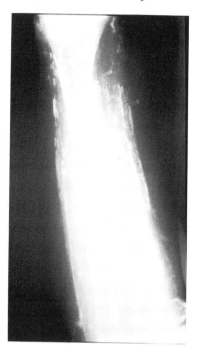

Fig. 4.6 Radiograph of the thigh of a patient with dermatomyositis demonstrating extensive subcutaneous, fascial and muscle calcification in several planes. (Reprinted from the American College of Rheumatology ARA Clinical Slide Set, with permission.)

gangrene due to ischemia are, fortunately, rare. Digital vasculitis without Raynaud's phenomenon has been cited as a clue to an underlying malignancy.

Renal involvement is uncommon, but five patients with PM were reported to develop proteinuria, an abnormal urine sediment and focal or mesangial proliferative glomerulonephritis on renal biopsy[77]. As noted above, acute renal failure secondary to myoglobinuria has been noted, but is rare[45].

Autoimmune hypothyroidism is associated with inflammatory myopathy[31], and Evans syndrome (autoimmune hemolytic anemia and thrombocytopenia) has been reported in one patient with DM[78].

SERUM AUTOANTIBODIES

An important development in our understanding of the diffuse connective tissue diseases has been the identification of serum autoantibodies which define clinically homogeneous patient subsets. In myositis, at least 80% of patients have recognizable autoantibodies to nuclear and/or cytoplasmic antigens, and approximately half of them have antibodies not found in non-myositis patients (so-called myositis-specific antibodies or MSA, Table 4.5). Autoantibodies which occur in patients with other connective tissue diseases may also be seen in myositis patients; they are termed myositis-associated rather than myositis-specific. Multiple MSA are rarely detected in the same patient.

Anti-Jo1 is the most frequently identified MSA. This antibody is detected in approximately 20% of myositis patients and is the most common of the group of anti-aminoacyl-tRNA synthetases[79]. These antibodies are directed against the enzymes that catalyze the binding of an amino acid to its cognate transfer RNA in the process of protein biosynthesis (Table 4.6). Anti-Jo-1 is itself directed against histidyl-tRNA synthetase. Interestingly, patients with this autoantibody are often anti-nuclear antibody negative because the enzyme (antigen) is cytoplasmic in location. The onset of illness in these patients is often acute, with any combination of findings, including myositis, interstitial lung disease, arthritis, Raynaud's phenomenon, fever and 'mechanics hands'. There is a strong immunogenetic association of anti-Jo-1 antibody with HLA-DR3 and DRw52. Response to therapy in this subset is only fair, with frequent relapse and a guarded prognosis with 5-year survival of less than 70%.

Antibodies to signal recognition particle (SRP) identify a second subgroup of myositis patients with MSA[80]. SRP is a cytoplasmic particle that binds to the signal sequence of

Table 4.5 Myositis-specific and myositis-associated antibodies

Antibody	Antigen	Prevalence in myositis (%)	Onset of disease	Clinical features	Response to therapy	Prognosis	HLA associations
Anti-synthetases (see Table 4.6)	t RNA synthesis	30–40	Acute	Fever, Raynaud's, arthritis, ILD*, 'mechanics hands'	Fair to moderate; frequent flares	Poor; 70% 5-year survival	DR3 DRw52
Antibodies to non-synthetase cytoplasmic antigens							
Anti-SRP	Signal recognition particle	4	Very acute	Myalgias, severe weakness, no rash, cardiac complications	Poor	Very poor; 25% 5-year survival	DRw52 DR5
Anti-Mas	Unidentified t RNA	1	Acute	Alcoholism	§	§	DRw53 DR4
Anti-Fer	Elongation factor 1α (protein synthesis)	<1	§	Nodular myositis	§	§	?
Anti-KJ	Unidentified translation factor	<1	§	PM, ILD, Raynaud's[‡]	§	§	DRw52
Anti-nuclear antibodies							
Anti-Mi-2	Nuclear protein complex	5–10	Acute	DM, severe rash, rare in PM	Good; (rash may persist)	Good, nearly 100% 5-year survival	DRw52 DR7
Anti-56 kDa	Ribonucleoprotein complex	80–90	←——— Common in all subgroups of myositis ———→				
Myositis-associated antibodies							
Anti-PM-Scl	Nucleolar protein complex	5–10	Subacute	Myositis/systemic sclerosis overlap, arthritis	Good	Good	DR3
Anti-U1RNP	U1 small nuclear ribonucleoprotein	10–15	Subacute	MCTD[‡], SLE	Good	Good	?
anti-Ku	DNA-binding proteins	<5	?	PM/systemic sclerosis overlap, SLE	Good	Good	?

* ILD = interstitial lung disease.
§ Inadequate number of patients reported.
‡ MCTD = mixed connective tissue disease.

Table 4.6 The anti-aminoacyl-tRNA synthetases and their antibodies in myositis

Antibody	Antigen (synthetase)	Prevalence in myositis (%)
Anti-Jo-1	Histidyl-tRNA	20–30
Anti-PL-7	Threonyl-tRNA	<5
Anti-PL-12	Alanyl-tRNA	<5
Anti-OJ	Isoleucyl-tRNA	<5
Anti-EJ	Glycyl-tRNA	<5

newly-formed proteins, and is involved in translocation of the protein into endoplasmic reticulum. Anti-SRP patients represent 5% of all myositis patients and have an acute, fulminant onset of severe muscle weakness without rash. In contrast to patients with the 'anti-synthetase syndrome', these patients do not have an increase in ILD, arthritis or Raynaud's phenomenon. Instead, they have greater than expected cardiac complications and an immunogenetic association with HLA-DR5. Anti-SRP patients have little responsiveness to corticosteroids and other forms of therapy and a very poor prognosis (25% 5-year survival)[81].

The third category of MSA includes anti-Mi-2, which is also found in only 5–10% of myositis patients and is characterized by the classic and often severe rash of DM[82]. Patients in all clinical subgroups of DM including adult, childhood, overlap (with SLE) and even malignancy-related myositis have been reported to have anti-Mi-2. These persons have no anti-synthetase or anti-SRP antibody clinical associations and in general have a good response to therapy (except for the rash) and a favorable prognosis. They have an increased frequency of the HLA-DR7 allele.

Two other myositis-associated autoantibodies worthy of mention are anti-PM-Sc1 and anti-U1RNP. The former is an antinuclear antibody which identifies another subset of patients with myositis, systemic sclerosis or an overlap of these two disorders.

They appear to have a good prognosis for survival[29]. This antibody is strongly associated with HLA-DR3. Anti-U1RNP is a serologic marker for so-called 'mixed connective tissue disease'. This antibody generally predicts a more benign progression of myopathy. The other MSA and their typical associated clinical features are noted in Table 4.5.

Overall, specific clinical features and prognosis in myositis patients correlate better with MSA than with clinical classification categories[8]. The importance of these autoantibodies in disease pathogenesis is supported by their association with the particular disease subsets, selective response against particular antigens, consistent immunogenetic associations and the occasional reported variation of antibody titer with disease activity[12].

ETIOLOGY AND PATHOGENESIS

The etiology of the inflammatory myopathies is unknown. However, there is considerable evidence that autoimmunity plays a major role. The association of myositis with many other autoimmune conditions is well-accepted. In a National Institutes of Health series, 60 of 315 (19%) patients with myositis had at least one other immunologic disease[31]. A summary of the immunologic abnormalities in PM/DM is presented in Table 4.7.

CELLULAR IMMUNITY

Several lines of evidence suggest that cellular immune mechanisms play a major role in the pathogenesis of myositis. Many studies have demonstrated alteration in the number and function of lymphocytes, while others have shown that mononuclear cells from patients with myositis not only respond to muscle antigens but also damage muscle cells *in vitro*[83]. The best evidence implicating cellular immunity comes from the detailed examination of the inflammatory cell infiltrate in

Table 4.7 Immunologic abnormalities in myositis

Cellular immunity
1. Inflammatory infiltrate consists of activated (DR+) T-cells and macrophages in close proximity to muscle cells
2. T-cells are cytotoxic to muscle fibers
3. Muscle fibers in myositis patients express class I and class II antigens
4. Peripheral blood mononuclear cells proliferate in response to autologous muscle
5. Trafficking of peripheral mononuclear cells to muscle
6. Increased expression of T-cell activation markers (e.g. interleukin-2 receptors) in peripheral blood

Humoral immunity
1. Higher ratio of CD4:CD8 cells in DM patients and close proximity of CD4+ cells to B-cells
2. Vascular endothelial changes with immunoglobulin and complement deposition in DM
3. Immune dysregulation as manifested by hyper-, hypo- and agammaglobulinemia in myositis patients
4. Presence of autoantibodies in serum of myositis patients (Tables 4.5 and 4.6)

muscle from patients with PM and DM. In a series of elegant experiments, Arahata and Engel have contributed greatly to our understanding of the mechanisms of muscle damage in myositis[84–88]. These investigators identified non-necrotic muscle fibers that were surrounded and invaded by mononuclear cells. Using monoclonal antibodies to surface markers, most of the invading cells were identified as activated, CD8$^+$ lymphocytes. Electron microscopy demonstrated that the CD8$^+$ cells adhered to muscle fibers and sent spike-like projections into the fibers. This specific attack also occurred in fibers where the surface membrane was intact, indicating a greater likelihood that this event is primary rather than secondary or non-specific. These findings were much more common in PM and IBM patients compared to those with DM. In a more recent study, Arahata emphasized the importance of antigen-specific, cell-mediated

immunity, and demonstrated that killer and natural killer cell activity did not play a major role in muscle damage[87]. On analysis of the CD8$^+$ T-cells in these PM and IBM biopsies, there were four times as many cytotoxic cells as suppressor cells among both surrounding and invading cells. Cytotoxic cells were even more abundant with increasing duration of disease. In summary, this evidence supports a cell-mediated, antigen-specific, cytotoxic attack on muscle in PM patients as a primary pathogenetic mechanism of muscle damage.

Other recently described features of disordered cellular immunity in myositis include abnormal peripheral mononuclear cell trafficking to muscle[89], increased expression of T-cell activation markers (interleukin-2 receptors) in the peripheral blood[90], and the induction of class II major histocompatibility complex antigen expression on cultured muscle cell surfaces by interferon gamma[91].

HUMORAL IMMUNITY

The immunologic mechanisms of tissue damage in DM patients are different than those in PM and IBM. B-cells are much more commonly identified in biopsy specimens. A higher CD4:CD8 ratio of infiltrating cells, the close proximity of CD4$^+$ cells to B-cells and the relative sparing of non-necrotic muscle fibers by lymphocytes all suggest that the primary pathogenetic mechanism of muscle damage in DM is humorally mediated[86]. The vasculature is clearly a target organ in both adult and childhood DM, with abundant evidence of endothelial cell injury and capillary obliteration. Earlier studies had demonstrated greater deposition of immunoglobulin in the muscle vasculature of childhood and adult DM as opposed to adult PM. More recently, complement activation has been detected, with deposition of the membrane attack complex (C5b-9) and C3 in the blood vessels of muscle biopsies from childhood DM and some adult DM patients but not in PM[92]. The end result of this vascular attack is an ischemic insult to muscle fibers leading to micro-infarction and subsequent perifascicular atrophy.

Beyond the biopsy findings in DM, the best evidence implicating humoral immune dysfunction is the presence of multiple autoantibodies directed against nuclear and/or cytoplasmic antigens in the serum of patients with inflammatory myopathy, see 'Clinical and laboratory manifestations' (above) and Tables 4.5 and 4.6. However, any role for these autoantibodies in the pathogenesis of disease remains speculative. That is, even in DM, where muscle injury appears to be humorally mediated, there is no evidence that MSA trigger the process of complement activation and subsequent blood vessel damage. Myositis-specific antibodies such as anti-Jo1 have not been found in muscle tissue. In fact, MSA are very infrequently identified in DM, particularly childhood DM, and it is the latter subset where humorally mediated vascular damage is most obvious.

Further evidence for humoral immune abnormalities in the inflammatory myopathies includes the finding of hypergammaglobulinemia and, rarely, hypo- or agammaglobulinemia in these patients. In addition, circulating immune complexes have been described in many cases of myositis.

ANIMAL MODELS AND THE ROLE OF VIRUSES

Animal models of myositis can be separated into two categories: spontaneously occurring disorders and induced models. Inflammatory myopathy develops spontaneously in collies and Shetland sheep dogs and includes dermatitis, symmetric distal muscle involvement with atrophy, characteristic myopathic EMG changes and histologic evidence of myositis with vasculitis[93]. Interestingly, elevation of serum muscle enzymes is not seen even in severe canine DM. In collies, DM is frequent and appears to be inherited as a dominant trait with variable penetrance[94]. The cutaneous lesions in collies include dermal inflammation and vasculitis, characteristically involving the face and areas susceptible to trauma.

Spontaneous PM has been reported in the South African rodent Mastomys (Praomys) natalensis[95]. These animals also develop thymoma and myocarditis, but are infrequently used for the investigation of inflammatory myopathy.

Induced myositis can be caused by immunization of laboratory animals (rabbits, guinea pigs) with muscle, so-called experimental autoimmune myositis (EAM). However, the disease is transient, requiring repeated injections to maintain inflammation, and there is no muscle weakness. Arthritis is often the dominant feature in these animals.

A viral etiology for the inflammatory myopathies is supported by the known association of viral infection leading to subsequent myositis. The picornaviruses are promising candidates since many members of this virus family cause myositis or myocarditis in laboratory animals, and some investigators have detected these viruses in the muscle of patients with inflammatory myopathy[37,96]. The group B Coxsackie viruses (CVB) are felt to be etiologically related to polymyositis and CVB RNA has been detected in the muscle of myositis patients[97]. A syndrome of chronic myositis followed CVB 1 infection in a susceptible strain of neonatal mice[98]. Following the initial acute muscle infection, these mice develop a chronic myositis involving proximal hindlimb muscles and demonstrate clinical weakness and electromyographic changes [96]. Using a sensitive and specific method based on polymerase chain reaction, Leff and colleagues failed to find direct evidence for the presence of several candidate viral nucleic acid sequences in muscle from 44 patients with active myositis and control muscle[99]. Encephalomyocarditis virus is an enterovirus known to induce a PM-like syndrome with elevated serum muscle enzymes and carditis in mice[100]. This condition occurs in adult mice, which makes investigative efforts simpler. The illness is dependent on the virus strain as well as the genetic makeup of the host, as all mouse strains are not susceptible.

The anti-Jo-1 antibody is directed against histidyl-tRNA synthetase, an enzyme which joins histidine to its transfer RNA in the process of normal protein synthesis. The genomic RNA of some picornaviruses have structural homology with tRNA. Thus, theoretically, in a virus-infected patient the synthetase enzyme could interact with and join histidine not only with the histidyl-tRNA but also with the viral RNA which resembles the human tRNA. A stable complex of the viral RNA and histidyl-tRNA synthetase may then form, be perceived as foreign and result in an autoimmune response leading to the anti-Jo-1 antibody[101]. An alternative autoimmune mechanism might simply involve antibodies being generated by the host against an infecting picornavirus with molecular mimicry resulting in the formation of the anti-Jo-1 antibody[38].

Various retroviruses may result in disease virtually identical to HIV-negative myositis without viral antigens in biopsy specimens, suggesting that retroviruses may precipitate the onset of an inflammatory myopathy[102]. Retroviruses known to have an association with PM include HIV-1, HTLV-1, human foamy retrovirus, simian retrovirus type 1 (SRV-1) and simian immunodeficiency virus (SIV).

OTHER INFECTIOUS AGENTS

Many other infectious agents, including some bacteria and many parasites, have been associated with chronic myopathy. Toxoplasma causes an inflammatory myopathy that is indistinguishable from PM, and one study has demonstrated that 50% of PM-DM patients have serum anti-toxoplasma IgM antibodies[103]. The significance of these auto-antibodies in disease pathogenesis remains unknown.

To summarize, the cause of inflammatory myopathy is unknown but presumably multifactorial. It is likely that individuals are genetically predisposed to react in an immunologically aberrant fashion to as yet unidentified viral or other environmental stimuli. The chronicity of disease and its obvious immunologic features implicate a disordered immune response that dominates after the initial insult.

TREATMENT OF THE INFLAMMATORY MYOPATHIES

GENERAL MANAGEMENT PRINCIPLES

One should exclude other diseases which present in a similar fashion to myositis such as endocrine myopathies, drug-induced myositis and atypical or late-onset dystrophies. It is essential for the physician to educate the patient regarding the disease process and natural history, and to provide reassurance concerning the threat of dependence and disability. One should be realistic, but optimistic, realizing that most patients do improve with treatment.

Although the timing of physical therapy remains controversial, the goal is to preserve muscle function, prevent disuse atrophy, which may occur with myositis-induced inactivity, and avoid joint contractures due to fibrotic healing of inflamed muscles. Some recommend bed rest during the acute phase of disease, while others emphasize the maintenance of function with passive range of motion exercises and the treatment of painful muscles with massage and moist heat[104]. Restoration of motion is especially important in childhood DM due to the high frequency of joint contractures in this patient subset. A standard approach is to delay physical therapy until after muscle enzymes have normalized (or are at least stable) and strength has improved before beginning active static and isometric exercises and range of motion followed by active isotonic exercises to increase strength and endurance[105]. More aggressive rehabilitative approaches have been recently reported. Five patients with active myositis receiving conventional treatment began an alternative program of resistive and non-resistive exercise during their rehabilitation[106]. Weekly assessment included manual muscle testing, muscle enzyme determination and measurement of peak isometric torque of the lower extremity muscles. Four of the five patients experienced an increase in strength and none had clinically significant CK elevations attributable to either exercise program. Another patient with active, stable PM received a 4-week isometric strengthening program and demonstrated a significant increase in strength with no sustained rise in creatine kinase[107]. Thus, a more aggressive rehabilitative approach in the setting of active myositis has not been responsible for causing an exacerbation of inflammation or further loss of muscle function.

INITIAL THERAPEUTIC CONSIDERATIONS

Assessing the impact of therapy in the inflammatory myopathies is difficult. Few studies have employed appropriate controlled, prospective techniques to study outcome in myositis patients. There is a need for the longitudinal analyses of large numbers of patients where therapeutic interventions are compared and drug-related morbidity and mortality are recorded. We are also limited in terms of adequate criteria to assess improvement or deterioration in the individual patient. The manual assessment of muscle strength is crude and the serum CK is helpful but often unpredictable as a measure of disease activity. Functional ability may be the most critical indicator of a therapeutic response, but an appropriate instrument that measures disability in myopathy patients must be established and validated. In general, the combined use of several of these disease assessment parameters is recommended to evaluate therapeutic efficacy in groups of treated patients.

During the course of myositis treatment, patients should be seen and evaluated at least monthly, at which time serum CK and manual muscle strength assessment are made. The severity of muscle weakness at each visit is recorded. In addition to the well-known method of assessing strength by grade[108], a rapid and reproducible method of lower extremity muscle strength has been tested and standardized for age and sex[109]. As a measure of upper extremity strength, a modified sphygmomanometer has been used to quantify shoulder abductor muscle strength[110].

CORTICOSTEROID THERAPY

Corticosteroids remain the agents of choice for the initial treatment of patients with myositis, although non-steroidal anti-inflammatory agents alone are occasionally used in very mild cases. We recommend beginning prednisone, 60–80 mg/day or the equivalent, given in divided doses, in the typical adult with active myositis. Children are treated with 1–2 mg/kg body weight per day. A lower initial prednisone dose may be tried in patients with less severe myositis. The high divided dose is continued until the serum CK level has fallen into the normal range, which generally occurs within 4–8 weeks[111]. Thereafter, prednisone is consolidated to a single daily dose or a lower total dose divided three times daily. The prednisone taper is continued on a monthly basis with a reduction in total dose that approximates 20–25% of the existing prednisone dose per month. Alternate methods of prednisone administration have been described[104]. Two approaches are illustrated in Figure 4.7.

With disease relapse, evidenced first by an increasing serum CK and then worsening weakness, the prednisone dose is increased or an immunosuppressive agent must be added. It is not necessary to raise the prednisone to the level that initiated treatment but only to that dose that effectively controls disease. Inherent in the management of myositis

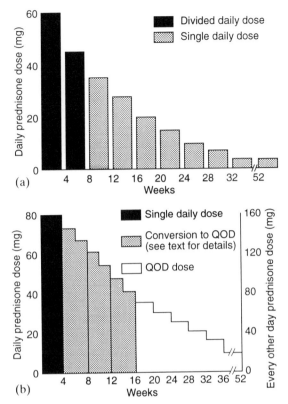

Fig. 4.7 Comparison of two different cortico-steroid treatment regimens in the management of myositis. The upper graph shows an initial 2-month course of divided dose corticosteroids followed by a tapering course of once daily prednisone. The lower graph approximates the administration of prednisone as recommended by Dalakas. An initial 80 mg/day single dose of prednisone is followed by a tapering scheme over 12 weeks to 80 mg qod (as outlined in the text). There is further reduction of the alternate-day dosage by 5–10 mg decrements every 3–4 weeks until a maintenance dose of 20 mg qod is reached.

patients is the realization that clinical improvement in muscle strength will lag behind CK normalization by weeks and even months. Patients should be reassured that if their CK becomes normal as the result of therapy, significant improvement in muscle strength will ensue shortly.

Another management problem, steroid myopathy, is suggested by continued or worsening proximal weakness involving predominantly the lower extremity at a time

when the serum CK level has improved or even normalized. In this setting, the clinician must not overtreat with prednisone due to the risk of additional serious corticosteroid-related side-effects. Steroid myopathy is completely reversible and should improve promptly with dose reduction or physical therapy intervention. Neck flexor weakness is unusual with steroid-related myopathy but is indicative of active disease.

Using the above method of dose reduction, a maintenance dosage of prednisone of 5–10 mg/day is often reached after about 6–8 months of therapy. Prolonged therapy may be necessary to control the disease and we generally do not recommend discontinuation of maintenance prednisone (i.e. a 5–10 mg daily dose) until active disease has been suppressed for one year or more.

One must be cautious not to rely solely on the serum CK as an indicator of disease activity. Some patients will continue to demonstrate mild to moderate CK elevations in the face of normal or at least stable muscle strength[112], and they should not receive continued high-dose prednisone based solely on muscle enzyme elevation. Conversely, some patients with a normal CK have been shown to have active myositis on muscle biopsy. This phenomenon appears more commonly in DM and an EMG or MRI may be helpful to document an active, inflammatory myopathy in such instances. In these cases, patients should be treated aggressively for active disease. The CK level may still be useful even though it fluctuates only within the normal range.

Dalakas suggests a potentially less toxic treatment regimen where prednisone is begun at 80–100 mg in a single daily dose for 3–4 weeks, then tapered over approximately 12 weeks to an alternate-day dose schedule of 80–100 mg by reducing the off-day dose by about 10 mg per week[104]. At this point there is further reduction of the alternate-day dosage by 5–10 mg decrements every 3–4 weeks until a maintenance dose of 20–25 mg every other day is reached. The patient is considered

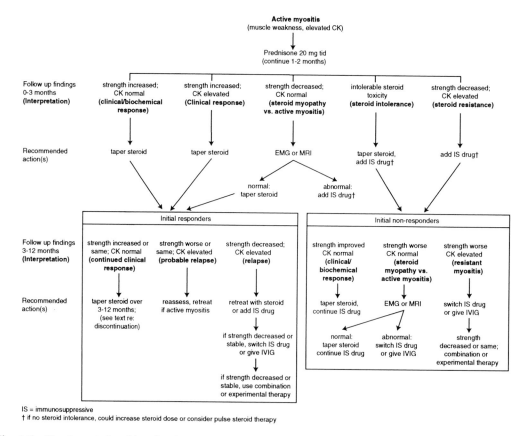

Fig. 4.8   Treatment algorithm for the management of inflammatory myopathy.

to be a prednisone failure if no improvement occurs by the time the 80–100 mg every other day dose schedule is reached (approximately 4 months of therapy).

In a retrospective study of 30 patients, we examined the relationship between serum CK, muscle strength and the method of prednisone administration[111]. Adherence to three principles predicted a favorable biochemical and clinical outcome in the treatment of myositis in these patients:

1. administration of a high initial (loading) corticosteroid dose – usually 60 mg/day;
2. continuation of the initial dose until or after the CK normalizes; and
3. a slow corticosteroid taper rate which averaged < 10 mg/month.

Other pitfalls include premature discontinuation of prednisone without appropriate low-dose maintenance therapy and early development of side-effects necessitating a rapid dose taper[104].

Although the use of high-dose intravenous pulse methylprednisolone has not been studied in adults, it can be used acutely in severe disease in an effort to keep the prednisone maintenance dose lower. Three of seven patients with childhood DM had an excellent response to pulse therapy with complete disease remission and no need for daily steroid therapy[112]. There are anecdotal reports that children treated with high-dose pulse therapy as their initial regimen had more rapid recovery of function and less soft-tissue calcification.

It is apparent from many studies that factors, such as infection, osteoporotic compression fracture and osteonecrosis, contribute significantly to pain and functional disability in steroid-treated myositis patients[111]. These unfortunate complications make the development of other immunosuppressive regimens essential in the management of inflammatory myopathy.

Assuming that corticosteroids are the initial form of treatment, any one of five distinct outcomes can occur within the first three months of therapy. An algorithm for management of myositis during this period and the subsequent 9 months is presented in Figure 4.8.

IMMUNOSUPPRESSIVE THERAPY

Most patients with inflammatory myopathy will respond in part to corticosteroid therapy alone. The addition of other immuno-suppressive agents is needed for disease control in the corticosteroid-resistant patient or one with rapid progression and serious visceral involvement, such as ILD. Also, these drugs act as steroid-sparing agents when unacceptable corticosteroid toxicity develops or unacceptably high steroid maintenance doses are required.

The first choice of most experts is methotrexate, which can be administered orally, subcutaneously or intramuscularly. The starting oral dose is 7.5–10 mg weekly, which is increased weekly by 2.5 mg increments to a maximum tolerated dose of 15–25 mg weekly. Intravenous methotrexate is usually begun at 15–20 mg/week and may be increased to 30–50 mg/week. Prednisone is often tapered as the methotrexate is increased and the combination therapy is continued (at the lowest prednisone dose possible) until weakness and muscle enzymes normalize. At this point the dosage of methotrexate may be continued for several months and then slowly tapered, observing for clinical and biochemical disease flares. Twenty-five steroid-resistant or -intolerant patients were treated with oral

metho-trexate and 22 of 25 (88%) had stable or significantly increased strength while 43% were able to reduce their steroid dose[113]. Others have reported methotrexate efficacy using oral or higher dose intravenous regimens of 50 mg/week[114]. A recently published pediatric study retrospectively reviewed the clinical course of 16 children with recalcitrant DM who were treated with oral methotrexate (20 mg/m^2) in addition to prednisone[115]. Although toxicity or non-compliance forced discontinuation in 5 patients, this combination of drugs was remarkably effective in controlling myositis, even in cases where long-standing steroid resistant disease had been present. Relapse occurred in 5 patients after methotrexate discontinuation. Frequently reported side-effects include stomatitis, abdominal pain, nausea, anorexia, cytopenia, cough, bronchitis-like symptoms, transaminase elevation and infections. Less common side-effects include interstitial pneumonitis, hepatic fibrosis and perhaps osteopenia.

Azathioprine is recommended by some as the immunosuppressive agent of choice after prednisone[104]. In the only controlled, prospective, double-blind trial of an immunosuppressive agent in myositis, patients treated with azathioprine 2 mg/kg/day and prednisone showed improvement in functional ability at 1 and 3 years after initiating treatment, and required reduced corticosteroid maintenance doses compared to patients treated with prednisone alone[116]. Recommended doses for active disease are in the range of 100–200 mg/day orally and the dose may be reduced by 25 mg monthly to a maintenance of 50 mg/day after remission is achieved. Toxicity due to azathioprine includes gastrointestinal intolerance, leukopenia from bone marrow suppression, susceptibility to infection and the possibility of late development of malignancy. Azathioprine hypersensitivity that mimicked an acute exacerbation of DM has been reported[117].

The use of cyclophosphamide in myositis is

more controversial. It was ineffective in 11 patients when administered in a monthly intravenous pulse fashion, but the majority of the patients were unlikely responders with chronic, severe, refractory disease or inclusion body myositis[118]. Others have reported good results with intravenous cyclophosphamide[119,120]; in one study, 10 adult polymyositis patients treated with 500 mg intravenously every 1–3 weeks demonstrated no relapse up to 4 months after their last therapy[119].

Chlorambucil, an alkylating agent of the nitrogen mustard family, was used at a dose of 4 mg/day in 5 patients with DM refractory to prednisone, azathioprine and methotrexate[121]. Improvement occurred within 4–6 weeks in all 5 patients. Corticosteroids were eventually discontinued in 4, and 4 stopped chlorambucil after 13–30 months due to continued disease remission. Toxicity was minimal with transient leukopenia in 2 patients.

Refractory cases of myositis may be treated with combination chemotherapy. Both chlorambucil (6 mg/day) and cyclophosphamide (25–50 mg/day)[122] have been added to prednisone and methotrexate. These regimens include potentially oncogenic alkylating agents, but they should nevertheless be considered in severe cases of inflammatory myopathy with potential reversibility.

Cyclosporine is a potent immunomodulator that selectively blocks the synthesis of interleukin-2 by T-helper cells and inhibits the activation and proliferation of T-cells. Several case reports of its efficacy have been published[123,124]. The dose generally ranges from 5–10 mg/kg/day and beneficial effects appear more quickly (2–6 weeks) than with other immunosuppressive agents. All of 14 children with incomplete or poor responses to steroids and other immunosuppressive agents were successfully treated with cyclosporine 2.5–7.5 mg/kg/day with corticosteroid sparing and no toxicity[125]. In two additional recent reports, all of 7 cyclosporine-treated children with DM noted improvement of muscle strength, but return to normal

strength occurred in only 2 patients[126,127]. The side-effect profile includes nephrotoxicity, hypertension, hypertrichosis, gingival hypertrophy, anemia and the potential for lymphoproliferative malignancy. Nephrotoxicicy is most worrisome with various irreversible side-effects, such as vasculopathy, tubular damage and interstitial fibrosis.

INTRAVENOUS IMMUNE GAMMA GLOBULIN

Although extremely expensive, intravenous immunoglobulin (IVIG) therapy has been increasingly reported in a variety of autoimmune diseases including PM/DM. Its mechanism of action is unknown, but IgG may block Fc receptors on vascular walls, thus preventing the attachment of immune complexes. Fifteen patients with treatment-resistant DM were given high-dose IVIG (one 2 g/kg infusion monthly for 3 months) while continuing maintenance prednisone (mean 25 mg/day) in a randomized double-blind, placebo-controlled trial[128]. The IVIG patients had significant improvements in muscle strength and ADLs and, after crossover, 12 patients with severe disability improved to near normal function. Five responders had repeat muscle biopsies, demonstrating marked histologic improvement. In the largest study to date[129], 15 of 20 refractory myositis patients had improved CK levels and muscle strength after two different IVIG regimens, but assessment of patient improvement was not rigorous and long-term follow-up to assess lasting efficacy was lacking. Eleven childhood DM patients from two centers maintained or improved muscle strength after 6 months of treatment with IVIG[130]. A pilot study of 4 inclusion body myositis (IBM) patients treated with 2 monthly infusions of IVIG demonstrated improvement in 3[131]. In other case reports, HIV-1 associated PM responded to IVIG in a 60-year-old male[132] and was transiently effective in a case of chronic graft versus host disease-associated PM[133]. Only minor side-effects have been thus far noted in the above publications. In summary, intravenous immunoglobulin appears safe and effective for myositis but is very expensive, and its long-term effectiveness is not well established. Based on one hypothesized mechanism of action, it may be most effective for DM.

PLASMA EXCHANGE AND LEUKAPHERESIS

The goal of plasmapheresis is to reduce the amount of circulating antibody and cytokines, thus reducing the tissue deposition of im-munoglobulins. In an uncontrolled study, 32 of 35 (91%) previously unresponsive myositis patients improved and those with the highest serum CK and most clinically active disease responded best[134]. In a recent prospective study, 39 patients with definite PM or DM were randomly assigned to receive plasma exchange, leukapheresis, or sham apheresis. None of these treatments was effective in a 1-month 12-exchange double-blind trial[135]. Limitations of the study included the brief duration and the presence of poor prognostic antibodies in 26 patients with anti-synthetase or anti-SRP antibodies, both known to be associated with a poor prognosis. Two additional patients with refractory PM responded dramatically to a combination of plasma exchange and IVIG despite the failure of each administered separately in one of the patients[136].

OTHER THERAPIES

Total body irradiation (TBI) has been reported in a small number of patients with myositis who had life-threatening, severe disease [137,138]. Both transient benefit and un-responsiveness have been observed[137,138]. This experimental treatment for myositis should be restricted to patients with severe disease in whom all other therapies have failed.

Thymectomy may serve as an alternative to TBI and has been performed in a small number of patients with myositis[139]. One patient with severe DM underwent transternal thymectomy and within 4 weeks demon-strated improvement of muscle strength, rash and CK level. One year later the patient remained stable off all medication.

One patient with childhood DM was treated with extracorporeal photochemotherapy after corticosteroids and methotrexate failed. After 20 months of photopheresis, steroids were unnecessary, but the continued use of metho-trexate made it difficult to assess the indepen-dent effect of photopheresis[140]. We have seen one patient with scleroderma in overlap with an inflammatory myopathy whose myo-sitis progressed while receiving photophere-sis (unpublished observation).

TREATMENT OF INCLUSION BODY MYOSITIS

Thirty-two patients with biopsy features sug-gestive of IBM were retrospectively reviewed and grouped into three categories based on the treatment they had received. Improve-ment was assessed by muscle strength and functional capacity[141]. All four patients who received no therapy deteriorated. Of the 13 who received prednisone alone, only two noted transient benefit. In contrast, among 15 patients who received a combination of pred-nisone with another immunosuppressive agent, 5 had short-term benefit and 3 (prednisone and oral methotrexate) had pro-longed remission. Although the number of patients studied is small, and the design did not allow for patient matching regarding dis-ease duration, some support is provided for a more aggressive approach to IBM with combi-nation therapy.

OTHER TREATMENT-RELATED ISSUES

One hundred and thirteen adult PM, DM or IBM patients seen at the National Institutes of Health were retrospectively analyzed to identify factors associated with response to treatment[142]. The efficacy of each prednis-one, methotrexate and azathioprine drug trial was assessed using predefined clinical and laboratory criteria. Similar to past obser-vations, the investigators found that a prolonged delay between onset of weakness and initiation of treatment was associated with a poor outcome. No patient with a delay greater than 18 months responded completely to prednisone, whereas 34% treated within 3 months of symptom onset had a complete response. Patients could also be separated into prognostic groups according to clinical classification and serum autoantibodies. Those with IBM responded poorly to therapy, but more than half had some improvement from prednisone alone. PM patients had higher response rates to the first prednisone trial compared to IBM patients, but DM patients responded better than PM. Cancer or connective tissue disease-associated myositis patients did best, as the initial prednisone course failed in only one patient and 50% had complete responses. Patients with autoantibodies to the synthetases or signal recognition particle responded only partially to prednisone therapy alone. Methotrexate was more beneficial in men and in patients with anti-synthetase antibodies; it was considered to be superior to azathioprine in anti-synthetase patients not responding to prednisone.

The observations of this well-characterized patient cohort highlight some important management-related issues. First, clinical classification and serum autoantibody status of all inflammatory myopathy patients should be identified as soon as possible. In patients known to have less favorable clinical or auto-antibody prognostic profiles, one should consider initiating therapy with prednisone in combination with an immunosuppressive agent. Methotrexate is a reasonable choice but low-dose cyclosporine or combination chemotherapy is a consideration as well. This approach may not only lead to more rapid disease control, but also reduce the frequency of corticosteroid-related side-effects that contribute significantly to long-term disability.

TREATMENT OF EXTRAMUSCULAR MANIFESTATIONS OF MYOSITIS AND THEIR TREATMENT

The constitutional symptoms of fatigue and fever tend to respond quickly to the addition of corticosteroids, although fatigue may persist and fever recur with disease flares. Raynaud's phenomenon is most commonly found in the overlap subset of the inflammatory myopathies and its management is outlined in Chapter 6.

CUTANEOUS

The rash of DM may be particularly difficult to treat. Sunscreens are essential, and topical and oral corticosteroids and immunosuppressive drugs may lessen erythema but not eradicate the rash, which may be refractory and behave independently of the myositis. 'Mechanics hands' seem to fit in the same category, responding, but unreliably, to therapy of the underlying disease.

Hydroxychloroquine 200–400 mg daily, when added to the corticosteroid regimen in 7 patients, improved the rash and lessened the required steroid dose[143]. Quinacrine 100 mg daily is a second-line antimalarial agent used for the rash. We have used isotretinoin (0.5–1 mg/kg/day) in several patients with refractory rash with good results. This drug must not be used by pregnant women since major fetal abnormalities related to isotretinoin have been documented.

Once present, subcutaneous calcification tends to worsen over time at an unpredictable pace. There is no uniformly accepted form of therapy, except for surgical excision of deposits that interfere with musculoskeletal function. Proposed therapies include low-dose warfarin[144], aluminum hydroxide[145] and probenecid[146]. The local inflammatory reaction at the periphery of calcinotic masses often responds to a short (1–2 week) course of oral colchicine at 0.5–1.5 mg daily[147].

ARTICULAR

Inflammatory polyarthralgias and arthritis in a rheumatoid-like pattern of wrist, knee and small hand joint involvement often resolve when the myositis is treated with corticosteroids. However, the chronic deforming arthropathy associated with the anti-Jo1 anti-body may require remittive agents[59].

PULMONARY

The most severe intrinsic pulmonary problem is an aggressive, diffuse alveolitis. Of 14 consecutive patients with myositis seen at one center, 9 (64%) had ILD and only one had anti-Jo1 but the other anti-synthetases were not ascertained[148]. The response to cortico-steroids was poor and 6 patients (67%) died from respiratory failure. A second report described 3 cases of myositis with ILD (2 anti-Jo1 positive) in which the addition of cyclophosphamide to prednisone improved outcome[149]. When alveolitis with pro-gression of restrictive lung disease is encoun-tered, aggressive combined corticosteroid and immunosuppressive therapy is indicated.

CARDIAC

The electrocardiographic or cardiac wall motion abnormalities seen with myositis may resolve after treatment with high doses of pre-dnisone[70]. If global left ventricular dysfunc-tion is detected, myocarditis should be suspected regardless of how mild the coexist-ing skeletal muscle involvement may appear; aggressive immunosuppressive therapy is thus recommended. Symptomatic arrhyth-mias require appropriate pharmacologic therapy, heart block often leads to placement of a permanent pacemaker, and congestive heart failure is treated with diuretics and digi-talis[70]. Pericardial involvement (pericarditis or tamponade), although unusual in myositis, often responds to corticosteroid therapy.

GASTROINTESTINAL

Proximal dysphagia secondary to pharyngeal weakness may be a stubborn complication responding poorly to therapy. It may require tube feedings or even parenteral hyper-alimentation. When pharyngeal dysfunction occurs in the elderly individual it is a poor prognostic sign often associated with aspir-ation. Aggressive therapy to relieve the symp-toms of distal dysphagia and heartburn secondary to esophageal dysmotility and to prevent later esophageal stricture is indicated. Measures such as elevating the head of the bed on blocks, not reclining after meals and not eating before bedtime are helpful. Medi-cations such as antacids, H_2-receptor antagon-ists and omeprazole are useful as well. Prokinetic drugs have been inadequately studied to date. Nifedipine, which is ben-eficial for Raynaud's phenomenon, may wor-sen lower esophageal symptoms, and diltiazem may be a better choice for patients with pyrosis.

The treatment of malabsorption includes frequent small meals during the day, avoid-ance of medications that reduce smooth muscle contractility, replacement of fat-soluble vitamins, treatment of related vitamin B_{12} and iron deficiency, and rotating anti-biotics, such as ampicillin, tetracycline and metronidazole, to decrease upper small intes-tinal bacterial overgrowth. Theoretically, pro-kinetic drugs, including erythromycin, metaclopramide and cisapride, will stimulate small intestinal smooth muscle contraction.

The gastrointestinal vasculitis of childhood DM should be aggressively treated with ster-oids and/or immunosuppressive agents.

SURVIVAL AND PROGNOSIS

Because of both muscle weakness and in-volvement of numerous other organ systems, PM/DM may result in significant morbidity, functional disability and mortality. A number of clinical features that predict both good and poor outcomes and interventions that alter prognosis have been identified. These factors have been reviewed in detail[150].

PROBLEMS IN THE DETERMINATION OF PROGNOSIS

Assessment of prognosis has proved difficult because of the relative rarity of PM and the use of retrospective cross-sectional rather than prospective longitudinal data. Also, patients with late stages of disease and those examined early in their course have been inappropriately grouped and analyzed together by some authors. Another difficulty with the inflammatory myopathies is that they are truly a family of diseases in which distinctive subsets of patients exist. Clinical, laboratory, pathologic and immunologic data must all be taken into consideration in developing an improved classification system, which will then provide more meaningful insights into disease etiology, pathogenesis and potential intervention. Finally, objective criteria for severity, activity and improvement (or deterioration) in PM/DM are not well-defined, and disease and treatment-related morbidity have been inadequately distinguished from one another.

MORTALITY

Prior to 1950 and the availability of corticosteroids, a high proportion of patients with untreated PM/DM (up to 50%) died from disease-related complications. Ten subsequent representative studies are summarized in Table 4.8, separated according to the decade of entry of the average patient. There were four reports including 554 patients studied primarily during the 1950s and followed for a mean of 2.5–6.1 years[4,151–153]. Both corticosteroid-treated and untreated patients were included in these series. The mortality rate was remarkably similar at 28–36%. Factors associated with poor survival were older age at onset[4,152]; African American race[152]; malignancy[4,151,152]; rapid progression of weakness[151]; severe weakness [152,153]; overlap with other connective tissue diseases[4,153], especially scleroderma[151]; dysphagia[152,153] and pulmonary infiltration[152]. Aspiration pneumonia due to pharyngeal muscle dysfunction was the most frequent cause of lung disease[152].

In the 1960s, almost all patients were treated with corticosteroids. Three series described 265 patients followed for a mean of 1.8–5.0 years[113,154,155]. The case fatality rate was more variable in this time period, ranging from 14% in a large medical center referral population[113] to 40% in a small series of 20 patients in which children were excluded and therapy was begun a mean of 2.8 years after onset of symptoms. The latter study may not be representative for the above reasons. Poor prognostic signs continued to be older age[113,154]; associated malignancy[113,155]; delayed treatment[113,155]; and dysphagia [154]. There is some disagreement concerning the effect of another connective tissue disease on mortality in patients with myositis in overlap[113,155].

Three representative investigators publishing on patients seen during the 1970s have noted improved survival[156–158]. Among the combined 288 patients in these series, 56 (19%) died and the mortality rate varied only slightly from 17–23%. As expected, older age[156–158], malignancy[156] and delayed therapy[156,158] adversely influenced prognosis and, for the first time, cardiac involvement[156,157] and complications of corticosteroid and immunosuppressive therapy[158] were implicated. The reasons for improved survival in more recent times are uncertain, but may include earlier diagnosis, detection of milder cases, better general medical care and more judicious use of the necessary potent therapeutic agents.

This trend is supported by a mortality study in the USA from 1968 to 1978 which demonstrated a temporal increase in mean age at death in PM/DM[159]. These results probably indicate improved prognosis over time for all patients or selectively for childhood disease, but are also consistent with increased incidence in older persons. In the US mortality data, a synergistic interaction between sex and race was noted[159]. The highest mortality rates occurred in non-white females, parallel to the incidence pattern described above. The age at death was unimodal and, as expected, was lowest for non-white females[159].

Mortality in juvenile myositis before the introduction of corticosteroids was high, with at least one-third of children dying[160]. Over the last 20 years, survival in children has

Table 4.8 Morality and factors affecting prognosis in representative PM/DM series stratified by decade of patient entry

First author (year)	Dates of patient entry	Number of patients	Mean follow-up from entry (years)	Mortality rate	Factors associated with reduced survival
Rose (1966)[4]	1954–64	89	6.1	30%	Malignancy, other CTD[§], acute course
Winkelmann (1968)[151]	–1959	279	3.0	32%	Malignancy, scleroderma, rapid progression
Medsger (1971)[152]	1947–68	124	2.5[†]	36%	Pulmonary infiltrates, severe weakness, dysphagia, age >50, African American race
Carpenter (1977)[153]	1947–71	62	NS[‡]	45%	Dysphagia, severe weakness
Bohan (1977)[113]	1956–71	153	4.3	14%	Malignancy, older age, delayed treatment
Benbassat (1985)[154]	1956–76	92	1.8	32%	Dysphagia, older age, leukocytosis, fever, failure to induce remission, shorter disease duration
Riddoch (1975)[155]	1960–70	20	5	40%	(Excluded children, cancer, CTD)
Henriksson (1982)[156]	1967–78	107	5	23%	Malignancy, older age, delayed treatment, cardiac involvement
Hochberg (1986)[157]	1970–81	76	NS	17%	Age >45, cardiac involvement
Tymms (1985)[158]	1970–82	105	4	18%	Older age, delayed treatment

[§] CTD = connective tissue disease.
[†] median.
[‡] NS = not stated.
Revised from *Prognosis in the Rheumatic Diseases* (ed. N. Bellamy) with permission.

improved, but the prognosis remains extremely variable and difficult to predict. For example, in one published series 3 (7%) of 41 patients died, only one definitely due to DM[161]. In contrast, in a recent study of 28 children with DM, 5 (18%) died during treatment.

DISABILITY

Information on morbidity and functional disability from PM/DM is limited. From the time of their greatest weakness, most survivors of myositis experience considerable short-term and long-term improvement in functional status. In one series, 40 of 124 patients treated with prednisone had improved strength averaging one grade (five-grade scale) after a mean of 2.1 months[113]. In half of the 46 patients in this series who also received immunosuppressive medications, muscle strength improved similarly by an average of one grade. Initiated early, physiotherapy with passive range of motion and more rapid mobilization can prevent muscle and tendon shortening with contractures.

Maximum benefit from therapy occurs 3–5 years after beginning corticosteroid therapy [4]. In a 20-year follow-up of 118 patients, the average disability grade after 4 years corresponded to minimal atrophy or weakness in one or more muscle groups without functional impairment[9]. At study end two-thirds of 82 survivors had no functional disability. A small group (20%) still had active disease during follow-up, but many of them were so classified with a stable clinical picture and elevated serum muscle enzymes. Finally, in a report on 107 patients, 87% of those who improved with initial therapy had minimal or no disability at follow-up (mean 5 years), in contrast to only 9% of persons who were treatment failures[156]. Delay in initiating therapy resulted in poor functional outcome.

Virtually every patient treated with high-dose corticosteroids (in the range of 40 mg daily) for more than several months develops adverse effects. Immunosuppressive medications may also lead to severe side-effects, e.g. bone marrow suppression, gastrointestinal hemorrhage and hepatic toxicity. Drug toxicity in reported series ranges from 20–50%[111,131,156,162,163]. In a community-based study, when toxicity was compared between corticosteroid regimens, Cushing's syndrome, severe infection, compression fractures and new onset insulin-dependent diabetes mellitus all occurred more frequently and were more severe in the group treated with daily as opposed to alternate-day steroids[162]. In two other series, corticosteroid complications occurred in 32%[164] and 41%[158] and included osteonecrosis, peptic ulcer, cataracts, diabetes mellitus and septicemia. In our own retrospective series of 30 corticosteroid treated patients, 4 suffered osteoporotic fractures, 2 had osteonecrosis (5 different joints), 2 each had peptic ulcer, hypertension requiring treatment and diabetes, and 1 patient experienced a recrudescence of a *Mycobacterium tuberculosis* infection[111]. In a prospective longitudinal study of functional disability in a national cohort of 257 PM/DM patients, disability increased with disease duration and was most influenced by the initial disability index, which in turn was greatest among older patients and those who subsequently developed either osteonecrosis or osteoporotic spinal fractures[163].

Three distinct courses for juvenile dermatomyositis (JDMS) have been described, i.e. monocyclic, chronic polycyclic and chronic continuous[165]. No onset features predicted which children would experience a severe continuous illness. As noted above, a subgroup of patients with severe generalized vasculitis did poorly despite an optimal therapeutic regimen[166]. In 38 of 41 surviving children with JDMS followed 0.5–15 years, 25 were functionally normal, 11 were ambulatory and capable of normal activities with residual weakness or contractures, and 2 had severe disability with wheelchair dependence[161]. No patient had progressive muscle weakness or decreased physical function late in the illness (5–15 years after onset). In another study of 47 JDMS patients, 78% of children receiving prompt, high-dose corticosteroid therapy had good functional outcomes[166]. In contrast, British investigators believe that low-dose corticosteroids (1 mg/kg/day) for a brief period of time produces better outcome and fewer long-term iatrogenic complications in JDMS[167], while excessive doses of steroids and/or immunosuppressives are associated with severe functional disability[168]. Adverse effects of corticosteroid therapy commonly observed in JDMS patients include growth retardation, osteoporosis, osteonecrosis and cataracts.

Dermal and subcutaneous calcification (calcinosis) is reported in 20–50% of JDMS patients[23,161] and is a major source of chronic disability. An exception is the reduced proportion of patients who develop calcification when corticosteroids are administered very soon after disease onset[166]. In severe cases, an exoskeleton-like calcification results [166]. Calcinosis persists even after active disease remits and may cause focal atrophy of muscle and skin, leading to contractures[167] and both deep and superficial cutaneous ulcerations. Calcinotic lesions tend to progress inexorably. Other features leading to chronic disability in JDMS include arthritis and Raynaud's phenomenon[169].

Very little has been reported on the short- or long-term economic impact of myositis. No studies have been published on immediate or delayed loss of work, decrease in earning capacity, or costs of medical intervention for disease or treatment complications. An encouraging follow-up of 18 JDMS patients evaluated an average of 18.5 years after diagnosis found that they had high educational achievement, good employment status and little residual disability[169].

OTHER PROGNOSTIC FACTORS

There is no correlation between the initial serum CK level and the grade of disability or degree of weakness at disease presen-tation[9]. Histopathologic changes in muscle do not predict either survival[153] or spontaneous remission[151]. As noted above, a non-inflammatory, occlusive vascular lesion of muscular arteries identifies a severe subset of JDMS[170].

Pulmonary involvement in PM/DM has been recognized as a serious complication that may account for the majority of deaths [148,171]. A subset of patients with anti-Jo1 antibody has a high frequency of interstitial lung disease[65]. Histologic findings have been considered superior to radiographic or clinical features in predicting outcome[172]. A bronchiolitis obliterans with organizing pneumonia pattern on lung biopsy has a good outcome, while diffuse alveolar damage has a poor survival[172]. Nearly all patients who aspirate complain of pharyngeal dysphagia, a well-recognized predictor of poor outcome in myositis[65,152,153]. Ventilatory insufficiency due to weakness of respiratory muscles, typically associated with severe generalized muscle weakness, is present in 4–8% of PM/DM patients[4,9,65] and is often corticosteroid responsive[65]. Iatrogenic pulmonary complications include opportunistic infection, kyphosis with restrictive lung disease following vertebral compression fractures, and drug-induced interstitial pneumonitis from either methotrexate or cyclophosphamide.

Cardiac involvement is associated with persistently active and severe skeletal myositis and a poor prognosis in PM/DM[9,155,173]. Manifestations include EKG abnormalities such as conduction disturbances, arrhythmias, congestive heart failure, coronary arteritis and myocarditis[66,67,173,174]. Persistent elevation of the serum CK-MB isoenzyme fraction above 3% of the total CK correlates with cardiac involvement and has been associated with fatal congestive heart failure[173].

Serum autoantibodies have been found to be associated with certain clinical features, some of which are important for prognosis. These have been described earlier. Not enough is known as yet to accurately predict long-term outcome in serologic subgroups, but a retrospective analysis has suggested that autoantibody status is one of the factors that influences response to corticosteroid and immunosuppressive therapy[142].

FUTURE PERSPECTIVES

Reliable prognostic information is crucial for the managing physician, who must counsel the patient and family, anticipate disease complications and select an optimal therapeutic regimen. In the future, it will be necessary to plan careful prospective, longitudinal studies of incident cohorts of PM/DM patients, including clinical, laboratory, serologic and functional outcome data. The acquisition of such information will lead to important new concepts of disease classification and prognosis, and will more accurately direct clinical and laboratory investigators in studies of etiology, pathogenesis and therapy.

REFERENCES

1. Medsger, T. A., Jr., Dawson, W. N., Jr. and Masi, A. T. (1970) The epidemiology of polymyositis. *Am. J. Med.*, **48**, 715–23.
2. Kurland, L. T., Hauser, W. A., Ferguson, R. H. *et al.* (1969) Epidemiologic features of diffuse connective tissue disorders in Rochester, Minnesota, 1951–1967, with special reference to systemic lupus erythematosus. *Mayo Clin. Proc.*, **44**, 649–63.
3. Benbassat, J., Geffel, D. and Zlotnick, A. (1980) Epidemiology of polymyositis-dermatomyositis in Israel, 1960–1976. *Isr. J. Med. Sci.*, **16**, 197–200.
4. Rose, A. L. and Walton, J. N. (1966) Polymyositis: A survey of 89 cases with particular reference to treatment and prognosis. *Brain*, **89**, 747–68.
5. Oddis, C. V., Conte, C. G., Steen, V. D. *et al.* (1990) Incidence of PM-DM: A 20-year study of hospital diagnosed cases in Allegheny County, PA, 1963–1982. *J. Rheumatol.*, **17**, 1329–34.
6. Findlay, G. H., Whiting, D. A. and Simson, I. W. (1969) Dermatomyositis in the Transvaal and its occurrence in the Bantu. *S. Afr. Med. J.*, **43**, 694–7.
7. Koh, E. T., Seow, A., Ong, B. *et al.* (1993) Adult onset polymyositis/dermatomyositis: Clinical and laboratory features and treatment response in 75 patients. *Ann. Rheum. Dis.*, **52**, 857–61.
8. Bohan, A. and Peter, J. B. (1975) Polymyositis and dermatomyositis. *N. Engl. J. Med.*, **292**, 344–7, 403–7.
9. Devere, R. and Bradley, W. G. (1975) Polymyositis: Its presentation, morbidity and mortality. *Brain*, **98**, 637–66.
10. Kagen, L. J. (1993) Polymyositis/dermatomyositis, in *Arthritis and Allied Conditions*, 12th edn, (ed. D. J. McCarty), Lea & Febiger, Philadelphia, pp. 1225–52.
11. Dalakas, M. C. (1992) Clinical, immunopathologic and therapeutic considerations of inflammatory myopathies. *Clin. Neuropharmacol.*, **15**, 327–51.
12. Love, L. A., Leff, R. L., Fraser, D. D. *et al.* (1991) A new approach to the classification of idiopathic myopathy: Myositis-specific antibodies define useful homogeneous patient groups. *Medicine*, **70**, 360–74.
13. Hochberg, M. C. (1989) Epidemiology of polymyositis/dermatomyositis. *Mt Sinai. J. Med.*, **55**, 447–52.
14. Medsger, T. A., Jr. (1984) Polymyositis and dermatomyositis, in *Epidemiology of the Rheumatic Diseases*, (eds R. C. Lawrence and L. E. Schulman), Gower Medical Publishing, New York, pp. 176–80.
15. Araki, S., Uchino, M. and Yoshida, O. (1983) Epidemiologic study of multiple sclerosis, myasthenia gravis and polymyositis in the city of Kumamoto, Japan. *Clin. Neurol.*, **23**, 838–41.
16. Lyon, M. G., Bloch, D. A., Hollack, B. *et al.* (1989) Predisposing factors in polymyositis-dermatomyositis: Results of a nationwide survey. *J. Rheumatol.*, **16**, 1218–24.
17. Manta, P., Kalfakis, N. and Vassilopoulos, D. (1989) Evidence for seasonal variation in polymyositis. *Neuroepidemiol.*, **8**, 262–5.
18. Love, L. A., Burgess, S. H., Hill, P. C. *et al.* (1992) Geographical and seasonal clustering of idiopathic inflammatory myopathy (IIM) in groups defined by myositis-specific autoantibodies (MSA) (abstract). *Arth. Rheum.*, **35**(9), S40.
19. Love, L. A. and Miller, F. W. (1993) Noninfectious environmental agents associated with myopathies. *Curr. Opin. Rheumatol.*, **5**, 712–18.

20. Harati, Y., Niakan, E. and Bergman, E. W. (1986) Childhood dermatomyositis in monozygotic twins. *Neurology*, **36**, 721–3.

21. Leonhardt, T. (1961) Familial occurrence of collagen diseases. II. Progressive systemic sclerosis and dermatomyositis. *Acta Med. Scand.*, **169**, 735–42.

22. Walker, G. L., Mastaglia, F. L. and Roberts, D. F. (1982) A search for genetic influence in idiopathic inflammatory myopathy. *Acta Neurol. Scand.*, **66**, 432–3.

23. Pachman, L. M. and Cooke, N. (1980) Juvenile dermatomyositis: A clinical and immunologic study. *J. Pediatr.*, **96**, 226–34.

24. Hirsch, T. J., Enlow, R. W., Bias, W. B. *et al.* (1981) HLA-D related (DR) antigens in various kinds of myositis. *Hum. Immunol.*, **3**, 181–6.

25. Wilcox, C. B. (1977) HLA and serum complement in polymyositis. *Lancet*, **2**, 978–9.

26. Reed, A. M., Pachman, L. and Ober, C. (1991) Molecular genetic studies of major histocompatibility complex genes in children with juvenile dermatomyositis: Increased risk associated with HLA-DQA1*0501. *Hum. Immunol.*, **32**, 235–40.

27. Goldstein, R., Duvic, M., Targoff, I. N. *et al.* (1990) HLA-D region genes associated with autoantibody responses to histidyl-transfer RNA synthetase (Jo-1) and other translation related factors in myositis. *Arth. Rheum.*, **33**, 1240–8.

28. Genth, E., Mierau, R., Genetzly, P. *et al.* (1990) Immunogenetic associations of scleroderma-related antinuclear antibodies. *Arth. Rheum.*, **33**, 657–65.

29. Oddis, C. V., Okano, Y., Rudert, W. A. *et al.* (1992) Serum autoantibody to the nucleolar antigen PM-Scl: Clinical and immunogenetic associations. *Arth. Rheum.*, **35**, 1211–17.

30. Medsger, T. A., Jr. and Oddis, C. V. (1994) Inflammatory muscle disease: Clinical Features, in *Rheumatology*, (eds J. Klippel and P. Dieppe), Mosby Year Book Europe Ltd, section 6, 12.1–12.14.

31. Plotz, P. H., Dalakas, M., Leff, R. L. *et al.* (1989) Current concepts in the idiopathic inflammatory myopathies: Polymyositis, dermatomyositis and related disorders. NIH Conference. *Ann. Intern. Med.*, **111**, 143–57.

32. Rockerbie, N. R., Woo, T. Y., Callen, J. P. *et al.* (1989) Cutaneous changes of dermatomyositis precede muscle weakness. *J. Am. Acad. Dermatol.*, **20**, 629–32.

33. Dietzman, D. E., Schaller, J. G., Ray, G. *et al.* (1976) Acute myositis associated with influenza B infection. *Pediatrics*, **57**, 255–8.

34. Christensen, M. L., Pachman, L. M., Schneiderman, R. *et al.* (1986) Prevalence of Coxsackie B virus antibodies in patients with juvenile dermatomyositis. *Arth. Rheum.*, **29**, 1365–70.

35. Mease, P. J., Ochs, H. D. and Wedgewood, R. J. (1981) Successful treatment of ECHO virus meningoencephalitis and myositis-fasciitis with intravenous immune globulin therapy in a patient with X-linked agammaglobulinemia. *N. Engl. J. Med.*, **304**, 1278–81.

36. Gabbai, A. A., Schmidt, B., Castelo, A. *et al.* (1990) Muscle biopsy in AIDS and ARC: Analysis of 50 patients. *Muscle Nerve*, **13**, 508–15.

37. Yousef, G. E. Isenberg, D. A. and Mowbray, J. F. (1990) Detection of enterovirus specific RNA sequences in muscle biopsy specimens from patients with adult onset myositis. *J. Rheum. Dis.*, **49**, 310–15.

38. Kagen, L. J., Kimball, A. C. and Christian, C. L. (1974) Serologic evidence of toxoplasmosis among patients with polymyositis. *Am. J. Med.*, **56**, 186–91.

39. Schoenen, J., Sianard-Gainko, J., Carpentier, M. *et al.* (1989) Myositis during *Borrelia burgdorferi* infection (Lyme disease). *J. Neurol. Neurosurg. Psychiatry*, **52**, 1002–5.

40. Gibson, R. K., Rosenthal, S. J. and Lukert, B. P. (1984) Pyomyositis: Increasing recognition in temperate climates. *Am. J. Med.*, **77**, 768–72.

41. Morgan, G. L., McGuire, J. L. and Ochoa, J. (1981) Penicillamine-induced myositis in rheumatoid arthritis. *Muscle Nerve*, **4**, 137–40.

42. Kaufmann, L. D., Seidman, R. J. and Gruber, B. L. (1990) L-tryptophan associated eosinophilic perimyositis, neuritis, and fasciitis: A clinicopathologic and laboratory study of 25 patients. *Medicine*, **69**, 187–99.

43. Fudman, E. J. and Schnitzer, T. J. Dermatomyositis without creatine kinase elevation. *Am. J. Med.*, **80**, 329–32.

44. Kagen, L. J. and Aram, S. (1987) Creatine kinase activity inhibitor in sera from patients with muscle disease. *Arth. Rheum.*, **30**, 213–17.

45. Kessler, E., Weinberger, I. and Rosenfeld, J. B. (1972) Myoglobinuric acute renal failure in a case of dermatomyositis. *Israel J. Med. Sci.*, **8**, 978.

46. Lovece, S., Kagen, L. J. (1993) Sensitive rapid detection of myoglobin in serum of patients with myopathy by immunoturbidimetric assay. *J. Rheumatol.*, **20**, 1331–4.

47. Wu, A. H. B. and Perryman, M. B. (1992) Clinical application of muscle enzymes and proteins. *Curr. Opin. Rheumatol.*, **4**, 815–20.

48. Hernandez, R. J., Keim, D. R., Chenevert, T. L. *et al.* (1992) Fat-suppressed MR imaging of myositis. *Radiology*, **182**, 217–19.

49. Fraser, D. D., Frank, J. A., Dalakas, M. *et al.* (1991) Magnetic resonance imaging in idiopathic inflammatory myopathy. *J. Rheumatol.*, **18**, 1693–1700.

50. Hernandez, R. J., Sullivan, D. B., Chenevert, T. L. *et al.* (1993) Magnetic resonance imaging in children with dermatomyositis: Musculoskeletal finding and correlation with clinical and lab findings. *AJR*, **161**, 359–66.

51. Ganczarczyk, M. L., Lee, P. and Armstrong, S. K. (1988) Nailfold capillary microscopy in polymyositis and dermatomyositis. *Arth. Rheum.*, **31**, 116–19.

52. Fusade, L. T., Belanyi, P., Joly, P. *et al.* (1993) Subcutaneous changes in dermatomyositis. *Br. J. Dermatol.*, **128**, 451–3.

53. van Linthoudt, D., Gabay, C. and Ott, H. (1989) Vitiligo and polymyositis (letter). *Clin. Exp. Rheumatol.*, **7**, 334–5.

54. Commens, C., O'Neill, P. and Walker, G. (1990) Dermatomyositis associated with multifocal lipoatrophy. *J. Am. Acad. Dermatol.*, **22**, 966–9.

55. Stonecipher, M. R., Jorizzo, J. L., White, W. L. *et al.* (1993) Cutaneous changes of dermatomyositis in patients with normal muscle enzymes: Dermatomyositis sine myositis? *J. Am. Acad. Dermatol.*, **28**, 951–61.

56. Euwer, R. L. and Sontheimer, R. D. (1993) Amyopathic dermatomyositis: A review. *J. Invest. Dermatol.*, **100**, S124–7.

57. Schumacher, H. R., Schimmer, B., Gordon, G. V. *et al.* (1979) Articular manifestations of polymyositis and dermatomyositis. *Am. J. Med.*, **67**, 287–92.

58. Bunch, T. R., O'Duffy, J. D. and McLeod, R. A. (1976) Deforming arthritis of the hands in polymyositis. *Arth. Rheum.*, **19**, 243–8.

59. Oddis, C. V., Medsger, T. A., Jr. and Cooperstein, L. A. (1990) A subluxing arthropathy associated with the anti-Jo-1 antibody in polymyositis/dermatomyositis. *Arth. Rheum.*, **33**, 1640–5.

60. Braun, N., Arora, N. S. and Rochester, D. F. (1983) Respiratory muscle and pulmonary function in polymyositis and the proximal myopathies. *Thorax*, **38**, 616–23.

61. Martin, L. M., Chalmers, I. M., Dhingra, S. *et al.* (1985) Measurements of maximum respiratory pressures in polymyositis and dermatomyositis. *J. Rheumatol.*, **12**, 104–7.

62. Marguerie, C., Bunn, C. C., Beynon, H. L. C. *et al.* (1990) Polymyositis, pulmonary fibrosis and autoantibodies to aminoacyl-tRNA synthetase enzymes. *Q. J. Med.*, **77**, 1019–38.

63. Clawson, K. and Oddis, C. V. (1993) Adult respiratory distress syndrome (ARDS) in myositis patients with anti-Jo-1 antibody (abstract). *Arth. Rheum.*, **36**, S256.

64. Warrick, J. H., Bhalla, M., Schabel, S. I. *et al.* (1994) High resolution computed tomography in early scleroderma lung disease. *J. Rheumatol.*, **18**, in press.

65. Dickey, B. F. and Myers, A. R. (1984) Pulmonary disease in polymyositis/dermatomyositis. *Semin. Arth. Rheum.*, **14**, 60–76.

66. Haupt, H. M. and Hutchins, G. M. (1982) The heart and cardiac conducting system in polymyositis-dermatomyositis. *Am. J. Cardiol.*, **50**, 998–1006.

67. Kehoe, R. F., Bauerfeind, R., Tommaso, C. *et al.* (1981) Cardiac conduction defects in polymyositis. *Ann. Intern. Med.*, **94**, 41–3.

68. Pereira, R. M., Lerner, S. and Maeda, W. T. (1992) Pericardial tamponade in juvenile dermatomyositis. *Clin. Cardiol.*, **15**, 301–3.

69. Rossi, M. A. (1990) Endomyocardial fibrosis in dermatomyositis. *Int. J. Cardiol.*, **28**, 119–22.

70. Askari, A. D. (1988) The heart in polymyositis and dermatomyositis. *Mt Sinai J. Med. (NY)*, **55**, 479–82.

71. Larca, L. J., Coppola, J. T. and Honig, S. (1981) Creatine kinase MB isoenzyme in dermatomyositis: A noncardiac source. *Ann. Intern. Med.*, **94**, 341–3.

72. Kagen, L. J., Hochman, R. B. and Strong, E. W. (1985) Cricopharyngeal obstruction in inflammatory myopathy (polymyositis/dermatomyositis). *Arth. Rheum.*, **28**, 630–6.

73. Jacob, H., Berkowitz, D. and McDonald, E. (1983) The esophageal motility disorder of polymyositis: A prospective study. *Arch. Intern. Med.*, **143**, 2262–4.

74. Henriksson, K. G., Hallert, C., Norrby, K. *et al.* (1982) Polymyositis and adult coeliac disease. *Acta Neurol. Scand.*, **65**, 301–19.

75. Cohen, M. G., Nash, P. and Webb, J. (1986) Calcification is rare in adult-onset dermatomyositis. *Clin. Rheumatol.*, **5**, 512–16.

76. Blanc, C. E., White, S. J. and Braunstein, E.

M. (1984) Patterns of calcification in childhood dermatomyositis. *AJR*, **142**, 397–400.

77. Dyck, R. F., Katz, A. and Gordon, D. A. (1979) Glomerulonephritis associated with polymyositis. *J. Rheumatol.*, **6**, 336–44.

78. Hay, E. M., Makris, M. and Winfeld, J. (1990) Evans syndrome associated with dermatomyositis. *Ann. Rheum. Dis.*, **49**, 793–4.

79. Arnett, F. C., Hirsch, T. J., Bias, W. B. *et al.* (1981) The Jo-1 antibody system in myositis: Relationship to clinical features and HLA. *J. Rheumatol.*, **8**, 925–30.

80. Targoff, I. N., Johnson, A. E. and Miller, F. W. (1990) Antibody to signal recognition particle in polymyositis. *Arth. Rheum.*, **33**, 1361–70.

81. Miller, F. W. (1991) Humoral immunity and immunogenetics in the idiopathic inflammatory myopathies. *Curr. Opin. Rheumatol.*, **3**, 902–10.

82. Targoff, I. N. and Reichlin, M. (1985) The association between Mi-2 antibodies and dermatomyositis. *Arth. Rheum.*, **28**, 796–803.

83. Ytterberg, S. R. (1988) Cellular immunity in polymyositis and dermatomyositis. *Mt Sinai J. Med. (NY)*, **55**, 494–500.

84. Arahata, K. and Engel, A. G. (1984) Monoclonal antibody analysis of mononuclear cells in myopathies: 1. Quantitation of subsets according to diagnosis and sites of accumulation and demonstration of counts of muscle fibers invaded by T cells. *Ann. Neurol.*, **16**, 193–208.

85. Engel, A. G. and Arahata, K. (1984) Monoclonal antibody analysis of mononuclear cells in myopathies. 2. Phenotype of autoinvasive cells in polymyositis and inclusion body myositis. *Ann. Neurol.*, **16**, 209–15.

86. Arahata, K. and Engel, A. G. (1986) Monoclonal antibody analysis of mononuclear cells in myopathies.: 3. Immunoelectron microscopic aspects of cell-mediated muscle fiber injury. *Ann. Neurol.*, **19**, 112–25.

87. Arahata, K. and Engel, A. G. (1988) Monoclonal antibody analysis of mononuclear cells in myopathies: 4. Cell-mediated cytotoxicity and muscle fiber necrosis. *Ann. Neurol.*, **28**, 168–73.

88. Arahata, K. and Engel, A. G. (1988) Monoclonal antibody analysis of mononuclear cells in myopathies: 5. Identification and quantitation of T8$^+$ cytotoxic and T8$^+$ suppressor cells. *Ann. Neurol.*, **23**, 493–9.

89. Miller, F. W., Read, E. J., Carrasquillo, J. A. *et al.* (1988) Abnormal lymphocytes trafficking to muscle in patients with idiopathic inflammatory myopathies (abstract). *Arth. Rheum.*, **31**, S60.

90. Wolf, R. E. and Baethge, B. A. (1990) Interleukin-1, interleukin-2, and soluble interleukin-2 receptors in polymyositis. *Arth. Rheum.*, **33**, 1007–14.

91. Kalovidouris, A. E., Horn, C. A. and Plotkin, Z. (1991) Recombinant human interferon-gamma (IFN-γ) enhances T cell adhesion to cultured human muscle cells (abstract). *Arth. Rheum.*, **34**, S147.

92. Kissel, J. T., Mendell, J. R. and Rammohan, K. W. (1986) Microvascular deposition of complement membrane attack complex in dermatomyositis. *N. Engl. J. Med.*, **314**, 329–34.

93. Hargis, A. M., Prieur, D. J., Haupt, K. H. *et al.* (1986) Postmortem findings in four litters of dogs with familial canine dermatomyositis. *Am. J. Pathol.*, **123**, 480–96.

94. Haupt, K. H., Prieur, D. J., Moore, M. P. *et al.* (1985) Familial canine dermatomyositis: Clinical, electrodiagnostic and genetic studies. *Am. J. Vet. Res.*, **46**, 1861–9.

95. Snell, K. C., Stewart, H. L. (1975) Spontaneous disease in a closed colony of Praomys (mastomys) natalensis. *Bull. World Health Org.*, **52**, 645–50.

96. Strongwater, S. L., Dorovin-Zis, K., Ball, R. D. *et al.* (1984) A murine model of polymyositis induced by Coxsackie B1 (Tucson strain). *Arth. Rheum.*, **27**, 433–42.

97. Bowles, N. E., Dubowitz, V., Sewry, C. A. *et al.* (1987) Dermatomyositis, polymyositis and Coxsackie B-virus infection. *Lancet*, **1**, 1004–7.

98. Ray, C. G., Minnich, L. L. and Johnson, P. C. (1979) Selective polymyositis induced by Coxsackie B1 in mice. *J. Infect. Dis.*, **140**, 239–43.

99. Leff, R. L., Love, L. A., Miller, F. W. *et al.* (1992) Viruses in idiopathic inflammatory myopathy: Absence of candidate viral genomes in muscle. *Lancet*, **339**, 1192–5.

100. Miller, F. W., Love, L. A., Biswas, T. *et al.* (1987) Viral and host genetic factors influence encephalomyocarditis virus-induced polymyositis in adult mice. *Arth. Rheum.*, **30**, 549–56.

101. Mathews, M. B. and Bernstein, R. M. (1983) Myositis autoantibody inhibits histidyl-tRNA synthetase: A model for autoimmunity. *Nature*, **304**, 177–9.

102. Dalakas, M. (1991) Polymyositis, dermatomyositis, and inclusion body myositis. *N. Engl. J. Med.*, **325**, 1487–98.

103. Magid, S. K. and Kagen, L. J. (1983) Serologic evidence for acute toxoplasmosis in polymyositis-dermatomyositis. *Am. J. Med.,* **75**, 313–20.

104. Dalakas, M. C. (1989) Treatment of polymyositis and dermatomyositis. *Curr. Opin. Rheumatol.,* **1**, 443–9.

105. Hicks, J. E. (1988) Comprehensive rehabilitative management of patients with polymyositis and dermatomyositis, in *Polymyositis and Dermatomyositis*. Butterworths, Boston, pp. 293–318.

106. Escalante, A., Miller, L. and Beardmore, T. D.(1993) Resistive exercise in the rehabilitation of polymyositis/dermatomyositis. *J. Rheumatol.,* **20**, 1340–4.

107. Hicks, J. E., Miller, F. W., Plotz, P. *et al.* (1993) Isometric exercise increases strength and does not produce sustained creatine phosphokinase increases in a patient with polymyositis. *J. Rheumatol.,* 1399–401.

108. British Medical Research Council. (1976) *Aids to the Examination of the Peripheral Nervous System*, 2nd edn HMSO, London.

109. Csuka, M. and McCarty, D. J. (1985) Simple method for measurement of lower extremity muscle strength. *Am. J. Med.,* **78**, 77–81.

110. Helewa, A., Goldsmith, C. H. and Smythe, H. A. (1986) Patient, observer and instrument variation in the measurement of strength of shoulder abductor muscles in patients with rheumatoid arthritis using a modified sphygmomanometer. *J. Rheumatol.,* **13**, 1044–9.

111. Oddis, C. V. and Medsger, T. A., Jr. (1988) Relationship between serum creatine kinase level and corticosteroid therapy in polymyositis-dermatomyositis. *J. Rheumatol.,* **15**, 807–11.

112. Laxer, R. M., Stein, L. D. and Petty, R. E. (1987) Intravenous pulse methylprednisolone treatment of juvenile dermatomyositis. *Arth. Rheum.,* **30**, 328–34.

113. Bohan, A., Peter, J. B., Bowman, R. L. *et al.* (1977) A computer-assisted analysis of 153 patients with polymyositis and dermatomyositis. *Medicine,* **56**, 255–86.

114. Metzger, A. L., Bohan, A., Goldberg, L. S. *et al.* (1974) Polymyositis and dermatomyositis: Combined methotrexate and corticosteroid therapy. *Ann. Intern. Med.,* **81**, 182–9.

115. Miller, L. C., Sisson, B. A., Tucker, L. B. *et al.* (1992) Methotrexate treatment of recalcitrant childhood dermatomyositis. *Arth. Rheum.,* **35**, 1143–9.

116. Bunch, T. W. (1981) Prednisone and azathioprine for polymyositis: Long-term followup. *Arth. Rheum.,* **24**, 45–8.

117. Goldenberg, D. L. and Stor, R. A. (1975) Azathioprine hypersensitivity mimicking an acute exacerbation of dermatomyositis. *J. Rheumatol.,* **2**, 346–9.

118. Cronin, M. E., Miller, F. W., Hicks, J. E. *et al.* (1989) The failure of intravenous cyclophosphamide therapy in refractory idiopathic inflammatory myopathy. *J. Rheumatol.,* **16**, 1225–8.

119. Bombardieri, S., Hughes, G. R. V., Neri, R. *et al.* (1988) Cyclophosphamide in severe polymyositis. *Lancet,* **1**, 1138–9.

120. Leroy, J. P., Drosos, A. A., Yiannopoulos, D. I. *et al.* (1990) Intravenous pulse cyclophosphamide therapy in myositis and Sjögren's syndrome. *Arth. Rheum.,* **33**, 1579–81.

121. Sinoway, P. A. and Callen, J. P. (1993) Chlorambucil: An effective corticosteroid-sparing agent for patients with recalcitrant dermatomyositis. *Arth. Rheum.,* **36**, 319–24.

122. Cagnoli, M., Marchesoni, A. and Tosi, S. (1991) Combined steroid, methotrexate and chlorambucil therapy for steroid-resistant dermatomyositis. *Clin. Exp. Rheumatol.,* **9**, 658–9.

123. Lueck, C. J., Trend, P. and Swash, M. (1991) Cyclosporin in the management of polymyositis and dermatomyositis. *J. Neurol. Neurosurg. Psychiatr.,* **54**, 1007–8.

124. Mehregan, D. R. and Su, W. P. D. (1993) Cyclosporine treatment for dermatomyositis/polymyositis. *Cutis,* **51**, 59–61.

125. Heckmatt, J., Saunders, C., Peters, A. M. *et al.* (1989) Cyclosporin in juvenile dermatomyositis, *Lancet,* **1**, 1063–6.

126. Rawlings, D. J., Richardson, L., Szer, I. S. *et al.* (1992) Cyclosporine is safe and effective in refractory JRA and JDMS: Results of an open clinical trial (abstract). *Arth. Rheum.,* **35**, S188.

127. Pistoia, V., Buoncompagni, A., Scribanis, R. *et al.* (1993) Cyclosporin A in the treatment of juvenile chronic arthritis and childhood polymyositis-dermatomyositis: Results of a preliminary study. *Clin. Exp. Rheumatol.,* **11**, 203–8.

128. Dalakas, M. C., Illa, I., Dambrosia, J. M. *et al.* (1993) A controlled trial of high-dose intravenous immune globulin infusions as treat-

ment for dermatomyositis. *N. Engl. J. Med.*, **329**, 1993–2000.

129. Cherin, P., Herson, S., Wechsler, B. *et al.* (1991) Efficacy of intravenous gammaglobulin therapy in chronic refractory polymyositis and dermatomyositis: An open study with 20 adult patients. *Am. J. Med.*, **91**, 162–8.

130. Barron, K. S., Sher, M. R. and Silverman, E. D. (1992) Intravenous immunoglobulin therapy: Magic or black magic? *J. Rheumatol. suppl.*, **33**, 94–7.

131. Soueidan, S. A. and Dalakas, M. C. (1993) Treatment of inclusion-body myositis with high-dose intravenous immunoglobulin. *Neurology*, **43**, 876–9.

132. Viard, J. P., Vittecoq, D., Lacroix, C. *et al.* (1992) Response of HIV-1-associated polymyositis to intravenous immunoglobulin (letter). *Am. J. Med.*, **92**, 580–1.

133. Hanslik, T., Jaccard, A., Guillon, J. M. *et al.* (1993) Polymyositis and chronic graft-versus-host disease: Efficacy of intravenous gammaglobulin. *J. Am. Acad. Dermatol.*, **28**, 492–3.

134. Dau, P. C. (1981) Plasmapheresis in idiopathic inflammatory myopathy. *Arch. Neurol.*, **38**, 544–52.

135. Miller, F. W., Leitman, S. F., Cronin, M. E. *et al.* (1992) Controlled trial of plasma exchange and leukapheresis in polymyositis and dermatomyositis. *N. Engl. J. Med.*, **326**, 1380–4.

136. Herson, S. P. and Coutellier, A. (1992) The association of plasma exchange synchronized with intravenous gamma globulin therapy in severe intractable polymyositis (letter). *J. Rheumatol.*, **19**, 828–9.

137. Morgan, S. H., Bernstein, R. M., Coppen, J. *et al.* (1985) Total body irradiation and the course of polymyositis. *Arth. Rheum.*, **28**, 831–5.

138. Cherin, P., Herson, S., Coutellier, A. *et al.* (1992) Failure of total body irradiation in polymyositis: Report of three cases. *Br. J. Rheumatol.*, **31**, 282–3.

139. Cumming, W. J. K. (1989) Thymectomy in refractory dermatomyositis (letter). *Muscle & Nerve*, **12**, 424.

140. DeWilde, A., DiSpaltro, F. X., Geller, A. *et al.* (1992) Extracorporeal photochemotherapy as adjunctive treatment in juvenile dermatomyositis: A case report. *Arch. Dermatol.*, **128**, 1656.

141. Sayers, M. E., Chou, S. M. and Calabrese, L. H. (1992) Inclusion body myositis: Analysis of 32 cases. *J. Rheumatol.*, **19**, 1385–9.

142. Joffe, M. M., Love, L. A., Leff, R. L. *et al.* (1993) Drug therapy of the idiopathic inflammatory myopathies: Predictors of response to prednisone, azathioprine, and methotrexate and a comparison of their efficacy. *Am. J. med.*, **94**, 379–87.

143. Woo, T. Y., Callen, J. P., Voorhees, J. J. *et al.* (1984) Cutaneous lesions of dermatomyositis are improved by hydroxychloroquine. *J. Am. Acad. Dermatol.*, **10**, 592–600.

144. Berger, R. G., Featherstone, G. L., Raasch, R. H. *et al.* (1987) Treatment of calcinosis universalis with low-dose warfarin. *Am. J. Med.*, **83**, 72–6.

145. Wang, W., Lo, W., Wong, C. *et al.* (1988) Calcinosis cutis in juvenile dermatomyositis: Remarkable response to aluminium hydroxide therapy. *Arch. Dermatol.*, **124**, 1720–1.

146. Skuterud, E., Sydnes, O. A. and Haavik, T. K. (1981) Calcinosis in dermatomyositis treated with probenecid. *Scand. J. Rheumatol.*, **10**, 92–4.

147. Fuchs, D., Fruchter, L., Fishel, B. *et al.* (1986) Colchicine suppression of local inflammation due to calcinosis in dermatomyositis and progressive systemic sclerosis. *Clin. Rheumatol.*, **5**, 527–30.

148. Takizawa, H., Shiga, J., Moroi, Y. *et al.* (1987) Interstitial lung disease in dermatomyositis: Clinicopathological study. *J. Rheumatol.*, **14**, 102–7.

149. Janadi, M., Smith, C. D. and Karsh, J. (1989) Cyclophosphamide treatment of interstitial pulmonary fibrosis in polymyositis/dermatomyositis. *J. Rheumatol.*, **16**, 1592–6.

150. Oddis, C. V. and Medsger, T. A., Jr. (1991) Polymyositis-dermatomyositis, in *Prognosis in the Rheumatic Diseases*, (ed. N. Bellamy), Kluwer Academic Publishers, London, pp. 233–50.

151. Winkelmann, R. K. *et al.* (1968) Course of dermatomyositis-polymyositis: Comparison of untreated and cortisone-treated patients. *Mayo Clin. Proc.*, **43**, 545–6.

152. Medsger, T. A., Jr., Robinson, H. and Masi, A. T. (1971) Factors affecting survivorship in polymyositis: a life-table study of 124 patients. *Arth. Rheum.*, **14**, 249–58.

153. Carpenter, J. R., Bunch, T. W., Engel, A. G. *et al.* (1977) Survival in polymyositis: Corticosteroids and risk factors. *J. Rheumatol.*, **4**, 207–14.

154. Benbassat, J., Geffel, D., Larholt, K. *et al.* (1985) Prognostic factors in PM-DM: A com-

puter-assisted analysis of 92 cases. *Arth. Rheum.*, **28**, 249–55.

155. Riddoch, D. and Morgan-Hughes, J. A. (1975) Prognosis in adult polymyositis. *J. Neurol. Sci.*, **26**, 71–80.

156. Henriksson, K. G. and Sandstedt, P. (1982) Polymyositis-treatment and prognosis: A study of 107 patients. *Acta Neurol. Scandinav.*, **65**, 280–300.

157. Hochberg, M. C., Feldman, D. and Stevens, M. B. (1986) Adult onset polymyositis/dermatomyositis: An analysis of clinical and laboratory features and survival in 76 patients with a review of the literature. *Semin. Arth. Rheum.*, **15**, 168–78.

158. Tymms, K. E. and Webb, J. (1985) Dermato-polymyositis and other connective tissue diseases: A review of 105 cases. *J. Rheumatol.*, **12**, 1140–8.

159. Hochberg, M. C., Lopez-Acuna, D. and Gittelsohn, A. M. (1983) Mortality from polymyositis and dermatomyositis in the United States, 1968–1978. *Arth. Rheum.*, **26**, 1465–71.

160. Bitnum, C., Darvschnor, C. W. and Travis, L. B. (1964) Dermatomyositis. *J. Pediatr.*, **64**, 101–31.

161. Sullivan, D. B., Cassidy, J. T. and Petty, R. (1977) Dermatomyositis in the pediatric patient. *Arth. Rheum.*, **20**, 327–31.

162. Hoffman, G. S., Franck, W. A., Raddatz, D. A. *et al.* (1983) Presentation, treatment and prognosis of idiopathic inflammatory muscle disease in a rural hospital. *Am. J. Med.*, **75**, 433–8.

163. Clarke, A. E., Oddis, C. V. and Bloch, D. A. (1993) A longitudinal study of functional disability in a national cohort of polymyositis-dermatomyositis patients (abstract). *Arth. Rheum.*, **36**, S83.

164. Baron, M. and Small, P. (1985) Polymyositis/dermatomyositis: Clinical features and outcome in 22 patients. *J. Rheumatol.*, **12**, 283–6.

165. Spencer, C., Kornreich, H., Bernstein, B. *et al.* (1979) Three courses of juvenile dermatomyositis. *Arth. Rheum.*, **22**, 661–5.

166. Bowyer, S. L., Blane, C. E., Sullivan, D. B. *et al.* (1983) Childhood dermatomyositis: Factors predicting functional outcome and development of dystrophic calcification. *J. Pediatr.*, **103**, 882–8.

167. Miller, G., Heckmatt, J. Z. and Dubowitz, V. (1983) Drug treatment of juvenile dermatomyositis. *Arch. Dis. Child.*, **58**, 445–50.

168. Dubowitz, V. (1984) Prognostic factors in dermatomyositis (letter). *J. Pediatr.*, **105**, 336–7.

169. Chalmers, A., Sayson, R. and Walters, K. (1982) Juvenile dermatomyositis: Medical, social and economic status in adulthood. *Can. Med. Assoc. J.*, **126**, 31–3.

170. Spencer, C. H., Hanson, V., Singsen, B. H. *et al.* (1984) Course of treated juvenile dermatomyositis. *J. Pediatr.*, **105**, 399–408.

171. Arsura, E. L. and Greenberg, A. S. (1988) Adverse impact of interstitial pulmonary fibrosis on prognosis in polymyositis and dermatomyositis. *Semin. Arth. Rheum.*, **18**, 29–37.

172. Tazelaar, H. D., Viggiano, R. W., Pickersgill, J. *et al.* (1990) Interstitial lung disease in polymyositis and dermatomyositis: Clinical features and prognosis as correlated with histologic findings. *Am. Rev. Respir. Dis.*, **141**, 727–33.

173. Askari, A. D. (1984) Cardiac abnormalities in inflammatory myopathy. *Clin. Rheum. Dis.*, **10**, 131–49.

174. Denbow, C. E., Lie, J. T., Tancreli, R. G. *et al.* (1979) Cardiac involvement in polymyositis. A clinicopathologic study of 20 autopsied patients. *Arth. Rheum.*, **22**, 1088–92.

A. G. Tzioufas and H. M. Moutsopoulos

HISTORY – EPIDEMIOLOGY

Among autoimmune diseases, Sjögren's syndrome (SS) possesses a unique position, since it can manifest either alone (primary SS) or in association with almost all of the systemic autoimmune rheumatic diseases (secondary SS). Primary SS expresses a diverse clinical spectrum expanding from organ-specific autoimmune disorder (autoimmune exocrinopathy) to systemic disorder, affecting several organs. In a considerable number of patients it evolves to B-lymphocyte malignancy[1].

The disease was described first in 1888 by Hadden in an elderly woman with dry mouth and impaired lacrimal secretion. In 1933, H. Sjögren, a Swedish ophthalmologist, published a classical monograph in which 19 patients characterized by chronic inflammation and hyposecretion of the lacrimal and salivary glands, which resulted in keratoconjunctivitis sicca (KCS), xerostomia and rhinopharyngeolaryngitis were described as a syndrome. Thirteen of these patients also had a systemic disorder in which arthritis was present (Table 5.1). In 1961, the discovery by Anderson of autoantibodies SjD and SjT, in the sera of SS patients, pointed further to the systemic autoimmune nature of the disease. Two years later, Bunim and Talal described that SS patients have a higher incidence for developing malignant lymphoproliferative disorders, indicating that a common link between autoimmune diseases and lymphoid neoplasias might exist. In recent years, the application of molecular immunology techniques coupled with previous clinical knowledge have offered potential insights into the understanding of the pathogenetic mechanisms underlying SS.

SS is more prevalent in women (female-to-male ratio 9:1). Although it usually appears in the fourth and fifth decade of life, it has also been described in children [2–4]. SS is considered the second most frequently occurring autoimmune disease following rheumatoid arthritis due to its increased prevalence in other autoimmune diseases (mainly in RA) and in the elderly population. The prevalence of primary SS in the general population has not been well established until recently. This was due to the lack of uniform diagnostic criteria for SS, differences in diagnostic techniques, as well as differences in the reference values of the tests used for evaluating KCS and salivary gland involvement. When the recently proposed and validated questionnaire as well as the diagnostic criteria for SS were applied as suggested by the European Community concerted action[5], to 837 women in one village (total population 2500; age range from 18–90 years), it was found that the prevalence of definite and probable SS was 0.6% and 3%, respectively (unpublished observations).

In another epidemiological study performed in 705 randomly selected Swedish adults with a more limited age range (from

Connective Tissue Diseases. Edited by Jill J. F. Belch and Robert B. Zurier. Published in 1995 by Chapman & Hall, London. ISBN 0 412 48620 2

Table 5.1   Historical steps in Sjögren's syndrome (SS)

1. Presentation of the first patient	Haaden, 1888
2. Description of the benign lymphoepithelial lesion	Mickulitz, 1892
3. Description of SS in France	Gougerot, 1925
4. Clinical presentation of SS in 19 patients	Sjögren, 1933
5. Mickulitz disease and SS are identical	Morgan and Castleman, 1953
6. Discovery of the precipitating autoantibodies SjD and SjT (termed later as Ro/SSA and La/SSB)	Aderson, 1961
7. Increased frequency of lymphoma in SS	Bunim and Talal, 1963
8. Definition of SS and proposed criteria for the diagnosis	Bloch, 1965
9. Association of SS with HLA alloantigens	Mann, 1977
10. Differentiation of SS into primary and secondary form	Moutsopoulos, 1978

52–72 years), the calculated prevalence for the disease was found to be 2.7%[6]. In the same population, symptoms of dry eyes and dry mouth were correlated with elevated levels of anti-Ro/SSA and anti-La/SSB antibodies, as determined by an enzyme-linked immunosorbent assay[7].

PATHOGENETIC ASPECTS

The etiology of SS is still unknown and the underlying pathophysiologic mechanisms have not been clearly defined. Over the past two decades, intense research on the related immunopathology, autoimmunity, immunogenetics, viruses and oncogenes has further refined the concepts concerning the pathophysiology and pathogenesis of SS. In this regard, it now appears that certain environmental factors may induce SS in individuals with a given genetic background.

IMMUNOGENETICS

The suggestion of a genetic predisposition to SS has been strongly supported because of associations with major histocompatibility complex (MHC) antigens and multiple cases of familial clustering[8]. Family members of SS patients have higher prevalence of SS or other connective tissue disorders, and a higher prevalence of serological autoimmune abnormalities than age- and sex-matched controls.

Table 5.2   HLA-associations with SS

HLA-B8	Primary SS
HLA-DR3	Caucasian and Italian patients with SS
HLA-DR5	Greek patients with SS
HLA-DR11	Israeli patients with SS
HLA-DW53	Japanese patients with SS
HLA-DQW6 DQW2.1	Association with SS and anti-Ro/ SSA and La/SSB

Approximately 30–35% of patients with SS will report a family history of another relative with an autoimmune disorder[9].

Primary SS is associated with the HLA-B8 antigen[10]. HLA-DR3 has been reported in 50–80% of SS patients[11]. In a recent study, the linkage of HLA and primary SS in 16 multicase families (with primary SS in sibships and/or in more than one generation) was investigated. It was found that HLA-DR3 possessed a strong association with the disease and served as a major susceptibility factor for the expression of SS in these families[12]. The association, however, of HLA-DR3 and SS has been reported to be weaker than that of HLA-DR3 and anti-Ro/SSA autoantibody positivity coupled with SS[13]. Other associations of HLA-related antigens with the SS included DRW52, DRW53, DQ and complement levels[13].

The racial and ethnic origin of the patients

studied thus far further influences the association with the DR phenotype. In fact, SS is associated with DR3 in white Americans and Italians, DR5 in Greeks and DR11 in Israelis (Table 5.2). Given the linkage disequilibrium which exists between alleles of HLA loci, it is unclear whether the disease susceptibility is dependent on the associated allele or on a closely related gene. In fact, DQ and to a lesser extent DP alleles are tightly linked to DR[14]. These observations may be explained by the shared epitope hypothesis, which proposes that amino acid sequences of the hypervariable region of the DR gene are shared between different DR specificities, and thus influencing disease susceptibility[15]. The application of techniques from molecular biology have made it possible to gain insights into the association of autoimmune diseases with various HLA haplotypes in different patient populations. The use of these techniques have demonstrated that different allelic variants associated with a certain disease share particular sequences or epitopes which may contribute to disease susceptibility. In this regard, a DNA-sequence specific oligonucleotide probe typing and a sequence analysis of Israeli Jewish and Greek non-Jewish patients with SS has been currently carried out[16]. The DNA samples were amplified by the polymerase chain reaction (PCR) using specific primers for DRB1, DRB3, DQA, DQB, DPA and DPB regions. It was found that the majority of patients in both groups presented either DRB1*1101 or DRB1*1104 alleles, that were in a disequilibrium linkage with DRB1*0301 and DQA1*0501. Molecular analysis of DQB1 and DQA1 alleles found in American Caucasian and American Black SS patients revealed high frequencies of DQB1*0201 and DQA1*0501[17]. Therefore, the majority of SS patients, independent of racial and ethnic differences, carry a common allele, specifically the DQA1*0501 allele. This strongly suggests that it may be a determining factor in the predisposition of certain individuals to primary SS. Furthermore, it has been shown that a glutamine residue at position 34 of the outermost domain of the DQA1 chain and/or leukine at position 26 of the outermost domain of the DQB1 chain have a 'gene dosage' role in anti-Ro/SSA and anti-La/SSB antibody response[18]. The DQA1*0501 gene is one of the genes which possesses glutamine at position 34 and is found in the majority of anti-Ro/SSA and anti-La/SSB patients. Taken together, it appears very likely that the DQA1*501 molecule plays an important role in the development of SS.

VIRAL STUDIES IN SS

As discussed previously, autoimmune reactions against host tissues following viral infection have been reported in both humans and experimental animals. These can be triggered by different mechanisms acting separately or synergistically[18]. First, a viral infection may lead to a consistent neoantigen expression resulting in a chronic antigenic stimulation. Secondly, viral antigens may have structural similarities with host antigens leading to the production of autoantibodies and/or cytotoxic T-cell clones through a mechanism of molecular mimicry. Finally, a persistent viral infection may alter the synthesis of certain cytokines at DNA level (i.e. IL-2 by the tax gene of HTLV-I[19]), raising a chronic T-cell dependent reaction. For these reasons, viruses have long been suspected of being major contributing factors in SS.

The first two viruses which were implicated in the pathogenesis of SS were the cytomegalovirus (CMV) and Epstein-Barr virus (EBV). They are both DNA viruses and both may produce chronic infection. CMV can infect many organs and among them the salivary glands are prime targets[20]. In one study, anti-CMV antibodies of both IgG and IgM classes were found in the serum of patients with primary SS, using an enzyme linked immunosorbent assay[21] although others have not confirmed these results[22]. EBV is a ubiquitous herpes virus which remains latent in the stomatopharyngeal cavity in immunologically intact humans[23]. Almost everyone becomes infected, mostly subclinically, with EBV before the age of 25. Primary EBV infection starts in the pharyngeal epithelium, which is permissive for virus replication. EBV soon spreads to subepithelial B-lymphocytes where it establishes latent infection. EBV replication also occurs in the salivary glands during primary infection[24]. This virus may play a role in SS, since antibodies to the EBV capsid antigen are more frequently found in SS patients[22] and EBV is a potent polyclonal activator of B-cells that can induce autoantibodies *in vitro*[25]. One of them, the anti-La/SSB antibody found in sera of SS patients, precipitates a cytoplasmic protein which is complexed with EBV and encodes small RNAs termed EBER 1 and EBER 2[26]. Recently, EBV DNA has been detected in the salivary gland biopsies in 50% of SS patients by *in situ* hybridization and PCR[27]. Although the role of EBV in activating B-lymphocytes is well known and the presence of EBV in SS patients is well established, at present one cannot postulate whether infection of salivary glands cells by this virus may initiate the autoimmune process in SS.

Recently, it has been reported that the hepatitis C virus (HCV) may produce a chronic lymphocytic sialadenitis, which resembles the one observed in SS. In fact, more than 50% of patients infected with HCV had histologic changes compatible with SS in their minor salivary glands, as compared to only 5% in controls[28]. On the other hand, SS patients do not present antibodies to HCV in their sera[29].

Recent experimental data suggests that retroviruses may be responsible for the initiation of the autoimmune damage in SS (Table 5.3). Transgenic mice bearing the tax gene from human T-cell leukemia/lymphoma virus type I (HTLV-I) produce three disease phenotypes. These affect the thymus (thymic atrophy), the nerve sheath (tumors arising from the nerve sheath) and the salivary gland. The

Table 5.3 Retroviral implication in the pathogenesis of SS

Antibodies to P_{24} protein of HIV-1 in sera of SS patients

Type A retrovirus after coculture of minor salivary glands with a lymphoblastoid cell line

Endogenous retroviral sequences (HRES-1) in minor salivary glands

Reaction of epithelial cytoplasmic protein of minor salivary glands, with monoclonal antibody to P_{19} gag protein of HTLV-1

Autoimmune exocrinopathy in transgenic mice bearing the tax gene of HTLV-1

---

histopathological picture in the salivary glands resembles that of primary SS with, initially, the epithelial cells proliferating, followed by a gradual infiltration of lymphocytes and plasma cells and, finally, a gradual destruction of the acini[30]. The extent of the histopathological change in the various glands of these transgenic mice correlated directly with the concentration of the tax protein expressed in the nuclei of the epithelial cells. The tax protein is a trans-acting gene activator, which in transfected T-lymphocytes increases the expression of the gene for IL-2, the IL-2 receptor, IL-3 (which is responsible for B-cell growth) and granulocyte/monocyte colony stimulated factor. It is clear from this study that the changes in the salivary gland are a direct result of the expression of the tax gene. Another report has shown that EBV and adult T-cell leukemia derived factor (ADF) were present in the salivary glands in 10 out of 11 patients with SS[31]. ADF has been isolated from HTLV-I infected T-cells and enhances the expression of IL-2 receptor on T-cells, suggesting the possibility of an autocrine mechanism in the progression of adult T-cell leukemia. HTLV-I was not detected in these samples. In another study, minor salivary gland biopsies of patients with SS associated with other connective tissue diseases, were examined with three monoclonal antibodies to core (gag) proteins to HTLV-I and two monoclonal antibodies to HIV-1. Sections from 31% of the patients with SS contained an epithelial cytoplasmic protein which was reactive with a monoclonal antibody to the P_{19} group specific antigen of HTLV-1. The antigen was also detected in a lower percentage in patients with secondary SS[32]. Experiments with affinity purified rabbit antibodies to the P_{25} protein of HTLV-related endogenous sequences (HRES-1) showed that this antigen is distinct from the HRES-1, although the open reading frame of HRES-1 has a similar sequence to the P_{19} gag of HIV-1[33]. In another study, however, 30% of SS patients had serum antibodies that reacted with the capsid antigen P_{24} of HIV. Healthy individuals matched for age, presented 1–4% of such autoantibodies in their sera[34].

In another study, a putative virus infecting the salivary glands of SS patients has been identified from the extracts of SS lip biopsies after coculture with the lymphoblastoid cell line RH9. A type A retroviral particle has been demonstrated in 2 of 6 patients studied. This particle is distinguishable from the HIV particles by several physicochemical and ultrastructural criteria[35]. Infected T-cell lines by this retrovirus, expressed less CD4, IL-6 receptor and IL-2, but more HLA-DR as compared with non-infected cells. In addition, these cells displayed impaired protein kinase C (PKC) activation and calcium mobilization, suggesting a possible involvement of this retrovirus in abnormal signal transduction of T-cells[36].

Indirect evidence supportive of viral infection in SS include the presence of autoantigen La/SSB on epithelial cell membranes and the aberrant expression of the c-myc oncogene in the same cells. The concentration of La/SSB antigen is strongly increased in the nuclei of virally infected cell lines and is also present in the cytoplasm and cell membrane of these cells[37]. Increased concentration of La/SSB antigen in the nuclei and cytoplasm was observed in acinic cells of patients with primary and secondary SS. This aberrant

immunostaining pattern was not observed in healthy control subjects and rheumatoid arthritis (RA) patients without SS[38, 39]. La/SSB antigen has also been detected in the cytoplasm and on the cell membrane of conjunctival epithelial cells of SS patients, but not in normal controls[40].

C-myc proto-oncogene is involved in the pathogenesis of Burkitt's lymphoma caused by EBV. Patients with SS and other autoimmune disorders were found to have a significantly increased expression of c-myc mRNA in peripheral blood mononuclear cells without, however, any evidence for abnormal forms such as these with a deletion, rearrangement or amplification of this proto-oncogene. Thus, increased expression of the c-myc proto-oncogene in peripheral blood lymphocytes may be considered as a marker of lymphocyte activation in these patients[41].

C-myc mRNA expression in minor salivary glands of SS patients has been demonstrated by using an *in situ* hybridization technique with a specific c-myc oligonucleotide probe[42]. None of the labial minor salivary gland tissues of normal individuals, RA and sarcoidosis patients have presented this picture. Immunostaining analysis of the hybridized tissue with monoclonal antibodies and correlation with the clinicoserological and histological picture of the patients showed that the proto-oncogene is probably expressed on the acinar epithelial cells and its appearance is strongly correlated with the disease duration of the patients, as well as with the intensity of the T-cell infiltration. It is not known, yet, whether this aberrant c-myc expression in the epithelial cells is a primary phenomenon resulting from a viral infection or whether it is an epiphenomenon attributed to cytokine or cytokine-like molecules. However, the selective c-myc expression suggests the former rather than the latter.

All the above findings have some implications concerning the pathogenesis of primary SS. Retroviral infection could cause significant changes in the behavior of the epithelial cells of exocrine glands, such as *de novo* expression of HLA-DR antigens, expression of autoantigen (i.e. La/SSB) on their surface and heightened expression of lymphocytic adhesion molecules on the proximal endothelium. Therefore, retroviral infection of exocrine cells in subjects with a susceptible genetic and environmental substratum may predispose the glands to the infiltration of immunocytes and development of a localized response with all the pathological consequences.

AUTOANTIBODIES AND LYMPHOCYTE FUNCTION

The two major autoimmune phenomena observed in SS patients are the B-lymphocyte hyperactivity (which is expressed either as polyclonal B-cell activation and/or oligomonoclonal B-cell expansion) and the focal lymphoplasmacytic infiltrates of the exocrine glands[1].

POLYCLONAL B-CELL ACTIVATION

The most common serologic finding in SS is hypergammaglobulinemia. The elevated immunoglobulin levels in SS patients contain a number of autoantibodies which recognize 'organ-specific' antigens (Table 5.4) and 'non-organ-specific antigens'. The latter are of particular importance to understand pathogenetic mechanisms. There are antibodies directed against immunoglobulins (rheumatoid factor (RF)), nuclear antigen (antinuclear antibodies (ANAs)) and to extractable cellular antigens Ro/SSA and La/SSB.

Table 5.4   Organ-specific autoantibodies in SS

Autoantibody to	Per cent
Salivary ducts	10–70%
Pancreatic duct cells	6–33%
Gastric mucosa	5–15%
Thyroid cells	50%

Table 5.5   Clinical associations of anti-Ro/SSA and anti-La/SSB autoantibodies. The large discrepancies are due to the different assay methods used in different studies

Disease	Anti-Ro/SSA	Anti-La/SSB
	Per cent positive	
Sjögren's syndrome	38–96%	25–87%
Systemic lupus erythematosus	12–69%	10–45%
Rheumatoid arthritis	15–28%	0–22%
Polymyositis	9–18%	0–18%
Controls	2–18%	0–8%

The most common autoantibodies to cellular antigens in SS patients are directed against the two ribonucleoprotein antigens known as Ro/SSA and La/SSB. These autoantibodies are present in SS, but they can also be found in other autoimmune diseases, particularly in SLE (Chapter 2 Table 5.5). These antibodies have stimulated a great interest in the immunology of SS, since their response demonstrate a remarkable strength and persistence, they have a limited disease association and are related to the genetic background.

Autoantibodies to Ro/SSA recognize a ribonucleoprotein particle composed of the cytoplasmic (hY)RNAs and two protein components[43]. The intracellular role of RoRNP is not yet clearly defined. It seems that it possesses nuclear (transcription, processing and transport) and cytoplasmic (translation and storage of processed mRNA) functions. It is possible that different RoRNPs are involved in different intracellular processes[44].

The 60 kDa protein, consisting of 538 amino acids, was considered the main autoimmune target, since Ro/SSA autoimmune sera did not recognize hY-RNAs alone using agar precipitation techniques and immunoblots. Most of the anti-Ro/SSA positive sera reacted with two different proteins, 60 kDa and 52 kDa respectively[45]. Affinity purified anti-52 kDa antibody immunoprecipitates hY-RNA from

Table 5.6 Molecular characteristics of Ro/SSA and La/SSB autoantigens

	Ro/SSA	*La/SSB*
Molecular weight of the protein	52 and 60 kDa	48 kDa
Aminoacid content	538 for the 60 kDa	408 kDa
	475 for the 52 kDa	
RNAs in conjunction	Cytoplasmic (hY$_{1,3,4,5}$)	7SRNA, 5srRNA, tRNA, U$_6$RNA, RoANAs, viral RNAs (EBER-1, EBER-2)
Chromosome location	?	2
Cell function	Translation and storage of processed mRNA	Transcription and maturation of RNA-polymerase III transcripts
Linear epitopes shared with other protein	Vesicular stomatitis virus N-protein (the 60 kDa protein)	Gag protein feline sarcoma virus Human cardiac myosin (B chain)

HeLa cell extracts, demonstrating that 52 kDa protein is also a component of the RNP complex. Peptide mapping studies showed that 60 kDa, 52 kDa and the 48 kDa La/SSB proteins are distinct intracellular proteins. Furthermore, affinity purification studies in autoimmune sera containing anti-Ro/SSA and La/SSB antibodies revealed different, non-cross reacting antibodies directed to these components. Analysis of the antigenic epitopes of the 60 kDa Ro patients using affinity purified anti-Ro antibodies against synthetic peptides, showed many immunogenic epitopes. Among them, a major immunogenic region had sequence identity in 8 aminoacids with the nuclear capsid protein of the vesicular stomatitis virus[46]. Autoantibodies to the 52 kDa component are frequently found in serum of more than 80% of SS patients, while antibodies to 60 kDa component are observed more often in serum of SLE patients[47].

La/SSB antigen is also a ribonucleoprotein particle associated with all RNA polymerase III transcripts including hY-RNAs. Therefore, a subpopulation of La/SSB particles may be complexed with Ro/SSA. Moreover, La/SSB is associated with U1 RNA (an RNA polymerase III transcript) and several other viral transcripts[45]. The LaRNP is primarily located in the nucleus. This localization and the association with newly synthesized RNA polymerase III transcripts led to the suggestion that La participates in the transcription, maturation and nuclear export of the transcripts. Genomic clones revealed that human La/SSB gene is localized on chromosome 2, and codes for a protein composed of 408 aminoacid residues with a calculated molecular weight of 47 kDa. The molecule contains in the N-terminal side an RNA-binding protein consensus motif. Comparative analysis of this region with 29 RNA-binding domains of several other proteins showed that La/SSB is a member of a large family of RNA-binding proteins that included the 70 kDa and B/B″ proteins of snRNPs and the Ro/SSA 60 kDa protein [45,48]. Autoantibodies to La/SSB are directed against epitopes located on the N-terminal and C-terminal half of the molecule (termed X and Y, respectively). There are at least two autoepitopes on domain X and three autoepitopes on domain Y[45,49]. However, further work is needed to define with higher resolution and accuracy these autoepitopes. The molecular characteristics of Ro/SSA and La/SSB autoantigens are shown in Table 5.6.

The mechanisms governing the autoimmune response to these antigens remain unknown. It seems, however, that this is an antigen-driven reaction, since:

1. a co-ordinated expression of different anti-La/SSB population exists;
2. human autoantibodies react preferentially with human antigens; and
3. most sera contain multiple epitopes of the antigens[44].

Furthermore, it is not yet clear how the antigens trigger the immune system. The onset of the immune response can be accomplished by two different means. First, it can be done by the mechanism of molecular mimicry. There is evidence to suggest that regions of both Ro/SSA and La/SSB proteins have sequences identical with viral proteins (Table 5.6). Furthermore, the immune response to La/SSB in mice is different from the autoimmune response in humans. This could be attributed to the differences of the two immune systems, but it could also be explained by the fact that the La/SSB protein itself is not involved in the onset of the immune response. Secondly, as mentioned in the previous section, the La antigen is able to translocate to the epithelial cell membrane after virus infection. Hence, the antigen is exposed to the immune system and after binding to HLA class II proteins, an autoimmune response might be induced[44].

The presence of anti-Ro/SSA and anti-La/SSB autoantibodies is associated with certain clinical manifestations of primary SS. In fact, these antibodies correlate with earlier disease onset, recurrent parotid gland enlargement, as well as with splenomegaly/lymphadenopathy and vasculitis. In addition, the incidence of these antibodies correlates with the intensity of the minor salivary gland infiltration[50]. Recently, it was demonstrated that the total number of immunoglobulin containing plasma cells in labial salivary glands of SS patients with serum anti-La/SSB autoantibodies is significantly greater than in SS patients without these autoantibodies[38]. Such a relationship between the total number of plasma cells and the presence of ANA, RF and anti-Ro/SSA antibodies was not found.

OLIGO-MONOCLONAL B-CELL EXPANSION

Several cases of SS patients with malignant lymphoma or systemic disease were shown to have circulating monoclonal immunoglobulins. A systematic study of serum and urine from unselected patients with primary SS, using a high resolution agarose electrophoresis technique combined with immunofixation, demonstrated that approximately 80% of the patients with extraglandular (systemic) disease had monoclonal light chains or immunoglobulins in their serum[51]. Furthermore, all patients excreted monoclonal light chains in the urine. In contrast, only 25% of the patients with disease limited to the exocrine glands had monoclonal light chains or immunoglobulins in their serum, while 43% of these patients excreted light chains in urine[52]. In the case of lymphoma development, the level of urinary free light chains may correlate with disease activity[53]. Furthermore, one-third of patients with primary SS have cryoglobulins in their serum. These are mixed cryoglobulins containing an IgMκ monoclonal RF. The presence of the cryoglobulins was associated with a higher prevalence of extraglandular disease and autoantibodies to Ro/SSA and RF, as compared to patients without cryoglobulins[54]. These findings suggest that patients with SS express monoclonal immunoglobulins in the circulation along with polyclonal B-cell activation very early in the disease course. Monoclonality is observed more often in SS patients with systemic extraglandular disease. The latter is of particular interest, since SS patients with extraglandular manifestations are at a higher risk for developing malignancy[55]. In fact, type II cryoglobulinemia has been shown to correlate with lymphoma in SS patients, suggesting that mixed monoclonal cryoglobulinemia may serve as prognostic factor for lymphoma development in SS (unpublished findings).

The observation that the activated B-lymphocyte is located in the salivary glands, in association with other possible promoting neoplastic mechanisms in the salivary gland lesion (e.g. the absence of NK cells), prompted studies for the detection of monoclonal B-cell subsets which were responsible for the production of monoclonal immunoglobulins in the minor salivary gland infiltrates of SS patients. The presence of a monoclonal B-cell population was demonstrated by immunophenotyping and immunogenotyping studies. Using the peroxidase-antiperoxidase (PAP) bridge technique for the detection of intracytoplasmic immunoglobulins in the salivary gland lymphocyte infiltrates, it was demonstrated that 7 to 12 SS patients with circulating IgMκ monoclonal cryoglobulins also had in their minor salivary glands a ratio of κ to λ light chain positive plasma cells greater than 3. The above immunohistologic picture is consistent with the existence of a monoclonal plasma cell subpopulation. In contrast, none of the SS patients without cryoglobulins or with polyclonal cryoglobulins (type III) had a ratio of κ to λ positive plasma cells greater than 3, suggesting a polyclonal plasma cell pattern in the minor salivary glands[56]. In another study, it was demonstrated by restriction fragment length polymorphism (RFLP) that 5 out of 9 SS patients with circulating monoclonal immunoglobulins had oligoclonal immunoglobulin gene rearrangements in their salivary gland lymphocytes with the κ gene in four patients and λ gene in 1. Two additional SS patients revealed oligoclonal rearrangements of the β chain of the T-cell antigen receptor gene. Three of the SS patients with immunoglobulin gene rearrangements developed non-Hodgkin's lymphoma 2–8 years after the initial biopsy[57]. The above data support the speculation that the salivary glands in SS patients may serve as the initial site of B-cell neoplastic transformation. However, B-cells from other organs, such as the peripheral blood and bone marrow, must be carefully evaluated for the presence of transformed B-cells.

In order to delineate the origin and the mechanisms of monoclonal RF production, several studies concentrated on the idiotypes of RFs. Monoclonal RFs have been shown to extensively share cross reactive idiotypes[58, 59]. Fifty per cent of monoclonal RFs reacted with the 17.109 monoclonal antibody. The 17.109 idiotype is κ light chain specific and is encoded by the Humkv 325 germ line gene which belongs to the V_{KIIIb} subgroup[60, 61].

Some cross-reactive idiotypes may be common in SS and RA[62, 63], while others, such as 17.109, are found only in RFs from SS patients[64]. In fact, 12 out of 15 monoclonal RFs from patients with SS reacted with the 17.109 anti-idiotype. B-cells containing immunoglobulins reactive with the 17.109 monoclonal antibody were detected in the salivary gland biopsies in 11 out of 12 SS patients at high frequencies. In one patient with pre-existing SS who developed non-Hodgkin's lymphoma, the malignant cell producing the RF paraprotein reacted with the anti-17.109 monoclonal antibody[64]. Further analysis of the 17.109 bearing idiotype B-cells in the salivary gland of SS patients revealed a multiclonal origin in which somatic mutations accumulated in a non-random fashion, strongly suggesting an antigenic and T-cell driven process in the expansion of these cells[61].

A polyclonal anti-idiotypic antibody raised in a rabbit against a monoclonal IgMκ RF from the cryoglobulin of one patient with SS reacted with the sera of two-thirds of SS patients and one-fourth of rheumatoid arthritis patients. The cross-reactive idiotype levels were significantly higher in SS patients with monoclonal expansion of the B-cells in the minor salivary gland infiltrates and in patients with monoclonal type II cryoglobulinemia[65]. Family studies of 17.109 and polyclonal rabbit anti-idiotype showed that the idiotypes are not inherited, but they may be present on immunoglobulins of first degree family members of SS probands who also present autoimmune serologic abnormalities, such as antinuclear antibodies or RF[66]. These findings suggest that immunoglobulins bearing the cross-reactive idiotypes of monoclonal RFs are probably required during the disease process by antigenic or T-cell driven mechanisms.

In order to address whether cross reactive idiotypes may serve as markers for lymphoproliferation in SS, comparative studies of three cross-reactive idiotypes, in SS patients were performed. It was shown that these are expressed very early in the clinical spectrum of SS and their prevalence increases as the disease evolves. Finally, the presence of 17.109 and G-6 (a VHI associated cross reactive idiotype) were mainly found in SS patients with lymphoma, suggesting that these idiotypic determinants may serve as markers for lymphoma development in SS (unpublished findings).

LYMPHOCYTIC FUNCTION

During the last 20 years, intense research in different laboratories has attempted to assess the number, function and communication of the peripheral blood immunocytes; studies have not yet provided any definite conclusions. In fact, the absolute number of the peripheral blood total lymphocytes, T- and B-cells of SS patients, do not differ substantially from that observed in normal individuals[67]. Studies of T-lymphocyte subsets in SS revealed inconclusive results. Although, decreased numbers of T-helper cells (CD4$^+$) and T-suppressor cells (CD8$^+$) have been reported[68], this finding has not been substantiated by other investigators[69]. At the same time, studies evaluating the immunopathologic lesion of the affected exocrine glands, although indirect, indicated that the majority of the infiltrating lymphocytes were T-cells and that the B-cells in the lesion were activated.

The explosion of molecular biology techniques, including the use of monoclonal antibodies and nucleic acid probes, heralded a more precise understanding of the immunopathologic lesion in the exocrine glands of SS patients. Several immunopathologic studies using monoclonal antibodies against specific lymphocyte markers have evaluated the composition of round cell infiltrates in the labial salivary glands of primary SS patients. All studies agree that the majority of the infiltrating lymphocytes are T-cells, while B-lymphocytes constitute one-fourth to one-fifth of the round cells. Monocytes, macrophages, as well as NK cells, are less than 5%[70]. Further analysis of the T-lymphocyte subpopulations have demonstrated that 60% to 70% of the T-lymphocytes bear the CD4 phenotype, and that the majority of them exhibit the memory/inducer marker (CD45 RO). Almost all infiltrating T-cells express the $\alpha\beta$ T-cell receptor[71]. Analysis of the TCR repertoire of the infiltrating T-lymphocytes from minor salivary gland biopsies of SS patients by a quantitative polymerase chain reaction, revealed that the repertoire of the TCR V$_\beta$ gene was not restricted; however V$_{\beta2}$ and V$_{\beta13}$ were predominantly expressed in the infiltrates of SS patients[72]. Interestingly, V$_{\beta2}$ and V$_{\beta13}$ positive T-cells can be stimulated either by minor lymphocyte (MLs) determinants or bacterial toxins, the so-called superantigens[73]. Thus, exposure of lymphocytes to these molecules (e.g. after a bacterial infection) may lead to the stimulation and expansion of T-cells expressing these two genes. In this regard, the junctional sequences of cDVA encoding, the V$_{\beta2}$ and V$_{\beta13}$ genes of TCR, from T-lymphocytes infiltrating the minor salivary glands of SS patients were investigated[74]. Despite the fact that V$_{\beta2}$ and V$_{\beta13}$ positive T-cells were polyclonal, the junctional usage was found to be restricted, supporting the notion that autoreactive T-cells that contribute to the immunopathologic lesion in SS are of oligoclonal origin.

The activation status of T-cells was evaluated by searching for membrane expression of HLA class II molecules, interleukin-2 receptor (IL-2r), the lymphocyte function associated antigen-1 (LFA-1) and the interleukin-2 (IL-2) production[70, 71]. On the other hand, none of the tissue lymphocytes were positive for IL-2 and IL-2r when monoclonal antibodies were used. In contrast, studies using *in situ* hybridization with oligonucleotide mRNA probes was evident for both IL-2 and IL-2r in the infiltrating lymphocytes of the labial salivary glands of pSS patients (Skopouli, F.N., personal communication).

B-lymphocytes infiltrating the labial salivary glands are activated, since they are able to produce increased amounts of immunoglobulins with autoantibody activity[75]. In addition, evaluation of the isotypes of intracytoplasmic immunoglobulins of the plasma cells infiltrating the salivary glands of SS patients with an immunoperoxidase technique, showed that the IgG and IgM isotype predominates, in contrast to the plasma cells of the normal salivary glands, where the IgA isotype is dominant[76]. This observation prompted some investigators to support that the quantitation of cells containing IgA and IgG intracytoplasmic immunoglobulins may serve as diagnostic criterion with high specificity and sensitivity[77].

THE IMMUNOPATHOLOGIC LESION

From the above data, it is clear that both lymphocyte compartments are activated in the tissue lesion of pSS, while the professional antigen presenting cell (monocyte-macrophage) is poorly represented. Therefore, the specific question which arises is: 'which cell plays the role of the antigen presenting cell?'

Several studies suggest that the glandular or acinar epithelial cell may play the role of the antigen presenting cell. Histopathologic studies in new cases of SS showed that the focal lymphocytic infiltrates start around the ducts. Furthermore, by staining the labial salivary glands with anti-class II HLA monoclonal antibodies, it was shown that the ductal and acinar epithelial cells inappropriately express these molecules. Since γ-interferon has

Table 5.7 Immunologic abnormalities in minor salivary glands of SS

Cell compartment	Characteristics
T-lymphocytes	HLA-DR expression
	Cytokine production
	Adhesion molecule expression
B-lymphocytes	Production of immunoglobulin
	Immunoglobulin class switching
Epithelial cells	Inappropriate HLA-DR expression
	C-myc protooncogene expression
	Cytokine production
	Autoantigen expression

been shown to induce expression of both histocompatibility antigen classes on the surface of epithelial and other cells, and since this is produced in abundance by the activated T-cell of the lesion, one is faced with the chicken and egg problem, that is, whether the HLA-DR expression and possible antigen presentation by epithelial cells predates or is a consequence of the lymphocytic infiltration. Subsequent observations, however, suggest that the HLA class II molecule expression may play a more fundamental role. In this regard, studying proto-oncogene mRNA expression in the minor salivary glands of SS patients, it was observed that the c-myc, in contrast to c-fos and c-jun, was expressed not by the activated lymphocytes, but by the epithelial glandular cells. Since the expression of the c-myc is so restricted, this phenomenon cannot be attributed to microenvironmental factors[42].

Furthermore, acinar epithelial cells co-express accessory adhesion molecules[78] and autoantigens, which in conjunction with class II antigen expression may potentially prime an autoimmune response. In fact, translocation and membrane localization of the nuclear antigen La/SSB has been observed in conjunctival epithelial cells of SS patients[40] (Table 5.7). In addition, the infiltrating lymphocytes express a diverse array of cell adhesion molecules (LFA-1, LAF-3, CD2,

LFA-3), while the intercellular adhesion molecule 1 (ICAM-1) was expressed on acinar epithelial cells adjacent to sites of intense inflammation. The synthesis of ICAM-1 is up-regulated in the epithelial cells in the presence of IFN-γ (which is found in abundance in the salivary glands of SS)[79]. These adhesion molecules belong to a group of proteins known as integrins and play a significant role in cell-to-cell interactions[80]. Their presence may foster cellular interactions and promote the chronic inflammatory response.

The proinflammatory cytokines IL-1 and IL-6 play an important role in the autoimmune process. These cytokines orchestrate the complex processes of immune reaction and inflammation. IL-1 (produced mainly by the macrophages/monocytes) induces the production of IL-6 in different cell types including fibroblasts and endothelial cells. In some instances, the IL-1 action on IL-6 production is augmented by the presence of IFN-γ and TNF-a[81]. The above findings indicate the central role of macrophage/monocyte in many autoimmune diseases (e.g. RA). In SS, however, the macrophage is poorly represented. In this regard, evaluation of IL-1$_\beta$ and IL-6 in labial salivary glands of SS patients with oligonucleotide probes and *in situ* hybridization technique, demonstrated that the mRNA of these cytokines are found in both the infiltrating lymphocytes and the epithelial cells (Skopouli, F.N., personal communication). Therefore, the production of proinflammatory cytokines by the epithelial cells adds further to the hypothesis that these cells may play a role in the priming of the immune response in the immunopathologic lesion of SS.

These changes of epithelial cells in SS, suggest an *in situ* immune response with the epithelial cell probably playing the role of an antigen presenting cell. As a consequence, T-cells may be attracted, become activated and secrete various cytokines, which stimulate B-lymphocytes to secrete antibodies.

CLINICAL PICTURE

In most patients with SS, the disease shows a rather slow and benign course. The most common clinical manifestations of primary SS are: sicca manifestations (dry eyes, dry mouth and vaginal dryness), arthralgia and arthritis, fatigue, Raynaud's phenomenon, myalgia, and major salivary gland enlargement[1]. The initial manifestations can be non-specific and usually in 8–10 years the initial symptoms progress into a full-blown development of the syndrome[2]. Extraglandular manifestations can be seen in one-third of the patients and include pulmonary involvement, renal involvement, hepatogastrointestinal involvement and lymphadenopathy. Finally, approximately 5% of the SS patients may develop a B-cell neoplasia (lymphoma or Waldenstorm's macroglobulinemia).

GLANDULAR INVOLVEMENT

Oral component

Xerostomia (dry mouth) is one of the hallmarks of SS. The oral manifestations may be subtle or overt, where complaints center around mouth soreness, burning sensation, difficulty in swallowing, change in taste, trouble with speech, acceleration of developing oral carries and problems in wearing complete dentures.

Extraorally, parotid gland and/or submandibular gland enlargement with or without inflammation is a frequent finding in SS patients (approximately 70%). Most patients manifest bilateral involvement of the salivary glands, but may initially present with unilateral pain, swelling and/or erythema[1].

Intraoral involvement in SS is manifested by dry mucosa, atrophy of the filiform papillae of the tongue, dental carries and, in some cases, *Candida* overgrowth on the oral mucosa.

For the evaluation of dry mouth, several tests with variable sensitivity and specificity have been used. Salivary flow rates can be measured clinically for whole saliva or for separate secretions from the parotid or submandibular and sublingual glands, with or without stimulation. Patients with clinically overt SS are presented with reduced salivary flow rates. However, flow measurements depend on many factors, such as the age, sex, drugs therapy and time of day, and there is a wide range of flow rates among normal individuals[82]. Therefore, it is difficult to give diagnostic thresholds for the sialometric tests.

Sialography is a radiocontrast method of assessing anatomical changes in the salivary gland duct system. When this method is used in SS patients various degrees of sialectases are observed[83]. It may cause pain and swelling of the parotid glands and sometimes allergic reactions to radio-opaque material. In addition, if the contrast medium extravasates beyond the duct system, a severe granulomatous reaction can be seen. Some studies suggest that the sialography is not sensitive and not specific[84]. In another study, however, sialography with water soluble media was applied in 84 patients with primary and secondary SS. The method was correlated with the minor salivary gland biopsy, as well as the clinical and serologic picture of the patients. The method was shown to be as sensitive and specific as the labial salivary gland biopsy. Furthermore, hypergammaglobulinemia, anti-Ro(SSA) antibodies, extraglandular manifestations and parotid swelling were all correlated with both sialographic and histologic abnormalities, suggesting that both tests are useful for the evaluation of salivary gland involvement in SS[85].

Scintigraphy provides a functional evaluation of all the salivary glands, by observing the rate and density of ^{99m}Tc sodium pertechnetate uptake and time of appearance in the mouth during a 60 minute period after intravenous injection. In SS patients the uptake of the label by the glands and secretion of labeled saliva in the mouth is delayed or absent. Abnormal scintigraphy correlates

with the reduced salivary flow, the sialographic picture and the intensity of minor salivary gland lymphocytic infiltrates[83]. In a recent study of 320 patients with oral dryness who had primary SS, secondary SS, graft-versus-host disease and other autoimmune diseases, it was found that scintigraphy revealed high sensitivity, but not well established disease specificity[86]. The limited discriminatory value of salivary gland scintigraphy for the diagnosis of primary SS was further supported by others[87].

Chemical and immunological parameters in saliva of SS patients have been examined extensively in the past. So far, the results are conflicting and controversial and seem to be of limited diagnostic value[88].

Ocular involvement

Ocular involvement is the second major glandular manifestation of SS. Diminished tear secretion leads to the destruction of corneal and bulbar conjunctival epithelium termed keratoconjunctivitis sicca (KCS). KCS in SS can be asymptomatic for years before symptoms appear[89]. When symptoms begin, patients may note a feeling of grittiness or sandy-like sensation when they arise in the morning. They often experience 'ropey' or thickened conjunctival secretions. Chronic uveitis can also be seen in SS as a result of KCS[90]. Acute iritis (posterior uveitis), however, due to immune complexes, is very rare and responds well to treatment with cyclosporine and cyclophosphamide[91].

The confirmation of KCS is performed by tests which evaluate the quantity and quality of tears. The Schirmer's tear test is used for the evaluation of tear secretion (plate 5). The test is performed with strips of filter paper 30 mm in length. The strip is slipped beneath the inferior eye lid, with the remainder of the paper hanging out. After 5 minutes the wetting length of the paper is measured. Wetting of less than 5 mm per 5 minutes is a strong indication for diminished secretion. However, there is no consensus in the literature concerning this threshold value, while presence of decreased tear secretion is not diagnostic of KCS.

KCS can be easily diagnosed using rose bengal staining. Rose bengal is an aniline which stains the devitalized or damaged epithelium of both the cornea and conjunctiva. Slit lamp examination after rose bengal staining shows a punctuate of filamentary keratitis. Tear break-up time is another useful parameter. A drop of fluorescein is instilled and the time between the last blink and appearance of dark, non-fluorescent areas in the tear film is measured. An overlap rapid break-up of the tear film, when not seen consistently over the same area and indicating a local surface irregularity, points toward either a mucin or lipid layer abnormality[89].

Other tests, such as lactoferrin and lysozyme concentration (which are usually diminished or absent), have been shown to be sensitive, but they are less easily done in clinical practice.

Other glandular involvement

Apart from the eyes and mouth, other mucous membranes as well as the skin may exhibit dryness. Nasal dryness with crusting, vaginal dryness with dyspareunia, cheilitis and xerosis (dry skin) have been described. Patients with dry skin frequently experience dermal stinging and itching.

Salivary gland pathology

The salivary glands are the best studied organs in SS since they are affected in almost all patients and are readily accessible. The most characteristic histological feature of major salivary glands is the benign lymphoepithelial lesion (BLEL), which is also termed as myoepithelial sialadenitis[92,93]. The development of a benign lymphoepithelial lesion begins with focal lymphocytic infiltrates,

especially around the ducts, and progresses to totally replacement of glandular parenchyma by the infiltrate. Lymphoid follicles with germinal centers may or may not be present. The lymphocytic infiltration is often associated with hyperplasia and metaplasia of ductal epithelium, resulting in the epimyoepithelial islands that characterize the established myoepithelial sialadenitis[92]. The epimyoepithelial islands are infiltrated by lymphocytes. In the later stages, hyalin material can be found in the epimyoepithelial islands. The cellular composition of epimyoepithelial islands is heterogeneous and may change during the development of the lesion.

The need for a practical and easy way to assess the salivary component of SS led to the introduction of labial minor salivary gland biopsy. The histopathologic characteristics of the biopsy of the minor salivary glands include:

1. lymphocytic focus, which is defined as an aggregate consisting of at least 50 lymphocytes and histiocytes; and
2. the consistent presence of these foci in all or most of the glands in the specimen.

The lymphocytic foci are often localized around or in the vicinity of the intralobular ducts. Plasma cells are often present in the periphery of a lymphocytic focus, as well as diffusely distributed between acini and in fibrous tissue. In the larger lymphocytic foci, germinal center formation can be often seen and sometimes there are so many large foci that confluence occurs. Epimyoepithelial islands occur very rarely in the minor salivary glands[94]. When epimyoepithelial islands are present in the labial salivary glands together with multinucleate giant cells, the differential diagnosis with sarcoidosis may be very difficult. In these cases, immunohistochemical staining for muramidase may reveal the correct diagnosis, as epithelioid cells contain muramidase, while the cells in the epimyoepithelial islands do not contain this enzyme[92, 95].

Several semiquantitative and qualitative

Table 5.8 Clinical forms of pulmonary involvement in SS

Xerotrachea
Small airways obstruction
Interstitial lung disease
Mediastinal or paratracheal lymphadenopathy
    (pseudolymphoma or lymphoma)
Pleural effusions (SS associated with RA or SLE)

---

methods have been applied for the assessment of minor salivary gland biopsies[94, 96]. The 'lymphocytic focus score' is defined as the number of lymphocytic foci per 4 mm² salivary gland tissue and was introduced to quantify the grade of the focal lymphocytic sialadenitis. A focus score greater than one is used as diagnostic threshold value for SS.

In conclusion, biopsy of minor salivary glands can be confirmatory for SS, if it is obtained through normal appearing mucosa, includes 5–10 glands, is separated from the surrounding connective tissue and shows focal lymphocytic infiltrates in most of the glands in the specimen with a focus score above the chosen diagnostic threshold.

EXTRAGLANDULAR MANIFESTATIONS

Arthritis

Joint symptoms and signs, such as arthralgias, myalgias, morning stiffness and synovitis, can be seen in 70% of patients. In some cases, it can precede the sicca manifestations. Chronic polyarthritis is rare and sometimes can lead to Jacoud's arthropathy[97]. In contrast to RA, radiographs of the hand usually do not reveal pathological changes[98, 99].

Raynaud's phenomenon

This is found in 35% of SS patients. It precedes sicca manifestations in approximately 40% of the patients and follows a pleomorphic course. In some patients it disappears during the course of SS, in some others the frequency of attack decreases, while in more than 50% of the patients it remains the same. Patients with the primary syndrome and Raynaud's phenomenon present with swollen hands, but in contrast to those with scleroderma, they do not experience digital ulcers and telangiectasias are not seen. Radiographs of the hands of these patients may show small tissue calcifications[100]. A small proportion of SS patients with long standing Raynaud's phenomenon may present antibodies to centromere[101].

Pulmonary involvement

Manifestations from the respiratory tract and the mediastinum are polymorphic (Table 5.8). These are usually mild and referred mostly to the small and large airways. They can present with a range of symptoms from dry cough secondary to dryness of the tracheobronchial mucosa (xerotrachea) to dyspnea from interstitial disease or airway obstruction[102]. The chest roentgenogram is often abnormal showing an interstitital pattern.

Interstitial disease in SS was thought to be a very common manifestation. A further analysis of the pulmonary involvement, however, by function tests revealed that the pathology is related to the bronchi, causing mild obstruction and pO_2 reduction. These findings were confirmed by CT scan and transbronchial biospy which disclosed peribronchial lymphocytic infiltrates (Papiris, S., personal communication). Pseudolymphoma or frank lymphoma should always be suspected when lung nodules or hilar and/or mediastinal lymphadenopathy are found on chest radiographs[102].

There are differences in respiratory manifestations between the primary and secondary syndrome. In the latter, the respiratory involvement is a reflection of the primary rheumatic disorders. In fact, pleuritis is usually found in SS associated with other rheumatic disorders and not in primary SS.

Gastrointestinal and hepatobiliary

Patients with SS often complain of dysphagia, nausea and epigastric pain. These symptoms are due to oesophageal dismotility and chronic atrophic lymphocytic gastritis. In addition, patients with SS have hypopepsinogenemia, an elevated serum gastrin, low levels of serum vitamin B_{12}, and antibodies to parietal cells[103].

Subclinical pancreatic involvement is a rather common finding, as illustrated by the fact that hyperamylasemia of pancreatic origin is found in one-quarter of patients with the syndrome[104].

The association of SS with chronic liver disease has been well established over the past years. Patients often present with hepatomegaly (25–28%)[103], and antimitochondrial antibodies (AMA) (5%). Liver enzymes and alkaline phosphatase are usually elevated in approximately 70% of SS patients with AMA and liver biopsy discloses in most of them a picture of mild primary biliary cirrhosis (Skopouli, F.N., personal communication). There is also a high incidence of SS in patients with primary biliary cirrhosis: sicca manifestations have been described in approximately half of a group of patients with primary biliary cirrhosis; among these, 10% had severe clinical features of mouth and eye dryness[105].

Renal involvement

Overt kidney disease is found in approximately 10% of patients with SS[106], while approximately 35% have an abnormal urine acidification test. Interstitial disease is the most common renal histopathologic finding. Most of the patients present with hyposthenuria and hypokalemic, hyperchloremic distal tubular acidosis before classical sicca manifestations are apparent. Distal tubular acidosis can be silent or can present with recurrent renal colic and/or hypokalemic muscular weakness. Untreated renal tubular acidosis

leads to renal stones, nephrocalcinosis and compromised renal function[107]. Less commonly, these patients have proximal tubular acidosis with Fanconi's syndrome.

Glomerulonephritis has been described in few SS patients. All cases have been associated with circulating immune complexes, mixed cryoglobulinemia, low levels of complement and clinical symptoms of extraglandular involvement with signs of small vessel vasculitis. Pathologic changes on renal biopsy included changes of membranous, membranoproliferative and proliferative glomerulonephritis[106].

Vasculitis

Systemic vasculitis in SS may be manifested by small, medium and, rarely, large vessel involvement. The most common clinical findings of vasculitis are skin involvement (palpable or non-palpable purpura and urticaria) and peripheral neuropathy. Other organ manifestations have been also demonstrated in SS patients including central nervous system (CNS), lungs, kidneys, GI tract, pancreas, liver, spleen and salivary glands[108]. There are two distinct histopathologic types of inflammatory vascular disease in primary SS: first, neutrophilic inflammatory vascular disease and, secondly, mononuclear inflammatory vascular disease. Both types of vasculitic involvement may result in end organ damage. The former has been associated with seropositivity for anti-Ro(SSA), anti-La(SSB) antibodies and RF. The mononuclear inflammatory vascular disease, however, is associated with seronegativity for these antibodies. These differences imply varying immunopathogenetic mechanisms for the two clinically similar manifestations of the disease where the mononuclear seronegative form of the disease may be a precursor for the seropositive neutrophilic 'phase' of the vasculitic process in SS[108].

In another classification of vascular involvement[109], the small-vessel vasculitis was of the hypersensitivity type, i.e. leucocytoclastic and lymphocytic, while the medium-vessel vasculitis was acute necrotizing, mimicking polyarteritis nodosa, without, however, the formation of aneurysms. Endarteritis obliterans was seen in patients with a long-standing history of vasculitis.

Neuromuscular involvement

Neurological manifestations of SS from the peripheral nervous system are well documented. Signs and symptoms from sensory, motor, autonomic and spinal ganglia are present with moderate severity in the form of symmetric or asymmetric sensory or sensory-motor polyneuropathy. Trigeminal sensory neuropathy, carpal tunnel syndrome, mononeuritis multiplex and sensory gangliopathy have been described[110,111]. Tonic pupil, as a result of parasympathetic denervation of the sphincter muscle, has been also reported.

Involvement of the CNS in the syndrome is a matter of considerable controversy. Over the last decade some investigators have described a high proportion of CNS involvement, which before had been internationally unrecognized[112]. They found that this disease was multifocal, recurrent and progressive. The clinical signs included focal lesions, i.e. hemiparesis, unilateral loss of vision, focal epilepsy and transverse myelitis. Some patients presented with diffuse brain injury, expressed as aseptic meningoencephalitis and progressive encephalopathy which leads to dementia. Furthermore, they described a recurrent neurologic syndrome resembling multiple sclerosis. Magnetic resonance imaging and cerebrospinal fluid analysis revealed changes identical to multiple sclerosis. On the other hand, others have failed to demonstrate severe CNS involvement in 55 patients with primary SS and 50 with secondary[113]. Eighteen of these patients had mild neurological abnormalities confined to the secondary syndrome. All were characteristics of the underlying rheumatoid disorders. A study of 63 consecutive patients with primary SS revealed that 17 had a mild sensory or sensorimotor neuropathy, while one patient with past history of hypertension had a mild cerebrovascular episode[114], suggesting that peripheral neuropathy is a rather common finding in SS, whereas CNS disease must be rare. Furthermore, evaluation of multiple sclerosis patients for the presence of SS, revealed that only two out of 252 patients had the signs and symptoms associated with SS[115,116].

Many patients with the primary syndrome complain of myalgias but muscle enzymes are usually normal or only slightly elevated. Severe polymyositis, with extensive necrosis of muscle fibers and invasion of macrophages into the affected muscle, have been described in SS[117].

Other manifestations

Overt autoimmune thyroiditis has been described in some cases of primary SS patients. Subclinical autoimmune thyroid disease as illustrated by the presence of antithyroid antibodies and altered thyroid function has been demonstrated in 50% of SS patients [118].

Mild normochronic and normocytic anemia is a common finding in SS patients, while leukopenia and thrombocytopenia are relatively rare features. Elevated erythrocyte sedimentation rate is found in approximately 70% of SS patients. In contrast, C-reactive protein is not detected in primary SS patients but in patients with SS and RA[119].

Lymphoproliferative disease

Patients with SS have a 44 times greater relative risk of developing lymphoma, compared with age, sex-, race-matched normal controls. The autoimmune disorder may precede the development of lymphoma by up to 20 years[55]. Certain extraglandular manifestations, such as splenomegaly, lymphadenopathy, as well as parotid swelling, are obtained more often in patients predisposed to lymphoma. Lymphomas may affect salivary glands or major parenchymal organs, such as the lungs, the kidneys or the gastrointestinal tract. Immunohistological studies in biopsies of such patients with lymphoma show that these are primarily of B-cell origin, usually expressing IgMκ in their cytoplasm[120]. The lymphomas are of two major types, either composed of highly undifferentiated B-cells or well-differentiated immunocytomas. Lymphomas may differ by location and grading. In our patient population, among 8 lymphomas in SS patients, 6 were low-grade immunocytomas, and 2 intermediate grade non-Hodgkin's lymphomas. Five of the immunocytomas affected the minor salivary or lacrimal glands. Two of patients with immunocytomas showed spontaneous regression, while 2 others (1 with immunocytoma and 1 with an intermediate grade) developed high-grade lymphoma 3 and 5 years later[121]. Therefore, the clinical picture of SS lymphoma appears to be diverse, suggesting that the therapeutic approach should be guided according to the stage and the grade of the disease.

Some of the patients develop a clinical picture of malignancy, which, however, cannot be classified as truly malignant, even using modern molecular pathology techniques, such as immunophenotyping and immunogenotyping. The term 'pseudolymphoma' has been applied to such cases[120]. The course of these patients is variable. Some of them respond to corticosteroid and immunosuppressive drug therapy, while some later develop a frank malignant lymphoma.

SECONDARY SS

Sicca manifestations can be found in other autoimmune diseases, such as RA, systemic lupus erythematosus (SLE) and progressive systemic sclerosis. With a smaller prevalence, SS manifestations have been described in polymyositis, polyarteritis nodosa, primary biliary cirrhosis and mixed connective tissue disease[1].

The prevalence of clinically overt SS in patients with RA is around 5%. Using a special questionnaire, however, 20% of RA patients complain of dry eyes and/or xerostomia[122]. The diagnosis of RA, precedes usually the diagnosis of SS by many years. Patients with RA and SS present usually with KCS, while parotid or other major salivary gland enlargement is uncommon, compared with primary SS. In addition, extraglandular features of primary SS, such as lymphadenopathy, renal involvement and Raynaud's phenomenon are quite uncommon in SS associated with RA[123].

Patients with primary SS and those with SLE may have similar disease manifestations, such as arthralgias, rash, peripheral neuropathy and glomerulopnehritis. These observations prompted Heaton to conclude that SS was a benign form of SLE[124]. Patients with SLE and secondary SS, however, usually present with more prominent symptoms and signs of SLE. The diagnosis is usually histological, where approximately 10% of SLE patients have lymphocytic infiltrates in their minor salivary gland biopsy. It should be noted, however, that the lymphocytic infiltrates in SLE patients with SS are perivascular and not periductular as in primary SS patients[125].

Sicca complaints of dry eyes and mouth are found in approximately 20% of unselected patients with systemic sclerosis[126]. Subjective xerostomia could be due to fibrosis of the exocrine glands. In fact, minor salivary gland biopsies of 44 unselected scleroderma patients showed that 38% had fibrosis, while only 22% had lymphocytic adenitis comparable with SS[127]. A very high incidence of SS has also been described in patients with the limited form of scleroderma (previously called CREST)[128].

DIAGNOSIS – DIFFERENTIAL DIAGNOSIS

Since the initial definition and the proposed

Table 5.9 Preliminary criteria for the classification of Sjögren's syndrome

1. Ocular symptoms.
   A positive response to at least 1 of the following 3 questions:
   (a) Have you had daily, persistent, troublesome dry eyes for more than 3 months?
   (b) Do you have a recurrent sensation of sandy or gravel feeling in the eyes?
   (c) Do you use tear substitutes more than 3 times a day?

2. Oral symptoms.
   A positive response to at least 1 of the following 3 questions:
   (a) Have you had a daily feeling of dry mouth for more than 3 months?
   (b) Have you had recurrent or persistently swollen salivary glands as an adult?
   (c) Do you frequently drink liquids to aid in swallowing dry foods?

3. Ocular signs.
   Objective evidence of ocular involvement determined on the basis of a positive result on at least 1
   of the following 2 tests:
   (a) Schirmer-1 test (≤ 5 mm in 5 minutes)
   (b) Rose bengal score (≥ 4, according to the van Bijsterveld scoring system)

4. Histopathologic findings.
   Focus score ≥ 1 on minor salivary gland biopsy (focus defined as an agglomeration of at least 50
   mononuclear cells, focus score defined as the number of foci/4 mm^2 of glandular tissue).

5. Salivary gland involvement.
   Objective evidence of salivary gland involvement, determined on the basis of a positive result on at
   least 1 of the following 3 tests:
   (a) Salivary scintigraphy
   (b) Parotid sialography
   (c) Unstimulated salivary flow (≤ 1.5 ml in 15 minutes)

6. Autoantibodies.
   Presence of at least 1 of the following autoantibodies in the serum:

   Antibodies to Ro/SSA or La/SSB antigens or antinuclear antibodies or rheumatoid factor.

A patient is considered as having probable SS if 3 of 6 criteria are present and as definite SS if 4 of 6
criteria are present.

Modified from [5].

criteria of SS by Bloch *et al.* in 1965[129], several sets of criteria have been used for the diagnosis of SS by different study groups. As a result, patients with SS had often been missed at diagnosis, or classified incorrectly due to both the great variability at disease presentation and to the lack of well-defined and commonly accepted diagnostic criteria.

Recently, a prospective concerted action involving 26 centers from 12 European countries conducted a study with a goal to set validated criteria for the diagnosis of SS[5]. The study resulted in:

1. the validation of a simple six-item questionnaire for determination of dry eyes and mouth, useful for the initial screening for SS; and
2. the definition of a new set of criteria for SS (Table 5.9).

The sensitivity and specificity of both questionnaire and diagnostic criteria were determined, exhibiting a good discrimination between patients and controls. Hence, using this set of criteria, a general agreement can be reached on the diagnosis of SS.

Table 5.10   Differential diagnosis of SS, sarcoidosis and HIV infection

Characteristics	SS	Sarcoidosis	HIV infection
Gender	Mostly women	Invariable	Mostly men
Autoantibodies to Ro/ SSA-La/SSB	Present	Absent	Absent
Minor salivary gland pathology	CD4$^+$ T-cell infiltrates	Granulomas	CD8$^+$ lymphocytosis
HLA associations	B$_8$/DR3	Unknown	DR5

Differential diagnoses must be considered of the diseases responsible for KCS, xerostomia and parotid gland enlargement. Sarcoidosis, is one of the diseases which can mimic the clinical picture of SS[130]. However, there is a lack of autoantibodies to Ro/SSA or La/SSB, and sometimes the minor salivary gland biopsy reveals non-caseating granulomas (Table 5.10). Other medical conditions which can mimic SS are hyperlipoproteinemias (types II, IV and V), chronic graft-versus-host disease, amyloidosis and more recently, patients with HIV infection. In fact, sicca manifestations with parotid gland enlargement, pulmonary involvement and lymphadenopathy, have been reported in patients with HIV infection. These patients had an increased prevalence of HLA-DR5 alloantigen. HIV has been detected in labial salivary gland lymphocytes in 2 out of 6 patients with HIV infection, but the two diseases seems to be different, since patients with HIV infection have no autoantibodies to Ro/SSA and La/SSB antigens and the lymphocytic infiltrates in the salivary glands are not as prominent as in SS and consist of CD8$^+$ T-cells (Table 5.10)[131].

THERAPY-PROGNOSIS

SS is a chronic, multisystem disease. Therefore, patients with SS should be regularly followed for significant functional deterioration, signs of disease complications and significant changes in the course of the disease.

Sicca manifestations are of unknown etiology. Hence, treatment of SS is aimed at symptomatic relief and limiting the damaging local effects of chronic xerostomia and keratoconjunctivitis sicca by substitution of the missing secretions (reviewed in[132]).

KCS is treated with fluid replacement supplied as often as necessary. To replace deficient tears, there are several readily available ophthalmic preparations (Tearisol; Liquifilm; 0.5% methylcellulose; Hypo Tears). In severe cases, it may be necessary for patients to use these as often as every 30 minutes. If corneal ulceration is present, eye-patching and boric acid ointment is recommended. Certain drugs which may further deteriorate lacrimal and salivary hypofunction, such as diuretics, antihypertensive drugs and antidepressants, should be avoided. The low levels of humidity in air-conditioned environments, as well as windy or dry climates, must be avoided. Soft contact lenses may help to protect the cornea, especially in the presence of filaments. However, the lenses themselves require wetting and the patients must be followed very carefully due to the increased risk of infection.

Treatment of xerostomia is difficult. Stimulation of salivary flow by sugar-free, highly flavored lozenges has been found to be rather helpful. Most patients carry water and use sugarless lemon drops or chewing gum. These must be sugar free, because of the risk of rampant dental carries. Adequate oral hygiene after meals is a prerequisite for the prevention of dental disease. Topical oral treatment with stannous fluoride enhances dental mineralization and retards damage to tooth surfaces. In cases of rapidly progressive dental disease, fluoride can be directly applied to the teeth from plastic trays that are used at night. Propionic acid gels may be used to treat vaginal dryness. Bromhexine given orally at high doses (48 mg/d) has been suggested to improve sicca manifestations. However, frequent ingestion of fluids, particularly with meals, is often the best solution[132].

Preliminary studies showed that hydroxychloroquine, which is efficacious and safe in other autoimmune diseases, may be useful in treating Sjögren's patients. A dose of 200 mg/d partially corrects hypergammaglobulinemia, and decreases IgG antibodies to La/SSB antigen. Furthermore, hydroxychloroquine treatment decreases the erythrocyte sedimentation rate and increases the hemoglobin levels[133].

Corticosteroids (prednisolone 0.5–1 mg/kg/d) or other immunosuppressive agents (i.e. cyclophosphamide) are indicated in treatment of life-threatening extraglandular manifestations, particularly when renal or severe pulmonary involvement and systemic vasculitis has been defined.

In conclusion, SS remains an incurable disease without a single therapeutic approach which can change its natural course. The prognosis of the disease depends on the extension and type of the systemic features and the appearance of lymphoma. The treatment and prognosis of malignant lymphoma, depends on the histologic type, the location and the extension. Decision-making with regard to chemotherapy and/or radiotherapy, should be guided by experienced oncologists.

REFERENCES

1. Moutsopoulos, H. M., Chused, T. M., Mann, D. L. *et al.* (1980) Sjögren's syndrome (sicca syndrome): current issues. *Ann. Int. Med.*, **92**, 212–26.
2. Pavlidis, N. A., Karsh, J. and Moutsopoulos, H. M. (1982) The clinical picture of primary Sjögren's syndrome: a retrospective study. *J. Rheumatol*, **9**, 685–90.
3. Deprettere, A. J., Van Acker, K. J., De Clerck, L. S. *et al.* (1988) Diagnosis of Sjögren's syndrome in children. *AJDC*, **142**, 1185–7.
4. Siamopoulou-Mavridou, A., Drosos, A. A. and Andonopoulos, A. P. (1989) Sjögren's syndrome in childhood: report of two cases. *Eur. J. Pediatr.*, **148**, 523–4.
5. Vitali, C., Bombardieri, S., Moutsopoulos, H. M. *et al.* (1992) Preliminary criteria for the classification of Sjögren's syndrome: Results of a prospective concerted action supported by the European Community. *Arth. Rheum.*, **36**, 340–8.
6. Jacobsson, L. T. H., Axell, T. E., Hansen, B. U. *et al.* (1989) Dry eyes or mouth – an epidemiological study in Swedish adults, with special reference to primary Sjögren's syndrome. *J. Autoimmunity*, **2**, 521–7.
7. Jacobsson, L., Hansen, B. U., Manthorpe, R. *et al.* (1992) Association of dry eyes and dry mouth with anti-Ro/SSA and anti-La/SSB autoantibodies in normal adults. *Arth. Rheum.*, **35**, 1492–1501.
8. Arnett, F. C., Bias, W. B., Reveille, J. D. (1989) Genetic studies in Sjögren's syndrome and systemic lupus erythematosus. *J. Autoimmunity*, **2**, 403–13.
9. Reveille, J. D., Wilson, R. W., Provost, T. T. *et al.* (1984) Primary Sjögren's syndrome and other autoimmune disease in families. Prevalence and immunogenetic studies in six kindreds. *Ann. Int. Med.*, **101**, 748–56.
10. Fey, K. H., Terasaki, P. I., Moutsopoulos, H. M. *et al.* (1976) Association of Sjögren's syndrome with HLA-B8. *Arth. Rheum.*, **19**, 883–6.
11. Chused, T. M., Kassan, S. S., Opelz, G., Moutsopoulos, H. M., Terasaki, P. I. (1977) Sjögren's syndrome associated with HLA-DW3. *N. Eng. J. Med.*, **296**, 895–7.
12. Foster, H., Stephenson, A., Walker, D. *et al.* (1993) Linkage studies of HLA and primary Sjögren's syndrome in multicase families. *Arth. Rheum.*, **36**, 473–84.
13. Arnett, F. C. (1991) Immunogenetics of the connective tissue diseases, in *Molecular Autoimmunity*, (ed. N. Talal), Academic Press, New York, pp. 31–51.
14. Navarette, C., Jaraquemada, D., Fainboin, L. *et al.* (1985) Genetic and functional relationships of the HLA-DR and HLA-DQ antigens. *Immunogenetics*, **21**, 97–101.

15. Gregerson, P. K., Silver, J. and Winchester, R. J. (1987) The shared epitope hypothesis. An approach to understanding the molecular genetics of susceptibility to rheumatoid arthritis. *Arth. Rheum.*, **30**, 1205–13.

16. Tambur, A. R., Friedmann, A., Safirmann, C. *et al.* (1993) Molecular analysis of HLA class II genes in primary Sjögren's syndrome: a study of Israeli and Greek non-Jewish patients. *Human Immunol.*, **36**, 235–42.

17. Reveille, J. D., Macteod, M. J., Whittington, K. *et al.* (1991) Specific amino acid residues in the second hypervariable region of HLA-DQA_1 and DQB_1 chain genes promote the Ro(SSA)/La(SSB) autoantibody responses. *J. Immunol.*, **146**, 3871–5.

18. Moutsopoulos, H. M. and Papadopoulos, G. K. (1992) Possible viral implication in the pathogenesis of Sjögren's syndrome. *Eur. J. Med.*, **4**, 219–23.

19. Rosenberg, Z. F. and Fauci, A. S. (1991) Immunopathologic mechanisms of human immunodeficiency virus (HIV) infection, in *The Human Retroviruses*, (eds R. C. Gallo and J. Jay), Academic Press, London, pp. 141–61.

20. Hudson, J., Chanther, J., Lok, L. *et al.* (1979) Model systems for analysis of latent CMV infection. *Can. J. Microbiol*, **25**, 245–50.

21. Shillitoe, E. J., Daniels, T. E., Whitcher, J. P. *et al.* (1982) Antibody to cytomegalovirus in patients with Sjögren's syndrome as detected by enzyme-linked immunosorbent assay. *Arth. Rheum.*, **25**, 260–5.

22. Venables, P. J. W., Oss, M. G. R., Charles, P. J. *et al.* (1985) A seroepidemiological study of cytomegalovirus and Epstein-Barr virus in rheumatoid arthritis and sicca syndrome. *Ann. Rheum.*, **44**, 742–6.

23. Chang, R. S., Lewis, J. L. and Abilgaard, C. F. (1973) Prevalence of oropharyngeal excreters of leukocyte-transforming agents among a human population. *N. Eng. J. Med.*, **289**, 1325–9.

24. Wolf, H., Haus, M. and Wilmes, E. (1984) Persistence of Epstein-Barr virus in the parotid gland. *J. Virol.*, **51**, 795–8.

25. Slaufhter, A., Carson, D. A., Jensen, F. C. *et al.* (1978) *In vitro* effects of Epstein–Barr virus on peripheral blood mononuclear cells from patients with rheumatoid arthritis and normal subjects. *J. Exp. Med.*, **148**, 1429–34.

26. Lerner, M. P., Andrews, N. C., Miller, G. *et al.* (1981) Two small RNAs encoded by Epstein–Barr virus and complexed with protein are precipitated by antibodies from patients with systemic lupus erythematosus. *Proc. Natl. Acad. Sci. (USA)*, **78**, 805–9.

27. Mariette, X., Gozlan, J., Clerk, D. *et al.* (1991) Detection of Epstein–Barr virus DNA by *in situ* hybridization and polymerase chain reaction in salivary gland biopsy specimens from patients with Sjögren's syndrome. *Am. J. Med.*, **90**, 286–94.

28. Haddad, J., Deny, P., Munz-Gothiel, C. *et al.* (1992) Lymphocytic sialadenitis of Sjögren's syndrome associated with chronic hepatitis C virus liver disease. *Lancet*, **339**, 321–3.

29. Vitali, C., Sciuto, M., Neri, R. *et al.* (1992) Anti-hepatitis C virus antibodies in primary Sjögren's syndrome: false positive results are related to hyper-γ-globulinemia. *Clin. Exp. Rheumatol.*, **10**, 103–4.

30. Green, J. B., Hinricks, S. H., Vogen, J. *et al.* (1989) Exocrinopathy resembling Sjögren's syndrome in HTLV-I tax transgenic mice. *Nature*, **341**, 72–4.

31. Saito, I., Nishimura, S., Kudo, I. *et al.* (1991) Adult T-cell leukemia-derived factor (ADF) in Sjögren's syndrome (Abstract). *Clin, Exp. Rheumatol*, **9**, 336.

32. Shattles, W. R., Brookes, S. M., Venables, P. J. W. *et al.* (1992) Expression of antigen reactive with a monoclonal antibody to HTLV-1 p19 in salivary glands in Sjögren's syndrome. *Clin. Exp. Immunol.*, **89**, 46–51.

33. Perk, A., Rosenblat, J. D., Chen, I. S. Y. *et al.* (1989) Detection and cloning of new HTLV-related endogenous sequences in man. *Nucl. Acids Res.*, **17**, 6841–54.

34. Talal, N., Dauphinee, M. J., Dang, H. *et al.* (1990) Detection of serum antibodies to retroviral proteins in patients with primary Sjögren's syndrome (autoimmune exocrinopathy). *Arth. Rheum.*, **33**, 774–81.

35. Garry, R. F., Fermin, C. D., Hart, D. J. *et al.* (1990) Detection of a human intracisternal A-type retroviral particle antigenically related to HIV. *Science*, **250**, 1127–9.

36. Flescher, E., Dauphinee, M. J., Fossum, D. *et al.* (1992) Signal transduction in Sjögren's syndrome T cells. Abnormalities associated with a newly described human A-type retrovirus. *Arth. Rheum.*, **35**, 1068–74.

37. Baboonian, C., Venables, P. J. W., Booth, J. *et al.* (1989) Virus infection induces redistribution and membrane localization of the nuclear antigen La(SSB): a possible mechanism

for autoimmunity. *Clin. Exp. Immunol.*, **78**, 454–9.

38. Bodeutsch, C., De Wilde, P. C. M., Kater, L. *et al.* (1992) Quantitative immunohistologic criteria are superior to the lymphocytic focus score criterion for the diagnosis of Sjögren's syndrome. *Arth. Rheum.*, **35**, 1075–87.

39. Bodeutsch, C., De Wilde, P., Van Den Hoogen, F. *et al.* (1992) Overexpression of La/SS-B antigen in labial salivary glands of patients with Sjögren's syndrome. *Clin. Rheumatol.*, **11**, 122 (Abstract).

40. Yannopoulos, D. I., Roncin, S., Lamour, A. *et al.* (1992) Conjunctival epithelial cells from patients with Sjögren's syndrome inappropriately express major histocompatibility complex molecules; La(SSB) antigen, and heat-shock proteins. *J. Clin. Immunol.*, **12**, 259–65.

41. Boumpas, D. T., Eleftheriades, E. G., Molina, R. *et al.* (1990) C-myc proto-oncogene expression in peripheral blood mononuclear cells from patients with primary Sjögren's syndrome. *Arth. Rheum.*, **33**, 49–56.

42. Skopouli, F. N., Kousvelari, E. E., Mertz, P. *et al.* (1992) C-myc mRNA expression in minor salivary glands of patients with Sjögren's syndrome. *J. Rheum.*, **19**, 693–9.

43. Wolin, S. L. and Steitz, J. A. (1984) The Ro small cytoplasmic ribonucleoproteins: identification of the antigenic protein and its binding site on the Ro RNAs. *Proc. Natl. Acad. Sci. (USA)*, **81**, 1996–2000.

44. Slobbe, R. L., Pruijn, G. J. M. and Van Venrooij, W. J. (1991) Ro(SSA) and La(SSB) ribonucleoprotein complexes: structure, function and antigenicity. *Ann. Med. Interne*, **142**, 592–600.

45. Chan, E. K. L. and Tan, E. M. (1989) Epitopic targets for autoantibodies in systemic lupus erythematosus and Sjögren's syndrome. *Curr. Opin. Rheumatol.*, **1**, 376–81.

46. Scofield, R. H. and Harley, J. B. (1991) Autoantigenicity of Ro/SSA antigen is related to a nucleocapsid protein of vesicular stomatitis virus. *Proc. Natl. Acad. Sci. (USA)*, **88**, 3343–7.

47. Ben-Chetrit, E., Fox, R. I. and Tan, E. M. (1990) Dissociation of immune response to the SS-A (Ro) 52-kD and 60-kD polypeptides in systemic lupus erythematosus and Sjögren's syndrome. *Arth. Rheum.*, **33**, 349–55.

48. Chambers, J. C., Kenan, D., Martin, B. J. *et al.* (1988) Genomic structure and amino acid sequence domains of the human La autoantigen. *J. Biol. Chem.*, **263**, 18043–051.

49. St. Clair, E. W., Burch, J. A., Ward, M. M. *et al.* (1988) Analysis of autoantibody binding to different regions of the human La antigen expressed in recombinant fusion proteins. *J. Immunol.*, **141**, 4173–80.

50. Manoussakis, M. N., Tzioufas, A. G., Pange, P. J. E. *et al.* (1986) Serological profiles in subgroups of patients with Sjögren's syndrome. *Scand. J. Rheum.*, **61**, (suppl), 89–92.

51. Moutsopoulos, H. M., Steinberg, A. D., Fauci, A. S. *et al.* (1983) High incidence of free monoclonal labda light chains in the sera of patients with Sjögren's syndrome. *J. Immunol.*, **130**, 2263–5.

52. Moutsopoulos, H. M., Costello, R., Drosos, A. A. *et al.* (1985) Demonstration and identification of monoclonal proteins in the urine of patients with Sjögren's syndrome. *Ann. Rheum. Dis.*, **44**, 109–12.

53. Walters, M. T., Stevenson, F. K., Hervert, A. *et al.* (1986) Urinary monoclonal free light chains in primary Sjögren's syndrome: an aid to the diagnosis of malignant lymphoma. *Ann. Rheum. Dis.*, **45**, 210–19.

54. Tzioufas, A. G., Manoussakis, M. N., Costello, R. *et al.* (1986) Cryoglobulinemia in autoimmune rheumatic disease; evidence of circulating monoclonal cryoglobulins in patients with primary Sjögren's syndrome. *Arth. Rheum.*, **29**, 1098–104.

55. Kassan, S. S., Thomas, T., Moutsopoulos, H. M. *et al.* (1978) Increased risk of lymphoma in sicca syndrome. *Ann. Intern. Med.*, **89**, 888–92.

56. Moutsopoulos, H. M., Tzioufas, A. G., Bai, M. *et al.* (1990) Primary Sjögren's syndrome: serum monoclonality is associated with a monoclonal B cell subset infiltrating the minor salivary glands. *Ann. Rheum. Dis.*, **49**, 929–31.

57. Freimark, B., Fantozzi, R., Bone, R. *et al.* (1989) Detection of clonally expanded salivary gland lymphocytes in Sjögren's syndrome. *Arth. Rheum.*, **32**, 859–69.

58. Kunkel, H. G., Angello, V., Joslin, F. G. *et al.* (1973) Cross-idiotypic specificity among monoclonal IgM proteins with anti-gammaglobulin activity. *J. Exp. Med.*, **331**, 42.

59. Agnelo, V., Arbetter, A., Ibanez, A. *et al.* (1980) Evidence for a subset of rheumatoid factors that cross react with DNA-histone and have a distinct cross-idiotype. *J. Exp. Med.*, **151**, 1514–27.

60. Carson, D. A. and Fong, S. (1983) A common

idiotype on human rheumatoid factors identified by a hybridoma antibody. *Molec. Immunol.*, **20**, 1081–7.

61. Kipps, T. J., Tomhave, E., Chen, P. P. *et al.* (1989) Molecular characterization of a major autoantibody associated cross-reactive idiotype in Sjögren's syndrome and rheumatoid factor associated cross reactive idiotype. *J. Immunol.*, **142**, 4261–8.

62. Mageed, R. A., Dearlove, M., Goodall, D. M. *et al.* (1986) Immunogenic and antigenic epitopes of immunoglobulins, XVII-monoclonal antibodies reactive with common and restricted idiotypes to the heavy chain of human rheumatoid factors. *Rheumatol. Int.*, **6**, 179–83.

63. Gharavi, A. E., Patel, E. M., Hughes, G. R. V. *et al.* (1985) Common IgA and IgM rheumatoid factors idiotypes in autoimmune diseases. *Ann. Rheum. Dis.*, **44**, 155–8.

64. Fox, R. I., Chen, P., Carson, D. A. *et al.* (1986) Expression of a cross-reactive idiotype on rheumatoid factor in patients with Sjögren's syndrome. *J. Immunol.*, **136**, 477–83.

65. Katsikis, P. D., Youinou, P. Y., Galanopoulou, V. *et al.* (1990) Monoclonal process in primary Sjögren's syndrome and rheumatoid factor associated cross reactive idiotype. *Clin. Exp. Immunol.*, **82**, 509–14.

66. Tzioufas, A. G., Boumba, D. S., Skopouli, F. N. *et al.* (1992) Inheritance of monoclonal rheumatoid factor cross-reactive idiotypes in primary Sjögren's syndrome (pSS). Comparative study of a rabbit polyclonal anti-idiotype and 17109 monoclonal anti-idiotype. *Eur. J. Clin. Invest.*, **22**, 475–81.

67. Moutsopoulos, H. M. and Fauci, A. S. (1980) Immunoregulation in Sjögren's syndrome. Influence of serum factors on T-cell subpopulation. *J. Clin. Invest.*, **65**, 519–28.

68. Bakshi, A., Miyasaka, N., Kavathas, P. *et al.* (1983) Lymphocyte subsets in Sjögren's syndrome: a quantitative analysis using monoclonal antibodies and the fluorescence-activated cell sorter. *J. Clin. Lab. Immunol.*, **10**, 63–9.

69. Fox, R. I., Robinson, C. A., Curd, J. G. *et al.* (1986) Sjögren's syndrome. Proposed criteria for classification. *Arth. Rheum.*, **29**, 577–85.

70. Moutsopoulos, H. M. and Talal, N. (1987) Immunologic abnormalities in Sjögren's syndrome, in *Sjögren's Syndrome. Clinical and Immunological Aspects*, (eds N. Talal, H. M. Moutsopoulos, S. S. Kassan), Springer-Verlag, pp. 258–65.

71. Skopouli, F. N., Fox, P. C., Galanopoulou, V. *et al.* (1991) T-cell subpopulations in the labial minor salivary gland histopathological lesion of Sjögren's syndrome. *J. Rheum.*, **18**, 210–14.

72. Sumida, T., Yonaha, F., Maeda, T. *et al.* (1992) T-cell receptor repertoire of infiltrating T-cells in lips of Sjögren's syndrome patients. *J. Clin. Invest.*, **89**, 681–5.

73. Kappler, J., Kotzin, B., Herron, L. *et al.* (1989) V_β specific stimulation of human T cells by staphylococcal toxins. *Science*, **244**, 811–13.

74. Youaha, F., Sumida, T., Maeda, T. *et al.* (1992) Restricted junctional usage of T cell receptor $V_{\beta 2}$ and $V_{\beta 13}$ genes, which are overpresented on infiltrating T cells in the lips of patients with Sjögren's syndrome. *Arth. Rheum.*, **35**, 1362–6.

75. Anderson, L. G., Cummings, N. A., Asofsky, R. *et al.* (1972) Salivary gland immunoglobulin and rheumatoid factor synthesis in Sjögren's syndrome: natural history and response to treatment. *Am. J. Med.*, **49**, 49–54.

76. Lane, H. C., Callihan, T. R., Jaffe, E. S. *et al.* (1983) Presence of intracytoplasmic IgG in the lymphocytic infiltrates of the minor salivary glands of patients with primary Sjögren's syndrome. *Clin. Exp. Rheumatol.*, **1**, 237–9.

77. Bodeuitsch, C., de Wilde, P. C. M., Kater, L. (1992) Quantitative immunohistologic criteria are superior to the lymphocytic focus score criterion for the diagnosis of Sjögren's syndrome. *Arth. Rheum.*, **35**, 1075–87.

78. St. Clair, E. W., Angellilo, J. C. and Signer, K. H. (1992) Expression of cell adhesion molecules in the salivary gland microenvironment of Sjögren's syndrome. *Arth. Rheum.*, **35**, 62–6.

79. Singer, K. H., Harden, E. A., Robertson, A. L. *et al.* (1985) *In vitro* growth and phenotypic characterization of mesodermal-derived and epithelial components of normal and abnormal human thymes. *Human. Immunol.*, **13**, 161–76.

80. Springer, T. A. (1990) Adhesion receptors of the immune system. *Nature*, **346**, 425–34.

81. Bendtzen, K. (1989) Immune hormones (cytokines); pathogenetic role in autoimmune rheumatic and endocrine diseases. *Autoimmunity*, **2**, 177–89.

82. Skopouli, F. N., Siouna-Fatourou, H. I., Ziciadis, C. *et al.* (1989) Evaluation of unstimulated whole saliva flow rate and stimulated parotid flow as confirmatory tests for xerostomia. *Clin. Exp. Rheumatol.*, **7**, 127–9.

83. Daniels, T. E. and Talal, N. (1987) Diagnosis and differential diagnosis of Sjögren's syndrome, in *Sjögren's syndrome. Clinical and Immunological Aspects* (eds N. Talal, H. M. Moutsopoulos, S. S. Kassan), Berlin, Springer-Verlag, p. 193–9.

84. Moutsopoulos, H. M. and Talal, N. (1989) New developments in Sjögren's syndrome. *Curr. Opin. Rheumatol.*, **1**, 332–8.

85. Vitali, C., Tavoni, A., Simi, U. *et al.* (1988) Parotid sialography and minor salivary gland biopsy in the diagnosis of Sjögren's syndrome: a comparative study of 84 patients. *J. Rheumatol.*, **15**, 262–7.

86. Parrago, G., Rain, G. D., Brochierion, C. *et al.* (1987) Scintigraphy of the salivary glands in Sjögren's syndrome. *J. Clin. Pathol.*, **40**, 1463–7.

87. Markusse, H. M., Pillay, M. and Breedveld, F. C. (1993) The diagnostic value of salivary gland scintigraphy in patients suspected of primary Sjögren's syndrome. *Br. J. Rheumatol.*, (in press).

88. Baum, B. J. and Fox, P. C. (1987) Chemistry in saliva. In *Sjögren's Syndrome. Clinical and Immunological Aspects* (eds N. Talal, H. M. Moutsopoulos, S. S. Kassan), Berlin, Springer-Verlag, pp. 35–40.

89. Kincaid, M. C. (1987) The eye in Sjögren's syndrome, in *Sjögren's Syndrome. Clinical and Immunological Aspects* (eds N. Talal, H. M. Moutsopoulos, S. S. Kassan), Berlin, Springer-Verlag, pp. 35–40.

90. Rosenbaum, J. T. and Bennett, R. M. (1987) Chronic anterior and posterior uveitis and primary Sjögren's syndrome. *Am. J. Ophthalmol.*, **104**, 345–52.

91. Bridges, A. J. and Burns, R. P. (1992) Acute iritis associated with primary Sjögren's syndrome and high titer anti Ro/SSA and anti La/SSB antibodies. Treatment with combination immunosuppressive therapy. *Arth. Rheum.*, **35**, 560–4.

92. Daniels, T. E. (1991) Benign lymphoepithelial lesion and Sjögren's syndrome, in *Surgical Pathology of the Salivary Glands* (eds G. L. Ellis, P. L. Auclair, D. R. Gnepp), Philadelphia, WB Saunders Company, pp. 528–43.

93. Schmidt, V., Helbron, D. and Lennert, K. (1982) Development of malignant lymphoma in myoepithelial sialadenitis (Sjögren's syndrome). *Pathol. Anat.*, **395**, 11–43.

94. Daniels, T. E. Aufdemorte, T. H. B. and Greenspan, J. S. (1987) Histopathology of Sjögren's syndrome, in Sjögren's Syndrome. Clinical and Immunological Aspects, (eds N. Talal, H. M. Moutsopoulos, S. S. Kassan), Berlin, Springer-Verlag, pp. 258–65.

95. De Wilde, P. C. M., Sllotweg, P. J., Hene, R. J. *et al.* (1984) Multinucleate giant cells in sublabial salivary gland tissue in Sjögren's syndrome. A diagnostic pitfall. *Virchows Arch. [Pathol. Anat]*, **403**, 247–56.

96. Daniels, T. E. (1984) Labial salivary biopsy in Sjögren's syndrome: assessment as a diagnostic criterion in 362 suspected cases. *Arth. Rheum.*, **27**, 147–56.

97. Maini, R. N. (1987) The relationship of Sjögren's syndrome to rheumatoid arthritis, in *Sjögren's Syndrome. Clinical and Immunological Aspects* (eds N. Talal, H. M. Moutsopoulos, S. S. Kassan), Berlin, Springer-Verlag, pp. 165–76.

98. Castro-Poltronieri, A. and Alacron-Segovia, D. (1983) Articular manifestation of primary Sjögren's syndrome. *J. Rheumatol.*, **10**, 485–8.

99. Tsampoulas, C. G., Skopouli, F. N., Sartoris, D. J. *et al.* (1980) Hand radiographic changes in patients with primary and secondary Sjögren's syndrome. *Scand. J. Rheumatol.*, **15**, 333–9.

100. Skopouli, F. N., Talal, N. Galanopoulou, V. *et al.* (1990) Raynaud's phenomenon in primary Sjögren's syndrome. *J. Rheumatol*, **17**, 618–20.

101. Vlachoyiannopoulos, P. G., Drosos, A. A., Wiik, A. *et al.* (1993) Patients with anticentromere antibodies: clinical features, diagnosis and evolution. *Br. J. Rheumatol.*, **32**, 297–301.

102. Constantopoulos, S. H., Tsianos, E. B. and Moutsopoulos, H. M. (1992) Pulmonary and gastrointestinal manifestations of Sjögren's syndrome. *Rheum. Dis. Clin. N. Am.*, **18**(3), 617–35.

103. Trevino, H., Tsianos, E. B. and Schenker, S. (1987) Gastrointestinal and hepatobiliary features in Sjögren's syndrome, in *Sjögren's Syndrome. Clinical and Immunological Aspects* (eds N. Talal, H. M. Moutsopoulos, S. S. Kassan), Berlin, Springer-Verlag, pp. 89–95.

104. Tsianos, E. B., Tzioufas, A. G., Kita, M. D. *et al.* (1984) Serum isoamylases in patients with autoimmune rheumatic diseases. *Clin. Exp. Rheumatol.*, **2**, 235–8.

105. Tsianos, E. B., Hoofnagle, J. H., Fox, P. C. *et al.* (1990). Sjögren's syndrome in patients with primary biliary cirrhosis. *Hepatology*, **11**, 730–4.

106. Kassan, S. S. and Talal, N. (1987) Renal disease with Sjögren's syndrome, in *Sjögren's Syndrome. Clinical and Immunological Aspects* (eds N. Talal, H. M. Moutsopoulos, S. S. Kassan), Berlin, Springer-Verlag, pp. 96–101.

107. Moutsopoulos, H. M., Cledes, J., Skopouli, F. N. *et al.* (1991) Nephrocalcinosis in Sjögren's syndrome: a late sequela of renal tubular acidosis. *J. Int. Med.*, **230**, 187–91.

108. Alexander, E. L. (1987) Inflammatory vascular disease in Sjögren's syndrome, in *Sjögren's Syndrome. Clinical and Immunological Aspects*, (eds N. Talal, H. M. Moutsopoulos, S. S. Kassan), Berlin, Springer-Verlag, pp. 102–24.

109. Tsokos, M., Lazarou, S. A. and Moutsopoulos, H. M. (1987) Vasculitis in primary Sjögren's syndrome. Histological classification and clinical presentation. *Am. J. Clin. Pathol.*, **88**, 26–31.

110. Onley, R. K. (1992) Neuropathies in connective tissue disease. *Muscle and Nerve*, **15**, 531–42.

111. Mellgren, S. I., Conn, D. L., Stevens, J. C. *et al.* (1989) Peripheral neuropathy in primary Sjögren's syndrome. *Neurology*, **39**, 390–4.

112. Alexander, E. L. (1987) Neuromuscular complications of primary Sjögren's syndrome, *Sjögren's Syndrome. Clinical and Immunological Aspects*, (eds N. Talal, H. M. Moutsopoulos, S. S. Kassan), Berlin, Springer-Verlag, pp. 61–82.

113. Andonopoulos, A. P., Lagos, G., Drosos, A. A. *et al.* (1990) The spectrum of neurological involvement in Sjögren's syndrome. *Br. J. Rheum.*, **29**, 21–3.

114. Binder, A., Snaith, M. L. and Isenberg, D. (1988) Sjögren's syndrome: a study of its neurological complications. *Br. J. Rheum.*, **27**, 275–80.

115. Noseworthy, H. J., Bass, B. H., Vandervoort, M. K. *et al.* (1989) The prevalence of primary Sjögren's syndrome in a multiple sclerosis population. *Ann. Neurol.*, **29**, 95–8.

116. Miro, J., Pena-Sagredo, J. L., Bercano, J. *et al.* (1990) Prevalence of primary Sjögren's syndrome in patients with multiple sclerosis. *Ann. Neurol.*, **27**, 582–4.

117. Leroy, J. P., Drosos, A. A., Yiannopoulos, D. I. *et al.* (1990) Intravenous pulse cyclophosphamide therapy in myositis and Sjögren's syndrome. *Arth. Rheum.*, **33**, 1579–81.

118. Karsh, J., Pavlidis, N., Neitraub, B. D. *et al.*

(1980) Thyroid disease in Sjögren's syndrome. *Arth. Rheum.*, **23**, 1326–9.

119. Moutsopoulos, H. M., Elkon, K. B., Mavridis, A. K., *et al.* (1983) Serum C-reactive protein in primary Sjögren's syndrome. *Clin. Exp. Rheumatol.*, **1**, 57–8.

120. Tzioufas, A. G., Moutsopoulos, H. M. and Talal, N. (1987) Lymphoid malignancy and monoclonal proteins, in *Sjögren's Syncrome. Clinical and Immunological Aspects* (eds N. Talal, H. M. Moutsopoulos, S. S. Kassan). Berlin, Springer-Verlag, pp. 129–36.

121. Pavlidis, N. A., Drosos, A. A., Papadimitriou, C. *et al.* (1992) Lymphoma in Sjögren's syndrome. *Med. Ped. Oncology*, **20**, 279–83.

122. Andonopoulos, A. P., Drosos, A. A., Skopouli, F. N. *et al.* (1987) Secondary Sjögren's syndrome in rheumatoid arthritis. *J. Rheumatol.*, **1**, 1098–103.

123. Moutsopoulos, H. M., Webber, B. L., Vlagopoulos, T. P. *et al.* (1979) Differences in the clinical manifestations of sicca syndrome in the presence and absence of rheumatoid arthritis. *Am. J. Med.*, **66**, 733–5.

124. Heaton, J. M. (1959) Sjögren's syndrome and systemic lupus erythematosus. *Br. Med. J.*, **1**, 466–9.

125. Skopouli, F. N., Siouna-Fatourou, H., Dimou, G. S. *et al.* (1991) Histologic lesion in labial salivary glands of patients with systemic lupus erythematosus. *Oral. Surg. Oral Med. Oral Pathol.*, **72**, 208–12.

126. Medsger, T. A. (1987) Sjögren's syndrome and systemic sclerosis (scleroderma), in *Sjögren's Syndrome. Clinical and Immunological Aspects* (eds N. Talal, H. M. Moutsopoulos, S. S. Kassan), Berlin, Springer-Verlag, pp. 182–7.

127. Andonopoulos, A. P., Drosos, A. A., Skopouli, F. N. *et al.* (1989) Secondary Sjögren's syndrome in rheumatoid arthritis and progressive systemic sclerosis. A comparative study. *Clin. Exp. Rheumatol.*, **7**, 203–5.

128. Drosos, A. A., Pennec, Y. L., Elisaf, M., Lamour, A. *et al.* (1991) Sjögren's syndrome in patients with the CREST variant of progressive systemic scleroderma. *J. Rheumatol.*, **18**, 1685–8.

129. Bloch, K. J., Buchanan, W. W., Wohl, M. J. *et al.* (1965) Sjögren's syndrome: a clinical pathological and serological study of sixty-two cases. *Medicine* (Baltimore) **44**, 187–231.

130. Drosos, A. A., Constantopoulos, S. H., Psychos, D. *et al.* (1989) The forgotten cause of

sicca complex; sarcoidosis. *J. Rheumatol.*, **16**, 1548–51.

131. Itescu, S., Brancato, L. J., Buxbaum, J. *et al.* (1990) A diffuse infiltrative CD8 lymphocytosis syndrome in human immunodeficiency virus (HIV) infection: a host immune response associated with HLA-DR5. *Ann. Int. Med.*, **112**, 3–10.

132. Talal, N. and Moutsopoulos, H. M. (1987) Treatment of Sjögren's syndrome, in *Sjögren's Syndrome. Clinical and Immunological Aspects* (eds N. Talal, H. M. Moutsopoulos, S. S. Kassan), Berlin, Springer-Verlag, pp. 291–5.

133. Fox, R. I., Chan, E., Benton, L. *et al.* (1988) Treatment of primary Sjögren's syndrome with hydroxychloroquine. *Am. J. Med.*, **85** (Suppl 4A), 62–7.

J. J. F. Belch and C. Maple

INTRODUCTION

In 1862 Maurice Raynaud defined this syndrome which now bears his name[1]. He described episodic ischemia of the digits provoked by cold and emotion. It manifests clinically by a tri-phasic color change: pallor, cyanosis and rubor: vasospasm in the digits leads to the pallor (Figure 6.1); subsequent venostasis – the cyanosis; and hyperemia following return of blood flow is responsible for the rubor. Raynaud's original definition requires some modification today, since it is now known that a full tri-phasic color change is not necessary for the diagnosis to be made. A history of cold-induced blanching alone or with subsequent reactive hyperemia may reflect significant underlying vasospasm. Furthermore cold and emotion are not the only stimuli which provide attacks – chemicals including tobacco[2], hormones[3] and trauma have also been implicated.

Raynaud's phenomenon (RP) is a common disorder affecting between 20–30% of the female population[4]. Although it is mild and benign in most cases, it can be severe and, in a small number of cases, threaten the viability of the digits. Although its existence has been recognized for over 130 years, there is still a lack of understanding of the etiology and pathophysiology of the condition. This has led to difficulties in the treatment of the condition and in the prediction of its prognosis. Recently, extensive research has, however, improved our diagnostic ability and is enabling a greater understanding of the condition.

NOMENCLATURE: RAYNAUD'S PHENOMENON, SYNDROME OR DISEASE?

Inconsistency in the terminology used to describe Raynaud's attacks has been one of the main problems for the clinician involved in the management of RP. Raynaud's phenomenon is the general term used by Europeans to describe cold-related digital vasospasm. It is subdivided according to the presence or absence of an associated disorder: Raynaud's syndrome (RS) is the term used if there is an associated disorder and primary Raynaud's disease (RD), if there is not. This European classification, however, is not globally accepted. Australasia and the USA tend to use the term phenomenon (Chapters 3 and 4). A further difficulty with nomenclature is that an associated disorder may not be apparent at the time of initial presentation, and RP may precede any subsequent systemic illness by more than 20 years[5].

ASSOCIATED DISORDERS

As many as 50% of the patients referred to hospital with vasospasm have an associated systemic disease, i.e. RS[6]. This is not surprising as one of the early markers for RS is severity of symptoms[7], hence these patients

Connective Tissue Diseases. Edited by Jill J. F. Belch and Robert B. Zurier. Published in 1995 by Chapman & Hall, London.
ISBN 0 412 48620 2

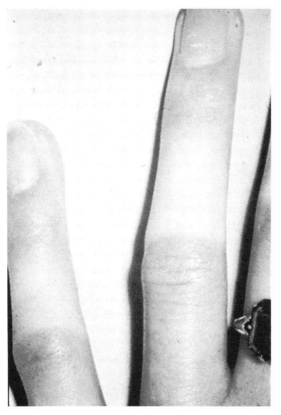

Fig. 6.1 A typical Raynauds attack.

are more likely to be referred to a hospital specialist. There is thus a higher proportion of RS in the hospital population than in general practice. Conditions associated with RS are listed in Table 6.1.

The connective tissue disorders (CTDs) are the most commonly associated disorders especially systemic sclerosis (SSc), mixed connective tissue disease (MCTD) but also systemic lupus erythematosus, Sjögren's syndrome, polymyositis and dermatomyositis[8]. RS occurs in rheumatoid arthritis and hyperviscosity syndromes in a percentage similar to that seen in the normal population (10%); however, the symptoms tend to be more severe.

Atherosclerosis is a common cause of RS in patients whose symptoms develop after the age of 60 years[9]. Thromboangiitis obliterans

(Buerger's disease) should also be considered in smokers who present in their 40s with RP.

Occupational-induced RP should also be considered in young male patients. Occupational RP can have many etiologies. Workers exposed to polyvinylchloride (PVC) can develop RP of occupational origin and vasospasm can occur in ammunition workers outside their place of work when the vasodilatory effects of nitrates are removed. Vibration white finger disease (VWF) is the most common form of occupational RS[6]. As its name suggests, VWF occurs in workers exposed to vibrating machines, such as chain saws, pneumatic grinders and buffs. It is estimated that about half of all workers using vibrating equipment can develop RS, although resolution of the symptoms may occur in 25% if a job change is effected early in the course of the disease, i.e. before achieving grade 2 on the Taylor–Pelmear scale of classification[10]. Clinicians previously thought that the vibration damage was limited to the hands in this form of RS. However, vasospasm in the toes has recently been described[11]. The development of occupational RP can also be associated with the long-term exposure to cold, and occurs in those who work with fish or in frozen food processing factories.

Many other conditions are associated with RS and the challenge of this condition is in differentiating between primary RD and secondary RS. Furthermore, early detection of those who may progress to the development of CTD is important, so that the correct management may be introduced early in the disease process.

CLINICAL PRESENTATION

RP is nine times more common in women than in men and has an overall prevalence in the population of approximately 10%. It may, however, have an increased prevalence in the younger age groups affecting as many as 20–30% of young women[4]. There is also a

Table 6.1   Conditions associated with Raynaud's syndrome (incidence %)

Connective tissue disorders
Systemic sclerosis (90%)
Systemic lupus erythematosus
Rheumatoid arthritis (10–15%)
Mixed connective tissue disease
Sjögren's syndrome
Dermatomyositis/polymyositis

Drugs
Egotamine and other migraine therapies
Beta blockers
Cytotoxics
Cyclosporin
Bromocriptine
Sulphasalazine

Occupation related
Vinyl chloride disease
Vibration white finger disease
Ammunition workers (outside work)
Frozen food packers

Obstructive
Thoracic outlet syndrome (e.g. cervical rib)
Atherosclerosis (especially thrombangiitis obliterans)
Micro-emboli

Metabolic and other
Endocrine (e.g. hypothyroidism)
Cryoglobulinemia
Malignancy
Uremia
Hepatitis B antigenemia
Reflex sympathetic dystrophy
Arteriovenous fistula

familial predisposition which is more marked if the age of onset is less than 30 years[8].

The diagnosis Raynaud's phenomenon requires the presence of episodic ischemia of the extremities producing blanching. This may be the presenting symptom of the patient or it may be elucidated during careful history taking. Occasionally, patients do not notice the pallor and it is the painful reactive hyperemia which causes their symptoms. In these patients digital blood pressure measurement before and after a cold challenge will often help to clarify the diagnosis. Patients who only report purple/blue discoloration of the digits on exposure to cold have acrocyanosis.

Although RP symptoms are characteristically located in the fingers and toes, similar symptoms can be observed in the ears lobes and the tip of the nose. The patient with RP may also suffer vasospasm in other areas, the so-called 'systemic vasospasm' (Table 6.2). Studies have shown an association between RP and migraine headaches and with non-specific or musculoskeletal chest pain[12].

Vasospasm in the lungs has also been documented with a reduction in the lung defusing capacity after the induction of digital vasospasm by a cold challenge[13]. Coronary artery spasm[14] may also occur in these patients. Indeed, the myocardial contraction band necrosis seen in patients with CTDs may result from RP of the intramural vessels. Furthermore, the esophageal symptoms which are present in an estimated 75% of patients with RS and the CTD SSc[15], may well be due to esophageal vasospasm, as reduction in esophageal blood flow has been detected in patients with RP following a cold challenge with a subsequent delay in re-warming time[16]. Patients with RP also have evidence of a prolonged reduction in retinal blood flow following cold challenge to the hands[17]. With this evidence of vasospasm in the heart, lung, esophagus and retina it is interesting to speculate that abnormalities of the vasculature may exist throughout the entire patient. They may contribute to the wide spectrum of symptoms seen in patients

Table 6.2   The systemic nature of Raynaud's phenomenon

Periphery	Fingers	
	Toes	
	Earlobes	
	Nose	
Gastrointestinal tract	Tongue	
	Esophagus	
Respiratory tract	Pulmonary vasculature	
Cardiovascular system	Cardiac vessels	(angina)
	Peripheral vessels	(essential hypertension)
	Cerebral vessels	(migraine)
Central nervous system	Retina	
Genitourinary tract	Kidney	(renal lesions)
	Uterine vessels	(infertility)
		(abortion)
		(pregnancy induced hypertension)
	Vasovasorum	(impotence)

with RP, such as pregnancy-induced hypertension, infertility, hypertension and impotence.

THE DIAGNOSIS OF RAYNAUD'S PHENOMENON

In the majority of cases, the diagnosis of RP can be made from the clinical history. A history of digital blanching on exposure to cold with or without cyanosis or rubor in the absence of clinical evidence of obstructive vascular disease allows the diagnosis of RP to be made. It is only rarely that objective measures of blood flow are needed, e.g. when the patient is unable to give a clear history, or in the presence of occlusive vascular disease when the contribution of vasospasm to the clinical problem needs to be determined. Significant occlusive vascular disease is likely if the systolic pressure of one arm is significantly lower than the other ($\geqslant$15 mm of mercury difference). If both appear low then formal arm blood flow measurements should be carried out.

There are many different techniques which can be used to measure blood flow to the digits. However, satisfactory standards of measurement have not yet been adequately established due to their variation in healthy individuals, especially after a cold challenge. In clinical practice, measurement of digital systolic blood pressure following local cooling of the hand in cool water at a temperature of approximately 15°C is widely used due to its simplicity. A drop in the pressure of more than 30 mmHg is usually considered significant[18]. This technique, however, will give a number of false negatives unless the following five precautions are observed:

1. To avoid recording a poor flow prior to the start of the test the patient must be warm and vasodilated before the first pressure recordings. The best way to obtain this is by leaving the patient to acclimatize in a temperature-stable laboratory for a period of half an hour.

2. Poor flow can also occur at the time of ovulation in women[3]. Assessment should be avoided mid-cycle in premenopausal women.

3. Drug-induced vasodilatation can also lead to a failure to detect a pressure drop. All vasoactive medication should be stopped 24 hours prior to testing, should such testing be considered necessary.

4. Tests carried out shortly after a Raynaud's

attack will also fail to produce a significant pressure drop as the cold challenge cannot overcome the ischemia induced reactive hyperemia.

5. Additionally, if the patient comes in from a warm environment, the body itself is warm and this protects the patient from developing vasospasm if digital cooling is used in isolation. Total body cooling in an environmental chamber may also be required during the summer months.

The digital systolic blood pressure measurements are most commonly made using strain gauge plethysmography. The disadvantages of this test are that considerable skill on the part of the operator is required, its measurement is discontinuous so that it cannot assess changes in flow and in fingers with fibrosed subcutaneous tissue as in the CTDs blood flow can be difficult to measure. Conversely, the technique is also inadequate for measuring high blood flow. Photoplethysmography can also be used, furthermore the advent of more sophisticated and sensitive Doppler ultrasound equipment makes it possible to measure the pressure at which the return of flow occurs by this method.

Thermography uses skin temperature as an indication of finger blood flow. However, skin temperature is not only dependent on blood flow but also receives a contribution from venous and arterial blood and results must be interpreted with caution.

Laser Doppler flowmetry has become popular for evaluating the skin microcirculation[19]. The nature of the signal detected is related almost exclusively to the velocity and number of moving red blood cells. Measurement occurs directly and continuously with a short response time and it is a non-invasive technique. This makes it ideally suited for measuring changes in microcirculatory flow. The same precautions apply to this technique as for the digital systolic blood pressure estimation, however, and

furthermore a temperature controlled environment is required.

Radioisotope clearance methods, where the patient is given an injection of a radioactive preparation over the area of measurement, can also be used. However, varying injection depth and tissue damage caused by the injection are potential sources of error. Additionally, the method is costly and the procedure is, by necessity, invasive[18].

Each of the above techniques, apart from the first, require sophisticated equipment and although they can be usefully employed in RP there are numerous drawbacks. Unless one is involved in clinical trials where accurate assessment of flow is required, measurement of the digital systolic blood pressures before and after cold challenge is usually sufficient for the diagnosis to be made.

RAYNAUD'S PHENOMENON AS A PRECURSOR OF CONNECTIVE TISSUE DISEASE

Once the diagnosis of RP is confirmed, a search for associated disorders should be undertaken. As RP is a common condition such a programme should be simple, relatively cheap, sensitive and non-invasive (Table 6.3). A detailed history is essential. Those with an obvious associated disorder will be easily detected, but difficulties arise in the early diagnosis of CTD or in predicting those likely to progress to CTD. Early studies suggest progression to CTD occurs in between 24%[20] to 50%[21] of cases. At present, the frequency with which secondary conditions are recognized varies widely with reported studies and may depend in part on the thoroughness with which the search for an associated disorder is undertaken, on the stage of development of the RP at the time seen and on clinician referral patterns. This latter aspect is clearly illustrated by Edwards and Porter[22]. In 1976 the authors reported an incidence of RS of 81% in their population of 100 RP patients. By 1988 the study

Table 6.3 Investigation of Raynaud's phenomenon

1. History	(include drug history)
2. Examination	
3. Laboratory tests	Full blood count (including white cell count and platelet count)
Hematology	Erythrocyte sedimentation rate/plasma and viscosity von Willebrand factor*
	Cryoglobulin/cryofibrinogen*
Biochemistry	Serum electrolytes
	Thyroid function tests
Immunopathology	Auto antibodies RA-latex
	Antinuclear factor
	Anticentromere antibody
	Antitopoisomerase antibody
Urinalysis	
4. Radiology	Chest X-ray* (first line if uni-lateral Raynaud's in hands)
5. Vascular assessment	+/− Cold challenge
	Strain gauge or photoplethysmography
	Laser Doppler flowmetry*
	Thermography*
6. Capillary microscopy	

* Second line tests.

population had grown to 615 patients, but the percentage of those with RS had fallen to 46%. The authors commented that in the early years of their studies the patients were only referred if severely symptomatic. As the authors' interest in RP became more widely recognized, more patients with milder symptoms were referred.

The early detection of a CTD in a patient with RP can be difficult, but recently more clearly defined pointers have been described which have strong links with disease progression and these are important in the management of the patient with RP. There are three areas which should be evaluated:

1. clinical features;
2. microscopic nailfold examination; and
3. laboratory tests.

CLINICAL FEATURES

The occurrence of certain clinical features suggests a high probability of disease progression (Table 6.4). The American Rheumatism Association criteria for the various CTDs

Table 6.4 Features which may differentiate syndrome from disease

Raynaud's syndrome	*Raynaud's disease*
Older age group	Younger age group
Children (<10 years)	
Attacks in 1 or 2 fingers initially	Four fingers affected and often symmetrical
Year-round attacks	Cold weather only
Any feature of CTD	Vasospasm in isolation
No family history	Family history
Anemia (normochromic) (macrocytic)	Normal hemoglobin or microcytic anemia
Autoantibodies present	
Basal fibrosis on chest X-ray	
Abnormal capillaroscopy	No visible nailfold capillaries

have high specificity but low sensitivity[23]. Therefore, patients who present with isolated features of CTD will not fulfil the ARA criteria;

nevertheless, these RP patients are more likely to develop a CTD than those without such symptoms[6]. In particular, digital ulceration, sclerodactyly and pitting scars over the finger pulp are strongly associated with later CTD development. Thus any features of CTD occurring in association with RP should alert the clinician.

The severity of the RP is said to be a strong indicator of progression to CTD[7]. Age of onset of RP may also be important. RP is a frequent finding in young women in their teens and 20s and most have primary RD[4]. Those presenting for the first time in their third and fourth decades are more at risk of developing RS[24]. In patients with RP onset at age 60 years or above, 80% will have an associated disorder though in this older age group the majority of cases are secondary to atherosclerosis[9]. Conversely, RP occurring in very young children, though rare, is usually due to an underlying CTD[25]. It is also of interest that those patients who do develop the CTD SSc, but whose symptoms are preceded by RP spanning many years, are much more likely to develop the limited form of SSc formerly 'CREST syndrome'. Those presenting with SSc within a year of onset of RP tend to have diffuse SSc. Other suspicious symptoms which should perhaps alert the clinician are the occurrence of chilblains in adults, the occurrence of severe attacks persisting throughout the summer months and an asymmetrical color change with a few digits involved initially. Questions relating to the patient's occupation or cold exposure will often, particularly in men, allow a diagnosis of VWF to be made, but it is important to remember that various 'female-associated' appliances, such as floor-polishers and industrial sewing machines, can have similar effects on the microvasculature. Drug history is equally important and it should be noted that even the cardioselective beta blockers produce a degree of peripheral vasoconstriction (Table 6.1).

A full physical examination is, of course,

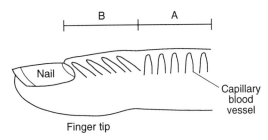

Fig. 6.2 Schematic representation of abnormal nail fold vessels.

essential. Not only to assess the above, but also to gauge the presence of obstructive vascular disease and search for signs of associated autoimmune conditions, such as thyroid dysfunction and vitiligo.

NAILFOLD CAPILLAROSCOPY

Particular attention should be paid to the microscopic examination of the nailfolds. Direct observation of the nailfold capillaries dates back to the early 1900s. Recent refinements have permitted photographic recordings of the rows of horizontal capillary loops at the nailfold just above the cuticle[26]. However, the clinician can examine the nailfold vessels as part of her/his routine clinical workup using a simple ophthalmoscope at the highest power. Normally, no vessels can be seen but patients with RP likely to progress to a CTD have abnormally dilated nailfold capillary loops (Figure 6.2). Although detection of such vessels is one of the most sensitive markers for disease progression, it should be noted that these abnormal vessels can appear in other microangiopathic states, such as diabetes mellitus and after trauma.

LABORATORY TESTS

Laboratory tests should include routine blood biochemistry, including thyroid hormone, levels as hypothyroidism is associated with RP. A full blood count should be carried out. The normochromic, normocytic anemia of a chronic disorder can be found in RS or iron deficiency anemia in a young woman which augments the symptoms of primary RD. A macrocytosis may reflect an associated auto-immune disorder. The ESR or plasma viscosity is usually normal in RD, but may be elevated in RS. It should be noted, however, that there may be some impairment of the acute-phase response in SSc[27] resulting in a normal ESR or plasma viscosity. Urinalysis and serum electrolytes will help to detect early renal disease in CTD or diabetes and a chest X-ray will determine whether a bony cervical rib is present or basal lung fibrosis which may be seen early in CTD. Care should be taken to remember that a fibrous cervical rib can still produce significant vascular occlusion and should be considered when the Raynaud's affects the upper limb alone and is associated with motor and sensory impairment.

Improvements in the techniques for anti-nuclear antibody determination have sub-stantially increased the usefulness of this approach in RP. While a mildly affected patient presenting to the GP does not require testing, those patients severe enough to re-quire consideration for hospital referral should have an immunopathological screen. The core tests for RP of suspected immuno-pathological origin are rheumatoid factor titer for detection of early rheumatoid arthritis, antinuclear antibody for systemic lupus erythematosus, anticentimere antibody for limited SSc and anti-topoisomerase antibody (formally scleroderma 70 antibody) for diffuse SSc[28]. The latter two autoantibodies have recently been shown to be very useful prog-nostic indicators, especially when used in conjunction with capillaroscopy[29] predic-ting almost 90% of those destined to develop SSc. While none of the above are entirely specific nor, indeed, fully sensitive, they pro-vide a good framework for the early diagnosis of the rheumatic disorders.

The endothelial product factor VIII von Willebrand factor antigen (VWF) is released in large quantities by damaged endothelium. It is elevated in RS, but normal in RD and may have a predictive value in the evolution or regression of disease[30]. This still requires further evaluation.

Both cryoglobulinemia and cryofibrino-genemia, where cold-precipitated proteins are detected, are rare disorders. Both allow the precipitation of large molecules in the cool digital circulation and thus can cause RP. However, they should not be tested for during the initial screen unless there is a high index of clinical suspicion.

Thus, while the vasospasm itself may be obvious, the investigations for an associated disorder are more complex. However, the importance of early detection of an underlying disorder cannot be underestimated. The diag-nosis of a CTD has implications for future screening and follow-up in hospital out-patient clinics. The diagnosis of an occu-pational disorder may have important financial consequences for the patient in terms of compensation awards, and progression of the disorder may be prevented by a change in occupation. Further lifestyle changes directed by the careful evaluation of an RP patient can also provide a significant benefit, e.g. the withdrawal of some anti-migraine drugs, beta blockade and their substitution with a vaso-dilating beta blocker or other alternative treat-ment.

PATHOPHYSIOLOGY OF RAYNAUD'S PHENOMENON

Maurice Raynaud postulated hyper-reactivity of the sympathetic nervous system in RP causing an increase in the vasoconstrictor response to cold[1]. This theory is supported by the fact that emotional stimuli can provoke attacks and lumbar sympathectomy can ameliorate symptoms in the lower limb. Lewis, however, preferred a 'local fault' theory suggesting that cold hypersensitivity of the precapillary resistance vessels caused the symptoms[31]. Subsequent work has shown that many of Lewis' findings may be related to abnormalities of the peripheral sympathetic nervous system[32–34].

These are three factors which should be considered as having etiological importance in RP:

1. neurogenic mechanisms;
2. blood and blood vessel wall interactions; and
3. abnormalities of the immunological and inflammatory responses.

NEUROGENIC MECHANISMS

Most work in this area has focused on the peripheral sympathetic nervous system. Abnormalities described include increased alpha-adrenergic receptor sensitivity and/or density[33] and also an increase in the responsiveness of beta presynaptic-receptors in the peripheral vessels of the RS patient[34].

Whether there is a role for the central sympathetic system is unknown. Support for its involvement comes from work showing that local vibration of one hand induces vasoconstriction of the other, which is abolished by proximal nerve blockade[35]. It is further supported by the finding that body cooling, inducing central nervous system mediated vasoconstriction, may produce vasospasm in the absence of local digital cooling[36]. Other studies, however, while showing changes in sympathetic activity following cooling, have failed to show any differences between patients with RP and control subjects. Fagius and Blumer showed an increase in sympathetic activity in the right hand in subjects whose left hand was immersed in ice water with no significant differences between patients and control subjects[37]. Increased levels of adrenaline and nor-adrenaline have been measured following mental stress and cold stimulus, again however, with no differences being detected between patients and

control subjects[38]. Thus, although abnormalities of the nervous system probably exist in RP, they are at present not clearly defined.

One new finding relates to a potential dysfunction of the calcitonin gene-related peptide-dependent neurovascular axis. Calcitonin gene-related peptide (CGRP) is a potent vasodilator and a pilot study has suggested that digital skin CGRP-containing neurones may be decreased in RP when compared to normal subjects[39].

BLOOD AND BLOOD VESSEL WALL INTERACTIONS

The changes in blood vessel tone described above do not, however, explain all the features of RP. In particular, it cannot explain the systemic nature of RP with its wide-spread effects on blood flow affecting many organs, when control of blood flow to all organs is not regulated by the same mechanism. It is, therefore, likely that blood-borne factors are also involved. Flow in the microcirculation depends not only on the size of the blood vessel lumen, but also on the integrity of the endothelium and the various cellular elements and plasma factors in the blood.

The endothelium is a functioning organ releasing important chemicals such as prostacyclin (PGI_2), a potent antiplatelet agent and vasodilator. PGI_2 may be elevated in the early stages of vascular disease[40], although in the later stages PGI_2 stimulating factor may be decreased[41], facilitating platelet aggregation and vasoconstriction. As discussed above, the damaged endothelium releases vWF, which can have prothrombotic effects via its participation in the coagulation cascade and in mediating platelet aggregation. Endothelin, another endothelial product, causes vasoconstriction and elevated baseline plasma levels have been reported in RP which are further increased by cold challenge[42]. Other manifestations of endothelial dysfunction have been detected in RP, such as impaired

fibrinolysis with reduction in tissue plasminogen activator levels and increased plasminogen activator inhibitor[43].

The cellular components of blood may also
be abnormal in RP. The platelet is more
aggregable releasing increased amounts of the
vasoconstrictor and platelet aggregant thromboxane A_2 (TXA_2) and other platelet release
products[44] (Chapter 1). The red blood cell
(RBC) appears generally less deformable in RP
and the cold temperature in association with
the acidosis present in cold ulcerated fingers
will further increase RBC stiffness[45]. Hard
red cells can thus occlude the microcirculation
and these may augment a vasospastic attack.
An important role has also been claimed for
the white blood cell (WBC) in maintaining
flow in the small vessels[46]. Polymorphonuclear leucocyte activation with increased
release of prothrombotic free radicals and
increased white cell aggregation has been
reported in RP and these may also contribute
to the decreased flow seen in this disorder[47].

It should be noted that RD patients do not
show these blood and endothelial abnormalities while the majority of RS patients do.
Interestingly, this is true for both CTD associated RS and that associated with VWF[48].
Thus, while these changes are likely to be a
consequence of the RP rather than a cause,
they may augment the symptoms of vasospasm and their attenuation is an important
feature in the pharmacological management
of RP.

IMMUNOLOGICAL AND INFLAMMATORY RESPONSES

More conventionally the WBC has been considered to be important as the producer and
modifier of the inflammatory and immune
responses. The endothelium is also involved
in these processes by the production of vasoactive agents, growth factors and growth
inhibitors. Disordered immune/inflammatory
responses occur in the majority of severe cases
of RS via their association with the CTDs[28],
but also in VWF which has no clear immune/
inflammatory basis[47]. Tumor necrosis
factor, lymphotoxin, phagocytes, macrophages and T-cell derived proteins, along
with immune complex deposition in the
vessel wall, are all likely to be involved in the
vascular damage seen in RS[49].

TREATMENT OF RAYNAUD'S PHENOMENON

As yet, there is no cure for RP and it is only
possible to ameliorate the symptoms. With
the apparent diverse pathophysiology of the
disorder, treatment must be aimed at one or
several of the mechanisms which have been
implicated. As our knowledge of the pathophysiology improves so will our management
of the condition. A diagram giving a suggested scheme for the management of RP is
shown in Figure 6.3.

SUPPORTIVE MEASURES

Much can be done in the first instance for
patients with mild disease without recourse to
pharmacological agents. Many patients are
apprehensive about their disease, reassurance
is often required and information regarding
both their disease and any local self-help
groups is often gratefully received. These
groups provide information booklets about
various disorders associated with RP which
can be requested by both doctor and patient. It
is also important to advise patients on protecting themselves from the cold. Achieving this
without becoming a hermit is difficult, but
practical solutions to the problem do exist.
Again, the self-help groups have informative
guidance booklets on how to keep warm.

Smoking is known to provoke attacks in
susceptible people[2] and therefore advice
about stopping smoking should always be
given. This also applies to passive smoking
and patients and their relatives should be
aware of this and advised accordingly. A
change in occupation is sometimes required in

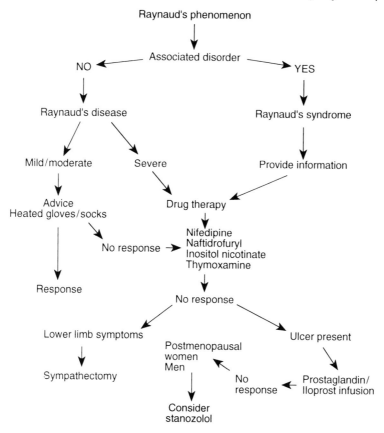

Fig. 6.3 Suggested flow chart for the management of Raynaud's phenomenon.

patients suffering from vibration white finger and other occupation-related causes of RP. Occasionally, however, modification of the work habit may be all that is needed. The withdrawal of drugs known to be associated with RP can also be useful (e.g. beta blockers). It has been suggested that the oral contraceptive pill is implicated in provoking attacks but, in our experience, need only be discontinued if there is a clear association with development of vasospasm. Hormone replacement therapy (HRT) is not contra-indicated by the presence of RP in a patient, as HRT may protect women against the development of vascular disease in general[50]. Some well-motivated people may benefit from bio-feedback techniques[51] with the suggestion that bio-feedback induced

vasodilatation is mediated through a non-neural decrease in beta-adrenergic stimulation[52].

Electrically heated gloves and socks are the perfect solution for some patients. A rechargeable battery fixed on a belt provides up to three hours of warmth and the wires can be concealed beneath the clothing to give a normal appearance (Figure 6.4). They can be a little bulky and heavy for the elderly, however, and they may be difficult to obtain on prescription due to budget constraints. Irritation of ulcers by the added heat has been an infrequent problem. Chemical handwarmers obtained from local chemists and sports shops provide a satisfactory alternative source of heat. These come in both disposable and

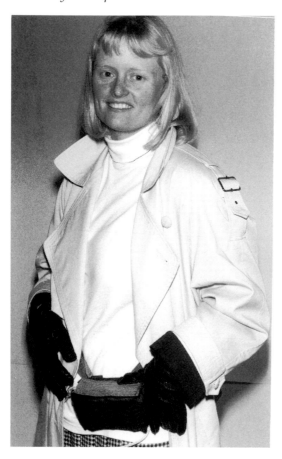

Fig. 6.4 Electrically heated gloves.

reusable forms. The reusable handwarmers are 'primed' by boiling or by heating in a microwave oven. They are then carried in the pocket until needed when they can be activated by finger pressure over a designated spot. 'Comfort shoes' obtained from surgical appliance departments can also be useful. The padded soles keep the feet warm and relieve the pressure on the toes which can result in vasospasm. Pressure is well recognized as causing vasospasm by the patients and they generally learn to avoid such things as carrying hand-held plastic shopping bags. It is, however, less well recognized that properly designed padded footwear can relieve pressure over the digital arteries and spread the

pressure more evenly throughout the foot, thus attenuating the vasospastic symptoms.

Good wound care of ulcers should also be undertaken. Any ulcer that is moist should be swabbed and cultured. A major pitfall in the management of digital ulceration in severe RP is the failure of the clinician to detect infection. Significant infection can be present even in the absence of warmth, erythema and pus formation since blood flow to initiate these responses is impaired. One should consider a trial of antibiotics in all cases prior to considering amputation of the digit. The organisms detected are usually staphylococcus, but infection by less-common organisms also can occur.

PHARMACOTHERAPY

If symptoms are severe and recurrent it is likely that some form of drug therapy will be required to reduce both the severity and frequency of attacks.

Calcium channel blockers

These are the most frequently described drugs for RP. Nifedipine is now the treatment of choice for symptoms of Raynaud's phenomenon. Its mechanism of action in RP though predominantly vasodilatatory has antiplatelet[53] and possibly other antithrombotic actions too[54]. Its use, however, is limited by the vasodilatory side-effects to which the RP patient appears very susceptible. These include dizziness, palpitations, headache, flushing and ankle swelling. To attenuate these side-effects, the patient should use the slow release or 'retard' preparation, commencing at 10 mg twice a day, increasing to three times a day and then after two weeks to 20 mg twice a day, further increasing to three times a day if required. The vasodilatory side-effects usually disappear with continued treatment so unless they are intolerable the patient should persevere for 7–10 days before discontinuing the therapy. It has not, however, been passed for use in pregnancy and the patient must be advised to avoid pregnancy when this drug is prescribed. If side-effects require discontinuation, two options are possible. The first option is to use other calcium channel antagonists, such as amilodipine[55] diltiazem[56)] and isradipine[57]. A controlled multi-center double-blind study of nicardipine showed a decrease in the number of vasospastic attacks but failed to show a change in the severity of the spasm or in the cold-induced reactive hyperemia test[58]. Verapamil has been found to be ineffective. Secondly, if chronic ankle swelling has necessitated the discontinuation of nifedipine, nifedipine capsules can be used as a rescue medication during a severe spasm attack[59], the capsule can be pierced with a pin or crushed by the teeth and placed below the tongue.

Other vasodilators

The use of other vasodilators in RP remains controversial as most studies have been uncontrolled. Four compounds do, however, merit consideration. Inositol nicotinate[60] has produced encouraging results in mild to moderate RP. The drug may take up to 3 months to produce an effect and should, therefore, be given for at least this period of time. Similarly, the use of naftidrofuryl[61] may produce benefit over the same time period as may oxpentifylline[62]. Although these drugs are known vasodilators, their action in RP may be through other mechanisms. These potential mechanisms may include modification of some of the rheological abnormalities mentioned earlier. Thymoxamine the selective alpha-1 blocker[63] may also be tried initially for a period of 2 weeks. A trial of these treatments given in sufficient dosages for a sufficient period of time may be worthwhile. It is unusual, however, for the more severely affected patient to benefit from these treatments most of which will have been prescribed by the GP before hospital referral. Thus in such a population simple vasodilators are often ineffective with the limiting factor being the development of side-effects at high dosage.

Manipulation of the arachidonic acid cascade

Manipulation of the body's own of vasodilatory prostaglandin (PG) production has also been evaluated as a treatment option. Dietary supplementation with evening primrose oil rich in the essential fatty acid gamma-linolenic acid (GLA) leads to increased production of dihomogammalinolenic acid (DGLA). Similarly, fish oil is high in eicosapentanoic acid (EPA) and docosahexenoic acid (DHA). These substances all stimulate increased production of the anti-platelet/vasodilator prostaglandins while inhibiting production of many pro-inflammatory vasoconstrictor mediators. There have been few studies directed at such treatments, however[64], and both need to be given in full dose, that is, evening primrose oil 12×500 mg capsules a day or fish oil 10×7 mg capsules a day for at least 3 months before being deemed ineffective. Disappointingly, in controlled studies, only a mild response has been detected and RP is not a licensed indication for their use.

Inhibition of the cyclo-oxygenase enzyme by non-steroidal anti-inflammatory agents (NSAIs) produces a significant anti-platelet effect. However, a study of acetylsalicyclic acid together with dypiridamole in patients with RP failed to show any clinical benefit[65].

Specific inhibition of the enzyme thromboxane synthetase results in a decrease in TXA_2 formation and promotes vasodilatation and platelet disaggregation; nevertheless, studies of such compounds have been disappointing[66]. Recent developments of drugs which combine thromboxane synthetase inhibition with thromboxane receptor site blockade may prove more promising[67].

Prostaglandin therapy

Discovery of the prostaglandins (PG), the metabolic products of essential fatty acids (EFAs), opened up new therapeutic approaches to RP. PGE_1 and PGI_2 both have potent vasodilatory and anti-platelet properties, whereas TXA_2 has opposite actions[68]. It is possible to manipulate the balance of these chemicals in favor of anti-thrombotic and vasodilatory effects. PGE_1 treatment has to be given intravenously (IV) often through a central line with an incremental dosage regime up to a maximum of 7.5 ng/kg/minute[69]. Although 10 ng/kg/minute was used in earlier studies, vasodilatory side-effects such as headache, flushing and hypotension persuaded later workers to lower the dosage. Most studies suggest a benefit from a 72-hour IV infusion of PGE_1 in RS and to aid wound healing following surgery. However, it is probably unhelpful in RD[70].

Prostacyclin also requires intravenous administration, but this can be through a peripheral vein[71]. A careful watch over the drip site should still be kept to avoid the pronounced inflammatory response seen after infusion into the tissues. PGI_2 is best given using a 6–8 hour infusion, intermittently over 3–5 days. Further infusion can be given thereafter on a daily basis if ulceration persists. The dose is also incremental, increasing from 1 ng/kg/minute to a maximum of between 5–7.5 ng/kg/minute. The dosage should be titrated to side-effects which are also vasodilatory. In general, women have more severe side-effects than men[72]. The intermittent regime described above appears to prevent tachyphylaxis of the platelet to the effects of the PG and rebound platelet aggregation after discontinuing the infusion[73]. Blood pressure and pulse should be measured during the time of increasing dose.

The beneficial effects of these PG infusions may last outwith the infusion time. In our experience, the persistence of the effect ranges from 1 week to 6 months, when repetition of the infusion is required. The anti-platelet effects of PGI_2 do not persist past the termination of the infusion by more than 2–3 hours[74]. Similarly, the clinical effects of vasodilatation, such as headache and flushing, pass off quickly after the end of the infusion. At the time of the first reporting of this prolonged benefit, it was common to read of an unexplained 'cyto-protective' effect. This term has been poorly defined but it has been used by many authors to explain the long-term beneficial effects of the vasodilatory prostaglandins. Sinzinger *et al.*[75] went some way to providing an explanation in their study of labelled platelets in patients with arterial atherosclerosis. Prior to treatment the labelled platelets became adherent to atherosclerotic plaques. PGI_2 decreased the platelet adhesion and this was maintained long after the infusion had been terminated. It is possible therefore, to speculate that the PGs may facilitate endothelial repair thereby breaking the vicious cycle of endothelial cell damage and altered blood flow. PGI_2 attenuates WBC activity and such an alteration in neutrophil and lymphocyte function might well be important in the provision of this therapeutic response seen with the prostaglandins[76].

As yet neither PGE_1 or PGI_2 are licensed as treatments for RP, nor is iloprost, a PGI_2 analogue, which may also be beneficial in RP[76]. Whereas both E_1 and I_2 are unstable, iloprost is not and this makes it easier to handle despite still requiring IV administration. Iloprost produced a significant decrease in duration and severity of vasospastic attacks over 6 weeks[77,78]. In one large study, the dose of 2 ng/kg/minute given over 8 hours for 5 days appeared effective with some vasodilatory side-effects. A subsequent study[79] compared the above regime to 0.5 ng/kg/minute and found both regimes to be equally effective in decreasing the frequency duration and severity of vasospastic attacks. Ulcer healing occurred to a similar degree in both treatment groups. As expected the low dose was associated with fewer side-effects and was better tolerated by the patients. Another study, which is of clinical relevance, was carried out by Radmaker *et al.*[80] where iloprost was compared to nifedipine treatment. Both treatments effectively reduced attacks and it was suggested that nifedepine was less effective in healing digital ulcers and additionally produced more side-effects. Despite iloprost's efficacy as a treatment and its equipotency with nifedipine, it still remains a second choice treatment because of its mode of administration, which requires hospital administration and the fact that it is not yet registered for use in RP.

Fibrinolytic agents and others affecting blood rheology

Parenteral administration of low molecular weight dextran or ancrod, a defibrinating agent, have been reported to alleviate RP. However, the need to monitor blood coagulation and the development of antibodies to ancrod limits their application. Likewise, troxerutin, an agent affecting red cell deformability, has been shown to be useful in one small study. However, no convincing work has been carried out using any of the above agents.

Stanozalol is an anabolic steroid that increases fibrinolysis and the results obtained with this compound are possibly more persuasive[81]. The drug is given in a dose of 5 mg twice a day and the beneficial effects can take up to 3 months to become apparent. Side-effects can be severe, however, and include an elevation of liver enzymes, virilization in women and dyspepsia. This agent is now rarely employed and then only in post-menopausal women or males who have normal liver function tests.

Future pharmacological agents

Although the intravenously administered PGs may be useful, their intravenous administration makes them less than satisfactory. This is particularly so for PGE_1 which may require infusion through a central line. This is an invasive procedure involving the risk of pneumothorax, a complication best avoided in patients at risk of developing pulmonary fibrosis in association with SSc. A novel solution incorporating PGE_1 into lipid microspheres, given as a bolus intravenously through a peripheral vein daily for 4 weeks, has been developed. In a multi-center, double-blind, placebo-controlled study[82] no objective measures of blood flow could be carried out. However, in the 135 patients with CTD associated RS a significant improvement in clinically detected ulcer healing occurred after lipo-PGE_1 treatment.

Studies of the orally active PGI_2 analogue cicaprost proved disappointing[83] although a recent pilot study of oral iloprost was perhaps more encouraging[84] as were the results obtained from the study of oral limaprost[85]. Transdermal prostaglandins proved popular with the RS patient as well as providing both subjective and objective improvement in the disorder[86].

Plasma serotonin has been shown to be increased in RS, possibly reflecting increased platelet aggregation and it may contribute to vasoconstriction. Ketanserin, a serotonin antagonist with mild alpha-1 adrenergic antagonistic effects, may be useful in RP. This was demonstrated in a large multicenter study of 222 patients with both RD and RS[87]. Unfortunately again, due to the multicenter nature of the study, objective tests of blood flow could not be measured. However, a Swiss study detected objective improvements in capillary blood flow in patients treated with this agent, suggesting that ketanserin may be a drug for the future[88]. Disappointingly the potassium channel opener, pinacidil, has shown no benefit over placebo in a small study comparing the agent to nifedipine[89].

Patients with RD may have a hypersensitivity to the potent, endogenous vasodilator CGRP. A pilot study of infused CGRP in patients with RD produced an increase in hand/skin blood flow throughout the duration of the infusion which persisted for 3 days after termination of the infusion[90]. Similarly L-arginine, a substrate for the potent endothelial vasodilator nitric oxide, has also been shown to have both vasodilatory effects and induce increased tissue plasminogen activator levels in patients with RP[91]. This may prove to be an important area for study in the future.

SURGICAL MANAGEMENT

Sympathectomy

Upper limb sympathectomy gives a high relapse rate and an especially poor response in RS. It is, therefore, no longer indicated for RP of the upper limb. It should be noted, however, that the more selective laparoscopic thoracic sympathectomy operation has not yet been assessed in RP although it is possible that it will fail in the same way. The same may not be so for the more localized digital sympathectomy where early work has produced encouraging results[92]. Long-term follow-up assessments are, however, essential in view of the subsequent failure of conventional upper limb sympathectomy. In contrast, sympathectomy still has an important role in the treatment of RP affecting the feet when results may be rewarding. Lumbar sympathectomy is usually carried out using needle injection of phenol into the ganglia rather than open operation.

Amputation

Very occasionally, in order to alleviate pain or intractable gangrene, it becomes necessary to amputate the digit. Fortunately, today, this is an uncommon occurrence. Usually it becomes necessary after long-term medical treatment has failed to salvage the digit. It is always important to instruct the patient to present early to the clinic. In systemic sclerosis where skin tightening over the finger pulp causes ischemia, operations to remove part of the terminal phalanx to relieve pressure may also be useful.

Other surgical procedures

Any local pressure on the arterial supply to the limb should be removed if possible. This includes the removal of cervical ribs and fibrous bands. Although these are relatively rare causes of RP, they should be considered particularly when the RP is unilateral or affects the hands only.

PLASMAPHORESIS

The use of this therapeutic option is now declining since the advent of the prostaglandins. Its beneficial effects may result from the alteration of platelet, WBC and RBC behavior. Blood viscosity is also lowered and immune complexes are removed[93]. However, this form of treatment produces only limited success, is time consuming and expensive. It is not a cure and requires repetition at a later date. Consequently, plasma exchange is reserved for patients with severe intractable ulceration and at the present time the prostaglandins are replacing this function.

CONCLUSION

RP is a common condition and until recently its management has been difficult. However, as research in the field continues and our knowledge of the pathogenesis of the disorder improves so has our management and diagnostic techniques. With the help of a careful clinical history and examination and a selection of specific blood tests, it is now possible to correctly diagnose RP, to assess the likelihood of progression to an associated disorder and institute helpful medical treatment. Although a cure is not available, many patients with RP can achieve a satisfactory amelioration of their symptoms. Finally, it should be remembered that the prognosis of RS is determined by that of the underlying disorder which also must be detected, monitored and treated.

ACKNOWLEDGEMENTS

JB receives support from the Sir John Fisher Foundation and the Raynaud's and Scleroderma Association. CM is an Arthritis and Rheumatism Council Clinical Research Fellow.

REFERENCES

1. Raynaud, M. (1862) *D'Asphyxre et de la gangrene symetriques des extremities*, Paris. (Trans. Thomas Barlow, London. New Syndenham Soc. 1988.)
2. Goodfield, M. J. D., Hume, A. and Rowell, N. R. (1990) The acute effects of cigarette smoking on cutaneous blood flow in smoking and non-smoking subjects with and without Raynaud's phenomenon. *Br. J. Rheumatol.*, **29**, 89–91.
3. Lafferty, K., De Trafford, J. C., Potter, C. *et al.* (1985) Reflex vascular responses in the finger to contralateral thermal stimuli during the normal menstrual cycle: a hormonal basis to Raynaud's phenomenon? *Clin. Sci.*, **68**, 10–5.
4. Fitzgerald, O., Hess, E. V., O'Connor, G. T. *et al.* (1988) Prospective study of the evolution of Raynaud's phenomenon. *Am. J. Med.*, **84**, 718–26.
5. Kallenberg, C. G. M., Waida, A. A., Hoet, M. H. *et al.* (1988) Development of connective tissue disease presenting with Raynaud's phenomenon: a 6 year follow-up with emphasis on predictive value of auto antibodies as detected by immunoblotting. *Ann. Rheum. Dis.*, **4**, 634–41.
6. Belch, J. J. F. B. (1990) Raynaud's phenomenon. *Curr. Opin. Rheumatol.*, **2**, 937–41.
7. Kallenberg, C. G., Waida, A. A. and Hoet, M. T. (1980) Systemic involvement and immunological findings in patients presenting with Raynaud's phenomenon. *Am. J. Med.*, **69**, 675–80.
8. Porter, J. M., Bardona, E. J., Baur, G. M. *et al.* (1976) The clinical significance of Raynaud's syndrome. *Surgery*, **80**, 756–64.
9. Friedman, E., Taylor, L. M. and Porter, J. M. (1988) Late onset of Raynaud's syndrome: diagnostic and thereputic considerations. *Geriatrics*, **43**, 59–70.
10. Taylor, W. (1989) The hand-arm vibration syndrome, secondary Raynaud's phenomenon of occupational origin. *Proc. Royal Coll. Physicians, Edinburgh*, **19**, 7–14.
11. Hedlund, U. (1989) Raynaud's phenomenon of fingers and toes of miners exposed to local and whole-body vibration and cold. *Int. Arch. Occup. Envirn. Health*, **61**, 457–61.
12. O'Keefe, S. T., Tsapatsaris, N. P., Beetham, W. P. Jnr. (1992) Increased prevelence of migraine and chest pain in patients with primary Raynaud's disease. *Ann. Int. Med.*, **116**(12 pt. 1), 985–9.
13. Baron, M., Feiglin, D., Hyland, R. (1983) Gallium lung scans in progressive systemic sclerosis. *Arth. Rheum.*, **26**, 967–74.
14. Kahan, A., Devaux, J. Y., Amor, B. *et al.* (1986) Nifedipine and thallium-201 myocardial perfusion in progressive systemic sclerosis. *N. Engl. J. Med.*, **314**(22), 1397–402.
15. McKenzie, J., Belch, J. J. F., Land, D. *et al.* (1988) Oesophageal ischaemia in motility disorders associated with chest pain. *Lancet*, 8611, 596–9.
16. Belch, J. J. F., Land, D., Park, R. H. R. *et al.* (1988) Decreased oesophageal blood flow in patients with Raynaud's phenomenon. *Br. J. Rheumatol.*, **27**, 426–30.
17. Salmenson, B. D., Rebman, J., Sinclair, S. H. *et al.* (1992) Macular capillary haemodynamic changes associated with Raynaud's phenomenon. *Opthalmology*, **99**(6), 914–9.
18. Lau, C. (1993) Haemostatic abnormalities in Raynaud's phenomenon and the potential for treatment with manipulation of the arachidomic acid pathway, (MD Thesis), University of Dundee.
19. Kristensen, J. K., Engelhart, M. and Nielsen, T. (1983) Laser-Doppler measurement of digital blood flow regulation in normals and in patients with Raynaud's phenomenon. *Acta Derm.* (Stockh) **63**, 43–47.
20. Gifford, R. W. and Hines, E. A. (1957) Raynaud's disease among young women and girls. *Circulation*, **16**, 1012–21.
21. Porter, J. M., Rivers, S. P., Anderson, C. J. *et al.* (1981) Evaluation and management of patients with Raynaud's syndrome. *Am. J. Surg.*, **142**, 183–9.
22. Edwards, J. M. and Porter, J. M. (1990) Associated disease in patient with Raynaud's syndrome. *Vasc. Med. Rev.*, **1**, 51–8.
23. LeRoy, E. C. and Medsger, T. A. Jr. (1992) Raynaud's phenomenon: a proposal for

classification. *Clin. Exp. Rheumatol.*, **10**, 485–8.

24. Kallenberg, C. G. M. (1990) Early detection of connective tissue disease in patients with Raynaud's phenomenon. *Rheum. Dis. Clin. North Am.*, **16**, 11–30.

25. Duffy, C. M., Laxer, R. M., Lee, P. *et al.* (1989) Raynaud's syndrome in childhood. *J. Pediat.*, **114**, 73–8.

26. Maricq, H. R. (1988) Raynaud's phenomenon and microvascular abnormalities in scleroderma (systemic sclerosis), in *Systemic Sclerosis: Scleroderma* (eds M. I. V. Jayson, C. M. Black). London: J. Wiley & Sons Ltd, pp. 151–66.

27. Whicher, J. T., Bell, A. M., Martin, M. F. R. *et al.* (1984) Prostaglandins cause an increase in serum acute-phase proteins in man, which is diminished in systemic sclerosis. *Clin. Sci.*, **66**, 165–71.

28. Cruz, M., Mejia, G., Lavalle, C. *et al.* (1988) Antinuclear antibodies in scleroderma, mixed connective tissue disease and primary Raynaud's phenomenon. *Clin. Rheumatol.*, **7**, 80–6.

29. Weiner, E. S., Hildebrandt, S., Senscal, J. L. *et al.* (1991) Prognostic significance of anticentromere antibody and antitopoisomerase I antibody in Raynaud's disease: A prospective study. *Arth. Rheum.*, **34**(1), 68–77.

30. Lau, C. S., McLaren, M. and Belch, J. J. F. (1991) Factor VIII von Willebrand Factor Antigen levels correlate with symptom severity in patients with Raynaud's phenomenon. *Br. J. Rheumatol.*, **30**, 433–6.

31. Lewis, T. (1938) The pathological changes in the arteries supplying the fingers in warm-handed people and in cases of so-called Raynaud's disease. *Clin. Sci.*, **3**, 288–311.

32. Walmsley, D. and Goodfeed, M. J. D. (1990) Evidence for abnormal peripherally mediated vascular response to temperature in Raynaud's phenomenon. *Br. J. Rheumatol.*, **29**, 181–4.

33. Freedman, R. R., Sabharwal, S. C., Desai, N. *et al.* (1980) Increased alpha adrenergic responsiveness in idiopathic Raynaud's. *Am. J. Med.*, **69**, 675–80.

34. Brotzu, G., Carboni, M. G., Falshi, S. *et al.* (1984) Altered regulator mechanism of presynaptic adrenergic nerves: a new pathophysiological hypothesis in Raynaud's disease. *Microvasc. Res.*, **27**, 110–13.

35. Olsen, N. and Petring, O. U. (1988) Vibration elicited vasoconstrictor reflex in Raynaud's phenomenon. *Br. J. Ind. Med.*, **45**, 413–19.

36. Carter, S. A., Dean, E. and Kroeger, E. A. (1988) Apparent finger systolic pressure during cooling in patients with Raynaud's syndrome. *Circulation*, **77**(5), 988–96.

37. Fagius, J. and Blumberg, H. (1985) Sympathetic outflow in the hand in patient with Raynaud's phenomen on. *Cardiovasc. Res.*, **19**, 249–53.

38. Marasini, B., Biondi, M. L., Mollica, R. *et al.* (1991) Cold induced changes in plasma norepinephrine, epinephrine and dopamine concentrations in patients with Raynaud's phenomenon. *Eur. J. Clin. Chem. Biochem.*, **29**(2), 111–14.

39. Bunker, C. B., Terenghi, G., Springall, D. R. *et al.* (1990) Deficiency of calcitonin generelated peptide in Raynaud's phenomenon. *Lancet*, **336**, 1530–3.

40. Kinney, E. L. and Demers, L. M. (1981) Plasma 6 keto PGF_1^α concentration in Raynaud's phenomenon. *Prostagland. Med.*, **7**, 389–93.

41. Holt, C. M., Moult, J., Lindsey, N. *et al.* (1989) Prostacyclin production by human umbilical vein endothelium in response to serum from patient with systemic sclerosis. *Br. J. Rheumatol.*, **28**, 216–20.

42. Zamora, M. R., O'Brien, R. F., Rutherford, R. B. *et al.* (1990) Serum endothelin-1 concentrations and cold provocation in primary Raynaud's phenomenon. *Lancet*, **336**, 1144–7.

43. Jarret, P. E. M., Morland, M. and Browes, N. L. (1978) Treatment of Raynaud's syndrome by fibrinolytic enhancement, in *Progress in Chemical Fibrinolysis and Thrombosis*, Vol. 3, (eds J. F. Davidson and R. M. Rowan), New York, Raven Press, pp. 521–8.

44. Belch, J. J. F., Drury, J., Flannigan, P. *et al.* (1987) Abnormal biochemical and cellular parameters in the blood of patients with Raynaud's phenomenon. *Scott. Med. J.*, **32**, 12–14.

45. Belch, J. J. F., McLaren, M., Anderson, J. *et al.* (1985) Increased prostacyclin metabolites and decreased red cell deformability in patients with systemic sclerosis and Raynaud's syndrome. *Prostagland Leuk. Med.*, **17**, 1–9.

46. Belch, J. J. F. B. (1990) The role of the white blood cell in arterial disease. *Blood Coag. Firbinol.*, **1**, 183–92.

47. Lau, C. S., O'Dowd, A. and Belch, J. J. F. (1992) White blood cell activation in Raynaud's phenomenon of systemic sclerosis and vibration induced white finger syndrome. *Ann. Rheum. Dis.*, **51**, 249–52.

48. Belch, J. J. F., McLaren, M., Chopra, M. *et al.* (1989) Coagulation and haemorheological abnormalities in patient with vibration white

finger, in *The Assessment and Associated Problems of Vibration White Finger (VWF)*, (eds T. C. Aw, R. A. Cooke, J. M. Harrington), University of Sheffield Press, Sheffield, pp. 18–28.

49. Kahaleh, M. B., Smith, E. A., Soma, Y. *et al.* (1988) Effect of lymphotoxin and tumour necrosis factor on endothelial and connective tissue cell growth and function. *Clin. Immunol. Immunopathol.*, **49**, 261–72.

50. Vanderbroucke, J. P. (1991) Postmenopausal oestrogen and cardioprotection. *Lancet*, **337**, 833–4.

51. Freedmann, R. R., Ianni, P. and Wenig, P. (1983) Behavioural treatment of Raynaud's disease. *J. Consult. Clin. Psy.*, **51**(4), 539–49.

52. Freedman, R. R., Keegan, D., Migaly, P. *et al.* (1991) Plasma catecholamines during behavioural treatments for Raynaud's disease. *Psychosom. Med.*, **53**, 433–9.

53. Rademaker, M., Meyrick Thomas, R. H., Kirby, J. D. *et al.* (1992) The anti-platelet effect of nifedipine in patients with systemic sclerosis. *Clin. Exp. Rheumatol.*, **10**(1), 57–62.

54. Malamet, R., Wise, R. A. and Ettinger, W. H. (1985) Nifedipine in the treatment of Raynaud's phenomenon – evidence for inhibition of platelet activation. *Am. J. Med.*, **78**(4), 602–8.

55. La Civita, L., Pitano, N., Rossi, M. *et al.* (1993) Amlodipine in the treatment of Raynaud's phenomenon. *Br. J. Rheumatol.*, **32**(6), 524–5.

56. Rhedda, A., McCans, J., Willan, A. R. *et al.* (1985) A double bind placebo controlled crossover randomized trial of diltiazem in Raynaud's phenomenon. *J. Rheumatol.*, **12**(4), 724–7.

57. Leppert, J., Jonasson, T., Nilsson, H. *et al.* (1989) The effect of isradipine, a new calcium-channel antagonist, in patients with primary Raynaud's phenomenon: a single-blind dose-response study. *Cardiovasc. Drugs Ther.*, **3**(3), 397–401.

58. French Cooperative Multicenter Group for Raynaud's Phenomenon (1991) Controlled multicenter double-blind trial of nicardipine in the treatment of primary Raynaud's phenomenon. *Am. Heart J.*, **122**, 352–5.

59. Weber, A. and Bounameaux, H. (1990) Effects of low dose nifedipine on a cold provocation test in patients with Raynaud's disease. *J. Cardiovasc. Pharmacol.*, **15**, 853–5.

60. Sunderland, G. T., Belch, J. J. F., Sturrock, R. D. *et al.* (1988) A double blind randomised placebo controlled trial of Hexopal in primary Raynaud's disease. *Clin. Rheumatol.*, **7**(1), 46–9.

61. Nilsen, K. H. (1979) Effects of naftidrofuryl on microcirculatory cold sensitivity in Raynaud's phenomenon. *Br. Med. J.*, **1**, 10–21.

62. Neirotti, M., Longo, F., Molaschi, M. *et al.* (1987) Functional vascular disorders: treatment with oxpentofylline. *Angiology*, **38**(8), 575–80.

63. Grigg, M. J., Nicolaides, A. N., Papadakis *et al.* (1989) The efficacy of thymoxamine in Raynaud's phenomenon. *Eur. J. Vasc. Surg.*, **3**, 309–13.

64. Belch, J. J. F., Shaw, B., O'Dowd, A. *et al.* (1985) Evening primrose oil (Efamol) in the treatment of Raynaud's phenomenon: a double blind study. *Thromb. Haemost.*, **54**(2), 490–4.

65. Van der Meer, J., Wouda, A. A., Kallenberg, C. G. M. *et al.* (1987) A double-blind controlled trial of low dose acetylsalicylic acid and dipyridamole in the treatment of Raynaud's phenomenon. *VASA*, **18**, 71–4.

66. Belch, J. J. F., Cormie, J., Newman, P. *et al.* (1983) Dazoxiben, a thromboxane synthetase inhibitor, in the treatment of Raynaud's syndrome: a double blind trial. *Br. J. Clin. Pharmacol.*, **15**, 1135–65.

67. Lau, C. S., Khan, F., McLaren, M. *et al.* (1991) The effects of thromboxane receptor blockade on platelet aggregation and digital skin blood flow in patients with secondary Raynaud's syndrome. *Rheumatol. Int.*, **11**, 163–8.

68. Belch, J. J. F. (1989) Eicosanoids and rheumatology: inflammatory and vascular aspects. *Prostaglands, Leuk. and Essential Fatty Acid Rev.*, **36**(4), 219–34.

69. Clifford, P. C., Martin, M. F. R., Sheddon, E. J. *et al.* (1980) Treatment of vasospastic disease with prostaglandin, E_1. *Br. Med. J.*, **281**, 1031–4.

70. Pardy, B. J. and Eastcott, H. H. G. (1983) Prostaglandin therapy in severe limb ischaemia. *World J. Surg.*, **7**, 353–62.

71. Belch, J. J. F., Drury, J. K., Capell, H. *et al.* (1983) Intermittent epoprostenol (prostacyclin) infusion in patients with Raynaud's syndrome – a double-blind controlled trial. *Lancet*, **8320**, 313–5.

72. Belch, J. J. F., McKay, A., McArdle, B. *et al.* (1983) A double blind study of the effect of prostacyclin infusion in severe peripheral vascular disease. *Lancet*, **8320**, 315–7.

73. Sinzinger, H., Silberbauer, K., Horsch, A. K. *et al.* (1981) Decreased sensitivity of human platelets to PGI_2 during long-term intra-arterial prostacyclin infusion in patient with peripheral vascular disease – a rebound phenomenon? *Prostaglandins*, **21**, 49–51.

74. O'Grady, J., Warington, S., Mote, M. J. *et al.* (1980) Effects of intravenous infusion of prostaglandin (PGI$_2$) in man. *Prostaglandins*, **19**, 319–32.

75. Sinzinger, H., Fitscha, P. and Kaliman, J. (1985) The optimal PGI$_2$ infusion time as judged by autologous platelet – labelling in patients with active atherosclerosis, in *Prostaglandins and Other Eicosanoids in the Cardiovascular System*, (ed. K. Schror), Basel, Karger, pp. 358–64.

76. Belch, J. J. F. B., Saniabadi, A., Dickson, R. *et al.* (1987) Effect of Iloprost (ZK 36374) on white cell behaviour, in *Prostacyclin and Its Stable Analogue Iloprost*, (eds R. J. Gryglewski and G. Stock), Berlin, Springer-Verlag, pp. 97–102.

77. Yardumian, D. A., Isenberg, D. A., Rustin, M. *et al.* (1988) Successful treatment of Raynaud's syndrome with iloprost, a chemically stable prostacyclin analogue. *Br. J. Rheumatol.*, **27**, 220–6.

78. Wigley, F. M., Wise, R. A., Siebold, J. R. *et al.* (1994) Intravenous iloprost infusion in patients with Raynaud phenomenon secondary to systemic sclerosis. A multicentre, placebo-controlled, double-blind study. *Ann. Intern. Med.*, **120**(3), 199–206.

79. Torley, H. I., Madhok, R., Capell, H. A. *et al.* (1991) A double blind randomised multicenter comparison of 2 doses of intravenous iloprost in the treatment of Raynaud's phenomenon secondary to connective tissue disease. *Ann. Rheum. Dis.*, **50**(11), 800–4.

80. Rademaker, M., Cooke, E. D., Almond, N. E. *et al.* (1989) Comparison of intravenous infusions of iloprost and oral nifedipine in treatment of Raynaud's phenomenon in patients with systemic sclerosis: a double blind randomised study. *Br. Med. J.*, **298**, 561–4.

81. Jarrett, P. E. M., Browse, M. and Browse, N. L. (1978) Treatment of Raynaud's phenomenon by fibrinolytic enhancement. *Br. Med. J.*, **ii**, 523–5.

82. Mizushima, Y., Shiokawa, Y., Homma, M. *et al.* (1987) A multicenter double blind controlled study of lipo-PGE$_1$, PGE$_1$ incorporated in lipid microspheres, in peripheral vascular disease secondary to connective tissue disorders. *J. Rheumatol.*, **14**, 97–103.

83. Lau, C. S., McLaren, M., Saniabadi, A. *et al.* (1991) The pharmacological effects of cicaprost, an oral prostacyclin analogue, in patients with Raynaud's syndrome secondary to systemic sclerosis – a preliminary study. *Clin. Exp. Rheumatol.*, **9**, 271–3.

84. Belch, J. J. F., Lau, C. S., Murphy, E. *et al.* (1992) A pilot study of oral iloprost, a prostacyclin analogue, in patients with Raynaud's syndrome and systemic sclerosis. *Br. J. Rheumatol.*, **31**, 55.

85. Murai, C., Sasaki, T., Osaki, H. *et al.* (1989) Oral limaprost for Raynaud's phenomenon (Letter). *Lancet*, 1218.

86. Belch, J. J. F. B., Shaw, B., Sturrock, R. D. *et al.* (1985) Double-blind trial of CL115,347, a transdermally absorbed prostaglandin E$_2$ analogue, in treatment of Raynaud's phenomenon. *Lancet*, 1180–83.

87. Coffman, J. D., Clement, D. L., Creager, M. A. *et al.* (1989) International study of ketanserin in Raynaud's phenomenon. *Am. J. Med.*, **87**, 264–8.

88. Gasser, P. (1991) Reduction in capillary blood cell velocity in nailfold capillaries to nifedipine and ketanserin in patients with vasospastic disease. *J. Int. Med. Res.*, **19**(1), 24–31.

89. Dopeling, E. C. and Smit, A. J. (1992) Assessment of pinacidil in patients with primary Raynaud's phenomenon. *Vasa*(Supp) **34**, 34–7.

90. Shawket, S., Dickerson, C., Hazleman, B. *et al.* (1991) Prolonged effect of CGRP in Raynaud's patients: a double-blind randomised comparison with prostacyclin. *Br. J. Clin. Pharmacol.*, **32**, 209–13.

91. Agostoni, A., Marasini, R., Biondi, M. L. *et al.* (1991) L-Arginine therapy in Raynaud's phenomenon? *Int. J. Clin. Lab. Res.*, **21**(2), 202–3.

92. El-Gammal, T. A. and Blair, W. F. (1991) Digital periarterial sympathectomy for ischaemic digital pain and ulcers. *J. Hand. Surg.*, **16**, 382–5.

93. O'Reilly, M. J. G. (1981) Plasma exchange therapy in Raynaud's phenomenon. *Viscositas*, **2**, 1–2.

G. C. Sharp and R. W. Hoffman

HISTORICAL OVERVIEW

Over an eight–year period of observation at Stanford University (1961–9) in a clinic in which patients with a spectrum of rheumatic diseases were seen, an interesting group of patients was observed whose serum showed very high titers of antinuclear antibodies by complement fixation which persisted through periods of active disease and clinical remission. This was in contrast to many patients with systemic lupus erythematosus (SLE) in whom antinuclear antibody titers declined or became negative during clinical remissions. When the clinical characteristics of these patients were examined in detail, it was noted that they did not fit the traditional disease classifications, but had a disease pattern combining features of SLE, polymyositis and scleroderma and, therefore, were referred to as having mixed connective tissue disease (MCTD).

In order to clarify the nature of the MCTD autoantibody pattern, a very sensitive passive hemagglutination (PHA) test was developed, and all of these sera had extremely high titers of antibodies (frequently >1:1 000 000) directed against an extractable nuclear antigen (ENA) which Holman had described earlier[1]. Enzyme digestion studies using the PHA method further revealed that these sera were reacting with an RNase- and trypsin-sensitive component of the crude ENA. Fluorescent antinuclear antibody (FANA) analyses

performed by Tan on these MCTD sera revealed high titers with speckled patterns which were eliminated by RNase treatment of the tissue sections[1]. These findings suggested that the circulating antibody in MCTD had a specificity for a nuclear ribonucleoprotein (RNP) antigen. Sera of about 50% of patients with typical SLE also contained antibodies to ENA which were usually present at a lower titer and often were of the RNase-resistant specificity of the Smith (Sm) antigen. Antibodies to native DNA and Sm, serological markers for SLE, were rarely detected in MCTD. Because of their similar clinical features and characteristic serological pattern, it was proposed that MCTD might represent a distinct rheumatic disease syndrome. The initial 25 patients reported with MCTD appeared to have an excellent response to corticosteroid therapy and a favorable prognosis[1].

In the early 1970s, double immunodiffusion (Ouchterlony) analyses in several laboratories showed that a precipitation system in addition to the PHA method can be used to detect antibodies reacting with ENA (2–4). Thus, it became clear that ENA contains at least two immunologically distinct antigenic components, the RNase- and trypsin-sensitive RNP antigen and the RNase- and trypsin-resistant Sm antigen. Using well-characterized reference sera, the Ouchterlony test provides a more definitive identification of RNP and Sm antibodies. However, the PHA

Connective Tissue Diseases. Edited by Jill J. F. Belch and Robert B. Zurier. Published in 1995 by Chapman & Hall, London. ISBN 0 412 48620 2

method with titers before and after RNase is also very useful because it is much more sensitive and quantitative[5]. The PHA test is also 100- to 1000-fold more sensitive than the FANA test. Therefore, the FANA may not be adequate as a screening test early in the course of MCTD when the antibody titer may be at a low level[6].

During the decade following the initial report of MCTD, studies in most centers showed that the serological pattern of very high titers of RNP antibodies and no Sm antibodies is most frequently associated with MCTD, is uncommon in patients with SLE or systemic sclerosis and is very rare in other rheumatic diseases[2,4,5,7,8]; however, one laboratory reported that this serological pattern occurred with some frequency in SLE[3]. There is general agreement that Sm antibodies, usually in association with lower titers of RNP antibodies, are most commonly found in SLE[5,7].

CLINICAL FEATURES OF MCTD

GENERAL FEATURES

As patients with MCTD have been followed over a longer period of time, it has become clear that this disease, like other connective tissue diseases, evolves over time. It is unusual to see all the typical overlapping clinical features early in the course of MCTD. More commonly in the early phase, patients are apt to have minimal symptoms, such as Raynaud's phenomenon, easy fatigability, arthralgias, myalgias and swollen hands, which are insufficient to make a definitive diagnosis. This constellation of findings has been referred to by some as an undifferentiated connective tissue disease (UCTD). In some patients, this mild syndrome may persist for years. Other patients may develop additional manifestations, resulting in a diagnosis of MCTD (8–12). Thus, prospective longitudinal studies are much more likely to reflect an accurate assessment of the evolving connective

tissue disease than cross-sectional studies or retrospective reviews of medical records.

In our prospective, longitudinal study at the University of Missouri-Columbia[11], 60% of 34 patients with high titers of RNP antibody initially had more limited clinical involvement and were thought to have rheumatoid arthritis, scleroderma, polymyositis, SLE or a UCTD. At their most recent medical evaluation, 91% had demonstrated typical overlapping features of MCTD, while 9% remained undifferentiated. In another prospective, long-term study in Sweden, on initial evaluation 17 out of 23 patients with high anti-RNP titers did not fulfill criteria for any defined connective tissue disease while at the end of the study with the appearance of new organ manifestations 17 out of 23 fulfilled criteria for MCTD[12]. Less frequently the typical overlapping disease pattern is fully expressed when the patients first come to medical attention, or there is an acute onset of MCTD which may present with high fever, acute arthritis, inflammatory myositis, serositis, aseptic meningitis or digital gangrene[1,8,11,13].

The prevalence of MCTD in caucasians is unknown. In our experience, which is likely to be biased toward referrals of MCTD patients, MCTD occurs as frequently as scleroderma, more commonly than polymyositis, and less frequently than SLE[14]. MCTD has occurred in patients ranging from 4–80 years, with a mean of 37 years; approximately 80% of patients have been female[14]. In a nationwide epidemiological survey in Japan, the prevalence per 100 000 population of MCTD was 2.7 compared with 20.9 for SLE, 5.7 for scleroderma and 4.9 for polymyositis/dermatomyositis[15]. The female-to-male ratio of MCTD was 16:1. Although unusual, there are reports of a familial occurrence of MCTD[16].

In our longitudinal study[11], the most common clinical features of MCTD included Raynaud's phenomenon, polyarthritis, swollen hands or sclerodactyly, pulmonary disease, inflammatory myositis and esophageal hypomotility. Less-frequent findings included lymphadenopathy, alopecia, malar rash, serositis, cardiac disease, renal disease, anemia and leukopenia. Diffuse scleroderma developed in only one-fifth of these patients. In the prospective, longitudinal study of Lundberg and Hedfors of 32 patients with RNP antibodies, none of them fulfilled the criteria for diffuse systemic sclerosis[12]. The very high frequency of pulmonary disease detected in our systematic prospective study had not been noted in our initial report[1], perhaps because early in the course of the disease patients may lack symptoms of their pulmonary involvement. In our longitudinal study, clinical evidence of renal disease was noted in only 18%, and none developed renal failure[11]. In the follow-up study of the original MCTD series, only 1 patient had developed membranous glomerulonephritis[17], and in the Swedish prospective study glomerulonephritis was seen in only 1 patient, in association with a falling anti-RNP titer and a rising anti-DNA titer[12]. Thus, in contrast to SLE where renal and central nervous system disease are the most frequent serious disease complications (Chapter 2), our longitudinal study and other reports have revealed that pulmonary hypertension with proliferative vasculopathy is the most frequent cause of disease-related deaths in MCTD[11,13,18–20].

It appears that MCTD patients with RNP antibodies and patients with limited systemic sclerosis (SSc) who typically have anti-centromere antibodies are at a greater risk for developing pulmonary hypertension and proliferative vascular lesions with minimal fibrosis than are patients with classical SLE, scleroderma and polymyositis[11,18,21–25]. When it occurs in systemic sclerosis, pulmonary hypertension is usually associated with substantial interstitial pulmonary fibrosis[21]. Anticardiolipin antibodies have been noted in 68% and anti-RNP antibodies in 21% of SLE patients who develop pulmonary hypertension[26].

Three sets of diagnostic criteria for MCTD were proposed at the 1986 International Symposium on MCTD and Antinuclear Antibodies[27–29]. Major criteria included Raynaud's phenomenon, swollen hands or sclerodactyly, synovitis, myositis, pulmonary disease and high titer anti-RNP antibody. Preliminary evaluations of these criteria have shown a very high sensitivity and specificity [30,31].

Certain clinical and serologic characteristics distinguish MCTD from polymyositis and other polymyositis-scleroderma overlap syndromes. In a 10-year study believed to include most cases of myositis in the South Stockholm geographical area[32], the diagnostic criteria of Bohan and Peter were used to categorize patients as idiopathic polymyositis (n = 10), dermatomyositis (n = 6) and myositis associated with another connective tissue disease (n = 13). All 7 patients with RNP antibodies had myositis in association with other connective tissue disease features and fulfilled criteria for MCTD[31]. Myositis was rarely the initial manifestation but appeared during the disease course. The 6 other patients with myositis associated with other connective tissue disease features had a myositis-scleroderma overlap and were negative for RNP antibodies. PM-1 (PM-Scl) and Jo-1 autoantibodies are serological markers for a polymyositis-scleroderma overlap syndrome which may resemble MCTD[33,34]. These patients lack the SLE-like features of MCTD and are almost always negative for RNP antibodies.

The report of a follow-up evaluation of the original 25 MCTD patients[17] has been widely cited as showing evidence of a transition of the disease from MCTD to classical systemic sclerosis. In point of fact, the summary of the article by Nimelstein *et al.* states:

'Inflammatory disease manifestations, such as arthritis, serositis, fever and myositis, have become less frequent and, when present, less severe. They appear to have been responsive to corticosteroid treatment. Sclerodermatous manifestations

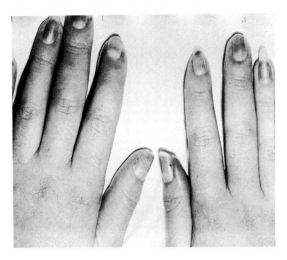

Fig. 7.1 Hands of a patient with MCTD prior to treatment, demonstrating the tapered or sausage appearance of the fingers. (From Sharp, G. C. *et al.* (1972) Mixed connective tissue disease – an apparently distinct rheumatic disease syndrome associated with a specific antibody to an extractable nuclear antigen (ENA). *Am. J. Med.*, **52**, 148, by permission of *The American Journal of Medicine*.)

such as sclerodactyly and esophageal disease were often unresponsive to corticosteroids and have persisted. This has resulted in a general evolution away from a 'mixed' clinical picture to that of a predominantly progressive systemic sclerosis. Renal disease has remained infrequent.'

Thus, from the follow-up evaluation of the original series[17] and in subsequent prospective, longitudinal studies[11,12] it appears that MCTD infrequently spontaneously evolves into diffuse systemic sclerosis.

Among the clinical transitions that have been noted to occur in MCTD, occasional patients transiently develop an illness that more resembles typical SLE with antibodies to Sm and/or DNA, higher levels of circulating immune complexes, glomerulonephritis and lupus-like skin lesions[14]. These findings were present in 4 MCTD patients who had defective reticuloendothelial systems (RES) clearance of immune complexes but not in 14

MCTD patients with lower levels of circulating immune complexes and normal RES clearance[35]. Perhaps the normal RES function in patients with more classic MCTD permits efficient clearance of immune complexes and precludes serious renal disease.

SPECIFIC MANIFESTATIONS

Mucocutaneous abnormalities

Raynaud's phenomenon is the most common finding and may precede other disease manifestations by months to years[1,4,5,8,9,36]. In over two-thirds of MCTD patients, it is accompanied by swollen hands and fingers resulting in a sausage appearance of the digits (Figure 7.1)[1,4,5,8,9,36]. Ischemic necrosis or ulcerations of the fingertips, common in scleroderma, are rare in MCTD[1,12]. Sclerodactyly is common, but diffuse sclerosis is much less frequent[1,5,11,12]. The initial observations that in some MCTD patients early edematous sclerodermatous manifestations resolved completely following corticosteroid therapy[1,17] and in a more recent longitudinal study diffuse scleroderma was transient and sclerodactyly was characterized by fluctuating severity[12] are in contrast to the usual course of the disease in patients with systemic sclerosis.

Lupus-like malar rashes and chronic discoid lesions are seen in about one-third of patients[1,5,8,9,11,37]. Other findings include nonscarring alopecia, 'squared' telangiectasia over the hands and face, periungual telangiectasia, violaceous discoloration of the eyelids and erythema over the knuckles that resemble dermatomyositis, calcinosis cutis and buccal and orogenital ulceration[13,38]. Skin biopsies have shown edema and increased dermal collagen content[1]. Immunofluorescent studies of skin biopsies in patients with MCTD have shown speckled intranuclear immunofluorescence of epidermal cells (raising the possibility of *in vivo* cellular penetration of anti-RNP antibodies)[39,40] and immunoglobulin deposits at the dermal-epidermal junction[1,9].

Joints

Polyarthralgias and stiffness are early symptoms in most MCTD patients, and three-quarters of them develop frank arthritis[1,5,8,41]. The arthritis is often non-deforming, but may resemble rheumatoid arthritis with ulnar deviation, swan neck and boutonniere deformities[1,13,41]. Rheumatoid-like changes were present in 30–35% in some studies, but were usually limited to involvement of the hands and wrists[14]. Radiographs may show a paucity of erosive disease; however, small, marginal erosions and even a more destructive arthritis including rib erosions may rarely be seen[12,41–45]. A flexor tenosynovitis may also contribute to hand deformities in MCTD[46]. Subcutaneous rheumatoid-like nodules are occasionally observed[1,12].

Muscles

Proximal muscle weakness, with or without tenderness, is frequent and may be severe in MCTD[1,4,5,13,47]. Serum levels of creatine kinase and aldolase may be markedly elevated, and electromyographic abnormalities and biopsy findings of muscle fiber degeneration and inflammatory changes similar to polymyositis may be seen. Even in patients with only mild muscular weakness, histochemical and immunofluorescent analyses may reveal perifascicular atrophy, type I fiber predominance and immunoglobulin deposition within normal-appearing vessels, within normal fibers, around or on the sarcoplasmic membrane, or within the perimysial connective tissues[47]. A study comparing myositis in MCTD patients with RNP antibodies with idiopathic polymyositis and dermatomyositis in patients negative for RNP antibodies noted milder histopathologic

muscle changes and more rapid improvement of muscle strength on lower doses of corticosteroids in the MCTD group[32]. The finding that infiltrating lymphocytes were confined to the endomysium in polymyositis and had a perimysial distribution in MCTD is of uncertain significance.

Esophagus

In a recent study of 61 patients with MCTD, lower esophageal sphincter (LES) pressure and amplitude of peristaltic pressures in the distal esophagus were significantly less than in normal controls[48]. Seventeen per cent of MCTD patients undergoing manometry had aperistalsis and 43% low-amplitude peristalsis of the distal esophagus. Among patients with abnormal peristalsis, 24% had no esophageal symptoms and 33% had normal cine esophagrams. Heartburn and dysphagia were the most common symptoms in this study. Mean upper esophageal sphincter (UES) pressures were also significantly less in MCTD patients than in normal controls[48]. Abnormal UES function may occur less frequently in scleroderma and may represent a distinguishing feature of MCTD[48]. In a comparative study, 91% of 17 patients with MCTD but only 20% of 14 patients with SLE had manometric abnormalities[49]. A statistically significant improvement in lower esophageal sphincter pressure (LES) was noted in 10 MCTD patients who received a mean of 67 weeks of corticosteroid therapy (average dose, 25 mg/day) for severe multisystem involvement[48]. This encouraging experience led to a trial of corticosteroid therapy in a MCTD patient who had an exacerbation of his disease characterized solely by marked UES and LES dysfunction and recurrent aspiration pneumonia[48]. His UES and LES dysfunction improved with the corticosteroid treatment and was associated with resolution of aspiration episodes. Histopathologic studies in MCTD and systemic sclerosis suggest that there may be differences in pathophysiology between these disorders, which make the former disorder more likely to respond to corticosteroid treatment[25].

Lungs

Pulmonary dysfunction is usually clinically silent in the early phases of MCTD and may go undetected unless systematic evaluations are performed. Although not appreciated in the initial report[1], subsequently it has become apparent that pulmonary involvement in MCTD may seriously compromise function, leading to exertional dyspnea and pulmonary hypertension, particularly in the later stages of disease[11,24,50,51]. In a prospective, longitudinal evaluation of 34 patients with MCTD, 85% were found to have evidence of pulmonary disease[11]. Dyspnea (58%) followed by bibasilar rales (42%) and pleuritic chest pain (40%) were the most frequent clinical findings; however, pulmonary involvement was also detected in 8 of 11 (73%) who had no pulmonary symptoms. The single breath diffusing capacity for carbon monoxide (DLCO), abnormal in 72%, was the most sensitive indicator of pulmonary disease. Chest roentgenographic abnormalities consisting of small, irregular opacities that involved predominantly the bases and middle regions were noted in 30%. Following corticosteroid and/or cyclophosphamide therapy, 45% had improvement of dyspnea on exertion for a measured distance, and over half of those with abnormal pulmonary function tests (PFTs) who were serially studied had improvement in their PFTs. In contrast to our prospective study, a retrospective review noted pleuropulmonary involvement in only 25% of 81 patients with MCTD[52]. Pulmonary hemorrhage and dysfunction of the diaphragm have occasionally been reported in MCTD[53–55]. Thus, pulmonary involvement in MCTD is common but may be clinically inapparent until far advanced.

In our longitudinal study, right heart catheterization was performed on 15 of 34 patients; 10 had elevated pulmonary vascular resistance and increased pulmonary artery pressure, but pulmonary wedge pressure was abnormal in only 1 patient. This 29% frequency of pulmonary hypertension probably reflects the referral of complicated patients to our Center since in a private rheumatology practice setting only 1 of 13 patients (8%) developed this complication[56]. A progressive decline in DLCO and severe capillary loop changes similar to those seen in SSc on nailfold capillaroscopy appear to identify MCTD patients who are at a greater risk for developing pulmonary hypertension[11]. In contrast to SSc in which pulmonary hypertension is usually associated with interstitial pulmonary fibrosis, pulmonary hypertension in MCTD is usually associated with proliferative vascular abnormalities with marked narrowing of the lumen of small and medium-sized pulmonary arteries and arterioles, but without significant interstitial fibrosis[11,18,21–25,51] (Figure 7.2). In 10 patients who had pulmonary hypertension associated with MCTD, l-SSc or d-SSc, treatment with oral nifedipine produced subjective improvement in dyspnea and a significant acute reduction in pulmonary vascular resistance which was sustained in all 6 patients who continued in a long-term study[57]. Thus, there appears to be a therapeutic rationale for identifying pulmonary disease and pulmonary hypertension in MCTD before major complications occur.

Heart

Pericarditis is the most frequent cardiac problem with a 10–43% incidence reported in MCTD and appears to be more frequent in children than in adults[1,8,10,13,25,50,58–60]. The pericarditis is usually responsive to corticosteroids[1,58]. In a prospective study of 38 adults with MCTD, pericarditis and/or pericardial effusion was detected in 11 patients, pulmonary hypertension was documented in 11 of 17 who underwent right heart

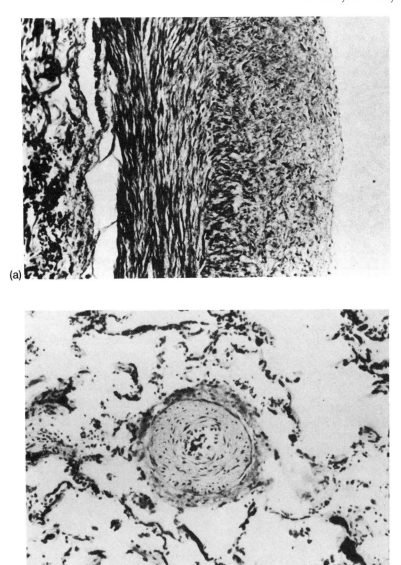

Fig. 7.2 **(a)** Cross-section of an intramural coronary artery in an 18-year-old woman with MCTD showing marked intimal hyperplasia and smooth muscle hypertrophy. Cellular elements in the intima are surrounded by a loose fibrillar connective tissue matrix. Acellular elements in the media (presumably mucopolysaccharides) are also quantitatively increased (hematoxylin and eosin stain, ×200). **(b)** Small pulmonary artery in the same patient showing intimal hyperplasia and smooth muscle hypertrophy without accompanying inflammation or pulmonary fibrosis, associated with severe pulmonary hypertension (hematoxylin and eosin stain, ×200). (From Alpert, M. A. *et al.* (1983) Cardiovascular manifestations of mixed connective tissue disease in adults. *Circulation*, **6**, 1182, by permission of the American Heart Association.)

cardiac catheterization, and mitral valve prolapse was identified in 10[58]. Electrocardiographic abnormalities included chamber enlargement/hypertrophy, conduction disturbances and arrhythmias. Myocarditis is being recognized with increasing frequency in MCTD[58,59,61]. Myocardial involvement may be due to inflammatory cell infiltrates and/or proliferative vasculopathy of the epicardial and intramural coronary arteries [22,23,25,58,61] (Figure 7.2). In a recent echocardiographic study, mitral valve prolapse was detected in 32% of patients with MCTD, 36% of patients with SLE, and 32% of patients with SSc compared with 10% in normal control subjects[62].

Kidneys

Longer follow-up now indicates that renal disease occurs in about 25% of patients with MCTD, and may be more frequent in children[8,11,12,20,63–65]. This is usually a membranous or focal glomerulonephritis[11,20,63,66]. Often it is asymptomatic, but it may result in a nephrotic syndrome[11,20,63]. The renal abnormalities responded well to corticosteroid therapy in our longitudinal study[11]. Diffuse proliferative glomerulonephritis is uncommon[14,20,67], and very rarely MCTD patients die of progressive renal failure[63]. Intramembranous, mesangial and subepithelial electron-dense deposits have been seen on electron microscopy[20,23,66]. Circulating immune complexes have been detected[68], but may be at a lower level than in SLE[35]. Efficient reticuloendothelial (RES) clearance of immune complexes may be related to the infrequency of severe glomerulonephritis in MCTD[35]. Proliferative vascular lesions similar to those seen in the lungs and other organs have been noted in renal vessels[11]. Occasional patients have died from a renovascular hypertensive crisis similar to the 'scleroderma kidney'[10,69]. The clinical and histologic findings suggest that vascular lesions may represent a more serious problem than glomerulonephritis in MCTD.

Nervous system

Neurological manifestations have been noted in about 10% of patients with MCTD[5,8,11–13,70], but were more common in two reports[12,70]. Trigeminal neuropathy is the most frequent neurological problem and occasionally has been an early feature in MCTD[5,71–73]. Vascular headaches have also been relatively common[74]. Headaches may also occur in conjunction with fever and signs of meningeal irritation due to an aseptic meningitis[71]. This must be distinguished from bacterial meningitis which can occur unexpectedly in MCTD patients who are otherwise healthy and not on medications that might compromise the immune system[75]. Central nervous system involvement with organic mental syndromes, seizures and encephalopathy have been much less frequently reported than in SLE[1,8,60,70]. Other neurological problems observed in MCTD include transverse myelitis, cauda equina syndrome, peripheral neuropathies, retinal vasculitis and cerebral infarction or hemorrhage, probably related to hypertension and atherosclerosis[1,8,37,60,70,71,76–78].

Miscellaneous clinical features

Sjögren's syndrome occurs frequently in MCTD and may be more common in children[25,79]. Hashimoto's thyroiditis and persistent hoarseness are occasionally observed[14]. Fever and lymphadenopathy are noted in about one-third of patients[1,5,9]. Lymph nodes may be massively enlarged suggesting a lymphoma, but when biopsied they reveal only lymphoid hyperplasia[1]. Hepatomegaly and splenomegaly may occur, but severe abnormalities of liver function are uncommon[1]. In addition to the esophageal abnormalities previously described, other much less frequent gastrointestinal manifestations have included intestinal hypomotility, dilatation, malabsorption, pseudodiverticula, sclerosis, serositis, perforation, pneumatosis cystoides intestinalis, secretory diarrhea and mesenteric vasculitis with bowel hemorrhage[8,13,43,80,81]. Acute pancreatitis and pancreatic pseudocyst, chronic active hepatitis and Budd–Chiari syndrome have also been described[48,82]. The information on pregnancy in MCTD is limited, and the results have been contradictory. One study showed a high risk of fetal loss and disease exacerbation, while in two studies the risk of fetal loss or maternal worsening of disease seemed slight[13,83,84].

LABORATORY FEATURES OF MCTD

Anemia and leukopenia are found in about one-third of patients with MCTD[1,5,11,13]. The anemia is usually consistent with the anemia of chronic inflammation[5,13]. A Coombs' test may be positive, but a frank hemolytic anemia is uncommon[1,13,85]. The observation of severe, sometimes fatal, infections with encapsulated organisms, such as pneumococcus and meningococcus, occurring in MCTD patients whose disease was inactive off corticosteroids and cytotoxic drugs led us to examine granulocyte function, which showed diminished chemotaxis[75]. Thrombocytopenia is uncommon in adults but appears to be more frequent in children with MCTD[1,5,8,86]. In a report of 14 children with MCTD, 6 had severe thrombocytopenia; two required splenectomy, and one died of an intracranial hemorrhage[8]. Thrombotic thrombocytopenic purpura and red cell aplasia are rarely seen in MCTD[87,88].

The majority of patients with MCTD have polyclonal hypergammaglobulinemia[1,5,13]. Rheumatoid agglutinins occur in over half of patients with MCTD, and their titers are often very high[5,11,13]. False-positive VDRL tests

have been noted in about 10% of patients[1,13], and anti-cardiolipin antibodies have been detected[19]. Serum complement levels are usually normal or only modestly reduced[1,5,9,13]. Antilymphocyte antibodies are much less frequently noted in MCTD than in SLE[89]. Circulating immune complexes have been associated with disease activity in MCTD, but their levels tend to be lower than in active SLE[35]

The typical serological findings in MCTD are a high titer (usually >1:1000) speckled FANA, very high titers (often >1:1 000 000) of antibody to the RNase-sensitive (RNP) component of ENA by hemagglutination, and anti-RNP antibodies by double immunodiffusion[1,5,11]. Antibodies to single-stranded DNA are frequently detected[13,90], but high anti-double stranded DNA titers and anti-Sm antibodies are rare and transient in MCTD, and their appearance is usually associated with a severe flare of SLE-like features [10,11,35]. Rarely, patients with clinical characteristics of MCTD will initially have no detectable anti-RNP antibodies, but will subsequently become positive, sometimes following corticosteroid therapy[1,5,10,91]. High titers of anti-RNP antibodies usually persist during periods of both active and inactive disease, but antibody levels may fall or become undetectable after many years in some patients who go into sustained remission[11,92].

Our earlier biochemical studies had shown a close physical association of the RNP and Sm antigens[93]. Subsequently, several laboratories, notably Lerner and Steitz and colleagues, have further elucidated the nature of the RNP and Sm antibodies[94,95]. Anti-Sm antibodies immunoprecipitate small nuclear RNA (snRNA)-protein complexes containing uridine-rich U1, U2, U4, U5 and U6 snRNAs, while anti-RNP antibodies immunoprecipitate U1 snRNA-protein complexes[96]. Immunoblotting studies revealed that anti-U1 RNP antibodies react with small nuclear ribonucleoprotein (snRNP) polypeptides with

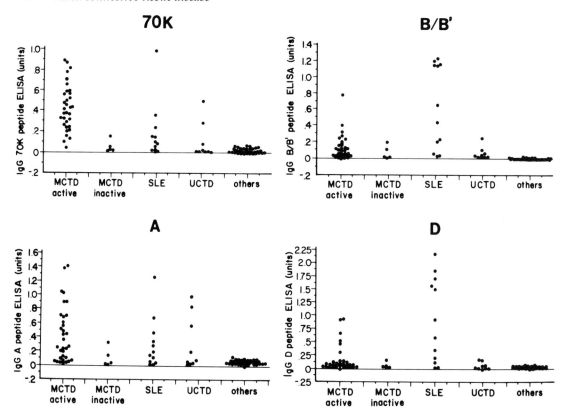

Fig. 7.3 Diagnosis in patients whose sera were tested for IgG reactivity with individual U1 snRNP polypeptides by ELISA. MCTD, mixed connective tissue disease; SLE, active systemic lupus erythematosus; UCTD, undifferentiated connective tissue disease; others, 14 patients negative for anti-RNP antibodies but positive for autoantibodies to other cellular components and 20 normal controls. Note that patients with active MCTD showed higher anti-70 K reactivity in the ELISA, than sera of patients with inactive MCTD, active SLE and UCTD. (From Takeda, Y. *et al.* (1989) Enzyme-linked immunosorbent assay using isolated (U) small nuclear ribonucleoprotein polypeptides as antigens to investigate the clinical significance of autoantibodies to these polypeptides. *Clin. Immunol. Immunopath.*, **50**, 213, by permission of Academic Press, Inc., Orlando.)

molecular weights (MW) 70 kDa (designated 70 K, previously referred to as 68 K), 33 kDa (A) and 22 kDa (C) while anti-Sm antibodies react with 28–29 kDa (B/B') and 16 kDa (D) polypeptides[92]. Takeda and colleagues more recently developed a very sensitive ELISA which permitted quantitation of autoantibodies to biochemically purified snRNPs [97].

As shown in Figure 7.3, while antibodies to the C polypeptides occur in both MCTD and SLE, it appears that antibodies to the 70 kDa

polypeptide are highly specific for MCTD and occur very rarely in SLE[92,97–100]. The fact that in immunoblotting anti-Sm antibodies may immunostain bands in the region of MW 70 000 (Sm-70 kDa) which are clearly distinct from the U1-snRNP-associated 70 kDa polypeptide[101] is not generally appreciated and may be the explanation for reports describing anti-U1 70 kDa antibodies in SLE. The U1 RNP gel-eluted 70 kDa polypeptide ELISA assay, therefore, is particularly useful since it does not measure antibodies reacting with Sm-70 kDa and is a quantitative assay[97,101]. Longitudinal studies demonstrated the persistence of U1 snRNP polypeptide autoantibody patterns for many years in MCTD and their subsequent disappearance in patients who were in prolonged remission[92,97].

More recent studies in our laboratory and elsewhere have shown that antibodies to U1 RNA occur quite frequently in MCTD and, of particular interest, rises in antibody level appear to correlate closely with disease flares[102]. Autoantibodies to the heterogeneous nuclear RNA (hnRNA) which is associated with the nuclear matrix have also been detected in MCTD[103,104].

HISTOPATHOLOGY AND IMMUNOPATHOLOGY

Brief mention of certain histopathologic findings has been included in the clinical description of MCTD in the previous section. In this section, the emphasis is on the most striking histopathologic findings and features that may distinguish MCTD from other connective tissue diseases.

The first comprehensive histopathologic investigation of MCTD was from a study group of 15 children with a median age at disease onset of 10.7 years[25]. This study, which included observations from three autopsies and five renal biopsies, emphasized the occurrence of widespread proliferative vascular lesions in MCTD. While earlier reports of MCTD had mentioned vascular changes, the histopathologic findings in this study were of particular interest because of the young age of the patients, short duration of disease and lack of corticosteroid treatment. From the three autopsies, 31 of 58 organs (53%) had intimal vascular change and 9 organs (16%) had medial hypertrophy in vessel walls. These obliterative vascular changes occurred in large vessels, such as the renal artery and aorta, and within small arterioles. The frequency and severity of this vasculopathy in

organs without overt evidence of clinical involvement was striking and included kidney, aorta, coronary vessels, lungs, myocardium and intestinal tract[25]. Inflammatory infiltration of blood vessels was not a prominent feature.

Similar proliferative vascular lesions have now been described in MCTD in adults and are of concern because vascular compromise may lead to organ failure and hemorrhage[11,24,51,105]. Characteristic findings in the lungs are intimal thickening with medial muscular hypertrophy of the pulmonary arteries and arterioles that is much more prominent than the minimal interstitial fibrosis that is present(Figure 7.2)[11]. This minimal fibrosis contrasts with the findings in systemic sclerosis in which the most characteristic histologic feature is diffuse interstitial fibrosis[21]. Ultrastructural analysis of pulmonary arterial lesions in MCTD has revealed an abundance of intimal ground substance, a disordered array of collagen fibers, perforated basal lamina, hypertrophy of muscle fibers in the media and increased fibroblast production of collagen[11]. Biochemical analyses of these lung specimens showed a selective increase of type III collagen synthesis, resulting in an abnormal type I/type III ratio[11]. This is in contrast to the lungs in SSc in which the type I/type III collagen ratio is identical to their proportions in normal lungs[106]. Thus, the presence of pulmonary hypertension in MCTD appears to be related to these proliferative vascular abnormalities with marked narrowing of the lumen of vessels without significant interstitial fibrosis[11,22].

Vascular abnormalities have also been described in both d-SSc and l-SSc[21]. However, the predilection for large vessel involvement, absence of fibrinoid change and minimal fibrosis in MCTD appear to distinguish it from scleroderma[11,25]. Although medial hypertrophy can be seen in l-SSc, it is much less prominent and there is often a decreased thickness with areas of focal medial atrophy [21], which appears to differ from MCTD in which medial hypertrophy is the rule[11]. The vasculopathy in MCTD has also been shown angiographically in digital, radial and ulnar arteries[107].

Other pathological changes of MCTD that may be unique include the extensive lymphocytic and plasmacytic inflammatory infiltration of the salivary glands, liver and gastrointestinal tract, widespread inflammatory myopathy and a distinctive replacement of the inner and outer muscle layers of the esophagus, pylorus and colon with a hyaline material which appears to be distinct from the type of muscle atrophy and fibrosis associated with systemic sclerosis[25].

The immunological abnormalities that have been identified in MCTD suggest that immune injury mechanisms may play a role in the pathogenesis of the disease. The persistence of extremely high titers of RNP antibodies for many years and marked polyclonal hypergammaglobulinemia are indicative of B-cell hyperactivity. One report estimated that RNP antibody constituted 33% of the total immunoglobulin in one case[108]. Perhaps this enormous quantity of circulating RNP antibodies in MCTD compared to other autoantibodies associated with other connective tissue diseases permits their penetration into living mononuclear cells as reported by Alarcón-Segovia[40]. It is still not resolved whether the direct speckled nuclear fluorescence noted in tissues from MCTD patients when they are incubated with fluoresceinated anti-human gammaglobulin is the result of *in vivo* penetration of cells by RNP antibodies or is an *in vitro* artifact due to high levels of RNP antibodies in the plasma entering cells during the processing of nonviable tissue[9,39,40].

Alarcón-Segovia has reported differences in immunoregulatory functions among MCTD, SLE, SSc rheumatoid arthritis and Sjögren's syndrome that support the concept that MCTD is a distinct entity[109]. MCTD patients often had lymphopenia and reduced total T-lymphocytes. T4, T8, and Tγ cells may all be diminished. In spite of increased numbers of

post-thymic precursor cells, spontaneously expanded suppression and concanavalin-A-induced suppression were both diminished. Natural killer cell function may be normal, and production of B-cell growth factor, B-cell differentiation factor, IL-1 and IL-2 was either normal or increased in MCTD. An immune regulatory imbalance resulting in increased T-cell help could result in B-cell stimulation with continuing production of anti-U1 RNP antibodies.

Circulating immune complexes have been noted during active disease in MCTD[35,68]. However, RES clearance of immune complexes is usually normal and, in contrast to active SLE, levels of immune complexes tend to be lower[35]. The minority of MCTD patients with abnormal RES clearance had higher levels of circulating immune complexes and a predominance of lupus-like disease with DNA and Sm antibodies, malar rash and glomerulonephritis[35]. Maintenance of normal RES function in patients with more classic MCTD may enable these patients to clear immune complexes efficiently and preclude serious renal damage. However, the lungs are more susceptible to injury in MCTD, perhaps because of the different nature of the circulating immune complexes; alternatively, the pulmonary disease could be due to other mechanisms. A solid-phase radioimmunoassay detected many U1 RNP-specific immune complexes in the pericardial fluid, but not in the serum of an MCTD patient with acute hemorrhagic pericarditis[110]. Locally formed U1 RNP immune complexes may have played a role in the development of pericarditis in this patient.

THE CONTROVERSY OF MCTD AS A DISTINCT DISEASE

Since the initial description of MCTD, a large number of studies from around the world have described various aspects of the disease. From these studies, a comprehensive description and clearer understanding of the evolution of the disease has emerged; these studies are reviewed above. Despite this large body of information, several investigators have challenged the existence of MCTD as a discrete entity. In essence, they would choose to classify such patients as SLE, SSc or undifferentiated connective tissue disease.

Over the past 20 years, MCTD has had both its proponents and detractors. In support of MCTD as a distinct entity is its wide recognition in numerous centers within the USA, as well as its recognition outside of the USA, particularly in Japan and Mexico. Does MCTD exist? Upon close critical inspection this is difficult to prove or disprove. The first problem resides in the inherent difficulty with any disease classification system where the etiology of the disease is unknown. In this context, the frequently overlapping and pleomorphic nature of most rheumatic diseases makes them subject to challenge. This is to say that the existence of any disease of unknown etiology is open to question and controversy. The widely recognized clinical syndromes classified as rheumatoid arthritis (RA), SLE, polymyositis and SSc may themselves not stand the test of time once their etiology is known. Further complexity arises when one examines the inherent problems with classification of syndromes. For example, a disease with a single etiology (e.g. Lyme disease) can cause multiple different clinical syndromes, while a single clinical syndrome (e.g. inflammatory polyarthritis) can have many etiologies. Yet despite these limitations, the categorization of diseases where there is incomplete knowledge does serve many useful purposes, such as providing a classification framework for research, treatment and prognosis. The fact that MCTD is characterized by distinct clinical, serologic and, more recently, immunogenetic characteristics, suggests that its recognition does currently serve a useful purpose.

Two potentially important factors to consider in the controversy over MCTD are variation in laboratory detection of autoantibodies and regional variation of disease. The first of these may influence the frequency of recognition and diagnosis of the disease, while the second may influence the true regional prevalence of the disease. Variation in testing of patients for specific antinuclear antibodies by different practitioners could be an important factor contributing to under-recognition of MCTD. In recent years, it has been observed that a substantial number of patients who ultimately develop MCTD initially have mild disease, the most common manifestations being arthralgia/arthritis, swollen hands, and Raynaud's phenomenon with high titer anti-U1-70 kDa autoantibodies (Table 7.1 and 7.2 and discussion below). If specific antinuclear antibody (ANA) testing is not performed on such patients, they may be classified as RA or UCTD without further evaluation for other subclinical manifestations of MCTD or anticipation that such clinical problems may develop. Furthermore, when persons not experienced in snRNP molecular biology perform ANA tests using commercial kits which may contain impure antigens, inaccurate conclusions may be drawn. Testing with sensitive and specific immunoblotting, immunoprecipitation methods or ELISA for measuring autoantibodies against individual snRNP polypeptide antigens is not widely available nor widely utilized. These may be important factors influencing recognition of MCTD.

A second major factor to consider is regional or geographic variation of disease. It has recently been reported that genetic factors influence autoantibody production and disease susceptibility; therefore, regional genetic variation could have a major influence on the incidence and prevalence of the disease in different areas of the world. Such genetic factors may account for the high prevalence of MCTD in Japan and Mexico, where the HLA-linked disease susceptibility gene HLA-DR4 is common in the population. Genetic variation could also contribute to the differences in recognition of MCTD between centers in the USA. It is also possible that there could be an

Table 7.1 Comparison of clinical features in anti-U1-70 kDa autoantibody-positive connective tissue disease patients and those in anti-U1-70 kDa autoantibody-negative systemic lupus erythematosus patients*

	Anti-U1-70 kDa autoantibody		
Clinical feature	Positive (n = 22)	Negative (n = 34)	P
Raynaud's phenomenon	21 (95)	11 (32)	<0.001
Hand swelling, observed	19 (86)	1 (3)	<0.001
Hand swelling, reported	19 (86)	5 (15)	<0.001
Esophageal hypomotility	15 (68)	0 (0)	<0.001
Gastroesophageal reflux	15 (68)	3 (9)	<0.001
Myositis	12 (55)	0 (0)	<0.001
Telangiectasias	11 (50)	5 (15)	<0.007
Sclerodactyly	10 (45)	0(0)	<0.001

* Values are the number (%). All clinical features in the database were compared between the two patient groups. Only those clinical features that were statistically significantly different after correction for multiple comparisons are shown. *P* values determined by Fisher's 2-tailed exact test.
(From Hoffman, R. W. *et al.* (1990) Human autoantibodies against the 70 kDa polypeptide of U1 small nuclear RNP are associated with HLA-DR4 among connective tissue disease patients. *Arth. Rheum.*, **33**, 666–73, by permission of J. B. Lippincott Company, Philadelphia).

environmental factor or environmental trigger which induces disease in a genetically susceptible host. An environmental trigger could have distinct geographic variation and thereby substantially influence the incidence and prevalence of the disease in different geographic areas.

Thus, perhaps many MCTD patients are not recognized or are currently classified as UCTD, RA, SLE or SSc. From a clinical viewpoint does proper recognition and classification of patients as MCTD have an important impact on patient care? Analysis of the existing data in point of fact does support the belief that recognition of MCTD is relevant and important to patient care. This topic is discussed further below in 'Management and prognosis'.

In our own work, we have taken the view that any clinical classification scheme can be considered arbitrary and flawed; thus, approaches have been sought to address basic scientific questions of clinical relevance, irrespective of the controversy of nosology.

These studies have focused on three areas: the immunobiology of anti-U1-70 kDa autoantibody production by human B-cells, the genetic basis of anti-U1-70 kDa autoantibody production, and T-cell regulation. Each of these will be reviewed below.

RECENT AUTOIMMUNE STUDIES

EPITOPE MAPPING OF HUMAN MCTD AND MRL/MP MOUSE AUTOANTIBODY REACTIONS WITH U1 RNP 70 kDa POLYPEPTIDE

Since recent studies have shown a high specificity of antibodies to the U1 RNP 70 kDa polypeptide for MCTD[97], we were interested in examining human serum autoimmune reactivity with that polypeptide through epitope mapping studies. Using a set of recombinant 70 kDa fusion proteins as antigen, ELISA and immunoblotting revealed that most human MCTD serum anti-70 kDa autoantibodies recognized a certain region of the U1 snRNP-associated 70 kDa polypeptide[111]. This region from amino acid residues 94–194 includes the 'RNA recognition motif', which is the U1 RNA-binding domain of the 70 kDa polypeptide[112]. Interestingly, MRL/Mp mice also develop circulating autoantibodies to U1 RNP and Sm antigens, and their anti-70 kDa reactivity is with this same RNA binding epitope region[111]. We have observed that pulmonary vascular lesions, previously reported in MRL mice[113], were particularly severe in mice with very high levels of anti-70 kDa antibodies; thus, these autoimmune mice appear to be analogous to patients with MCTD. Treatment of the MRL mice with monoclonal anti-CD4 lymphocyte antibodies eliminated the snRNP autoimmune serological responses as well as the pulmonary vascular and renal lesions that spontaneously develop in these animals[114]. If it can be shown that there are similarities in pathophysiologic mechanisms between the MRL/Mp mice and patients with MCTD, novel therapeutic approaches might be studied in these mice prior to clinical therapeutic trials.

IMMUNOGENETICS OF HLA AND IMMUNOGLOBULIN ALLOTYPE

Because of the controversy over disease classification and because recent studies have shown a strong association between HLA and the production of specific autoantibodies (such as SSA(Ro)/SSB(La))[115], Hoffman *et al.* have compared HLA phenotypes between anti-U1-70 kDa autoantibody-negative SLE patients (classified using the Revised ACR criteria for disease classification) versus anti-U1-70 kDa autoantibody-positive patients, irrespective of their clinical classification. Patients were classified into anti-U1-70 kDa autoantibody-positive versus negative using a highly specific ELISA. In this ELISA a recombinant U1-70 kDa fusion protein was used as the antigen. It was found that there were highly significant associations between

Table 7.2 Clinical manifestations of MCTD among anti-U1-70 kDa autoantibody-positive pediatric patients

	At onset (%)	Cumulative (%)
	N = 11	
Arthralgia/arthritis	11 (100)	11 (100)
Swollen hands	6 (55)	9 (82)
Raynaud's phenomenon	9 (82)	9 (82)
Abnormal diffusion capacity	3 (27)	9 (82)
Sclerodactyly	4 (36)	7 (64)
Abnormal esophageal motility*	3 (27)	6 (55)
Photosensitivity	5 (45)	6 (55)
Proximal muscle weakness	4 (36)	6 (55)
Pleural effusion	4 (36)	5 (45)
Lymphadenopathy	3 (27)	4 (36)
Cardiac disease	4 (36)	4 (36)
Dysphagia	3 (27)	4 (36)
Telangiectases	3 (27)	4 (36)
Malar erythema	2 (18)	3 (27)
Renal disease	0 (0)	3 (27)[†]
Rheumatoid nodules	2 (18)	2 (18)
Central nervous system disease	2 (18)	2 (18)

* Determined by cine esophagram, manometrics or both.
† Demonstrated by renal biopsy to be focal proliferative, membranous and diffuse proliferative glomerulonephritis, respectively, among these three patients.
(From Hoffman, R. W. *et al.* (1993) U1-70 kDa autantibody-positive mixed connective tissue disease in children: a longitudinal clinical and serologic analysis. *Arth. Rheum.*, **36**, 1599–1602, by permission of JB Lippincott Company, Philadelphia).

the presence of the U1-70 kDa autoantibody and the clinical findings of Raynaud's phenomenon, swollen hands, esophageal hypomotility, gastroesophageal reflux, myositis, telangiectasias and sclerodactyly (Table 7.1). It was found that the U1-70 kDa autoantibody-positive group appeared genetically distinct from the SLE group, based upon the high frequency of HLA-DR4 and HLA-DRw53 among the anti-U1-70 kDa autoantibody-positive group[100].

This work has recently been extended to include a similar study among pediatric

MCTD patients[116]. Eleven pediatric patients with anti-U1-70 kDa autoantibodies were followed longitudinally at the University of Missouri between 1970–90. Clinical features of these patients are summarized in Table 7.2. As shown in Table 7.2, these pediatric patients with anti-U1-70 kDa autoantibody demonstrated clinical manifestations similar to adult patients with anti-U1-70 kDa autoantibody-positive connective tissue disease: Raynaud's phenomenon, swollen hands, esophageal hypomotility, gastroesophageal reflux, myositis, telangiectasias and sclerodactyly. In addition, these patients shared similar immunogenetics with adult patients, with all patients studied possessing HLA-DR4 or HLA-DR2.

In an attempt to further characterize the molecular basis of the association of HLA with anti-U1-70 kDa autoantibodies, molecular genetic methods have been used to examine the genotypes of HLA-DR and DQ genes found among patients. The polymerase chain reaction (PCR) and a method recently developed for direct sequencing of PCR-amplified HLA genes, was used to characterize the HLA genotypes of patients. In a comprehensive analysis of HLA-DRB1, DRB5, DQA1 and DQB1 from 27 patients and controls, a shared epitope was identified within the HLA antigen binding groove, encoded by the amino acids FDYFYQA at positions 26, 28, 30–32, 70, and 73 respectively, of HLA-DRB1 (Figure 7.4). This shared epitope was found on select genotypes of HLA-DR4 and HLA-DR2. From these studies it was concluded that a common cluster of shared amino acids, or a so-called shared epitope, might be important in regulating an autoimmune response to the U1-70 kDa autoantigen[117].

Several studies from Europe, the USA, Mexico and Japan have independently reported association of HLA-DR4 or HLA-DR2 with the presence of autoantibodies to U1 RNP[100,117–120] or MCTD *per se*[118,121,122]. Taken together these data indicate that there is a genetic basis for the production of anti-U1-70 kDa and anti-U1 RNP autoantibodies. Together with clinical data from the study among anti-U1-70 kDa autoantibody-positive versus-negative CTD patients[100], a clear pattern appears to be emerging. Patients who are prone to develop anti-U1-70 kDa autoantibodies have distinct immunogenetics from those who develop other autoantibodies. Furthermore, the presence of certain autoantibodies appears to be linked to the presence of select clinical manifestations of disease, including Raynaud's phenomenon, swollen hands, esophageal hypomotility, gastroesophageal reflux, myositis, telangiectasias and sclerodactyly.

Other polymorphic genes which might be associated with the production of autoantibodies are those encoding the immunoglobulin heavy and light chain genes. Several studies have examined immunoglobulin allotypes to address the question of whether these genes are associated with MCTD[118,119]. Genth *et al.* have reported that the Gm 1,3;5,21 allotype was associated with anti-U1 RNP autoantibodies among German patients[119], and Black *et al.* have reported that the Gm 1,3;5,21 allotype was associated with anti-U1 RNP autoantibodies among patients from the UK[118]. Thus, it appears that there are complex interactions between multiple unlinked immune response regulating genes, which influence the production of autoantibodies reactive with the U1 RNP antigen.

HUMAN snRNP-REACTIVE T-CELLS

The association of anti-U1-70 kDa autoantibodies with HLA class II alleles suggests that T-cells may play a role in autoantibody production. Furthermore, these findings are compatible with an HLA-restricted, antigen-driven immune response. To investigate this possibility further, three groups have attempted to stimulate peripheral blood mononuclear cells (PBMC) from patients or normal blood donors with snRNP antigen and study their T-cell response[123–125]. It has been

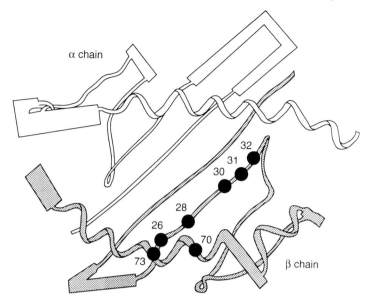

Fig. 7.4 Model of HLA-DR as deduced from X-ray crystallography. Amino acids in positions 26, 28, 30–32, 70 and 73 are shared by HLA-DR4- and HLA-DR2-positive MCTD patients. Amino acids at these positions are spatially related and form a pocket for antigen binding. The amino acid residues Phe, Asp, Tyr, Phe, Tyr, Gln, and Ala at positions 26, 28, 30–32, 70 and 73 form the shared epitope identified among anti-U1-70kDa autoantibody-positive patients. (From Kaneoka *et al.* (1992) Molecular genetic analysis of HLA-DR and HLA-DQ genes among anti-U1-70 kDa autoantibody positive connective tissue disease patients. *Arth. Rheum.*, **35**, 83–94, by permission of J. B. Lippincott Company, Philadelphia.)

recently reported by Hoffman *et al.* that human T-cell lines and clones reactive with snRNP autoantigens can be derived from MCTD and SLE patients, as well as healthy donors possessing the appropriate HLA-DR4 or HLA-DR2 responder genotypes[123]. Similar results have been independently reported by two other groups[124–125]. O'Brien *et al.* have reported that PBMC from MCTD patients proliferated to a U1-70 kDa fusion protein, and they mapped this to a T-cell epitope spanning 63 amino acids of the C-terminal protein of the 70 kDa polypeptide[125]. Wolff-Vorbeck *et al.* have reported generating a single human T-cell line from a healthy donor which was specific for U1-70 kDa and restricted in antigen presentation by HLA-DR4[124]. Taken together these data demonstrate that T-cells reactive with snRNP antigens can be isolated from MCTD patients who possess the appropriate genotypes. Such studies demonstrate that snRNP-

reactive T-cells can be generated *in vitro* and suggest that such cells *in vivo* could play a role in the immunopathogenesis of disease.

With regard to the original question 'does MCTD exist?' these data would appear to bring the question full circle. It appears that there are genetic factors which influence auto-antibody and autoreactive T-cell generation. Finally, the presence of such autoantibodies and autoreactive T-cells appears to be associated with the presence of a specific constellation of clinical manifestations of disease: Raynaud's phenomenon, swollen hands, esophageal hypomotility, gastroesophageal reflux, myositis, telangiectasias and sclerodactyly[100].

MODEL PROPOSED FOR DISEASE PROCESS

Based upon existing data, a working model of disease susceptibility and pathogenesis in

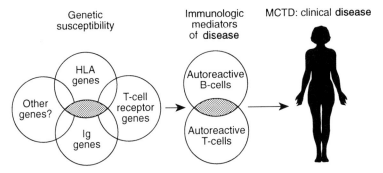

Fig. 7.5 In this proposed model for disease susceptibility HLA genes, immunoglobulin genes, T-cell receptor genes and other currently unidentified genes contribute to disease susceptibility.

MCTD can be proposed (Figure 7.5). While it is currently speculative, it appears reasonable to propose that an infectious agent or another triggering event may initiate disease in a susceptible host. It is clear that genetic susceptibility, linked to HLA, immunoglobulin genes and perhaps other genes, contributes to anti-U1-70 kDa autoantibody production. With regard to HLA and Ig allotypes which have been identified, genes encoding the disease-associated phenotypes are common in the population; therefore, additional factors must be considered in any model of disease susceptibility. Three alternative hypotheses are possible based upon existing data. First, an environmental factor(s) is necessary to cause disease in a genetically susceptible host. To date no such agent(s) has been identified; however, this remains one of the most attractive models. Secondly, a yet unidentified gene, such as that for a T-cell receptor polymorphism, interacts with HLA and Ig genes and the presence of multiple (at least three) unlinked genes is necessary for disease to occur. Thirdly, stochastic events influencing the immune system, such as those which occur in shaping the T-cell and B-cell repertoires, occur and are essential in causing disease in an individual patient.

MANAGEMENT AND PROGNOSIS

Lacking controlled, longitudinal evaluations, the treatment of MCTD is based on anecdotal information. Because the disease frequently undergoes transitions in its evolution, different treatments may be appropriate for the same patient over a period of time. In the original report of MCTD, the disease appeared to be responsive to corticosteroids and/or cyclophosphamide[1]. However, with longer observations and the recognition of severe complications of pulmonary disease, pulmonary hypertension and proliferative vascular lesions, it is now appreciated that the outcome is not always favorable[11,12].

In our prospective, longitudinal study in which almost all of the 34 patients had significant major organ system involvement requiring moderate to high doses of corticosteroids and/or cytotoxic drugs, about two-thirds responded favorably to treatment[11]. A good, long-term prognosis for some patients with MCTD is demonstrated by the 38% of these patients studied whose disease became inactive, including 10 who have been in a sustained remission (9 off all therapy) for 7–20 years (mean 16 years). Inflammatory changes, such as pleuritis, rash, pericarditis and myositis, are likely to respond to corticosteroids, while pulmonary and scleroderma-like features are less likely to respond. One-third of the patients in our long-term study had very severe disease, were less responsive to corticosteroids, and 4 patients died.

In our MCTD patients who are in prolonged remission following intensive corticosteroid

Table 7.3 Management of MCTD

Type of disease activity	Recommendations
Mild undifferentiated connective tissue disease (Raynaud's phenomenon, arthralgias, myalgias, fatigue, mild synovitis)	NSAIDs*, antimalarials, low-dose corticosteroids, avoid cold exposure, calcium channel blockers as tolerated if Raynaud's phenomenon is severe
Disease activity limited to erosive rheumatoid arthritis-like joint involvement	NSAIDs, antimalarials; low dose corticosteroids or methotrexate if more severe
Mild-moderate systemic lupus erythematosus-like involvement (rash, serositis, anemia, leukopenia, fever, lymphadenopathy)	Avoid sun exposure, topical corticosteroids, antimalarials, low to intermediate doses of corticosteroids
Systemic lupus erythematosus-like involvement of major organ systems (pericarditis, myocarditis, thrombocytopenia, glomerulonephritis, aseptic meningitis[†*]), myositis, progressive involvement of lung, dysfunction of upper esophageal sphincter with dysphagia and/or aspiration pneumonia	Moderate to high doses of corticosteroids depending on severity; add cytotoxic drug if steroid-dependent
Esophageal reflux without upper sphincter involvement	Raise head of bed, avoid caffeine, discontinue smoking, H2 blockers, H^+ proton pump blockers, metoclopramide; corticosteroids may be used if severe dysphagia related to lower esophageal involvement is not responsive to these conservative measures
Asymptomatic pulmonary hypertension	Right heart catheterization and monitoring pressures in response to therapeutic agents may be a guide to therapy; calcium channel blockers, angiotensin-converting enzyme inhibitors
Symptomatic pulmonary hypertension	Calcium channel blockers, angiotensin-converting enzyme inhibitors, corticosteroids, cyclophosphamide or other cytotoxic drugs

* NSAID = nonsteroidal anti-inflammatory drugs.
† Ibuprofen and Sulindac have been associated with a hypersensitivity aseptic meningitis in MCTD so NSAIDs should be discontinued.

and cytotoxic drug therapy, very sensitive immunoblotting and ELISA assays have revealed the eventual disappearance of serum anti-U1 RNP autoantibodies, including the anti-70 kDa snRNP reactivity which had usually persisted for years[92,97]. Whatever mechanisms are responsible for the sustained production of U1 RNP antibodies would seem to have been altered in these patients. This is in contrast to a group of 13 MCTD patients followed in the private rheumatology practice of Dr Jack Horn who had milder disease and were treated with either low doses of corticosteroids, or non-steroidal anti-inflammatory drugs (NSAIDs)[92]. The sera of these patients still showed anti-70 kDa and other U1 snRNP polypeptide reactivity after years of observation and mean follow-up time of 8.5 years, even though most had minimal disease activity and 5 were in remission.

Guidelines for management of specific clinical problems in MCTD are presented in Table 7.3. Mild, undifferentiated connective tissue disease features can often be managed without resorting to corticosteroids. If arthritis predominates without major organ system involvement, it can also frequently be managed conservatively with NSAIDs or antimalarials[41]; however, if bone erosions occur or the synovitis is more refractory, low doses of corticosteroids and/or methotrexate may be required. Mild SLE-like features usually respond to antimalarials or low doses of corticosteroids. Higher doses of corticosteroids may be required for treatment of more serious systemic involvement (e.g. pericarditis, myocarditis, myositis).

Studies of 10 patients treated for other manifestations of the disease suggested that esophageal function in MCTD may be responsive to corticosteroids[48]. One patient whose disease flare was confined to severe dysfunction of the upper esophageal sphincter (UES) and lower esophagus had improvement in UES function, esophageal motility and resolution of recurrent aspiration pneumonia following corticosteroid therapy[48]. Improvement in pulmonary diffusing capacity has also been observed in MCTD patients treated with corticosteroids[11].

It has become clear that certain clinical problems in MCTD (e.g. myositis, pulmonary disease, pulmonary hypertension) may be present for years before they become symptomatic[11]. Early treatment of myositis in MCTD may be successful with only moderate doses of corticosteroids[32]. Pulmonary hypertension, particularly if it is detected early, may respond to treatment with nifedipine[57]. During right heart catheterization, hemodynamic measurements can be made to try to determine which therapeutic agent (calcium channel blocker, angiotensin-converting enzyme inhibitor, etc.) may be most effective[57]. When pulmonary hypertension is severe, corticosteroids and cytotoxic agents have also been employed, but the responses have not always been favorable [11,50,51].

The initial report of MCTD suggested a favorable prognosis[1]. A less generally favorable prognosis, citing cardiac disease, severe thrombocytopenia, proliferative vascular lesions and renal disease, was first indicated in the pediatric literature[8,25]. Causes of death were pneumococcal or meningococcal infections in three and cerebral hemorrhage (secondary to thrombocytopenia) in one patient. In addition, the follow-up study of the initially reported MCTD patients stated that 8 patients had died and that scleroderma-like features had persisted while the inflammatory disease manifestations appeared to have responded to corticosteroid treatment[17]. However, 6 of the 8 deaths were not directly related to a rheumatic disorder[17]. Other long-term studies with sequential assessment have shown that the most frequent disease-related deaths are associated with proliferative vascular lesions, pulmonary hypertension, cor pulmonale, pericardial tamponade and sepsis, with perforated bowel, intravascular coagulation and renal failure less frequently noted.

The combined mortality rate from 7 long-term studies of MCTD (236 patients) was 13.6%, with a mean disease duration of 10 years[11,12,126]. The mortality rate of deaths directly related to the disease was 9.7%. Thus, the prognosis in MCTD is similar to that of SLE but better than that of systemic sclerosis.

In the summary of the follow-up report in 1980 by Nimelstein *et al.* of the original MCTD series it is stated:

'. . . within our present knowledge, treatment of patients classified as having MCTD or with antibodies to RNP should not be different from treatment of patients with SLE, PM or PSS with similar disease manifestations. At this time, determination of antibody to RNP has little practical clinical utility, though study of it and other auto-antibodies continues to be of investigative importance.'

Thirteen years later the accumulated evidence from continued investigations tends to refute these conclusions. It has been shown that

Table 7.4 Distinctive clinical, immunologic and genetic features of MCTD

1. Clinical: constellation of arthralgia/arthritis, swollen hands, Raynaud's phenomenon, abnormal esophageal motility, sclerodactyly, pulmonary hypertension.
2. B-cell responses: high titer U1 RNP antibodies and particularly anti-U1-70 kDa autoantibodies, typically in the absence of other autoantibodies.
3. Genetic: association with HLA-DR4 and shared epitope on HLA-DRB1 found on haplotypes bearing HLA-DR4 and HLA-DR2.
4. Immunoregulatory: T-cell: snRNP-reactive T-cells found in the peripheral blood of patients; immunoregulatory defects of T-cells differing from those of SLE and systemic sclerosis.
5. Immune complexes: lower levels of immune complexes found in the circulation than in SLE; more rapid RES clearance of immune complexes than from the circulation in SLE.
6. Histopathology: proliferative vasculopathy in the virtual absence of fibrosis and widespread lymphocytic and plasmacytic infiltrates.

high titers of anti-U1 RNP with anti-70 kDa antibodies are associated with a high risk of myositis, esophageal dysfunction, pulmonary disease and pulmonary hypertension, which can be detected by functional tests and biopsies early in MCTD when patients are still asymptomatic. Thus, this serologic pattern serves as a guide to the clinician to evaluate muscle enzymes, EMG, muscle biopsy, esophageal motility studies, pulmonary function tests and, depending on these results, an echocardiogram and possibly a right heart catheterization might be performed.

If abnormalities in these organ systems are detected, studies have shown that early therapeutic intervention may be indicated and may control the disease with shorter and/or more selective types of drug therapy than would be true if the disease were more advanced or due to a different connective tissue disease. Thus, early treatment of myositis in MCTD may be successful with lower doses of corticosteroids for a shorter duration than in the case of polymyositis[32]. Early pulmonary DLCO abnormalities and esophageal dysfunction in MCTD may respond to corticosteroid therapy[11,48] in contrast to systemic sclerosis, and early pulmonary hypertension in MCTD (in an asymptomatic phase) may be successfully treated with nifedipine[57], thus avoiding more severe symptomatic disease.

In terms of the clinician's overall management of the patient, the finding of a high titer of anti-70 kDa U1 RNP antibody and absence of Sm and DNA antibodies allows a focus on development of these more likely clinical problems rather than on CNS and renal disease complications more to be anticipated in SLE. Thus, despite the absence of controlled trials to guide therapy, a rational approach to treatment in MCTD can be formulated based upon careful, clinical and serologic evaluation of patients with systemic rheumatic diseases. Recognition of this distinct group of patients with MCTD has important implications for both management and prognosis (Table 7.4).

snRNP CELL BIOLOGY

In addition to their usefulness as markers of systemic rheumatic diseases, autoantibodies to snRNPs have also proven to be invaluable tools for the molecular characterization of snRNP antigens. A substantial number of snRNP antigens have now been molecularly cloned, including those encoding the U1-70 kDa polypeptide[127]. Structural analysis of cDNA clones encoding individual polypeptides has yielded interesting findings that may be relevant in the pathogenesis of autoimmunity. For example, it was shown that structural homology exists between U1-70 kDa and a retroviral p30^{gag} antigen[128]. These findings were provocative in that they implicated a possible retroviral etiology in MCTD. Subsequent epitope mapping studies, however, by Takeda *et al.* and others have demonstrated that the region shared with p30^{gag} is not the main epitope recognized by MCTD sera[111]. Future studies of this type may, however, lead to the identification of cross-reactive epitopes of clinical significance in the pathogenesis of MCTD.

Autoantibodies have also been described which recognize epitopes on U1 RNA stem loops. Thus, not only are protein components of snRNP recognized by autoantibodies, but RNA components of the complex are recognized as well[129]. Of particular clinical interest are recent studies that have reported that anti-U1 RNA antibody levels correlate with disease activity in MCTD[102].

Human antisera have also proved to be useful in basic cell biologic studies, such as in determining the intranuclear localization of snRNP antigen. These antisera have been used with double immunofluorescence and digital imaging techniques to characterize the intranuclear organization of the cell. They have also assisted in the co-localization analysis of intracellular antigens, such as Sm/U1snRNP[130].

FUTURE DIRECTIONS

Future studies from a number of research laboratories are currently focusing on further characterization of the fine specificities of B-cell and T-cell responses against snRNP antigens. Studies which are attempting to characterize T-cell clones and the basic biology of antigen recognition potentially could lead to clinical applications, such as of the use of synthetic peptides as therapeutic agents. Recent basic studies on mucosal immunity and studies demonstrating that the oral administration of antigenic peptide can modulate autoimmunity pose interesting new potential avenues of investigation using snRNP antigens as oral tolerogens.

Other areas of future promise include the use of targeted immunotherapy with monoclonal antibodies, and cytokine receptor antagonists as therapeutic agents. For example, humanized monoclonal antibodies, directed against cell surface receptors, such as CD4 or CD5, or against cytokines, may be useful as therapeutic agents to treat systemic rheumatic diseases, including MCTD (Chapter 15). Studies using humanized anti-CD4 monoclonal antibodies have shown promise in treating rheumatoid arthritis and systemic lupus erythematosus in clinical trials. Preliminary results have suggested that soluble receptors for various cytokines may have efficacy in immune-mediated disease. Another approach which holds potential promise is the use of monoclonal antibodies directed against the T-cell receptors of select receptor phenotypes. For example, if effector T-cells in MCTD use a restricted set of variable region genes, these could be targeted for depletion as a new therapeutic approach in MCTD. Precedent for the use of a limited set of T-cell receptor variable-region genes exists in multiple sclerosis, where selective TCR genes appear to predominate. Although multiple sclerosis may be the exception rather than the rule, we are currently examining the possibility that a limited set of T-cell receptor $V\beta$ or $V\alpha$ genes are used by auto-reactive T-cells in MCTD.

REFERENCES

1. Sharp, G. C., Irvin, W. S., Gould, R. G. *et al.* (1972) Mixed connective tissue disease. An apparently distinct rheumatic disease syndrome associated with a specific antibody to an extractable nuclear antigen (ENA). *Am. J. Med.*, **52**, 148–59.
2. Northway, J. S. and Tan, E. M. (1972) Differentiations of antinuclear antibodies giving speckled staining patterns in immnofluorescence. *Clin. Immunol. Immunopath.*, **1**, 140–54.
3. Reichlin, M. and Mattioli, M. (1972) Correlation of a precipitin reaction to an RNA protein antigen and low prevalence of nephritis in patients with systemic lupus erythematosus. *New Eng. J. Med.*, **286**, 908–11.
4. Parker, M. D. (1973) Ribonucleoprotein antibodies: frequencies and clinical significance in systemic lupus erythematosus, scleroderma and mixed connective tissue disease. *J. Lab. Clin. Med.*, **82**, 769–75.

5. Sharp, G. C., Irvin, W. S., May, C. M. *et al.* (1976) Association of antibodies to ribonucleoprotein and Sm antigens with mixed connective tissue disease, systemic lupus erythematosus and other rheumatic diseases. *New Eng. J. Med.,* **295**, 1149–54.

6. Bridges, A. J., Anderson, J. D., McKay, J. *et al.* (1993) Antinuclear antibody testing in a referral laboratory. *Lab. Med.,* **24**(6), 345–9.

7. Notman, D. D., Kurata, N. and Tan, E. M. (1975) Profiles of antinuclear antibodies in systemic rheumatic diseases. *Ann. Int. Med.,* **83**, 464–9.

8. Singsen, B. H., Kornreich, H. K., Koster-King, K. *et al.* (1977) Mixed connective tissue disease in childhood. A clinical and serologic survey. *J. Ped.,* **90**, 893–900.

9. Gilliam, J. N. and Prystowsky, S. D. (1977) Mixed connective tissue disease syndrome: The cutaneous manifestations of patients with epidermal nuclear staining and high titer antibody to RNase sensitive extractable nuclear antigen (ENA). *Arch. Derm.,* **113**, 583–7.

10. Grant, K. D., Adams, L. E. and Hess, E. V. (1981) Mixed connective tissue disease – a subset with sequential clinical and laboratory features. *J. Rheum.,* **8**, 587–98.

11. Sullivan, W. D., Hurst, D. J., Harmon, C. E. *et al.* (1984) A prospective evaluation emphasizing pulmonary involvement in patients with mixed connective tissue disease. *Medicine,* **63**, 92–107.

12. Lundberg, I. and Hedfors, E. (1991) Clinical course of patients with anti-RNP antibodies. A prospective study of 32 patients. *J. Rheum.,* **18**(10), 1511–19.

13. Bennett, R. M. and O'Connell, D. J. (1980) Mixed connective tissue disease: a clinicopathologic study of 20 cases. *Sem. Arth. Rheum.,* **10**, 25–51.

14. Sharp, G. C. and Singsen, B. H. (1993) Mixed connective tissue disease, in *Arthritis and Allied Conditions,* (eds D. J. McCarty and W. J. Koopman), Lea & Febiger, Philadelphia, pp. 1213–24.

15. Nakae, K., Furusawa, F., Kasukawa, R. *et al.* (1987) A nationwide epidemiological survey on diffuse collagen diseases: Estimation of prevalence rate in Japan, in *Mixed Connective Tissue Disease and Anti-nuclear Antibodies,* (eds R. Kasukawa and G. C. Sharp), Elsevier Science Publishers B. V., Amsterdam, pp. 9–13.

16. Horn, J. R., Kapur, J. J. and Walker, S. E. (1978) Mixed connective tissue disease in siblings. *Arth. Rheum.,* **21**, 709–14.

17. Nimelstein, S. H., Brody, S., McShane, D. *et al.* (1980) Mixed connective tissue disease: A subsequent evaluation of the original 25 patients. *Medicine,* **59**, 239–48.

18. Manthorpe, R., Elling, H., van der Meulen, J. T. *et al.* (1980) Two fatal cases of mixed connective tissue disease. Description of case histories terminating as progressive systemic sclerosis. *Scand. J. Rheum.,* **9**, 7–10.

19. Hainaut, P., Lavenne, E., Magy, J. M. *et al.* (1986) Circulating lupus type anticoagulant and pulmonary hypertension associated with mixed connective tissue disease. *Clin. Rheum.,* **5**, 96–101.

20. Kitridou, R. C., Akmal, M., Turkel, S. B. *et al.* (1986) Renal involvement in mixed connective tissue disease: a longitudinal clinicopathologic study. *Sem. Arth. Rheum.,* **16**, 135–45.

21. Salerni, R., Rodnan, G. P., Leon, D. F. *et al.* (1977) Pulmonary hypertension in the crest syndrome variant of progressive system sclerosis (scleroderma). *Ann. Int. Med.,* **86**, 394–9.

22. Hosoda, Y., Suzuki, Y., Takano, M. *et al.* (1987) Mixed connective tissue disease with pulmonary hypertension: A clinical and pathological study. *J. Rheum.,* **14**, 826–30.

23. Hosoda, Y. (1987) Review on pathology of mixed connective tissue disease, in *Mixed Connective Tissue Disease and Anti-nuclear Antibodies,* (eds R. Kasukawa and G. Sharp), Elsevier Science Publishers B. V., Amsterdam, pp. 281–90.

24. Jones, M. B., Osterholm, R. K., Wilson, R. B. *et al.* (1978) Fatal pulmonary hypertension and resolving immune-complex glomerulonephritis in mixed connective tissue disease. A case report and review of the literature. *Am. J. Med.,* **65**, 855–63.

25. Singsen, B. H., Swanson, V. L., Bernstein, B. H. *et al.* (1980) A histologic evaluation of mixed connective tissue disease in childhood. *Am. J. Med.,* **68**, 710–17.

26. Asherson, R. A., Higenbottam, T. W., Dinh Xuan, A. T. *et al.* (1990) Pulmonary hypertension in a lupus clinic: Experience with twenty-four patients. *J. Rheum.,* **17**, 1292–8.

27. Sharp, G. C. (1987) Diagnostic criteria for classification of MCTD, in *Mixed Connective Tissue Disease and Anti-nuclear Antibodies,* (eds R. Kasukawa and G. C. Sharp), Elsevier

Science Publishers B. V., Amsterdam, pp. 23–32.

28. Alarcón-Segovia, D. A. and Villarreal, M. (1987) Classification and diagnostic criteria for mixed connective tissue disease, in *Mixed Connective Tissue Disease and Anti-nuclear Antibodies*, (eds R. Kasukawa and G. C. Sharp), Elsevier Science Publishers B. V., Amsterdam, pp. 33–40.

29. Kasukawa, R., Tojo, T., Miyawaki, S. *et al.* (1987) Preliminary diagnostic criteria for classification of mixed connective tissue disease, in *Mixed Connective Tissue Disease and Anti-nuclear Antibodies*, (eds R. Kasukawa and G. C. Sharp, Elsevier Science Publishers B. V., Amsterdam, pp. 41–7.

30. Porter, J. F., Kingsland, L. C. III, Lindberg, D. A. B. *et al.* (1988) The A1/RHEUM knowledge-based computer consultant system in rheumatology: Performance in the diagnosis of 59 connective tissue disease patients from Japan. *Arth. Rheum.*, **31**, 219–26.

31. Alarcón-Segovia, D. and Cardiel, M. H. (1989) Comparison between 3 diagnostic criteria for mixed connective tissue disease. Study of 593 patients. *J. Rheum.*, **16**, 328–34.

32. Lundberg, I., Nennesmo, I. and Hedfors, E. (1992) A clinical, serological, and histopathological study of myositis patients with and without anti-RNP antibodies. *Sem. Arth. Rheum.*, **22**(2), 127–38.

33. Treadwell, E. L., Alspaugh, M. A., Wolfe, J. F. *et al.* (1984) Clinical relevance of PM-1 antibody and physiochemical characterization of PM-1 antigen. *J. Rheum.*, **11**, 658–62.

34. Wasicek, C. A., Reichlin, M., Montes, M. *et al.* (1984) Polymyositis and interstitial lung disease in the patient with the anti-Jo$_1$ prototype. *Am. J. Med.*, **76**, 538–44.

35. Frank, M. M., Lawley, T. J., Hamburger, M. I. *et al.* (1983) Immunoglobulin G Fc receptor-mediated clearance in autoimmune disease. *Ann. Int. Med.*, **98**, 206–18.

36. Rasmussen, E. K., Ullman, S., Hier-Madsen, M. *et al.* (1987) Clinical implications of ribonucleoprotein antibody. *Arch. Derm.*, **123**, 601–5.

37. Kappes, J. and Bennett, R. M. (1982) Cauda equina syndrome in a patient with high titer anti-RNP antibodies. *Arth. Rheum.*, **25**, 349–52.

38. Konttinen, Y. T., Tuominen, T. S., Piirainen, H. I. *et al.* (1990) Signs and symptoms in the masticatory system in ten patients with mixed connective tissue disease. *Scan. J. Rheum.*, **19**, 363–73.

39. Iwatsuki, K., Tagami, H., Imaizumi, S., *et al.* (1982) The speckled epidermal nuclear immunofluorescence of mixed connective tissue disease seems to develop as an in vitro phenomenon. *Br. J. Derm.*, **107**, 653–7.

40. Alarcón-Segovia, D., Ruiz-Arguelles, A. and Fishbein, E. (1979) Antibody penetration into living cells. I. Intranuclear immunoglobulin in peripheral blood mononuclear cells in mixed connective tissue disease and systemic lupus erythematosus. *Clin. Experi. Immunol.*, **35**, 364–75.

41. Bennett, R. M. and O'Connell, D. J. (1978) The arthritis of mixed connective tissue disease. *Ann. Rheum. Dis.*, **37**, 397–403.

42. Martinez-Cordero, E. and Lopez-Zepeda, J. (1990) Resorptive arthropathy and rib erosions in mixed connective tissue disease. *J. Rheum.*, **17**, 719–22.

43. O'Connell, D. J. and Bennett, R. M. (1977) Mixed connective tissue disease – clinical and radiological aspects of 20 cases. *Br. J. Radiol.*, **50**, 620–5.

44. Sargent, E. N., Turner, A. F. and Jacobson, G. (1969) Superior marginal rib defects: an etiologic classification. *Am. J. Roentgenol.*, **106**, 491–505.

45. Piirainen, H. I. (1990) Patients with arthritis and anti-U1-RNP antibodies: a 10-year follow-up. *Br. J. Rheum.*, **29**, 345–8.

46. Lewis, R. A., Adams, J. P., Gerber, N. L. *et al.* (1978) The hand in mixed connective tissue disease. *J. Hand Surg.*, **3**, 217–22.

47. Oxenhandler, R., Hart, M., Corman, L. *et al.* (1977) Pathology of skeletal muscle in mixed connective tissue disease. *Arth. Rheum.*, **20**, 985–8.

48. Marshall, J. B., Kretschmar, J. M., Gerhardt, D. C. *et al.* (1990) Gastrointestinal manifestations of mixed connective tissue disease. *Gastroenterology*, **98**, 1232–8.

49. Gutierrez, F., Valenzuela, J. E., Ehresmann, G. R. *et al.* (1982) Esophageal dysfunction in patients with mixed connective tissue disease and systemic lupus erythematosus. *Digest. Dis. Sci.*, **27**, 592–7.

50. Rosenberg, A. M., Petty, R. E., Cumming, G. R. *et al.* (1979) Pulmonary hypertension in a child with mixed connective tissue disease. *J. Rheumatol.*, **6**, 700–4.

51. Wiener-Kronish, J. P., Solinger, A. M., Warnock, M. S. *et al.* (1981) Severe pulmonary

involvement in mixed connective tissue disease. *Am. Rev. Respir. Dis.*, **124**, 499–503.

52. Udaya, B. S. and Prakash, M. D. (1985) Intrathoracic manifestations in mixed connective tissue disease. *Mayo Clin. Proc.*, **60**, 813–21.

53. Sanchez-Guerrero, J., Cesarman, G. and Alarcón-Segovia, D. (1989) Massive pulmonary hemorrhage in mixed connective tissue disease. *J. Rheumatol.*, **16**, 1132–4.

54. Germain, M. J. and Davidman, M. (1984) Pulmonary hemorrhage and acute renal failure in a patient with mixed connective tissue disease. *Am. J. Kid. Dis.*, **3**, 420–4.

55. Martens, J. and Demedts, M. (1982) Diaphragm dysfunction in mixed connective tissue disease. *Scan. J. Rheumatol.*, **11**, 165–7.

56. Horn, J. R. Personal Communication.

57. Alpert, M. A., Pressly, T. A., Mukerji, V. *et al.* (1991) Acute and long-term effects of Nifedipine on pulmonary and systemic hemodynamics in patients with pulmonary hypertension associated with diffuse systemic sclerosis, the CREST syndrome and mixed connective tissue disease. *Am. J. Cardiol.*, **68**, 1687–91.

58. Alpert, M. A., Goldberg, S. H., Singsen, B. H. *et al.* (1983) Cardiovascular manifestations of mixed connective tissue disease in adults. *Circulation*, **68**, 1182–93.

59. Oetgen, W. J., Mutter, M. L., Davia, J. E. *et al.* (1983) Cardiac abnormalities in mixed connective tissue disease. *Chest*, **2**, 185–8.

60. Cryer, P. F. and Kissane, J. M. (Eds.) (1978) Clinicopathologic Conference. Mixed connective tissue disease. *Am. J. Med.*, **65**, 833–42.

61. Lash, A. D., Wittman, A. L. and Quismorio, F. P., Jr. (1986) Myocarditis in mixed connective tissue disease: clinical and pathologic study of three cases and review of the literature. *Sem. Arth. Rheum.*, **15**, 288–96.

62. Comens, S. M., Alpert, M. D., Sharp, G. C. *et al.* (1989) Frequency of mitral valve prolapse in systemic lupus erythematosus, progressive systemic sclerosis and mixed connective tissue disease. *Am. J. Cardiol.*, **63**, 369–70.

63. Bennett, R. M. and Spargo, B. H. (1977) Immune complex nephropathy in mixed connective tissue disease. *Am. J. Med.*, **63**, 534–41.

64. Bresnihan, B., Bunn, C., Snaith, M. L. *et al.* (1977) Antiribonucleoprotein antibodies in connective tissue diseases: Estimation by counter-immunoelectrophoresis. *Br. Med. J.*, **1**, 610–1.

65. Rao, K. V., Berkseth, R. O., Crosson, J. E. *et al.* (1976) Immune complex nephritis in mixed connective tissue disease. *Ann. Intern. Med.*, **84**, 174–6.

66. Koboyashi, S., Nagase, M., Kimura, M. *et al.* (1985) Renal involvement in mixed connective tissue disease. *Am. J. Nephrol.*, **5**, 282–9.

67. Cohen, I. M., Swerdlin, A. H., Steinberg, S. M. *et al.* (1980) Mesangial proliferative glomerulonephritis in mixed connective tissue disease (MCTD). *Clin. Nephrol.*, **13**, 93–6.

68. Halla, J. T., Schronhenloher, R. E., Hardin, J. G. *et al.* (1978) Circulating immune complexes in mixed connective tissue disease (MCTD). *Arth. Rheum.*, **21**, 562–3.

69. Crapper, R. M., Dowling, J. P., Mackay, I. R. *et al.* (1987) Acute scleroderma in stable mixed connective tissue disease: treatment by plasmapheresis. *Austral. New Zealand J. Med.*, **17**, 327–9.

70. Bennett, R. M., Bong, D. M. and Spargo, B. H. (1978) Neuropsychiatric problems in mixed connective tissue disease. *Am. J. Med.*, **65**, 955–62.

71. Searles, R. P., Mladinich, E. K. and Messner, R. P. (1978) Isolated trigeminal sensory neuropathy: early manifestation of mixed connective tissue disease. *Neurol.*, **28**, 1286–9.

72. Varga, E., Field, E. A. and Tyldesley, W. R. (1990) Orofacial manifestations of mixed connective tissue disease. *Br. Dent. J.*, **168**, 330.

73. Vincent, R. M. and Van Houzen, R. N. (1980) Trigeminal sensory neuropathy and bilateral carpal tunnel syndrome: the initial manifestation of mixed connective tissue disease. *J. Neurol., Neurosurg. Psych.*, **43**, 458–60.

74. Bronshvas, M. M., Prystowsky, S. D. and Traviesa, D. C. (1978) Vascular headaches in mixed connective tissue disease. *Headache*, **18**, 154–60.

75. Hyslop, D. L., Singsen, B. H. and Sharp, G. C. (1986) Leukocyte function, infection and mortality in mixed connective tissue disease (MCTD). *Arth. Rheum.*, **29**, S64.

76. Weiss, T. D., Nelson, J. S., Woolsey, R. M. *et al.* (1978) Transverse myelitis in mixed connective tissue disease. *Arth. Rheum.*, **21**, 982–6.

77. Martyn, J. B., Wong, M. J. and Huang, S. H. (1988) Pulmonary and neuromuscular complications of mixed connective tissue disease: a report and review of the literature. *J. Rheumatol.*, **15**, 703–5.

78. Kraus, A., Cervantes, G., Borojas, E. *et al.*

(1985) Retinal vasculitis in mixed connective tissue disease. *J. Rheumatol.*, **12**, 1122–4.

79. Fraga, A., Gudino, J., Ramos-Niembro, F. *et al.* (1978) Mixed connective tissue disease in childhood. Relationship with Sjögren's syndrome. *Am. J. Dis. Child.*, **132**, 263–5.

80. Norman, D. A. and Fleischmann, R. M. (1978) Gastrointestinal systemic sclerosis in serologic mixed connective tissue disease. *Arth. Rheum.*, **21**, 811–19.

81. Lynn, J. T., Gossen, G., Miller, A. *et al.* (1984) Pneumatosis intestinalis in mixed connective tissue disease: two case reports and literature review. *Arth. Rheum.*, **27**, 1186–9.

82. Cosnes, J., Levy, R. A. and Darnis, F. (1980) Budd-Chiari syndrome in a patient with mixed connective tissue disease. *Dig. Dis. Sci.*, **25**, 467–9.

83. Lundberg, I. and Hedfors, E. (1991) Pregnancy outcome in patients with high titer anti-RNP antibodies. A retrospective study of 40 pregnancies. *J. Rheumatol.*, **18**, 359–62.

84. Kaufman, R. L. and Kitridou, R. C. (1982) Pregnancy in mixed connective tissue disease: comparison with systemic lupus erythematosus. *J. Rheumatol.*, **9**, 549–55.

85. Segond, P., Yeni, P., Jacquot, J. M. *et al.* (1978) Severe autoimmune anemia and thrombopenia in mixed connective tissue disease. *Arth. Rheum.*, **21**, 995–6.

86. de Rooij, D. J. R. A. M., van de Putte, L. B. A. and van Beusekom, H. J. (1982) Severe thrombocytopenia in mixed connective tissue disease. *Scan. J. Rheumatol.*, **11**, 184–6.

87. ter Borg, E.-J., Houtman, P. M., Kallenberg, C. G. M. *et al.* (1988) Thrombocytopenia and hemolytic anemia in a patient with mixed connective tissue disease due to thrombotic thrombocytopenic purpura. *J. Rheumatol.*, **15**, 1174–7.

88. Julkunen, H., Jantti, J. and Pettersson, T. (1989) Pure red cell aplasia in mixed connective tissue disease. *J. Rheumatol.*, **16**, 1385–6.

89. Diaz-Jouanen, E., Llorente, L., Ramos-Niembro, F. *et al.* (1977) Cold-reactive lymphocytotoxic antibodies in mixed connective tissue disease. *J. Rheumatol.*, **4**, 4–10.

90. Sharp, G. C., Irvin, W. S., LaRoque, R. L. *et al.* (1971) Association of autoantibodies to different nuclear antigens with clinical patterns of rheumatic disease and responsiveness to therapy. *J. Clin. Invest.*, **50**, 350–9.

91. Alarcón-Segovia, D. (1979) Mixed connective tissue disease: Appearance of antibodies to ribonucleoprotein following corticosteroid treatment. *J. Rheumatol.*, **6**, 694–9.

92. Pettersson, I., Wang, G., Smith, E. I. *et al.* (1986) The use of immunoblotting and immunoprecipitation of (U) small nuclear ribonucleoproteins in the analysis of sera of patients with mixed connective tissue disease and systemic lupus erythematosus. A cross-sectional, longitudinal study. *Arth. Rheum.*, **29**, 986–96.

93. Takano, M., Golden, S. S., Sharp, G. C. *et al.* (1981) Molecular relationships between two nuclear antigens, ribonucleoprotein and Sm: purification of active antigens and their biochemical characterization. *Biochemistry* **21**, 5929–36.

94. Lerner, M. R. and Steitz, J. A. (1979) Antibodies to small nuclear RNAs complexed with proteins are produced by patients with systemic lupus erythematosus. *Proc. Nat. Acad. Sci. USA.*, **76**, 5495–9.

95. Lerner, M. R., Boyle, J. A., Hardin, J. A. *et al.* (1981) Two novel classes of small ribonucleoproteins detected by antibodies associated with lupus erythematosus. *Science*, **211**, 400–2.

96. Pettersson, I., Hinterberger, M., Mimori, T. *et al.* (1984) The structure of mammalian small nuclear ribonucleoproteins: identification of multiple protein components reactive with anti-(U1) ribonucleoprotein and anti-Sm autoantibodies. *J. Bio. Chem.*, **259**, 5907–14.

97. Takeda, Y., Wang, G. S., Wang, R. J. *et al.* (1989) Enzyme-linked immunosorbent assay using isolated (U) small nuclear ribonucleoprotein polypeptides as antigens to investigate the clinical significance of autoantibodies to these polypeptides. *Clin. Immunol. Immunopath.*, **50**, 213–30.

98. Habets, W. J., de Rooij, D. J., Salden, M. H. *et al.* (1983) Antibodies against distinct nuclear matrix proteins are characteristic for mixed connective tissue disease. *Clin. Experi. Immunol.*, **54**, 265–76.

99. Habets, W. J., de Rooij, D. J., Hoet, M. H. *et al.* (1985) Quantitation of anti-RNP and anti-Sm antibodies in MCTD and SLE patients by immunoblotting. *Clin. Experi. Immunol.*, **59**, 457–66.

100. Hoffman, R. W., Rettenmaier, L. J., Takeda, Y. *et al.* (1990) Human autoantibodies against the 70-kd polypeptide of U1 small nuclear RNP are associated with HLA-DR4 among

connective tissue disease patients. *Arth. Rheum.*, **33**, 666–73.

101. Habets, W. J. A., Hoet, M. H., Sillekens, P. T. G. *et al.* (1989) Detection of autoantibodies in a quantitative immunoassay using recombinant ribonucleoprotein antigens. *Clin. Experi. Immunol.*, **76**, 172–7.

102. Hoet, R. M., Koornneef, I., de Rooij, D. J. *et al.* (1992) Changes in anti-U1 RNA antibody levels correlate with disease activity in patients with systemic lupus erythematosus overlap syndrome. *Arth. Rheum.*, **35**, 1202–10.

103. Fritzler, M. J., Ali, R. and Tan, E. M. (1984) Antibodies from patients with mixed connective tissue disease react with heterogeneous nuclear ribonucleoprotein or ribonucleic acid (hn RNP/RNA) of the nuclear matrix. *J. Immunol.*, **132**, 1216–22.

104. Salden, M. H. L., Van Eekelen, C. A. G., Habets, W. J. A. *et al.* (1982) Anti-nuclear matrix antibodies in mixed connective tissue disease. *Euro. J. Immunol.*, **12**, 783–6.

105. Cooke, C. L. and Lurie, H. I. (1977) Case report: Fatal gastrointestinal hemorrhage in mixed connective tissue disease. *Arth. Rheum.*, **20**, 1421–7.

106. Seyer, J. M., Kang, A. H., Rodnan, G. (1981) Investigation of type I and type III collagens of the lung in progressive systemic sclerosis. *Arth. Rheum.*, **24**, 625–31.

107. Peller, J. S., Garbor, G. T., Porter, J. M. *et al.* (1985) Angiographic findings in mixed connective tissue disease. *Arth. Rheum.*, **23**, 768–74.

108. Maddison, P. J. and Reichlin, M. (1977) Quantitation of precipitating antibodies to certain soluble nuclear antigens in SLE: their contribution to hypergammaglobulinemia. *Arth. Rheum.*, **20**, 819–24.

109. Alarcón-Segovia, D. (1987) Immunological abnormalities in mixed connective tissue disease, in *Mixed Connective Tissue Disease and Anti-nuclear Antibodies*, (eds R. Kasukawa and G. C. Sharp), Elsevier Science Publishers B. V., Amsterdam, pp. 189–96.

110. Negoro, N., Kanayama, Y., Yasuda, M. *et al.* (1987) Nuclear ribonucleoprotein immune complexes in pericardial fluid of a patient with mixed connective tissue disease. *Arth. Rheum.*, **30**, 97–101.

111. Takeda, Y., Nyman, U., Winkler, A. *et al.* (1991) Antigenic domains on the U1 small nuclear ribonucleoprotein-associated 70K polypeptide: A comparison of regions

selectively recognized by human and mouse autoantibodies and by monoclonal antibodies. *Clin. Immunol. Immunopath.*, **61**, 55–68.

112. Query, C. C., Bentley, R. C. and Keene, J. D. (1989) A common RNA recognition motif identified within a defined U-1 RNA binding domain of the 70K U1 snRNP protein. *Cell*, **57**, 89–101.

113. Sunderrajan, E. V., McKenzie, W. N., Lieske, T. R. *et al.* (1986) Pulmonary inflammation in autoimmune MRL/MP-1pr/1pr mice. *Am. J. Path.*, **124**, 353–62.

114. O'Sullivan, F. X., Ray, C. J., Takeda, Y. *et al.* (1991) Long term anti-CD4 treatment of MRL/1pr mice ameliorates immunopathology and lymphoproliferation but fails to suppress rheumatoid factor production. *Clin. Immunol. Immunopath.*, **61**, 421–35.

115. Harley, J. B., Sestak, A. L., Willis, L. G. *et al.* (1989) A model for disease heterogeneity in systemic lupus erythematosus. *Arth. Rheum.*, **32**, 826–36.

116. Hoffman, R. W., Cassidy, J. T., Takeda, Y. *et al.* (1993) U1-70 Kd autoantibody-positive mixed connective tissue disease in children: A longitudinal clinical and serologic analysis. *Arth. Rheum.*, **36**, 1599–1602.

117. Kaneoka, H., Hsu, K. C., Takeda, Y. *et al.* (1992) Molecular genetic analysis of HLA-DR and HLA-DQ genes among anti-U1-70-kd autoantibody positive connective tissue disease patients. *Arth. Rheum.*, **35**, 83–94.

118. Black, C. M., Maddison, P. J., Welsh, K. I. *et al.* (1988) HLA and Ig allotype in mixed connective tissue disease. *Arth. Rheum.*, **31**, 131–4.

119. Genth, E., Zarnowski, H., Mieru, R. *et al.* (1987) HLA-DR4 and Gm (1,3;5,21) are associated with U1-nRNP antibody positive connective tissue disease. *Ann. Rheum. Dis.*, **46**, 189–96.

120. Smolen, J. S., Klippel, J. H., Penner, E. *et al.* (1987) HLA-DR antigens in systemic lupus erythematosus: association with specificity of autoantibody responses to nuclear antigens. *Ann. Rheum. Dis.*, **46**, 457–62.

121. Granados, J. and Alarcón-Segovia, D. (1991) Immunogenetics of scleroderma and mixed connective tissue disease, in *The Immunogenetics of Autoimmune Diseases*, Vol. 2, (ed. N. R. Farid), CRC Press, Boca Raton, pp. 94–101.

122. Ruuska, P., Hämeenkorpi, R., Forsberg, S. *et al.* (1992) Differences in HLA antigens between patients with mixed connective tissue

disease and systemic lupus erythematosus. *Ann. Rheum. Dis.*, **51**, 52–5.

123. Hoffman, R. W., Takeda, Y., Sharp, G. C. *et al.* (1993) Human T cell clones reactive against U-small nuclear ribonucleoprotein autoantigens from connective tissue disease patients and healthy individuals. *J. Immunol.*, **151**, 6460–9.

124. Wolff-Vorbeck, G., Schlesier, M., Hackl, W. *et al.* (1989) A human T cell clone recognizing small nuclear ribonucleoproteins (UsnRNP), in *Molecular and Cell Biology of Autoantibodies and Autoimmunity*, (eds E. K. F. Bautz, J. R. Kalden, M. Homma and E. M. Tan), Springer-Verlag, Heidelberg, p. 106.

125. O'Brien, R. M., Cram, D. S., Coppel, R. L. *et al.* (1990) T-cell epitopes on the 70-kDa protein of the (U1)RNP complex in auto-immune rheumatologic disorders. *J. Auto-imm.*, **3**, 747–57.

126. Cassidy, J. T., Wortmann, D. W., Nelson, A. M. *et al.* (1991) Clinical outcome of children with mixed connective tissue disease (MCTD). Pediatric Rheumatology meeting, Park City, Utah, March 2–6.

127. Theissen, Hl, Etzerodt, M., Reuter, R. *et al.* (1986) Cloning of the human cDNA for the U1 RNA-associated 70K protein. *EMBO J.*, **5**, 3209–17.

128. Query, C. C. and Keene, J. D. (1987) A human autoimmune protein associated with U1 RNA contains a region of homology that is cross-reactive with retroviral p30^{gag} antigen. *Cell*, **51**, 211–20.

129. Deutscher, S. L. and Keene, J. D. (1988) A sequence-specific conformational epitope on U1 RNA is recognized by a unique autoantibody. *Proc. Nat. Acad. Sci. USA*, **85**, 3299–303.

130. Nyman, U., Hallman, H., Hadlaczky, G. *et al.* (1986) Intranuclear localization of snRNP antigens. *J. Cell Biol.*, **102**, 137–44.

C. A. Langford and R. M. McCallum

Vasculitis is a clinicopathologic entity characterized by blood vessel inflammation with resultant organ ischemia and injury. This inflammation may affect any vessel in the body and thus lead to a wide variety of clinical manifestations ranging from mild cutaneous disease to multisystem organ failure and death. Vasculitis can develop in conjunction with an underlying disorder (secondary vasculitis) or occur as an idiopathic (primary) process (Table 8.1)[1–3]. Within the spectrum of idiopathic vasculitis, individual vasculitic syndromes have been recognized which possess characteristic clinical and pathologic features. Although the vasculitic syndromes have a low incidence in the general population, literature review studies and longitudinal patient series have greatly expanded our understanding of these syndromes. This has lead to earlier diagnosis and treatment with an overall improvement in patient outcome.

CLASSIFICATION AND DIAGNOSTIC APPROACH

The classification and nosology of vaculitis has been a complex and changing process, owing largely to the degree of overlap among syndromes and the adaptations that have been necessary as our knowledge has grown. Individual vasculitic syndromes have previously been classified on the basis of histopathological or clinical features[1–7]. In 1990 the American College of Rheumatology published classification criteria for seven major vasculitic disorders[8]. While these provide a useful tool for uniformity in literature review and clinical research, they were not intended as guidelines for identifying a vasculitic disorder in an individual patient. The diagnosis of a specific vasculitic syndrome is best approached through a careful patient evaluation that combines pathological and clinical data[6]. Although inflammation can potentially occur in any vessel and organ system, distinctive patterns of disease may be observed which allow individual disorders to be identified. While there are similarities among the vasculitides, the identification of a specific syndrome is worth pursuing as it may have important implications for associated organ involvement, treatment options and prognosis.

The first step in the approach to vasculitis is its recognition within the differential diagnosis of any patient with unexplained multisystem disease, glomerulonephritis, pulmonary infiltrates, ischemic signs or symptoms, palpable purpura or other necrotic skin lesion, mononeuritis multiplex or fever[1,6]. Once a concern for vasculitis has been raised, the extent of clinical disease must be determined using information obtained from the history, physical examination and laboratory evaluation. Although laboratory tests are not diagnostic for vasculitis, they

Connective Tissue Diseases. Edited by Jill J. F. Belch and Robert B. Zurier. Published in 1995 by Chapman & Hall, London.
ISBN 0 412 48620 2

Table 8.1 The vasculitides

Idiopathic (primary) vasculitides
Polyarteritis nodosa
Churg-Strauss syndrome
Polyangiitis overlap syndrome
Wegener's granulomatosis
Lymphomatoid granulomatosis*
Henoch–Schönlein purpura
Takayasu's arteritis
Giant cell arteritis[†]
Isolated central nervous system vasculitis
Cogan's syndrome
Kawasaki disease[‡]

Secondary vasculitides
Drug-related vasculitis
Foreign protein related vasculitis
Vasculitis associated with infection
Vasculitis in malignancies
Hypocomplementemic urticarial vasculitis
Hypergammaglobulinemic purpura
Cryoglobulinemic vasculitis
Radiation vasculitis
Transplant vasculitis
Connective tissue disease associated vasculitis:
  Rheumatoid arthritis
  Systemic lupus erythematosus
  Sjögren's syndrome
  Scleroderma
  Spondyloarthropathies
  Dermatomyositis/polymyositis
  Sarcoidosis
  Relapsing polychondritis
  Antiphospholipid antibody syndrome
  Behçet's disease

* Now considered a lymphoproliferative rather than vasculitic process.
[†] Discussed in Chapter 10.
[‡] Discussed in Chapter 9.

provide important data about inflammatory activity and organ involvement. Serum electrolytes with blood urinary nitrogen (BUN) and creatinine, liver function tests (LFT), complete blood count (CBC) with differential, sedimentation rate (ESR), rheumatoid factor (RF), antinuclear antibodies (ANA), urinalysis, chest radiograph and electrocardiogram should be performed in all patients. The role of anti-neutrophil cytoplasmic antibodies (ANCA), which have been found in association with Wegener's granulomatosis, remains under investigation. Although these studies are useful, the diagnosis of vasculitis requires demonstration of vessel inflammation or damage, usually through angiography or biopsy. An abnormal angiogram can be diagnostic and in select patients may obviate the need for biopsy. Except in these cases, histologic documentation of vasculitis should be considered the rule and must be pursued aggressively prior to initiating treatment. Biopsies are best obtained from sites where there is clinical evidence of disease, as blind biopsies are typically of low yield[1,6].

PATHOPHYSIOLOGY

Immunological mechanisms are felt to play a major role in the pathogenesis of most of the vasculitic syndromes. Evidence in support of this has come from animal models of immune complex-mediated disease, immunologic studies in patients with vasculitis, and the response of vasculitis patients to immunosuppressive therapy[9]. The immune complex model remains foremost among the possible mechanisms of disease. In 1970, an association was noted between hepatitis B infection and polyarteritis nodosa[10,11]. In these patients, circulating and tissue-bound immune complexes containing hepatitis B surface antigen were demonstrated[12]. Evidence of immune complex circulation and deposition has since been found in several disorders including Churg–Strauss syndrome, Wegener's granulomatosis and Henoch–Schönlein purpura[9]. The immune complex model theorizes that immune complexes circulate and deposit in blood vessel walls provoking an inflammatory response, which ultimately results in vascular injury[3]. Cell-mediated immune injury and antibody-associated injury are other mechanisms which may play an important role in certain types of vasculitis[1,9,13]. Recent advances in molecular biology have provided exciting new insights into inflammatory mediators that may participate in vessel damage. Cytokines and adhesion molecules that are involved in normal lymphopoiesis and protective immune responses also appear to be mediators of pathogenic immune and inflammatory responses in vasculitic syndromes[9,13]. These studies have given rise to several possible mechanisms for vascular damage, which include roles for infectious agents and tumor cell-mediated vessel damage[9]. Research into the pathophysiology of these syndromes remains of key importance in both improving our understanding of these rare disorders and in developing new strategies for treatment.

TREATMENT PRINCIPLES

Although treatment for specific disorders will be discussed individually, some general comments regarding the use of corticosteroids and cyclophosphamide are warranted. Corticosteroids form the foundation of treatment for most vasculitic syndromes[3,5,6]. In the setting of acute illness, steroids are administered orally or intravenously at a dose of approximately 1 mg/kg/day given in three or four divided doses[5,6,14]. Although more efficacious, divided dose therapy has a profound suppressive effect on the hypothalamic-pituitary-adrenal axis and carries a high incidence of toxic side-effects[6,15]. After 3–7 days of divided-dose therapy, the steroid dose should be consolidated to a single morning dose and slowly tapered to the lowest effective dosage. Corticosteroids have many potential adverse affects, one of which is an increased risk of infection[5,15]. An association between corticosteroid usage and herpes zoster has been well documented[16]. Severe bacterial and fungal infections can also occur and appear to be more frequent at higher corticosteroid doses[5,15,16].

Cyclophosphamide is the cytotoxic drug of choice in the treatment of systemic vasculitis[3,5,6,14,16,17]. It should initially be administered at a dose of 2 mg/kg/day by daily oral route in combination with corticosteroids[5,6,14]. Fulminant vasculitis may require 4 mg/kg/day for 3 days followed by rapid dose reduction over the next 3-day period until a dose of 1–2 mg/kg/day is reached[5,6,14]. If the patient is unable to take oral medication or if gastrointestinal malabsorption is of concern, an equivalent daily dose can be administered intravenously. After the initial induction period, adjustments in cyclophosphamide dosing are based upon the peripheral leukocyte count. One of the most severe adverse effects is bone marrow suppression, specifically leukopenia, which typically begins 7–14 days after initiation of therapy[5,6,14]. Blood counts should be monitored every 1–3 days during this period and every week thereafter. The dosage of cyclophosphamide should be decreased or held if there are signs of decreasing white blood cell count or if the total leukocyte count falls below 3000–3500 per mm^3[5,6,14]. Corticosteroid tapering may lower the leukocyte count and necessitate reductions in the cyclophosphamide dose[5]. Changes in leukocyte count lag behind changes in cyclophosphamide dosing and generally follow the rule that 'this week's counts reflect last week's dose'[1,5]. Cytotoxic treatment is typically maintained for at least a year after the disappearance of active disease or until there is evidence of drug toxicity[5,6,14]. Although effective, cyclophosphamide is a potentially life-threatening drug. Patient understanding, follow-up with blood counts, and physician visits are important in protecting the patient from adverse effects. Inability of the patient to comply with these may be a reason for withholding cyclophosphamide treatment. Another potential cyclophosphamide toxicity is hemorrhagic cystitis, particularly with daily oral administration[5,16]. Adequate hydration is important in minimizing contact of the drug metabolites with the bladder epithelium in order to prevent irritation, inflammation and bleeding. If evidence of hematuria develops, cyclophosphamide should be withheld until this is fully evaluated. Cyclophosphamide has been associated with an increased risk for bladder carcinoma and hematologic malignancies. Other important adverse affects include sterility, nausea and hair loss[5,16]. Cyclophosphamide is a potent immunosuppressive agent and can predispose patients to life-threatening infections, particularly in the setting of neutropenia. Because of the risk of infection with both corticosteroids and cyclophosphamide, it is extremely important that infection be ruled out prior to beginning treatment. One particular instance where the question of concurrent infection often arises is in the setting of pulmonary infiltrates, where radiographic changes may represent infection or vasculitis. In this setting, an open lung biopsy with special stains and culture should be pursued prior to the initiation of therapy, both for diagnostic purposes and to rule out infection.

POLYARTERITIS NODOSA

One of the first complete reports in the literature of a vasculitic syndrome was made in 1866 by Kussmaul and Maier who described a nodular, inflammatory arterial disorder they called periarteritis nodosa[18]. In 1903 Ferrari presented the term polyarteritis nodosa (PAN), in recognition of both the multiplicity of vessel involvement and the transmural nature of the inflammatory process[19]. Initially, the diagnosis of polyarteritis encompassed multiple forms of vasculitis. Over the last several decades, however, distinctive clinical and pathological features have been recognized which have allowed polyarteritis to be categorized into different vasculitic syndromes[20]. Despite this, PAN is still recognized as a unique process characterized by a systemic, necrotizing vasculitis which involves the small- and medium-sized muscular arteries.

The prevalence of PAN has varied between 4.6 per 1 000 000 in England[21] to 77 per 1 000 000 in a hepatitis B hyperendemic Alaskan Eskimo population[22]. PAN is more prevalent in males at a ratio of 2 to 1[23–26]. The average age at diagnosis is 40–60 years, although PAN has been seen in both children and the elderly[1,23–27].

The observed frequency of specific organ involvement has varied greatly among studies (Table 8.2)[1,21,23–25,28,29]. Major contributing factors to this variability are differences in the inclusion criteria between studies and the inclusion of patients that may have other vasculitic syndromes[20]. Presenting symptoms are often non-specific and include malaise, myalgias, abdominal pain, weight loss, fever and neurologic symptoms [1,25,27,28]. Visceral involvement can develop simultaneously or may lag behind[27]. Clinical renal disease with proteinuria, active urinary sediment, and progressive renal insufficiency occurs in about 70% of patients, although acute renal failure is uncommon[27]. Hypertension is seen frequently and can be an important clue to the diagnosis of PAN[1,21,27,28]. Gastrointestinal involvement is common with symptoms of abdominal pain, nausea and vomiting. Acute events, such as hemorrhage, perforation or infarction, are rare but are associated with high mortality[1,21,24]. Liver abnormalities can occur and should raise the possibility of concurrent hepatitis B infection[21,28]. Cutaneous disease and mononeuritis multiplex are common and provide excellent sites for biopsy. Arthralgias with or without a non-deforming polyarthritis occur in 33–58% of patients[1,24,25,27–29]. Other important sites of involvement include the retina and testis[1,21,25,27,28]. Although believed to be rare, the true incidence of pulmonary involvement in PAN is controversial[20,27]. Several studies have found patients with evidence of asthma or pulmonary infiltrates. It is unclear, however, whether these patients indeed had PAN or instead had Churg–Strauss syndrome or Wegener's granulomatosis, where pulmonary involvement is common.

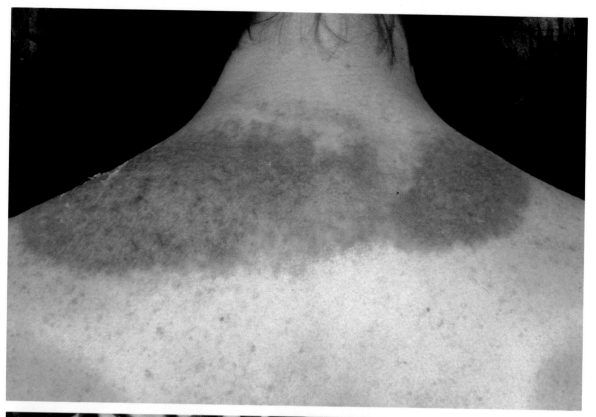

Plate 1 Photosensitive skin rash in a lupus patient.

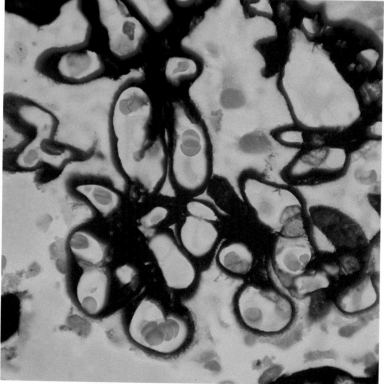

Plate 2 Kidney biopsy (silver stain) demonstrating changes of membranous nephropathy. This patient had a nephrotic syndrome but normal creatinine clearance. (Photograph courtesy of Dr E.M. Thompson, Hammersmith Hospital).

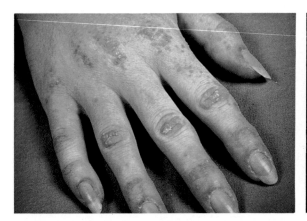

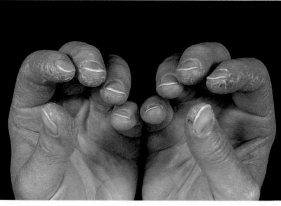

Plate 3 Gottron's papules. This erythematous, raised, scaly rash over the knuckles and dorsum of the hand is a common early cutaneous feature of dermatomyositis.

Plate 4 'Mechanic's hands'. Note the digital skin fissuring and cracking in this patient with myositis. (Reprinted from *Rheumatology*, (eds J. Klippel and P. Dieppe), (in press), with permission.)

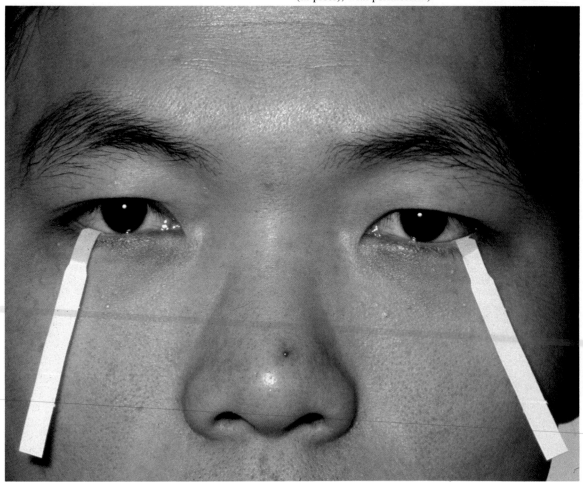

Plate 5 Schirmer's tear test.

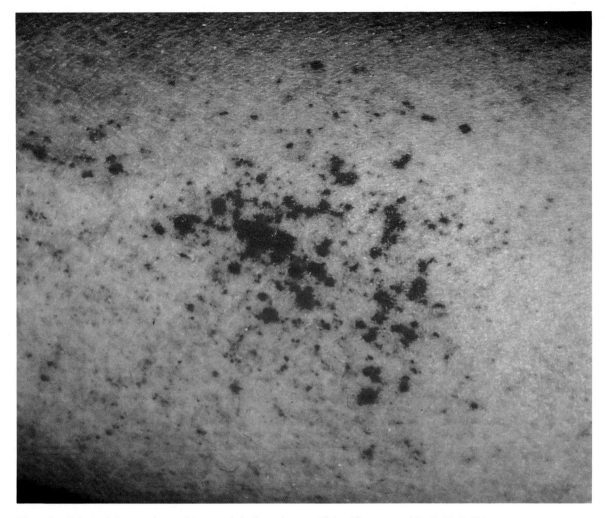

Plate 6 Skin rash in a patient with cryoglobulinemic vasculitis. (Courtesy of Dr R.Y. Ball.)

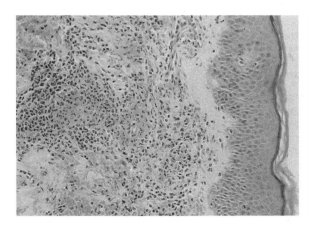

Plate 7 Skin biopsy from the same patient as Plate 6. There is a very dense dermal leucocyte infiltrate with leucocytoclasis and extravasation of erythrocytes. Hyaline thrombi are not seen. (Courtesy of Dr R.Y. Ball.)

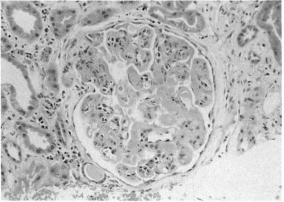

Plate 8 Renal biopsy from the same patient as Plate 6. There is prominent lobularity of the glomeruli. Hyaline thrombi are present in peripheral capillary loops. Hematoxylin and eosin stain. (Courtesy of Dr R.Y. Ball.)

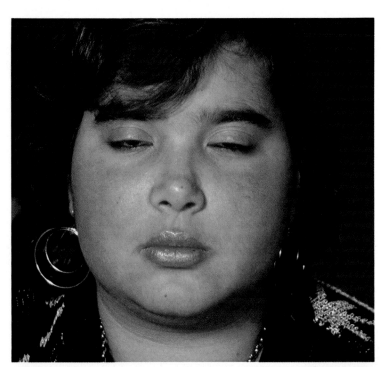

Plate 9   Typical systemic lupus erythematosus facial rash in a teenager presenting as hemolytic anemia.

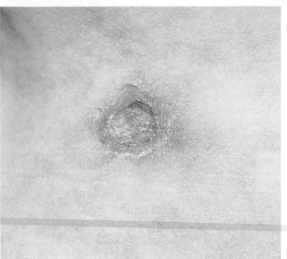

Plate 10   Ulceration over a calcinotic lesion in dermatomyositis.

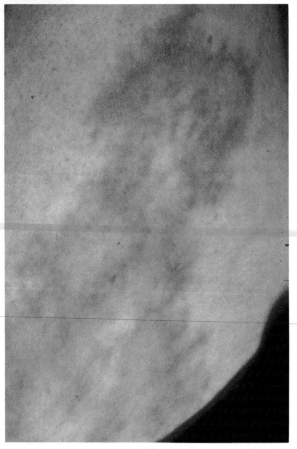

Plate 11   Cutaneous vasculitis looking like 'erythema abigne' some 3 weeks after a known streptococcal infection.

Table 8.2   Clinical features of polyarteritis nodosa*

Symptom or sign	% patients affected
Fever	36–76
Weight loss	30–71
Hypertension	25–70
Kidney	8–77
Gastrointestinal:	14–78
Abdominal pain	43–65
Cardiac	10–56
Nervous system:	
peripheral	23–60
central	3–41
Musculoskeletal:	
Arthralgia/arthritis	33–58
myalgia	8–77
Skin	28–65
Eye	1–47
Testicular pain	1–4

* Data compiled from references (1,21,23–25,28,29].

LABORATORY FINDINGS

Laboratory findings are non-specific and include anemia, leukocytosis and an elevated ESR[1,21,23–29]. Measurement of serum creatinine and urinalysis are important in evaluating renal function. A positive ANA or RF can be seen in 10–40% of patients [1,21,23,24,26,28,29]. Hepatitis B surface antigen and antibody should be sought in all patients with PAN. Angiography may be diagnostic for PAN with characteristic findings including saccular or fusiform aneurysms and arterial narrowing (Figure 8.1)[1,28]. Positive results are found most frequently in studies of the renal and celiac circulation, although there does not appear to be a correlation between these abnormalities and corresponding clinical involvement[28]. Aneurysms are seen at a frequency of 58–60% and are associated with severe hypertension, hepatitis B antigenemia and clinically severe disease[26,28]. The demonstration of aneurysms is suggestive but not pathognomonic of PAN as similar features may be seen in other disorders[28].

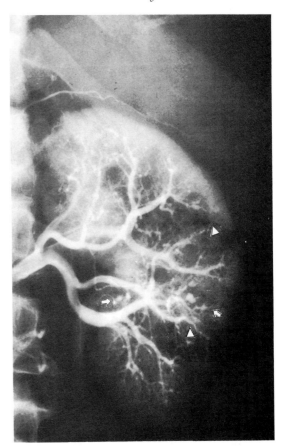

Fig. 8.1   Renal arteriogram in a patient with polyarteritis nodosa demonstrating aneurysms (arrows) and arterial narrowing (arrowheads).

Autopsy studies have found that organs may be histologically abnormal despite the absence of clinical disease[1]. The pathological changes of PAN consist of a focal but panmural necrotizing arteritis preferentially occurring at the vessel bifurcation of small- and medium-sized muscular arteries (Figure 8.2)[7,27]. Necrotizing vasculitis with fibrinoid necrosis is the hallmark acute-phase lesion of PAN[7]. The inflammatory process involves initial media destruction with an acute neutrophilic inflammatory response and fibroblastic proliferation extending to all layers. Lesions at all stages of progression and healing may be seen, which is a characteristic feature of PAN[1,7].

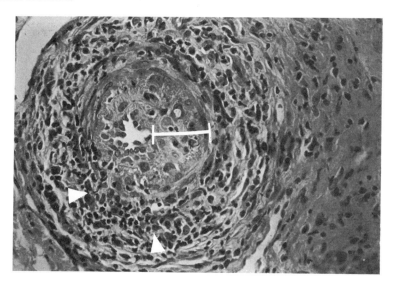

Fig. 8.2 Necrotizing arteritis with intimal proliferation (bar) and polymorphonuclear leukocyte inflammation (arrowheads).

Glomerular changes commonly include segmental necrosis and crescent formation[7,20,27,28].

DIAGNOSIS

PAN can be difficult to diagnose given its non-specific presentation, potential for diverse organ involvement, and low disease prevalence. The diagnosis of PAN is based upon the demonstration of vasculitis by angiography or biopsy. Angiography may be especially valuable in the setting of gastrointestinal abnormalities or when a potential biopsy site is unavailable or unreachable. Prior to biopsying the liver or kidney in patients suspected to have PAN, angiography should be considered as the predilection for aneurysms at these sites increases the risk of severe bleeding from a closed needle biopsy[1]. Biopsy sites that should be considered include muscle, skin, sural nerve, kidney, rectum and testis[1,7,20,21,23–27,30].

PROGNOSIS

The prognosis of PAN has greatly improved with the use of corticosteroids, extending the 5-year survival rate from 13% to 50–60% [21,23–25,29]. The majority of deaths are seen within the first year and are usually related to vasculitic manifestations or infectious complications of treatment[1,21,23,24,27]. Mortality occurring after one year of disease is often due to sequelae of vessel obliteration, such as myocardial infarction or cerebrovascular event[1,24,27].

TREATMENT

Glucocorticoids are the cornerstone of treatment in PAN with prednisone 1 mg/kg/day or the IV equivalent being given initially [1,24,27,29]. When the activity of the disease is controlled, the prednisone can be tapered to the lowest effective dosage necessary to control disease activity[24,27]. The length of time that therapy should be continued has not been determined and should be guided by the clinical status of the individual patient. Several reports have found concurrent cyclophosphamide and corticosteroid treatment superior to steroids alone[17,21,29,31]. One study did not find such an association

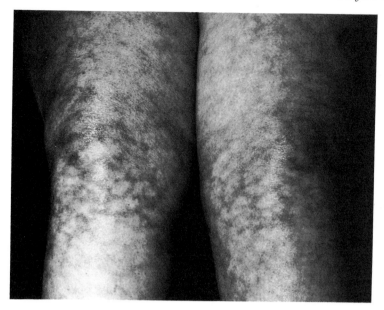

Fig. 8.3 Livedo reticularis as can be seen in both cutaneous and systemic polyarteritis nodosa.

although these patients were studied retrospectively with cyclophosphamide being given for more severe disease[24]. Nevertheless, the role of cyclophosphamide in the initial treatment of PAN has remained controversial. Concurrent cyclophosphamide at a dose of 2 mg/kg/day and corticosteroids should be strongly considered in patients who have severe disease, multiorgan involvement, or who have not responded to corticosteroid therapy[1]. Plasma exchange has not been found to be superior to steroids alone and is not recommended for the initial treatment of non-hepatitis B associated PAN[32,33]. Control of hypertension is important in protecting renal function, lessening the risk of aneurysm rupture and decreasing the rate of late mortality[1].

PAN VARIANTS

Two variants of PAN which deserve special mention are cutaneous PAN and PAN associated with heptatitis B. Cutaneous PAN is characterized by a necrotizing vasculitis of the small muscular arteries in subcutaneous tissue[1,34]. By definition, this is a localized process sparing the visceral arteries and is therefore not a systemic vasculitis[1]. The diagnosis is established by characteristic pathological findings on skin biopsy in conjunction with a negative systemic evaluation. It is important to recognize that similar lesions can be seen in systemic PAN and that cutaneous PAN should be considered a diagnosis of exclusion (Figure 8.3). As a rule, cutaneous PAN does not progress to systemic disease and follows a benign course with an excellent long-term outcome[1,34]. Hepatitis B surface antigen positivity has been found in 0–54% of patients with PAN[12]. There is emerging evidence that hepatitis C is also associated with PAN, although little is currently known about its clinical disease spectrum[35–37]. The time between infection with hepatitis B and the onset of PAN has varied between months and years. Patients frequently have subclinical hepatitis B and may not be aware that they are infected until the diagnosis of hepatitis B associated PAN[38].

There does not appear to be an association between the activity of the hepatitis and vasculitis[38]. Patients with hepatitis B associated PAN have been found to have a higher incidence of elevated LFTs and aneurysms but are otherwise clinically similar to non-hepatitis related PAN[12,38]. The presence of hepatitis B complicates treatment. Enhanced viral replication can occur during immunosuppression with the potential for progressive liver disease during treatment and even fulminant hepatitis upon therapy cessation[12,32]. Despite these concerns, the role of therapy is important as untreated hepatitis B associated PAN has a high mortality rate. Therapy has largely been the same as non-hepatitis related disease and there have been very few trials where the treatment of hepatitis B associated PAN has been examined specifically[32,39]. Plasma exchange in combination with steroids and antiviral therapy has been used with some success[32].

CHURG-STRAUSS SYNDROME

Churg-Strauss syndrome (CSS) is a unique systemic vasculitis associated with eosinophilia, asthma, and allergic rhinitis. In 1951, Churg and Strauss identified a group of patients initially felt to have PAN, who demonstrated similar findings of asthma, hypereosinophilia, necrotizing arteritis and extravascular lesions with an eosinophilic and granulomatous histology[40]. They proposed that this represented a distinct disease which they called 'allergic angiitis and allergic granulomatosis'. Although it is still referred to by this name, it has become more commonly known as Churg–Strauss syndrome.

Although no epidemiologic surveys are available, CSS is thought to be rare[1,41]. The age at onset for CSS is 15–69 with a median age of vasculitis of 38[42]. When all reported cases are combined there is a slight male predominance[1,42,43]. CSS has been said to be divided into three clinical phases: the prodrome, the eosinophilic phase, and the vasculitic phase[42,44]. Although this separation is helpful in approaching CSS, these phases are not clearly identifiable in all patients and may occur simultaneously. It is also important to note that histologic findings of eosinophilic infiltration, granulomas and vasculitis can be seen concurrently[44].

The prodromal phase consists of allergic disease which is one of the key features that distinguishes CSS from other forms of vasculitis. Allergic rhinitis is seen as the first feature of CSS in the majority of patients, with 70% developing symptoms during the course of their disease[44]. Allergic upper respiratory tract involvement can lead to nasal obstruction, recurrent sinusitis and nasal polyposis[42]. Asthma typically begins in adulthood and may precede the development of systemic vasculitis by up to 30 years[43]. Asthmatic symptoms are initially mild but will often increase with time[40]. The onset of vasculitis may bring about a dramatic improvement in asthmatic symptoms although exacerbations may also occur[42–44].

The eosinophilic phase is characterized by peripheral blood eosinophilia and eosinophilic tissue infiltrates. When seen as an isolated clinical phenomenon, the eosinophilic phase often involves the lung or gastrointestinal tract and may resemble Löffler's syndrome, chronic eosinophilic pneumonia or eosinophilic gastroenteritis respectively [44].

The onset of the vasculitic phase is often heralded by nonspecific systemic symptoms including fever, weight loss, leg cramps and malaise[42]. Symptoms of specific organ dysfunction are variable and may not be present for weeks to months. Cardiac involvement occurs in 25–62% of CSS patients and is the major cause of death[1,42]. Although the heart is often not affected until late in the course of disease, changes may progress rapidly and be difficult to reverse once established[44]. CSS may affect the heart in many ways but primarily causes an eosinophilic and granulomatous myocarditis, pericarditis and

Table 8.3 Clinical features of Churg-Strauss syndrome*

Symptom or sign	% of cases involved
Upper respiratory	
Allergic rhinitis	70
Pulmonary	
Asthma	100
Pulmonary infiltrates	72
Pleural effusion	29
Cardiac	
Congestive heart failure	47
Pericarditis	32
Cutaneous	
Purpura	48
Erythema/urticaria	35
Nodules	30
Nervous system	
Mononeuritis multiplex	66
Central nervous system	27
Gastrointestinal	
Abdominal pain	59
Diarrhea	33
Bleeding	18
Renal	
Hypertension	29
Mild/moderate	49
Renal failure	9
Musculoskeletal	
Myalgias	41
Arthralgias/arthritis	51

* Data adapted from [42].

coronary vasculitis[1,40,44]. Pulmonary infiltrates are a central feature of CSS and may be related to eosinophilic infiltration or a small vessel vasculitis. Patients rarely develop significant clinical renal disease, although the kidneys are frequently abnormal histologically[42–44]. The benign nature of the renal disease is an important distinguishing characteristic from the other systemic vasculitides[42]. Myalgias are common and can be associated with a granulomatous myositis [42]. Arthralgias and a non-destructive arthritis occur in conjunction with the vasculitic phase but can also be seen prodromally [42,43]. Other organ system involvement that should be carefully sought includes the peripheral nervous system, lower urinary tract and skin (Table 8.3)[40,42–45].

LABORATORY FINDINGS

Laboratory findings in CSS are non-specific. Peripheral blood eosinophilia may be seen in any phase of disease and is a hallmark of CSS. Eosinophilia may not be found in all patients due to prior steroid treatments for asthma or the wide and rapid fluctuation in the eosinophil count that can occur in this disorder[42,44]. Normalization of the eosinophil level in response to steroid treatment is a feature of CSS and distinguishes it from the hypereosinophilic syndrome where eosinophilia is frequently steroid resistant[42,44]. An association between the degree of eosinophilia and the activity of the vasculitic disease may be seen in some patients[42,43]. Anemia, leukocytosis, and increased ESR frequently accompany the vasculitic phase[42,43]. IgE levels may be elevated and RF positivity may be seen but is usually low in titer[42,43]. In contrast to PAN, no association has found between CSS and hepatitis B[42]. Chest radiograph is important in examining for pulmonary infiltrates which occur in 72% of patients[42]. These are typically transient and patchy without a specific predilection for any one region[42–44]. Nodular infiltrates can occur which rarely cavitate[42]. Pleural effusions and hilar adenopathy have also been reported. Eosinophilic infiltration and pulmonary vasculitis look identical on radiograph and therefore cannot be distinguished using this technique[42]. Electrocardiogram may be abnormal in >50% of patients and is especially important in monitoring for cardiac involvement[42]. Angiography may demonstrate areas of narrowing and aneurysm which can occur in CSS[42,44]. It has a relatively low diagnostic yield and should not be pursued as a primary test for diagnosis unless histologic proof is considered unobtainable [44].

Table 8.4 Comparative features of Wegener's granulomatosis, Churg-Strauss syndrome and polyarteritis nodosa

Feature	WG	CSS	PAN
Sex (male:female)	1:1	1.3:1	2:1
Blood vessel involvement	Sm. art. & veins med. art.	Sm. art. & veins med. art.	Sm. art. med. art.
Pathologic features	Granulomatous	Eosinophilic	Mixed cell
Ear/nose/throat	++++	+++	+
Pulmonary			
Infiltrates	++++	+++	+
Asthma	−	++++	+
Cardiac	+	+++	++
Gastrointestinal	−	+++	+++
Renal			
Involvement	+++	+++	+++
Renal failure	++	+	+
Nervous system			
Central nervous system	+	++	+
Peripheral nervous system	++	+++	+++
Cutaneous	++	+++	+++
Hypertension	+	++	++
Arthralgia/arthritis	+++	++	++
Ocular	+++	+	+
Lower urinary tract	−	++	++
Eosinophilia	+	++++	+
Hepatitis B surface antigenemia	−	−	++
Aneurysms	−	++	+++

Key: − = 0–1%; + = 1–10%; ++ = 10–50%; +++ = 50–80%; ++++ = >80%
WG = Wegener's granulomatosis
CSS = Churg-Strauss syndrome
PAN = polyarteritis nodosa

The three primary pathological features of CSS are tissue infiltration by eosinophils, formation of 'allergic granulomas' and necrotizing vasculitis. The allergic granuloma was first described by Churg and Strauss and represents an area of necrosis in a densely packed focus of eosinophils[40,44]. With time, the necrotic center becomes surrounded by epithelioid macrophages and giant cells and can heal to a non-specific, often calcified scar. The characteristic glomerular lesion of CSS is a focal segmental glomerulonephritis with necrotizing features[40,42,44]. Interstitial nephritis, granulomatous nodules and vasculitis may also be seen. The necrotizing vasculitis of CSS involves the small arteries and veins and, less frequently, the medium arteries[44]. Frequently, the inflammation includes prominent numbers of eosinophils which tend to form granulomas in and around the vessel wall[44].

DIAGNOSIS

Historically, the diagnosis of CSS has been based solely on histological criteria which require the demonstration of necrotizing vasculitis, tissue infiltration by eosinophils and extravascular granuloma[40]. In practice, however, few biopsy specimens contain all of these findings[44]. In order to increase the likelihood of identifying and diagnosing CSS, it has been proposed that the emphasis for diagnosis be shifted to include clinical features[42,44]. One study has recommended the following criteria:

1. asthma;
2. peripheral blood eosinophilia in excess of $1.5 \times 10^9/l$;
3. systemic vasculitis involving two or more extrapulmonary organs[42].

It should be emphasized that appropriate diagnosis still requires the demonstration of biopsy-proven vasculitis[46]. Open lung biopsy frequently does not demonstrate all of the histologic features of CSS but should be pursued before the institution of therapy if there is any question of infection. When there is evidence of clinical involvement, useful biopsy specimens may be obtained from the skin, muscle, sural nerve, prostate and kidney[1,40,42]. The differential diagnosis chiefly includes PAN, Wegener's granulomatosis, and the hypereosinophilic syndrome. Although these diseases frequently appear similar, CSS possesses unique clinical and histologic findings that allow its differentiation(Table 8.4)[43,44,46,47].

PROGNOSIS

The recent prognosis of CSS appears to have improved, likely due to improved recognition leading to earlier diagnosis and corticosteroid treatment[45]. In 1958, the mortality rate at 3 months was 50%[48], in contrast to a 5-year survival rate of 62% found in 1977[43]. Congestive heart failure and myocardial infarction are responsible for 48% of all deaths in CSS[42]. Other potential causes of death include cerebral hemorrhage, renal failure, gastrointestinal perforation or hemorrhage, status asthmaticus and respiratory failure [40,42–44]. Shortness of duration between the onset of asthma and the onset of vasculitis has been found to be an unfavorable prognostic sign[42,43]. With successful treatment, recovery from major organ involvement in the

vasculitic phase is often complete. Notable exceptions are peripheral nerve damage and hypertension, which may resolve slowly over time or continue indefinitely[42,43].

TREATMENT

The treatment of CSS has largely centered on the use of corticosteroids[42,43,49]. Active vasculitis is treated with prednisone 1 mg/kg/ day or the IV equivalent [42,44]. The role of immunosuppressive therapy in the treatment of CSS is currently unclear. Azathioprine and cyclophosphamide have been found to be of benefit in small studies but have not been investigated in a well-controlled fashion [17,32,33,42–44,50,51]. Patients with significant vasculitis, evidence of cardiac involvement or persistent disease activity despite high dose steroids should be managed aggressively with concurrent corticosteroids and an immunosuppressive agent[17,44,46]. Although no single agent has been specifically examined in CSS, the experience in Wegener's granulomatosis and PAN favors the use of cyclophosphamide 1–2 mg/kg/day in this setting[44,46]. Given the rapidity with which organ damage can occur, it has been argued that immunosuppressive therapy should be instituted concomitantly with steroids in all patients with CSS vasculitis[44]; however, this has remained controversial as many patients respond promptly to prednisone alone. Immunosuppressive agents may also be of benefit in maintenance therapy and in patients who are unable to taper their corticosteroid dosage to an acceptable level[42,44]. Plasma exchange has been studied in a mixed population of PAN and CSS patients and was not found to have significant therapeutic benefit[32,33].

POLYANGIITIS OVERLAP SYNDROME

Polyangiitis overlap syndrome represents a heterogenous group of disease entities possessing mixed features of several distinct

Table 8.5   Characteristics of the polyangiitis overlap syndrome*

Patient number	Overlapping syndromes
1	SNV – not classified
2	PAN and CSS
3	PAN and CSS
4	Temporal arteritis and PAN
5	PAN and CSS
6	Takayasu's arteritis and PAN
7	SNV – not classified
8	PAN and cutaneous vasculitis
9	HSP and PAN
10	Giant cell arteritis and CSS or WG
11	PAN and WG

SNV = systemic necrotizing vasculitis
PAN = polyarteritis nodosa
CSS = Churg–Strauss syndrome
HSP = Henoch–Schönlein purpura
WG = Wegener's granulomatosis
* Reproduced with permission from Leavitt, R. Y. and Fauci, A. S. (1986) Pulmonary vasculitis, *Am. Rev. Respir. Dis.*, **134**, 149–66.

vasculitic disorders[1,3,41,46,52]. These patients, by definition, have evidence of a systemic necrotizing vasculitis but do not manifest disease in such a way that would clearly place them into a specific diagnostic category. Patients with polyangiitis overlap syndrome may have overlapping features from different diseases, overlapping pathological findings, or atypical involvement that does not meet one specific disease syndrome (Table 8.5)[46,52]. The NIH has treated ten patients with polyangiitis overlap syndrome in a prospective manner[52]. The mean age of these patients was 25 years. Patients manifested a wide variety of clinical features. Cutaneous disease occurred most commonly with the lung and kidney also being frequently affected. All patients were treated with corticosteroids and cyclophosphamide, which were successful in bringing about disease remission.

Like other well-defined vasculitic syndromes, polyangiitis overlap syndrome has the potential to involve multiple organ systems and is a true systemic vasculitis. Although the prognosis of polyangiitis overlap syndrome is not known, the potential for serious organ damage and life-threatening disease exists[1,52]. Patients should be approached, both diagnostically and therapeutically, as if they had a well-defined vasculitic syndrome[1,52]. A careful history, physical examination and laboratory evaluation should be performed to define the extent of their systemic involvement. The diagnosis of polyangiitis overlap syndrome requires the demonstration of vasculitis which should be aggressively pursued by biopsy or angiography. Once the presence of a systemic necrotizing vasculitis has been ascertained and other diagnoses, specifically infection, have been ruled out, treatment should be initiated with corticosteroids and consideration for additional immunosuppressive agents.

WEGENER'S GRANULOMATOSIS

Wegener's granulomatosis is a form of vasculitis which chiefly involves the medium arteries and small arteries and veins of the upper and lower respiratory tract and kidneys. Although it is a systemic, necrotizing, granulomatous vasculitis, Wegener's granulomatosis (WG) is viewed as a distinct clinicopathological entity based upon its predilection for this 'classic triad' (upper respiratory, lung and kidney) of involvement. In addition to generalized disease, limited forms have been described that lack renal manifestations[53,54]. Over 50% of patients felt to have limited disease, however, have evidence of renal pathology by biopsy[55]. It is not clear that these patients follow a more benign course and many later develop generalized features[56]. Patients with limited forms of WG are, therefore, best viewed as presenting at the mild end of the disease spectrum and should be approached in the same manner as those with more generalized involvement.

Table 8.6 Symptoms and signs of Wegener's granulomatosis*

Symptom or sign	% onset	% total
Ear nose and throat	73	92
Sinusitis	50	85
Nasal disease	38	70
Otitis media	25	45
Hearing loss	15	42
Subglottic stenosis	1	18
Ear pain	8	15
Oral lesions	3	10
Pulmonary	45	85
Infiltrates	25	65
Nodules	24	58
Cough	19	46
Hemoptysis	11	30
Pleuritis	10	28
Kidney	18	75
Eye disease	12	52
Musculoskeletal	31	67
Fever	23	50
Cutaneous	13	46
Weight loss	15	35
Peripheral nervous system	1	15
Central nervous system	1	8
Pericarditis	2	6

* Data adapted from [16].

Table 8.7 Wegener's granulomatosis physical findings

Skin
  Papules
  Vesicles
  Palpable purpura
  Ulcers
  Subcutaneous nodules
Nasal
  Crusting exudate
  Mucosal erythema
  Septal perforation
  Saddle nose defect
  Sinus tenderness
Eye
  Proptosis
  Conjunctival erythema
  Scleral erythema
Oral
  Gingival ulceration
  Palatal ulcer
Otic
  Otitis media
  Decreased hearing
Pulmonary
  Abnormal chest auscultation
Joints
  Polyarthritis
Neurologic
  Foot or wrist drop
  Motor or sensory loss
General
  Fever
  Weight loss

Wegener's granulomatosis affects predominantly caucasians and has equal prevalence in men and women[16]. The mean age at onset is 41 years, but it has been reported in individuals from 3 months to 75 years of age[55].

The manifestations and severity of disease at presentation are variable (Table 8.6)[16]. Ninety per cent of patients present with upper and/or lower airway symptoms. In the absence of other systemic features, diagnosis may be delayed as these symptoms are frequently considered to be related to allergy or infection. Often, it is only after persistent or new symptoms develop and further evaluation ensues, that the diagnosis of WG is confirmed. Sinus disease is prominent with involvement of, in descending order of frequency, the maxillary, ethmoid, frontal and sphenoid sinuses[57]. Secondary infection occurs frequently, with *Staphylococcus aureus* being the most commonly cultured organism[14]. Lower airway symptoms occur frequently during the course of disease and include cough, hemoptysis or pleuritis. Renal involvement is unusual at the time of presentation although 75% of patients eventually develop glomerulonephritis[16]. Musculoskeletal symptoms may be seen in 67% of patients. This primarily consists of arthralgias or myalgias, although a non-deforming symmetrical synovitis of the small and large joints has been reported[16]. Other important sites

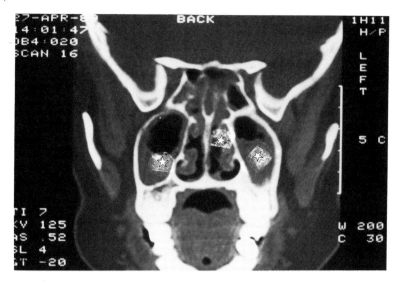

Fig. 8.4 Computed tomography of the sinuses showing mucosal thickening (stars) in a patient with Wegener's granulomatosis.

of involvement include the eye[58], skin[59–61], heart[14], central and peripheral nervous system[62]. Findings characteristic of WG on physical examination are non-specific, but when present, suggest the need for further evaluation, especially when seen in combination or as part of a systemic illness (Table 8.7).

LABORATORY FINDINGS

Laboratory findings typical of WG include leukocytosis, normochromic normocytic anemia and thrombocytosis[16]. Leukopenia in an untreated patient is not seen and distinguishes WG from other disorders[14,56]. Prior to treatment, an elevated ESR is seen in 80% of patients[16]. Although an increasing ESR may herald recurrent disease in the previously stable patient, it is more frequently indicative of infection[14]. A careful evaluation should, therefore, be performed before attributing changes in ESR to disease activity alone. Manifestations of renal involvement include microscopic or gross hematuria, proteinuria, red cell casts and/or elevated serum

BUN and creatinine. Circulating immune complexes and elevated serum immunoglobulins may be found. RF is positive in >50% of patients and ANA's are usually absent[16]. Sinus X-rays or computed tomography may show evidence of mucosal thickening, sinus opacification, or air fluid levels (Figure 8.4)[56]. Multiple, bilateral, nodular infiltrates that frequently cavitate are the most common finding on chest radiograph, although a wide range of abnormalities may be seen (Figure 8.5)[1,55,56,63,64]. Chest X-rays are abnormal at presentation with infiltrates, nodules, or both in 45% of patients[16].

In the early 1980s autoantibodies directed against the cytoplasmic components of neutrophils were detected in patients with segmental necrotizing glomerulonephritis and systemic vasculitis[65,66]. These antineutrophil cytoplasmic antibodies (ANCA) have since been found to be present in two distinct staining patterns, the c-ANCA (cytoplasmic staining) and the p-ANCA (perinuclear staining). The antigen bound by c-ANCA is a 29 kD neutral serine protease,

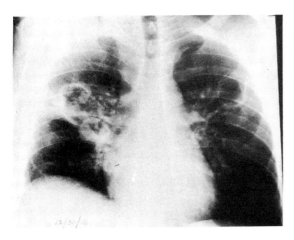

Fig. 8.5 Chest radiograph in a patient with Wegener's granulomatosis demonstrating bilateral nodular infiltrates with cavitation.

(Figure 8.6). In the NIH series, vasculitis and necrosis were seen in 89% of biopsy samples, granulomas and necrosis in 90% and combinations of granulomas and vasculitis as well as vasculitis, necrosis and granulomas in 91%[16]. The most common finding seen on renal biopsy is segmental necrotizing glomerulonephritis, which is present to varying degrees in 80% of specimens[77,78]. Vasculitis not related to the glomerulus is unusual and present in only 8% of biopsies. Skin specimens most commonly show a small vessel leukocytoclastic vasculitis, although dermal necrotizing granulomas or necrotizing vasculitis involving the larger dermal arteries or veins have been noted[16,61].

proteinase-3[67], while p-ANCA is reactive to myleoperoxidase, elastase, and other neutrophil enzymes[68]. Several institutions have found the presence of a positive c-ANCA to be highly specific and sensitive for WG[69–74]. Changes in ANCA titer have been reported to parallel disease activity[69,71–73], although recent data has not supported this correlation[74]. Although a positive c-ANCA should be regarded as suggestive of WG and prompt further evaluation, there is insufficient data at this time to fully judge its use as a diagnostic or monitoring tool. The diagnosis of WG and decision to treat should never be based upon the finding of a positive ANCA alone and, similarly, a negative ANCA should never be used to exclude disease.

Although the morphologic spectrum of disease is broad, the pathological hallmark of WG is a necrotizing, granulomatous vasculitis[7,75,76]. The vaculitis predominantly follows a pattern of fibrinoid necrosis with early infiltration of the vessels by polymorphonuclear leukocytes followed by mononuclear cells[1]. Pulmonary tissue may show any combination of vasculitis, necrosis and granuloma, and biopsy specimens will often not include all of these characteristic features

DIAGNOSIS

Although clinical features and laboratory findings may be suggestive of disease, a diagnosis of WG should only be made in combination with pathologic confirmation. Pulmonary tissue obtained via open lung biopsy offers the best opportunity to make an accurate diagnosis[1,16]. Transbronchial biopsy does not yield adequate tissue for diagnosis and has been found to be diagnostic for vasculitis <10% of the time[16]. Although head and neck tissue is more easily obtainable, characteristic pathologic features are found in <23% of biopsy specimens. Diagnostically useful tissue from the head and neck region is best obtained from, in decreasing order of frequency, the paranasal sinuses, nose and the subglottic region. Renal tissue, although frequently suggestive of WG, is rarely diagnostic. Many other disorders can be similar clinically and radiographically to WG (Tables 8.4 and 8.8)[1,55,57,61]. Of these, infection is an important consideration and one which can have fatal consequences when mistakenly treated with immunosuppressive therapy. It is therefore of extreme importance to pursue tissue diagnosis aggressively, both to confirm WG and rule out other disorders.

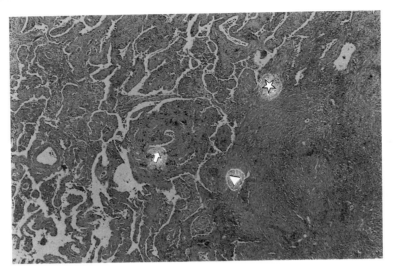

Fig. 8.6 Pulmonary parenchyma a patient with Wegener's granulomatosis demonstrating necrosis (star), granuloma (arrowhead) and vasculitis (arrow).

PROGNOSIS AND TREATMENT

Prior to the use of immunosuppressive therapy, WG was almost universally fatal. Renal disease was the major cause of death and continues to be the worst prognostic factor during the first year. Thereafter, glomerulonephritis does not seem to have distinct significance and lung involvement becomes the most important prognostic factor[79]. In 1958, WG had a mean survival of 5.2 months and a 93% mortality rate within 2 years[80]. The introduction of corticosteroids in the 1960s brought about occasional remissions but only improved the mean survival to 12.5 months[81]. A dramatic improvement in survival was found in the early 1970s when daily oral cyclophosphamide in combination with corticosteroids was introduced in the treatment of WG[14,16,55]. In the 1992 NIH report a marked improvement or partial remission was achieved in 91% of patients with complete remission in 75%[16]. An overall mortality rate of 20% was noted, 13% of which could be completely or partially attributed to WG. Despite this marked improvement in survival and remission, disease relapse and morbidity from both disease and treatment were noted. Fifty per cent of complete remissions were followed by one or more relapses which occurred 3 months to 16 years after achieving remission[16]. Despite these concerns, treatment with daily oral cyclophosphamide and corticosteroids remains the best-known means of achieving remission and prolonging survival, and it is the therapy of choice in the treatment of WG. Intermittent high-dose intravenous (pulse) cyclophosphamide plus corticosteroids improved disease but was not able to sustain remission[82,83]. Trimethoprim-sulfamethoxazole has been reported to be useful, although its efficacy has not been proven in prospective controlled trials[83–87]. Azathioprine has not been satisfactory in achieving remission but may have a role in maintaining remission in patients who are unable to continue cyclophosphamide[57,88]. Preliminary studies found cyclosporin A to be of benefit[89,90] and the use of methotrexate is currently under investigation[16,88]. Anecdotal use of nitrogen mustard, chlorambucil and apheresis has been reported[88].

Table 8.8 Differential diagnosis of Wegener's granulomatosis

Vasculitic disease
  Polyarteritis nodosa
  Henoch–Schönlein purpura
  Hypersensitivity angiitis
  Polyangiitis overlap syndrome
  Churg–Strauss syndrome
Connective tissue disease
  Systemic lupus erythematosus
  Scleroderma
  Dermatomyositis
  Sjögren's syndrome
  Behçet's syndrome
  Relapsing polychondritis
Granulomatous diseases
  Lymphomatoid granulomatosis
  Midline granuloma
  Sarcoidosis
  Berylliosis
  Bronchocentric granulomatosis
Mixed granulomatous and vasculitic diseases
  Löffler's syndrome
  Eosinophilic pneumonia
Infectious
  Tuberculosis
  Histoplasmosis
  Blastomycosis
  Coccidiomycosis
  Syphilis
  Streptococcus
  Leprosy
  Subacute bacterial endocarditis
Pulmonary-renal syndromes
  Goodpasture's syndrome
Neoplastic diseases
  Nasopharyngeal
  Lung
  Metastatic disease to above sites
  Hodgkin's lymphoma
  Non-Hodgkin's lymphoma
Miscellaneous
  Amyloidosis
  Uremic pleuritis/pneumonitis

LYMPHOMATOID GRANULOMATOSIS

Lymphomatoid granulomatosis is an incompletely understood angiocentric, angio-destructive process initially described by Leibow *et al.* in 1972[91]. As its name was chosen to suggest, this disease was initially thought to resemble both Wegener's granulomatosis and lymphoma. Since that time, much speculation and investigation has been undertaken regarding the nature of this disorder and it is increasingly recognized as a lymphoproliferative disease of T-cell origin with varying degrees of aggressiveness [92,93].

The disease prevalence is believed to be low and fewer than 300 cases have been reported. It is slightly male predominant with a mean age at onset of 48 years and a range of 7–85 years[91,94,95]. The lung is the primary site of involvement, although widespread organ infiltration can be seen (Figure 8.7). Cutaneous[96,97] and neurological manifestations also occur frequently[91,94,95]. In contrast to Wegener's granulomatosis, upper airway or clinical renal disease is unusual although the kidneys are often found to be histologically involved. Presenting symptoms are often nonspecific and include fever, malaise, weight loss and fatigue (Table 8.9)[94]. Respiratory complaints of cough, dyspnea or chest pain are the most common focal findings[94]. Arthralgias may be seen[91,94,98] and arthritis has been reported[99].

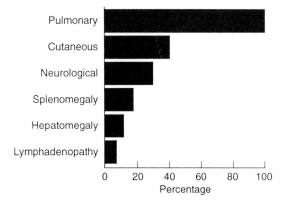

Fig. 8.7 Clinical organ system involvement in lymphomatoid granulomatosis (data adapted from[1]).

Table 8.9   Presenting symptoms and signs in lymphomatoid granulomatosis*

Symptom or sign	Percentage
Fever	57
Cough	53
Malaise	35
Weight loss	34
Dyspnea	28
Neurological dysfunction	21
Chest pain	13
Cutaneous lesion	11
Arthralgia	7
Myalgia	3
Gastrointestinal tract distress	3
Asymptomatic	3

* Reproduced with permission from Cupps, T. R., Fauci, A. S. (1981) *The Vasculitides*, W. B. Saunders, p. 89.

Lymphomatoid granulomatosis has no characteristic pattern of laboratory abnormalities. Leukocytosis can occur although a relative lymphocytosis may suggest malignancy[1,91,94]. Leukopenia has been seen in 20% of patients and when present is an important distinguishing feature from Wegener's granulomatosis[94]. Urinary sediment is usually normal and sedimentation rate is normal or minimally elevated[94]. Results of RF and ANA have not been consistently studied. Chest radiograph most commonly reveals bilateral, nodular infiltrates which typically involve the lower lung fields [91,94,95,98].

DIAGNOSIS

Diagnosis is made by biopsy. Given that benign and malignant disease can be seen simultaneously, it is essential to obtain as many biopsy samples as possible to assess for the presence of atypical cells[1,92]. Although lymphomatoid granulomatosis has been classified as a vasculitis, it is pathologically not a true vascular inflammation. Blood vessels are infiltrated and invaded in an angiocentric and angiodestructive manner by atypical

mononuclear cells (Figure 8.8). In contrast to Wegener's granulomatosis, the cells are mononuclear rather than polymorphonuclear leukocytes and consist primarily of atypical lymphocytes and plasma cells[46,91,94,95]. Necrosis can occur secondary to vessel obliteration and mitotic figures are present to varying degrees[1]. At autopsy, the lung is found to be involved in almost 100% of cases with the kidney being the second most frequently involved site[1,94]. In the kidney, the glomerulus is typically spared and the interstitial space infiltrated with pleomorphic, mononuclear cells. Lymphomatoid granulomatosis does not characteristically involve the lymph nodes, spleen or bone marrow[1].

It remains controversial whether lymphomatoid granulomatosis is a part of a spectrum extending from a benign lymphocytic angiitis and granulomatosis to a malignant neoplasm[1,3,98,100] or an actual lymphoma with varying degrees of aggressiveness[46,101,102]. Immunophenotypic studies have found the involved lymphocytes to be a mature T-cell phenotype with a predominance of T-helper cells[102,103]. These studies support the concept that these lesions represent a spectrum of post-thymic T-cell proliferation. Recently, the term angiocentric immunoproliferative lesion (AIL) has been proposed as an alternative to lymphomatoid granulomatosis[93]. This nomenclature conveys both the proliferative character of the lesion and its cytologic composition. A histologic grading system for AIL based upon the degree of cellular atypia has also been introduced, which has been found to be useful in subclassifying disease and predicting clinical course[102]. This system may be of benefit in the future for guiding clinical management, although further study will be required.

PROGNOSIS AND TREATMENT

Patient outcome in lymphomatoid granulomatosis has been historically poor[91,94,95]. In one study of 157 patients, 64% died, 94% of

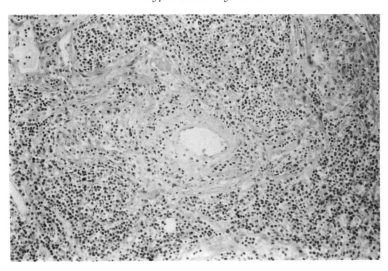

Fig. 8.8 Angiocentric mononuclear inflammation in a lung biopsy from a patient with lymphomatoid granulomatosis.

deaths occurred within 36 months and the mean survival was 11.3 months[94]. Deaths were most frequently secondary to destruction of pulmonary parenchyma, pulmonary hemorrhage or infectious complications[94]. Neurologic disease is a grave prognostic sign[94], although one study has found achievement of an initial complete remission[102] to be the most important prognostic indicator for ultimate survival. Progression to frank lymphoma is common and occurs in 12–47% of patients[91,94,100]. Given the rarity of this disease and confusion regarding its nature, information regarding therapy has largely been retrospective and anecdotal. At this time, there remains no well-established treatment of choice. Corticosteroids alone do not appear to provide consistent long-term benefit[95]. The use of cyclophosphamide and corticosteroids has been studied prospectively and was found to achieve complete remission in 7 out of 13 patients[100]. Recently, early treatment with more aggressive chemotherapeutic regimens has been proposed, especially in patients with higher degrees of cellular atypia[92,104,105]. Various combinations of cyclophosphamide, vincristine,

procarbazine, doxorubicin, chlorambucil, azathioprine and prednisone have been used with anecdotal success, although no one regimen has been consistently studied [3,92,94,95,98,104,105]. As this disease becomes better understood, further prospective investigation will be needed to determine optimal treatment regimens.

HYPERSENSITIVITY VASCULITIS – HENOCH–SCHÖNLEIN PURPURA (ALSO CHAPTER 12)

The classification of hypersensitivity vasculitis (HSV) is confusing. The term HSV was initially used to classify a group of disorders characterized by small vessel vasculitis that was believed to be precipitated by antigenic exposure[106]. It has become appreciated that such a mechanism of 'hypersensitivity' may play a role in the pathophysiology of many vasculitic syndromes, thus making the use of this term in conjunction with only certain disorders somewhat of a misnomer[1,3]. The term has nevertheless persisted and has even been further complicated by the synonymous use of the terms dermal necrotizing vasculitis,

Table 8.10   Syndromes associated with leukocytoclastic vasculitis

Exogenous precipitating events
  Drugs
  Foreign protein
  Infectious agents
Coexistent disease
  Connective tissue disease
    Rheumatoid arthritis
    Systemic lupus erythematosus
    Sjögren's syndrome
    Dermatomyositis/polymyositis
    Scleroderma
    Relapsing polychondritis
  Malignancy
  Cryoglobulinemia
  Hypocomplementemic urticarial vasculitis
  Hypergammaglobulinemic purpura
  Polyarteritis nodosa
  Subacute bacterial endocarditis
  Chronic active hepatitis
  Ulcerative colitis
  Retroperitoneal fibrosis
  Primary biliary cirrhosis
  Goodpasture's syndrome
Uncertain etiology
  Henoch–Schönlein purpura
  Idiopathic palpable purpura
  Erythema elevatum diutinum

allergic vasculitis and leukocytoclastic vasculitis[3,7,107–110]. Difficulty has also arisen in defining what disorders come under the category of HSV. Patients with HSV in response to an exogenous agent develop predominantly cutaneous involvement with histological evidence of small vessel inflammation and leukocytoclasis[1,7,107,108,110–112]. Similar skin and pathological changes can occur in association with a wide variety of disorders and, because of this, the term HSV has often been used to encompass all syndromes with these findings (Table 8.10) [1,3,107–110,112,113]. Despite the similarities, these other disorders can be very different with the potential for larger vessel inflammation, multiorgan involvement and a different prognosis and treatment

[1,3,7,107,113]. Although the disease spectrum should be considered in all patients with evidence of a cutaneous, leukocytoclastic vasculitis, the use of the term 'hypersensitivity vasculitis' seems best applied to vasculitis that occurs after exposure to an identifiable or strongly suspected sensitizing agent.

Henoch–Schönlein purpura (HSP) is a systemic small vessel vasculitis characterized by non-thrombocytopenic purpura with articular, gastrointestinal and renal manifestations. Although the syndrome is known most commonly as HSP, it is sometimes referred to as anaphylactoid purpura or Schönlein–Henoch purpura[114]. HSP has been considered to be a form of hypersensitivity vasculitis, although no clear provoking etiology has been identified[1,114,115]. An upper respiratory tract infection, unrelated to any one infectious agent, precedes the onset of HSP in 30–50% of patients[1,114–117]. Elevated levels of circulating IgA as well as the demonstration of vascular and renal IgA deposition suggest that HSP is an IgA immune complex-mediated disease[1,114,118].

HSP is predominantly a disease of children and is described further in Chapter 12. However, it has been observed in ages ranging from 6 months to 65 years. The median age of onset is 4 years with 75% of cases occurring before age 7[114,117]. HSP has a 3:2 male predominance and has a seasonal peak in the months of March through May[1,114–117,119,120].

Cutaneous involvement is almost universal and generally precedes the appearance of other disease manifestations. The lesions consist of areas of urticarial edema and petechial to maculopapular purpura[114,117,119]. They occur in a characteristic pattern over the buttocks and lower extremities, sparing the trunk and abdomen[1,115–117,119]. Edema affecting the face, scalp and distal extremities is common[117,119]. Arthralgias and periarticular edema occur in 70% of children, primarily affecting the ankles and knees[116–119]. Gastrointestinal (GI) symptoms are seen in 50–70% of patients and presumably result from edema and petechial hemorrhage in the bowel wall[1,117,119]. GI involvement can occasionally precede cutaneous and joint disease and mimic an acute abdominal emergency[114]. The most common symptoms are colicky abdominal pain and vomiting, although hemorrhage or life-threatening intussusception can occur[116,117]. The prevalence of renal disease has ranged from 20–100% in different studies, related in part to variations in patient populations and criteria for diagnosis[116–121]. Clinical expression may extend from transient isolated microscopic hematuria to acute or chronic renal insufficiency. Although hematuria has been seen as the presenting symptom, urinary abnormalities usually follow other manifestations within 4–8 weeks of disease onset[116,118,120]. Hematuria and proteinuria are the commonest urinary abnormalities [116–118,120,121]. An acute nephritis syndrome (hematuria plus two out of the following three: hypertension, oliguria, azotemia) with nephrotic syndrome occurs in severe cases and is correlated with a higher frequency of renal insufficiency[116,120,122].

Laboratory studies in HSP are non-specific and are primarily useful in ruling out other disorders and monitoring for evidence of renal involvement. Leukocytosis and elevated ESR may be seen[117]. CBC with platelet count and coagulation studies are important in the evaluation of cutaneous purpura. Stool guaiacs should be performed intermittently to look for evidence of occult blood loss. Urinalysis and serum creatinine measurements should be performed at the onset of illness and twice weekly until systemic signs have resolved[114]. Radiology studies may be necessary to evaluate the abdomen for evidence of intussusception[1].

The majority of pathological information comes from biopsies of the skin and kidney, as there have been few autopsy descriptions of HSP[114]. The cutaneous histology is that of a small vessel leukocytoclastic vasculitis involving the arterioles, venules and capillaries[1,114]. The principal glomerular lesion is a focal, proliferative glomerulonephritis [114,116–119,123–125]. However, abnormalities can span a range of severity from a minimal change pattern to a diffuse, proliferative glomerulonephritis with crescents [116,118]. Although renal biopsy is a useful tool in assessing the severity of disease, focal variation of the glomerular lesions limit its accuracy[116].

DIAGNOSIS

Difficulty with diagnosis is rarely encountered, except when other major sites of involvement precede the characteristic skin lesions[114]. The diagnosis is essentially clinical with laboratory studies being used to rule out other disorders. Renal biopsy is typically not needed for diagnosis but is used to assess disease severity and estimate prognosis[114]. Included in the differential of HSP is any cause of an acute abdomen, nephritis or purpura.

PROGNOSIS

The natural history of HSP has been difficult to assess as many series have come from selected populations in whom renal disease predominates. Although gastrointestinal (GI) complications can occur, renal involvement is the major determinant of outcome. The overall prognosis in HSP is good with a mortality rate of 1–3%[120]. End-stage renal failure has been estimated to occur in 2–5% of affected children and accounts for 15% of children put on dialysis programs[114,120,121]. Renal presentation and biopsy can provide helpful prognostic information, although these should not be regarded as precise measures of outcome[118,120,122]. Almost all patients who present with microscopic hematuria and 75% of those with hematuria and proteinuria will have normal renal function 2 years past disease onset. Those who have an acute nephritic presentation, particularly with nephrotic syndrome, have the worst outcome with < 50% having normal renal function and urinalyses 2 years later[116,118,120,122]. The percentage of glomeruli with crescents may also be a useful prognostic indicator [114,118,120,122]. Only 4% of patients progress to renal failure when <50% of the glomeruli have crescents. This rises to 25% with 50–75% crescents and in the setting of >75% crescents, two-thirds of patients eventually require dialysis[118,120]. Despite these guidelines, it is important to realize that HSP can be extremely variable and patients having severe clinical or biopsy abnormalities may make a full recovery and those with mild changes can progress to renal insufficiency[118,120]. Disease recurrence is seen in 25–40% of cases and largely consists of skin manifestations[114,116,117,120,122]. Deterioration or improvement may be seen most notably during the first 2–3 years following the resolution of the acute episode, although significant changes in outcome have also been seen after that time[118,122]. Regular follow-up with measurements of blood pressure and urinalysis is therefore extremely important for at least the first 5 years following an episode of HSP[116,122].

TREATMENT

Treatment is largely supportive as there is no therapy of proven benefit for the treatment of HSP nephritis[114,116,118,120,122]. Analgesia may alleviate joint and soft-tissue discomfort, although salicylates should be avoided given the risk of GI ulceration and platelet dysfunction[1]. Intestinal intussusception frequently requires surgical intervention[1,117,118]. Corticosteroids at a dose of prednisone 1–2 mg/kg/day may be useful in decreasing tissue edema, joint pain and abdominal discomfort[1,115,117,118]. Steroids are of no proven benefit in the treatment of skin or renal disease and do not shorten the duration of HSP[1,114–118,120,122]. There is no role for sustained use of corticosteroids as

they do not lessen the chance of recurrence[117]. Several immunosuppressive agents as well as plasmapheresis have been successfully used anecdotally, but remain of unproven efficacy[1,114–116,118,120,126].

Less is known about HSP in adults due to its low prevalence. The information that is available varies widely from finding it to be a disease process very similar to that which is seen in children[123,127,128] to a catastrophic illness with a high potential for renal failure[129]. HSP in adults appears to be more frequent in persons over 45[115,127,128]. Rash remains a feature in almost all patients but may occur more diffusely and have a higher propensity for necrosis[114,127,128]. Articular manifestations occur to the same degree as in children but may affect both large and small joints[127,128]. The incidence of GI manifestations is slightly lower in adults and intussusception is extremely rare[1,115,127,128]. Myocardial involvement may be seen, which is rare in children[115]. Although some studies have found renal disease to be worse in adults, this has not been a consistent finding[123,127–129]. The glomerular changes are similar to those found in children and crescents again appear to be a good estimator of prognosis[123–125]. The course of renal disease may be slower and more insidious in adults, making the role of close follow-up highly important[124,128]. The treatment of HSP is similar to that of children, although care should especially be taken in the management of hypertension as this may affect concurrent medical problems that can occur in the adult[115].

TAKAYASU'S ARTERITIS

Takayasu's arteritis is an inflammatory and obliterative arteritis which primarily affects the large elastic arteries. Although initially believed to be a disease of the aortic arch, it is now known to affect all levels of the aorta, its branches and the pulmonary arteries. Based upon the localization of lesions, as many as 24 different eponyms have been used to describe this entity during its history[130]. It is now appreciated that these all represent the same process that has come to be referred to most commonly in the Western literature as Takayasu's arteritis.

Takayasu's arteritis has a striking female predominance, affecting women 5–9 times more frequently than men[1,130–132]. It primarily presents between 10 and 29 years of age, although a range of 3–75 years has been reported[130–133]. Although initially thought to be a disease of the Orient, it is now recognized to affect all races and has a worldwide distribution[1]. The disease prevalence may vary among ethnic groups as numbers reported in clinical series from Japan, China and India exceed those seen in North America or Europe[134,135]. In a study of Olmstead County, Minnesota, the prevalence was estimated at 2.6 cases/million/year[135]. An association with tuberculosis has been reported although no direct causation has ever been proven[1,130,132–134,136].

The disease symptoms have been divided into two phases, the acute systemic, or pre-pulseless, phase and the chronic obliterative, or pulseless, phase. In reality, these phases are often not as clinically distinct as the names imply. The recognition of an acute phase has varied greatly in patient series, ranging from 13–63%[1,130,132,133,135,137]. The acute symptoms are often non-specific and consistent with a generalized inflammatory process. Features may include fatigue, malaise, weight loss and fever. Arthralgias and myalgias are common and synovitis of single and multiple joints has been described[133–135]. Acute symptoms may merge into chronic phase symptoms such that the two are inseparable. For this reason the interval of time between progression from the acute to chronic stages has been difficult to clearly estimate[1]. The symptoms of the chronic phase are a direct manifestation of the location of the arterial lesions (Table 8.11)[1,131–135,138]. Physical examination is important in the diagnosis and

Table 8.11 Symptoms and signs of Takayasu's arteritis

General
  Hypertension
Cardiac/pulmonary
  Chest pain
  Dyspnea
  Palpitations
  Myocardial infarction
  Congestive heart failure
  Hemoptysis
Extremities
  Claudication
  Raynaud's phenomenon
Cranial
  Syncope
  Dizziness
  Headache
  Visual disturbance
  Paresis
  Stroke
  Seizures
  Dementia
Cutaneous
  Erythema nodosum
  Pyoderma gangrenosum
Gastrointestinal
  Vomiting
  Diarrhea
  Abdominal pain
  Hemorrhage

monitoring of Takayasu's arteritis. Possible findings include diminished or absent arterial pulses, vascular bruits, hypertension, inequality of blood pressure between extremities and abnormalities on cardiac examination. Retinal arteriovenous anastomoses as were first reported by Takayasu are seen in less than one-third of patients but are meaningful when present[1,139].

LABORATORY STUDIES

Laboratory studies in Takayasu's arteritis reflect a systemic inflammatory disorder. The ESR is elevated in 75–100% of patients with active disease but tends to return to normal

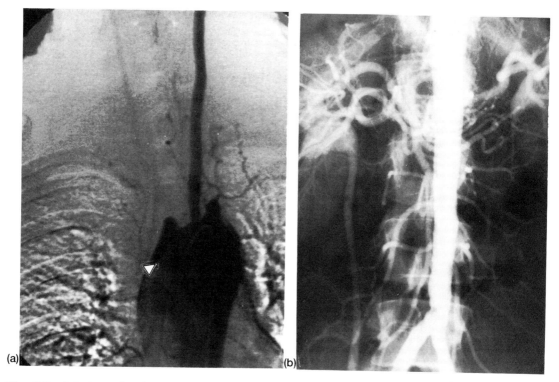

Fig. 8.9 Arteriography in a patient with Takayasu's arteritis revealing large vessel occlusions (a, arrowheads) and a 'rat-tail' appearance (b) of the distal abdominal aorta.

over time[131–133,135,139]. It has been felt to be a reliable index of inflammatory activity and has been used as an adjunct to monitor the effectiveness of therapy [131,133,135,136,139,140]. Improvement in disease, both symptomatically and angiographically, has been found to correlate with decline of the ESR[133,135,140–143]. Hematological studies often show mild anemia and/or leukocytosis[133,135,138,140]. RF and ANA are usually negative[1,134,135,138]. Circulating immune complexes may be present in up to 50% of cases but do not appear to correlate with disease activity or to be implicated as a causative factor[138]. Chest radiograph may be useful in evaluation for widening of the aortic shadow or mediastinum, pulmonary artery enlargement or cardiomegaly [1,131,132,135,144]. Preliminary studies have been inconsistent regarding the efficacy of

magnetic resonance imaging (MRI) of arterial wall thickness and MR angiography as diagnostic tools in Takayasu's arteritis[145–147]. Arteriography plays an important role in the diagnosis and evaluation of patients with Takayasu's arteritis. Angiographic findings can include vessel occlusion, stenosis, collateralization, aneurysm formation and irregularity (Figure 8.9)[1,130,135,137]. Elongate coarctations of the thoracic aorta frequently occur and are described as having a characteristic 'rat-tail' appearance (Figure 8.9) [130,131,137]. Total aortoarteriography is essential for defining the extent of vascular disease[133,135,137]. All levels of the aorta as well as its major branches may be involved (Table 8.12)[1,132–135,137,140]. Pulmonary artery involvement has been seen in up to 50% of those patients in whom it has been specifically sought[1,132,139,144].

Table 8.12 Arterial involvement in Takayasu's arteritis as determined by angiography*

Artery	Percentage
Subclavian	83
Descending aorta	58
Renal	56
Carotid	43
Ascending aorta	30
Abdominal aorta	20
Vertebral	19
Iliac	17
Innominate	16
Pulmonary	15
Mesenteric	15
Coronary	9
Femoral	8
Brachial	6

* Reproduced with permission from Cupps, T. R., Fauci, A. S. (1981) *The Vasculitides*, W. B. Saunders, p. 112.

Table 8.13 Differential diagnosis of Takayasu's arteritis

Infectious
  Syphilis
  Mycotic
  Rheumatic fever
Rheumatologic
  Ankylosing spondylitis
  Relapsing polychondritis
  Reiter's syndrome
  Temporal arteritis
  Cogan's syndrome
Vascular
  Atherosclerosis
  Congenital coarctation
  Buerger's disease
Miscellaneous
  Neurofibromatosis
  Ergotism
  Radiation fibrosis
  Traumatic stenosis

Two phases of histologic abnormality can be seen in Takayasu's arteritis[1,130,134,135]. The early phase is characterized by a granulomatous inflammation with patchy involvement of the vessel wall[130]. The cellular infiltrate is primarily lymphoplasmacytic with a variable number of giant cells and polymorphonuclear leukocytes[130,131]. The inflammation is most pronounced in the media but is also seen in the adventitia and vasa vasora[130]. As disease progresses, late changes occur characterized by intimal proliferation and fibrosis of the adventitia and media. The disease may escape histological recognition in this phase as the acute inflammation resolves and transmural sclerosis occurs[130].

DIAGNOSIS

The diagnosis of Takayasu's arteritis is chiefly made by combined data from history, physical examination and angiography[144]. The predilection for Takayasu's arteritis to affect young females is an important feature that often separates it from other diagnostic considerations (Table 8.13)[1,130,131,135,144].

PREGNANCY IN TAKAYASU'S ARTERITIS

As Takayasu's arteritis primarily affects women in their childbearing years, the safety of pregnancy is an important issue. Despite the obvious vascular concerns, Takayasu's arteritis is compatible with good maternal and fetal outcome[1,130,131,134,136,140,148,149]. Hypertension is the most common complicating feature and should be treated aggressively[148]. Fetal growth retardation has been observed and is likely affected by maternal vascular involvement, hypertension during pregnancy and pre-eclampsia[148–150]. There does not appear to be any increase in neonatal death or congenital abnormality[149]. Induction of labor or Cesarean section are not indicated for the disease *per se*[148]. Therefore, Takayasu's arteritis is not a contraindication to pregnancy, but close follow-up and careful management is important in optimizing a successful outcome for both mother and child[149].

PROGNOSIS

The prognosis of Takayasu's arteritis has been difficult to estimate but appears to be substantially determined by the presence and severity of complications[134,139,141,150]. Ischikawa has separated disease involvement into categories based upon the degree of complications that are present[139,150]. The major complications included Takayasu's retinopathy, secondary hypertension, aortic valve insufficiency and aortic/arterial aneurysm. Patients without or with only one mild to moderate complication were found to have a 5- and 10-year eventless survival of 97%[150]. In contrast, patients with one severe or multiple complications had a 72% 5-year and a 59% 10-year eventless survival rate[150]. Two North American studies have found excellent survival rates with 1 death in 52 patients [135,138]. Of note is that very few of these patients had severe disease and based upon Ishikawa's findings they would be expected to have a more favorable prognosis[134]. It is unclear whether the decline in disease severity seen in these more recent studies reflects genetic differences, changes in health care delivery practices, earlier diagnosis or a true beneficial role of early medical treatment[130,133,135]. Disease-related deaths usually occur from vascular complications, such as congestive heart failure, cerebrovascular events, myocardial infarction and aneurysm rupture[1,130–132,134,141,150].

TREATMENT

Although medical therapy has been found to bring about symptomatic improvement, its precise benefit on preservation of organ function and survival has been difficult to assess. Despite this, an aggressive approach to medical treatment during the acute inflammatory phase is supported by available data. Corticosteroids and cyclophosphamide have both been found to be effective in halting the angiographic progression of vascular lesions[138,142,143]. The use of such agents to interrupt inflammation prior to the establishment of vessel occlusion may lessen the development of disease complications and, in doing so, ultimately improve prognosis. In patients with active disease, treatment should be initiated with prednisone 1 mg/kg/day orally or the intravenous equivalent. If patients are clinically improved at 4 weeks attempts may be made to gradually taper the dose. The effectiveness of steroids has varied greatly in the literature with a range of 25–100% of patients receiving benefit[132–134,136,138,140,142,150]. In addition to angiographic stabilization, steroids have also been found to bring the return of pulses in some instances[133,135,140]. The use of cyclophosphamide has been reported with favorable results[138]. When there is continued evidence of disease activity or inability to taper steroids, institution of cyclophosphamide 1–2 mg/kg/day should be considered[138]. Methotrexate has been used anecdotally with success but has not been thoroughly studied to date[151–153]. Vasodilators, anticoagulants and non-steroidal anti-inflammatory agents have been used for relief of symptoms, but have not been investigated with regards to disease control [130,131,133,134]. Management of hypertension is important in decreasing comorbidity, although care should be taken to not bring about hypotension and decreased perfusion[1,134]. Therapeutic response is best assessed by improvement in symptoms, decline of ESR, improvement in physical examination parameters and serial angiographic studies[138]. The appropriate frequency of angiography has not been determined but should be considered at 6–12 months following treatment institution to guide therapy. Ultrasound and MRI have yielded favorable results in preliminary studies as another means of monitoring disease progression[145,154,155].

Surgical therapy can be useful to bypass stenosed or occluded segments that are producing significant ischemia. The most frequent indications may include bypasses for significant cranial vessel involvement, renal artery stenosis or symptomatic extremity vessel occlusion[156]. In carefully selected patients, the safety of surgery and the potential benefits have been found to be favorable, although the reported patency and complication rate have varied greatly [132,135,136,138,150,156,157]. It is recommended that vascular reconstruction be deferred until active inflammation is medically controlled for fear of aneurysm formation, suture failure or graft occlusion [131,134,135,150,156]. Preliminary reports using percutaneous angioplasty in Takayasu's arteritis have been favorable in select patients but will require further investigation[152,158].

ISOLATED CNS VASCULITIS

Isolated central nervous system (CNS) vasculitis (ICNSV) is a form of vasculitis localized to the vessels of the cranium and spinal cord. Our understanding and investigation of this disorder has been greatly complicated by the lack of specific symptoms, signs or tests by which it can be diagnosed. Further confusion has arisen secondary to its description in the literature under a variety of names, which are now believed to represent the same process. These have included granulomatous angiitis with a predilection for the CNS[159], granulomatous giant-cell angiitis of the CNS[160], cerebral granulomatous angiitis[161], granulomatous angiitis of the nervous system (GANS)[162], primary angiitis of the CNS[163] and ICNSV[1]. Although several reports have demonstrated histologic abnormalities in other organs, it is by definition clinically localized to the CNS, leading to the preference for its designation as ICNSV[1].

ICNSV is believed to be a rare disorder, although its true prevalence may be underestimated due to the difficulty in making a definitive diagnosis. The mean age at onset is 43 with a range of 3–78 years and there is a

Table 8.14 Symptoms and signs of isolated CNS Vasculitis*

Symptom or sign	Frequency (%)
Headache	65
Weakness	45
Confusion/psychiatric disorder	45
Nausea/vomiting	23
Aphasia/dysphasia	27
Seizure	20
Lethargy	18
Incoordination	18
Memory disturbance	17
Loss of consciousness	14
Numbness	9
Stiff neck	9
Hemiplegia/single limb paresis	48
Pathologic lower extremity reflexes	30
Cranial nerve disorder	29
Fever	20
Fundoscopic abnormalities	16
Myelopathy	8
Ataxia	6
Tremor	2

* Data adapted from [164].

slight male predominance at a 4:3 ratio of males to females[164].

Presenting symptoms are not readily distinguishable from those seen in other diseases associated with CNS ischemia[163]. Initial symptoms tend to be generalized and include headache, weakness and confusion (Table 8.14)[1,163–170]. Diffuse neurologic changes typically predominate early in the course of disease, with focal symptoms and signs developing later[1,163]. The clinical course may be rapidly progressive or wax and wane for prolonged periods of time[1,163]. In contrast to other forms of vasculitis, ICNSV is not associated with symptoms such as arthralgias, myalgias, fever or weight loss[1,163,165–167].

LABORATORY STUDIES

Laboratory studies are not useful in making a definitive diagnosis of ICNSV, but they do

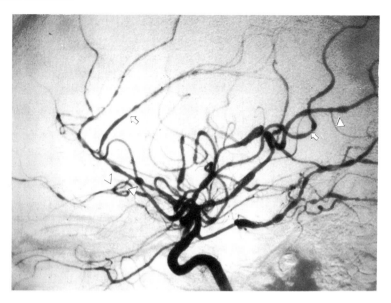

Fig. 8.10   Cerebral angiography in a patient with isolated CNS vasculitis showing a 'beaded' pattern with focal stenoses (arrows) and ectasia (arrowheads).

play an important role in excluding other disease processes. An elevated ESR was observed in 62% of patients combined from the literature[164], although a normal ESR has been found in several individual series[165–167]. Anemia has been seen in only 17% of patients with the remainder of hematologic parameters being normal[163,169]. RF, ANA and ANCA are typically absent[165,167,170]. Cerebrospinal fluid (CSF) is abnormal in a high percentage of patients with features including increased opening pressure, elevated protein, lymphocytic pleocytosis and normal glucose levels[163–167]. Completely normal CSF parameters may also be seen, however, and cannot be used to rule out vasculitis[1,170]. Electroencephalography is abnormal in 74% of cases, but is unfortunately highly non-specific[163,164]. Computed tomographic (CT) scans are often normal and even when there are changes, they are not of a unique, distinguishable pattern[163,165,166]. Preliminary studies using MRI have found it to be more sensitive than CT in identifying foci of infarction[164,170,171]. Although evidence of small vessel infarction is not specific for ICNSV, a negative MRI makes this diagnosis unlikely. Angiography has been felt to be the most useful diagnostic test in the evaluation of ICNSV and remains the initial invasive procedure of choice[163]. Abnormal angiograms have been observed in 82% of ICNSV patients, although normal studies have been seen in patients later found to have active vasculitis by biopsy or post/mortem examination[160,163,165,166,172]. The most specific or diagnostic change is that of alternating areas of focal stenosis and ectasia giving a 'sausage' or 'beaded' pattern (Figure 8.10)[1,163,167]. Other findings include focal vascular stenoses, abrupt termination and narrowing or irregularity of vessels [1,165,166,170]. Unlike PAN, aneurysms are rarely observed[163,167]. These changes are all non-specific and must always be interpreted in the context of the overall clinical picture. There are numerous examples of similar angiographic findings being due to atherosclerosis, emboli, infection, drugs and vasospasm[163,165,173,174]. In addition to providing diagnostic information, there has been evidence to suggest that angiography may be useful in following disease activity and guiding treatment[163,165,175].

Pathologically, the small- and medium-sized arteries are the most frequently affected, although any size artery or vein can be involved[1,163,169]. Inflammation is predominantly lymphocytic and monocytic with a variable degree of neutrophils, plasma cells, eosinophils and giant cells[163,170]. It is frequently a segmental, necrotizing or granulomatous vasculitis often accompanied by thrombosis[169]. Skip lesions are common and, for this reason, characteristic changes can be missed even on extensive biopsy specimens[163]. Every portion of the brain may be affected and there is no clear predominance in one area[170]. Significant vasculitis is rarely seen outside of the cranium, although the spinal cord, cranial nerves and temporal arteries can be rarely involved[164]. Histologic changes not associated with evidence of clinical disease have been seen in the lung and kidney[164].

DIAGNOSIS

The diagnosis of ICNSV remains largely one of exclusion as there is no one symptom, sign or test which can establish or rule out the diagnosis[1]. Diagnostic criteria for ICNSV have been proposed to aid in the determination of disease[163]. These have included:

1. CNS dysfunction that is unexplained by clinical, laboratory and neurologic investigation;
2. documentation by angiogram and/or biopsy of an arteritic process within the CNS; and
3. no evidence of a systemic vasculitis or other condition to which the angiographic or pathologic features could be secondary.

The role of brain biopsy in the evaluation of ICNSV remains controversial, although some authors advocate that biopsy evidence is essential to make a definitive diagnosis[164–166]. The widespread application of biopsy has been tempered not only by its invasive nature but also by the unreliability of demonstrating histologic vasculitis even in the setting of active disease. The optimum location for biopsy has not been determined, although one study has used the temporal tip[165]. It is believed that the yield of biopsy can be increased by obtaining samples of both parenchyma and leptomeningeal vessels[163–167]. Given the difficulty in obtaining diagnostic certainty with this disease, it is equally as important to rule out other possible etiologies. The differential diagnosis must be carefully considered in all cases and be used in deciding the appropriate tests to both support a diagnosis of ICNSV and to exclude other processes (Table 8.15)[1,163,164,168–170].

PROGNOSIS AND TREATMENT

The prognosis of ICNSV is poor and 60–70% of patients die within the first year following diagnosis[163,169]. No prospective trials have been done to determine a treatment regimen of choice. Corticosteroids alone have been of variable success, but there have been several well-documented cases of disease progression despite steroid therapy[1,167,172]. Azathioprine has been used anecdotally without clear benefit[176]. Several small series using combination therapy with corticosteroids and daily cyclophosphamide have demonstrated an improved patient outcome[1,163,167,172]. Although the efficacy of this regimen has not been proven in a large clinical trial, the overall poor prognosis supports the use of aggressive treatment in cases where the diagnosis of ICNSV has been adequately supported and other processes ruled out[177]. Many authors advocate initiation of combination therapy with cyclophosphamide and corticosteroids in patients with severe rapidly progressive disease or addition of cyclophosphamide to

Table 8.15 Differential diagnosis of isolated CNS vasculitis

Infective angiitis
  Bacterial, fungal, mycoplasmal
  Protozoal, rickettsial, viral
Systemic vasculitides that often affect the CNS
  Polyarteritis nodosa
  Churg–Strauss syndrome
  Giant–cell arteritis
  Takayasu's arteritis
  Wegener's granulomatosis
  Lymphomatoid granulomatosis
  Cogan's syndrome
  Henoch–Schönlein purpura
  Cryoglobulinemia
Rheumatic syndromes associated with CNS disease
  Systemic lupus erythematosus
  Progressive systemic sclerosis
  Mixed connective tissue disease
  Sjögren's syndrome
  Rheumatoid disease
  Juvenile rheumatoid arthritis
  Polymyositis/dermatomyositis
  Behçet's syndrome
  Ankylosing spondylitis
  Reiter syndrome
  Sarcoid angiitis
Drug related
  Allopurinol, ephedrine
  Amphetamines, cocaine, heroin
Malignancy related
  Hodgkin's lymphoma
  Non-Hodgkin's lymphoma
  Leukemia
  Metastatic small cell lung carcinoma
Vasculitis simulators
  Fibromuscular dysplasia
  Moyamoya disease
  Antiphospholipid syndrome
  Vasospasm or acute arterial hypertension
  Thrombotic thrombocytopenic purpura
  Cardiac myxoma embolism
  Sickle-cell anemia
  Radiation vasculopathy
  Acute meningoencephalitis
  Acute leukoencephalitis

steroids in patients with milder disease who fail to respond to steroids alone [163,167,170,172].

COGAN'S SYNDROME

Cogan's syndrome (CS) is an uncommon disorder characterized by acute interstitial keratitis and vestibuloauditory dysfunction. It was first recognized as a distinct clinico-pathologic entity by Cogan in 1945[178]. Since that time, literature reviews and small patient series have provided insight into the manifestations of this disease[179–182]. Previous reports have separated CS into 'typical' and 'atypical' subsets based upon the presence of interstitial keratitis versus other types of ocular inflammation[179]. This nomenclature has been found to be less useful than initially thought as patients with 'typical' disease can later go on to develop 'atypical' ocular features[181–183].

CS affects primarily young adults at an average age of 25 with a range of 5–63 years[179,180]. Men and women are believed to be affected equally. An antecedent upper respiratory tract infection occurs in 40–65% of CS patients, although the role of this in disease pathogenesis remains unclear [179,180].

Inflammatory eye disease and vestibulo-auditory dysfunction are the *sine qua non* of CS and occur simultaneously or with one slightly preceding the other[179]. Ocular symptoms can consist of blurred vision, photophobia, redness, lacrimation and pain[179–181]. In addition to interstitial keratitis, other sites of ocular inflammation may include conjunctivitis, iritis, scleritis/episcleritis or posterior segment involvement[182]. Careful and repetitive examination may be necessary as findings can be short lived. Vestibuloauditory symptoms are Meniere-like and consist of nausea, vomiting, vertigo and tinnitus associated with hearing loss[179–181]. Vestibular symptoms may be incapacitating on presentation but often resolve spontaneously. Loss

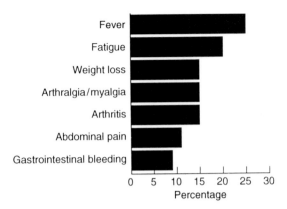

Fig. 8.11 Systemic manifestations of Cogan's syndrome.

of auditory acuity occurs frequently and is the major disabling sequelae in CS. Systemic symptoms are common and may include fever, weight loss, headache, arthralgias, arthritis and myalgias (Figure 8.11)[179–181]. A systemic necrotizing vasculitis is noted in 10–15% of CS patients[179–182]. Typically, the large vessels are primarily affected (Takayasu-like), although medium-vessel disease has been reported[182]. When present, vasculitis may be severe and associated with death. The other life-threatening feature in CS is aortic insufficiency (AI), which occurs secondary to inflammatory aortitis. This develops in 10% of patients and may be seen with other cardiac abnormalities including coronary arteritis, pericarditis, hypertrophy and arrhythmias[179–181]. Patients may present at any point of their disease with an asymptomatic murmur or develop signs of chest pain or dyspnea[179,180]. Careful physical examination and echocardiography should therefore be performed at regular intervals to monitor for the development of valvular changes[182].

LABORATORY FINDINGS

The most common laboratory abnormalities observed are an elevated ESR in 75–100% of patients, leukocytosis and anemia

[179,180,182]. Serologic studies are variable with low-titer RF and ANA being observed in <20% of patients and positive cryoglobulins in 23%[179,180]. Audiograms are almost always abnormal with losses typically noted at the extreme frequencies sparing the midrange. Echocardiography is useful in evaluating for aortic valvular abnormalities. In cases where vasculitis is suspected, confirmation by angiogram or biopsy must be pursued. Pathological changes in the cornea and cochlea include lymphocyte and plasma cell infiltration indicative of an inflammatory process[179,180]. It has been postulated that the ocular and otic manifestations are related to vasculitis, but this has never been histologically proven, and this is not felt to be the primary pathophysiology of CS[182].

DIAGNOSIS AND TREATMENT

The differential diagnosis for CS is especially important given the rarity of this condition and the need to consider early treatment (Table 8.16)[179–181]. CS can be confused with other diseases entities, particularly infectious diseases, Meniere's disease and rheumatic diseases. VDRL, FTA-abs, and tuberculin skin testing should be done in all patients to rule out syphilis and tuberculosis.

The natural history of CS is that of hearing loss and eye inflammation that is non-vision threatening. Ocular outcome is generally favorable with severe visual loss occurring in 4–5% of patients[179,180]. Deafness is a major cause of morbidity with moderate to profound hearing loss developing in 80–95% of untreated patients[179,181,182,184]. Interstitial keratitis and other forms of anterior segment inflammation are almost always responsive to topical corticosteroids [179,180,182,185,186]. Posterior segment involvement may require systemic corticosteroids or other forms of systemic immunosuppression[182,185]. Corneal transplant may be of benefit, although recurrent disease has been reported to occur in the transplant[179]. Co-ordinating care

Table 8.16   Differential diagnosis of Cogan's syndrome*

Infectious
  Congenital syphilis
  Acquired syphilis
  Lyme disease
  Chlamydia
  Virus
  Tuberculosis with streptomycin therapy
Vasculitis
  Polyarteritis nodosa
  Wegener's granulomatosis
  Temporal arteritis
  Takayasu's arteritis
Rheumatic diseases
  Rheumatoid arthritis
  Relapsing polychondritis
  Behçet's syndrome
Toxins
  3-methyl-1-pentyn-3-yl acid phthalate
  (whipcide)
  Cobalt
  Deferoxamine
Other
  Sarcoidosis
  Vogt–Koyanagi–Harada
  Meniere's disease with eye inflammation

* Reproduced with permission from McCallum, R. M. and Hayes, B. F. (1993) Cogan's syndrome, *Ocular Infection and Immunity*, Mosby-Year Book, 1993 (in publication)

with an ophthalmologist is important in detecting and following disease, as well as in making therapeutic decisions. Hearing loss in the patient with newly diagnosed CS is potentially responsive to systemic corticosteroids given at a dose of 1–2 mg/kg/day[179,182,184–186]. This appears to be of most benefit when begun early, preferably within the first 2 weeks of symptom onset[179,184]. Audiograms are useful as a means of quantitating hearing loss and measuring response to treatment. The duration of steroid treatment is unclear and hearing loss may recur in some patients once the steroid dose is tapered[179]. In patients who are unable to taper the steroids or who have progressive loss despite

steroid therapy, immunosuppressive agents, such as cyclophosphamide, methotrexate and azathioprine, have been used anecdotally with success[180,182,185]. When documented by angiography or tissue biopsy, systemic vasculitis should be treated with systemic steroids and immunosuppressive therapy. Large-vessel vasculitis has been treated with cyclosporin A and medium-vessel disease has been treated with cyclophosphamide [182,183,185,186]. However, when either drug is ineffective the other should be considered[182,185,186]. The development of AI, in the absence of other etiologies, suggests the presence of aortitis. After infection is ruled out by blood cultures, initiation of systemic steroids is indicated[182,183]. If AI develops while on corticosteroids, consideration should be given to beginning immunosuppressive therapy with cyclophosphamide [182–184]. Patients with AI must be followed closely by examination and echocardiography for evidence of vegetations and decreased left ventricular function. Aortic valve replacement is often required and may provide significant benefit [179,180,187].

SUMMARY

The vasculitides are a complex group of disorders. Although they share similar features of blood vessel inflammation and damage, the spectrum of disease varies widely. Since the description of vasculitis, there have been significant improvements in both diagnosis and treatment. Despite this, the vasculitic syndromes remain poorly understood and continue to have the potential for significant patient morbidity and mortality. Ongoing studies into disease pathophysiology with controlled diagnostic and therapeutic trials hold promise for a greater comprehension of these disorders and subsequent improvements in patient outcome.

The authors wish to thank Nancy Allen, MD, and E. William St. Clair, MD, for their generous contribution of clinical materials and, together with Cheryl Robertson, MD, their constructive reviews of this chapter.

REFERENCES

1. Cupps, T. R. and Fauci, A. S. (1981) *The Vasculitides*, W. B. Saunders, Philadelphia.
2. Churg, A. and Churg, J. (1991) Introduction, in *Systemic Vasculitides*, (eds A. Churg and J. Churg), Igaku-Shoin, New York, pp. 3–5.
3. Fauci, A. S., Haynes, B. F. and Katz, P. (1978) The spectrum of vasculitis: clinical, pathologic, immunologic, and therapeutic considerations. *Ann. Inter. Med.*, **89**, 660–76.
4. Lie, J. T. (1992) Vasculitis, 1815 to 1991: classification and diagnostic specificity. *J. Rheumatol.*, **19**, 83–9.
5. Fauci, A. S. and Leavitt, R. Y. (1988) Systemic vasculitis, in *Current Therapy in Allergy, Immunology and Rheumatology-3*, (eds L. M. Lichtenstein and A. S. Fauci), B. C. Decker, Philadelphia, pp. 149–55.
6. Haynes, B. F., Allen, N. B. and Fauci, A. S. (1986) Diagnostic and therapeutic approach to the patient with vasculitis. *Med. Clin. N. Am.*, **70**, 355–68.
7. Lie, J. T. (1990) Diagnostic histopathology of major systemic and pulmonary vasculitic syndromes. *Rheum. Dis. Clin. N. Am.*, **16**, 269–92.
8. Hunder, G. G., Arend, W. P., Bloch, D. A. *et al.* (1990) The American College of Rheumatology 1990 criteria for the classification of vasculitis: introduction. *Arth. Rheum.*, **33**, 1065–7.
9. Haynes, B. F. (1992) Vasculitis: pathogenic mechanisms of vessel damage, in *Inflammation: Basic Principles and Clinical Correlates*, 2nd edn, (eds J. I. Gallin, I. M. Goldstein and R. Snyderman), Raven Press Ltd., New York, pp. 921–41.
10. Gocke, D., Hsu, K. and Morgan, C. *et al.* (1970) Association between polyarteritis and australia antigen. *Lancet*, **2**, 1149–53.
11. Trepo, C. and Thivolet, J. (1970) Hepatitis associated antigen and periarteritis nodosa. *Vox Sang*, **19**, 410–11.
12. Johnson, R. J. and Couser, W. G. (1990) Hepatitis B infection and renal disease: clinical, immunopathogenetic and therapeutic considerations. *Kid. Inter.*, **37**, 663–76.
13. Savage, C. O. S. (1991) Pathogenesis of systemic vasculitis, in *Systemic Vasculitides*, (eds A. Churg and J. Churg), Igaku-Shoin, New York, pp. 7–30.
14. Fauci, A. S., Haynes, B. F., Katz, P. *et al.* (1983) Wegener's granulomatosis: prospective clinical and therapeutic experience with 85 patients for 21 years. *Ann. Int. Med.*, **98**, 76–85.
15. Haynes, B. F. (1992) Glucocorticoid therapy, in *Cecil Textbook of Medicine*, 19th edn, (eds J. B. Wyngaarden, L. H. Smith and J. C. Bennett), W. B. Saunders, Philadelphia, pp. 104–8.
16. Hoffman, G. S., Kerr, G. S., Leavitt, R. Y. *et al.* (1992) Wegener granulomatosis: an analysis of 158 patients. *Ann. Inter. Med.*, **116**, 488–98.
17. Fauci, A. S., Katz, P., Haynes, B. F. *et al.* (1979) Cyclophosphamide therapy of severe systemic necrotizing vasculitis. *N. Eng. J. Med.*, **301**, 235–8.
18. Kussmaul, A. and Maier, R. (1866) Uber eine bisher nicht beschreibene eigenthumliche Arterienerkrankung (Periarteritis nodosa), die mit Morbus Brightii und rapid fortschreitender allgemeiner Muskellahmung einhergeht. *Dtsch. Arch. Klin. Med.*, **1**, 484–517.
19. Ferrari, E. (1903) Uber Poly-arteritis acute nodosa (sogenannte Periarteritis nodosa) und ihre Beziehungen zur Polymyositis und Polyneuritis acuta. *Beitr. Pathol. Anat.*, **34**, 350–86.
20. Rosen, S., Falk, R. J. and Jeanette, J. C. (1990) Polyarteritis nodosa, including microscopic form and renal vasculitis, in *Systemic Vasculitides*, (eds A. Churg and J. Churg), Igaku-Shoin, New York, pp. 55–77.
21. Scott, D. G. I., Bacon, P. A., Elliott, P. J. *et al.* (1982) Systemic vasculitis in a district general hospital 1972–1980: clinical and laboratory features, classification and prognosis of 80 cases. *Q. J. Med.*, **203**, 292–311.
22. McMahon, B. J., Heyward, W. L., Templin, D. W. *et al.* (1989) Hepatitis B-associated polyarteritis nodosa in Alaskan Eskimos: clinical and epidemiologic features and long-term follow-up. *Hepatology*, **9**, 97–101.
23. Sack, M., Cassidy, J. T. and Bole, G. G. (1975) Prognostic factors in polyarteritis. *J. Rheumatol.*, **2**, 411–20.
24. Cohen, R. D., Conn, D. L. and Ilstrup, D. M. (1980) Clinical features, prognosis, and response to treatment in polyarteritis. *Mayo Clin. Proc.*, **55**, 146–55.
25. Frohnert, P. P. and Sheps, S. G. (1967) Long-term follow-up study of periarteritis nodosa. *Am. J. Med.*, **43**, 8–14.
26. Ewald, E. A., Griffin, D. and McCune, W. J.

(1987) Correlation of angiographic abnormalities with disease manifestations and disease severity in polyarteritis nodosa. *J. Rheumatol.*, **14**, 952–6.

27. Conn, D. L. (1990) Polyarteritis. *Rheum. Dis. Clin. N. Am.*, **16**, 341–62.

28. Travers, R. L., Allison, D. J., Brettle, R. P. *et al.* (1979) Polyarteritis nodosa: a clinical and angiographic analysis of 17 cases. *Sem. Arth. Rheum.*, **8**, 184–99.

29. Leib, E. S., Restivo, C. and Paulus, H. E. (1979) Immunosuppressive and corticosteroid therapy of polyarteritis nodosa. *Am. J. Med.*, **67**, 941–7.

30. Maxeiner, S. R., McDonald, J. R. and Kirklin, J. W. (1952) Muscle biopsy in the diagnosis of periarteritis nodosa. *Surg. Clin. N. Am.*, **32**, 1225–33.

31. Fauci, A. S., Doppman, J. L. and Wolff, S. M. (1978) Cyclophosphamide-induced remissions in advanced polyarteritis nodosa. *Am. J. Med.*, **64**, 890–4.

32. Guillevan, L., Lhote, F., Jarrousse, B. *et al.* (1992) Treatment of polyarteritis nodosa and Churg-Strauss syndrome: a meta-analysis of 3 prospective controlled trials including 182 patients over 12 years. *Annales Medicine Interne*, **143**, 405–16.

33. Guillevin, L., Fain, O., Lhote, F. *et al.* (1992) Lack of superiority of steroids plus plasma exchange to steroids alone in the treatment of polyarteritis nodosa and Churg-Strauss syndrome. *Arth. Rheum.*, **35**, 208–15.

34. Diaz-Perez, J. L. and Winkelmann, R. K. (1980) Cutaneous periarteritis nodosa: a study of 33 cases, in *Major Problems in Dermatology*, (eds K. Wolff and R. Winkelmann), W. B. Saunders, Philadelphia, pp. 273–84.

35. Cacoub, P., Lunel-Fabiani, F. and Du, L. T. H. (1992) Polyarteritis nodosa and hepatitis C virus infection. *Ann. Int. Med.*, **116**, 605–6.

36. Quint, L., Deny, P., Guillevin, L. *et al.* (1991) Hepatitis C prevalence in patients with polyarteritis nodosa prevalence in 38 patients. *Clin. Exp. Rheumatol.*, **9**, 253–7.

37. Carson, C. W., Conn, D. L., Czaja, A. J. *et al.* (1993) Frequency and significance of antibodies to hepatitis C virus in polyarteritis nodosa. *J. Rheumatol.*, **20**, 304–9.

38. Sergent, J. S., Lockshin, M. D., Christian, C. L. *et al.* (1976) Vasculitis with hepatitis B antigenemia: long-term observations in nine patients. *Medicine*, **55**, 1–18.

39. Inman, R. D. (1982) Rheumatic manifestations of hepatitis B virus infection. *Sem. Arth. Rheum.*, **11**, 406–20.

40. Churg, J., Strauss, L. (1951) Allergic granulomatosis, allergic angiitis, and periarteritis nodosa. *Am. J. Path.*, **27**, 277–301.

41. Michet, C. J. (1990) Epidemiology of vasculitis. *Rheum. Dis. Clin. N. Am.*, **16**, 261–8.

42. Lanham, J. G., Elkon, K. B., Pusey, C. D. *et al.* (1984) Systemic vasculitis with asthma and eosinophilia: a clinical approach to the Churg–Strauss syndrome. *Medicine*, **63**, 65–81.

43. Chumbley, L. C., Harrison, E. G. and DeRemee, R. A. (1977) Allergic granulomatosis and angiitis (Churg-Strauss syndrome). *Mayo Clin. Proc.*, **52**, 477–84.

44. Lanham, J. G. and Churg, J. (1991) Churg–Strauss syndrome, in *Systemic Vasculitides*, (eds A. Churg and J. Churg), Igaku-Shoin, New York, pp. 101–19.

45. Finan, M. C. and Winkelmann, R. K. (1983) The cutaneous extravascular necrotizing granuloma (Churg–Strauss granuloma) and systemic disease: a review of 27 cases. *Medicine*, **62**, 142–58.

46. Leavitt, R. Y. and Fauci, A. S. (1986) Pulmonary vasculitis. *Am. Rev. Respir. Dis.*, **134**, 149–66.

47. Yousem, S. A. and Hochholzer, L. (1989) Overlap syndromes: Wegener's granulomatosis and Churg–Strauss syndrome. *Sem. Respir. Med.*, **10**, 162–6.

48. Rose, G. A. and Spencer, H. (1957) Polyarteritis nodosa. *Q. J. Med.*, **26**, 43–81.

49. MacFadyen, R., Tron, V., Keshmiri, M. *et al.* (1987) Allergic angiitis of Churg and Strauss syndrome: response to pulse methylprednisolone. *Chest*, **91**, 629–31.

50. Cooper, B. J., Bacal, E. and Patterson, R. (1978) Allergic angiitis and granulomatosis: prolonged remission induced by combined prednisone-azathioprine therapy. *Arch. Int. Med.*, **138**, 367–71.

51. Chow, C-C., Li, E. K. M. and Lai, F. M-M. (1989) Allergic granulomatosis and angiitis (Churg–Strauss syndrome): response to 'pulse' intravenous cyclophosphamide. *Ann. Rheum. Dis.*, **48**, 605–8.

52. Leavitt, R. Y. and Fauci, A. S. (1986) Polyangiitis overlap syndrome: classification and prospective clinical experience. *Am. J. Med.*, **81**, 79–85.

53. Carrington, C. B. and Liebow, A. A. (1966) Limited form of Wegener granulomatosis. *Am. J. Med.*, **41**, 497–527.

54. Cassan, S. M., Coles, D. T. and Harrison, E. G. (1970) The concept of limited forms of Wegener's granulomatosis. *Am. J. Med.*, **49**, 366–79.

55. Fauci, A. S. and Wolff, S. M. (1973) Wegener's granulomatosis: studies in 18 patients and a review of the literature. *Medicine* (Baltimore), **52**, 535–61.

56. Specks, U. and DeRemee, R. A. (1990) Granulomatous vasculitis: Wegener's granulomatosis and Churg–Strauss syndrome. *Rheum. Dis. Clin. N. Am.*, **16**(2), 377–97.

57. Wolff, S. M., Fauci, A. S., Horn, R. G. *et al.* (1974) Wegener's granulomatosis. *Ann. Intern. Med.*, **81**, 513–25.

58. Haynes, B. F., Fishman, M. L., Fauci, A. S. *et al.* (1977) The ocular manifestations of Wegener's granulomatosis: fifteen years experience and review of the literature. *Am. J. Med.*, **63**, 131–41.

59. Reed, W. B., Jensen, A. K., Konwaler, B. E. *et al.* (1963) The cutaneous manifestations of Wegener's granulomatosis. *Acta Dermatol. Venereol.*, **43**, 250–64.

60. Hu, C-H., O'Loughlin, S. and Winkelmann, R. K. (1977) Cutaneous manifestations of Wegener's granulomatosis. *Arch. Dermatol.*, **113**, 175–82.

61. Cupps, T. R. and Fauci, A. S. (1980) Wegener's granulomatosis. *Inter. J. Dermatol.*, **19**, 76–80.

62. Drachman, D. A. (1963) Neurological complications of Wegener's granulomatosis. *Arch. Neurol.*, **8**, 145–55.

63. Farrelly, C. A. (1982) Wegener's granulomatosis: a radiological review of the pulmonary manifestations at initial presentation and during relapse. *Clin. Radiol.*, **33**, 545–51.

64. Gohel, V. K., Dalinka, M. K., Israel, H. L. *et al.* (1973) The radiological manifestations of Wegener's granulomatosis. *Br. J. Radiol.*, **46**, 427–32.

65. Davies, D. J., Moran, J. E., Niall, J. F. *et al.* (1982) Segmental necrotizing glomerulonephritis with antineutrophil antibody: possible arbovirus aetiology, *Br. Med. J.*, **285**, 606.

66. Hall, J. B., Wadham, B. McN., Wood, C. J. *et al.* (1984) Vasculitis and glomerulonephritis: a subgroup with an antineutrophil cytoplasmic antibody. *Australia and New Zealand J. Med.*, **14**, 277–8.

67. Nile, J. L., McCluskey, R. T., Ahmad, M. F. *et al.* (1989) Wegener's granulomatosis autoantigen is a novel neutrophil serine protease. *Blood*, **74**, 1888–93.

68. Cohen Tervaert, J. W., Goldschmeing, R., Elena, J. D. *et al.* (1990) Association of autoantibodies to myeloperoxidase with different forms of vasculitis. *Arth. Rheum.*, **33**, 1264–72.

69. Specks, U., Wheatley, C. L., McDonald, T. J. *et al.* (1989) Anticytoplasmic antibodies in the diagnosis and treatment of Wegener's granulomatosis. *Mayo Clin. Proc.*, **64**, 28–36.

70. Jeanette, J. C., Wilkman, A. S. and Falk, R. J. (1989) Anti-neutrophil cytoplasmic antibody-associated glomerulonephritis and vasculitis. *Am. J. Path.*, **135**, 921–30.

71. Van der Woude, F. J., Rasmussen, N., Lobatto, S. *et al.* (1985) Autoantibodies against neutrophils and monocytes: tool for diagnosis and marker of disease activity in Wegener granulomatosis. *Lancet*, **1**, 425–9.

72. Cohen Tervaert, J. W., van der Woude, F. J., Fauci, A. S. *et al.* (1989) Association between active Wegener granulomatosis and anticytoplasmic antibodies. *Arch. Inter. Med.*, **149**, 2461–5.

73. Nolle, B., Specks, U., Ludemann, J. *et al.* (1989) Anticytoplasmic autoantibodies: their immunodiagnostic value in Wegener's granulomastosis. *Ann. Inter. Med.*, **11**, 28–40.

74. Kerr, G. S., Fleisher, T. A., Hallahan, C. W. *et al.* (1993) Limited prognostic value of changes in antineutrophil cytoplasmic antibody titer in patients with Wegener's granulomatosis. *Arth. Rheum.*, **36**, 365–71.

75. Godman, G. C. and Churg, J. (1954) Wegener's granulomatosis, pathology and review of the literature. *Arch. Pathol.*, **58**, 533–53.

76. Lieberman, K. and Churg, A. (1991) Wegener's granulomatosis, in *Systemic Vasculitides*, (eds A. Churg and J. Churg), Igaku-Shoin, New York, pp. 79–99.

77. Horn, R. G., Fauci, A. S., Rosenthal, A. S. *et al.* (1974) Renal biopsy pathology in Wegener's granulomatosis. *Am. J. Pathol.*, **74**, 423–40.

78. Weiss, M. A. and Crissman, J. D. (1989) Renal pathologic features of Wegener's granulomatosis: a review. *Sem. Respir. Med.*, **10**, 141–8.

79. DeRemee, R. A., McDonald, T. J. and Weiland, L. H. (1987) Aspekte zur therapie und verlaufsbeobachtungen der Wegenerschen granulomatosis. *Med. Welt*, **38**, 470–3.

80. Walton, E. W. (1958) Giant-cell granuloma of

the respiratory tract (Wegener's granulomatosis). *Br. Med. J.*, **2**, 265–70.

81. Hollander, D. and Manning, R. T. (1967) The use of alkylating agents in the treatment of Wegener's granulomatosis. *Ann. Inter. Med.*, **67**, 393–8.

82. Hoffman, G. S., Leavitt, R. Y., Fleisher, T. A. *et al.* (1990) Treatment of Wegener's granulomatosis with intermittent high-dose intravenous cyclophosphamide. *Am. J. Med.*, **89**, 403–10.

83. Steppat, D. and Gross, W. L. (1989) Stage adapted treatment of Wegener's granulomatosis. *Klin Wochenschr*, **67**, 666–71.

84. De Remee, R. A., McDonald, T. J., Weiland, L. H. *et al.* (1985) Wegener's granulomatosis: observations on treatment with antimicrobial agents. *Mayo Clin. Proc.*, **60**, 27–32.

85. Israel, H. L. (1988) Sulfamethoxazole-trimethoprim therapy for Wegener's granulomatosis. *Arch. Inter. Med.*, **148**, 2293–5.

86. West, B. C., Todd, J. R. and King, J. W. (1987) Wegener's granulomatosis and trimethoprim-sulfamethoxazole: complete remission after a twenty-year course. *Ann. Intern. Med.*, **106**, 840–2.

87. Leavitt, R. Y., Hoffman, G. S. and Fauci, A. S. (1988) Response: the role of trimethoprim/sulfamethoxazole in the treatment of Wegener's granulomatosis. *Arth. Rheum.*, **31**, 1073–4.

88. Weiner, S. R. and Paulus, H. E. (1989) Treatment of Wegener's granulomatosis. *Sem. Respir. Med.*, **10**, 156–61.

89. Harley, N., Ihle, B. (1990) Wegener's granulomatosis use of cyclosporin A: a case report. *Australia and New Zealand J. Med.*, **20**, 71–3.

90. Allen, N. B., Caldwell, D. S., Rice, J. R. *et al.* (1993) Cyclosporin A therapy for Wegener's granulomatosis. *Advan. Exp. Med. Biol.*, **336**, 473–6.

91. Liebow, A. A., Carrington, C. R. B. and Friedman, P. J. (1972) Lymphomatoid granulomatosis. *Human Pathol.*, **3**, 457–536.

92. Letendre, L. (1989) Treatment of lymphomatoid granulomatosis: old and new perspectives. *Sem. Respir. Med.*, **10**, 178–81.

93. Jaffe, E. S. (1984) Pathologic and clinical spectrum of post-thymic T-cell malignancies. *Cancer Invest.*, **2**, 413–26.

94. Katzenstein, A-L.A., Carrington, C. B., Leibow, A. A. (1979) Lymphomatoid granulomatosis: a clinicopathologic study of 152 cases. *Cancer*, **43**, 360–73.

95. Saldana, M. J., Patchefsky, A. S., Israel, H. I. *et al.* (1977) Pulmonary angiitis and granulomatosis: the relationship between histological features, organ involvement and response to treatment. *Human Pathol.*, **8**, 391–409.

96. James, W. D., Odom, R. B., Katzenstein, A. A. (1981) Cutaneous manifestations of lymphomatoid granulomatosis. *Arch. Dermatol.*, **117**, 196–202.

97. Tong, M. M., Cooke, B. and Barnetson, R. S. (1992) Lymphomatoid granulomatosis. *J. Am. Acad. Dermatol.*, **27**, 872–6.

98. Israel, H. L., Patchefsky, A. S., Saldana, M. J. (1977) Wegener's granulomatosis, lymphomatoid granulomatosis and benign lymphocytic angiitis and granulomatosis of lung: recognition and treatment. *Ann. Intern. Med.*, **87**, 691–9.

99. Bergin, C., Stein, H. B., Boyko, W. *et al.* (1984) Lymphomatoid granulomatosis presenting as polyarthritis. *J. Rheumatol.*, **11**, 537–9.

100. Fauci, A. S., Haynes, B.F., Costa, J. *et al.* (1982) Lymphomatoid granulomatosis: prospective clinical and therapeutic experience over 10 years. *N. Engl. J. Med.*, **306**, 68–74.

101. Lie, J. T. (1989) Classification of pulmonary angiitis and granulomatosis: histopathologic perspectives. *Sem. Respir. Med.*, **10**, 111–21.

102. Jaffe, E. S., Lipford, E. H., Margolick, J. B. *et al.*(1989) Lymphomatoid granulomatosis and angiocentric lymphoma: a spectrum of post-thymic T-cell proliferations. *Sem. Respir. Med.*, **10**, 167–72.

103. Nichols, P. W., Koss, M., Levine, A. M. *et al.* (1982) Lymphomatoid granulomatosis: a T-cell disorder? *Am. J. Med.*, **72**, 467–71.

104. Drasga, R. E., Williams, S. D., Wills, E. R. *et al.* (1984) Lymphomatoid granulomatosis: successful treatment with CHOP combination chemotherapy. *Am. J. Clin. Oncology*, **6**, 75–80.

105. Jenkins, T. R. and Zaloznik, A. J. (1989) Lymphomatoid granulomatosis: a case for aggressive therapy. *Cancer*, **64**, 1362–5.

106. Zeek, P. M., Smith, C. C. and Weeter, J. C. (1948) Studies on periarteritis nodosa: the differentiation between the vascular lesions of periarteritis nodosa and of hypersensitivity. *Am. J. Pathol.*, **24**, 889–917.

107. Calabrese, L. H. and Clough, J. D. (1982) Hypersensitivity vasculitis group (HVG): a case-oriented review of a continuing clinical spectrum. *Cleveland Clin. Q.*, **49**, 17–42.

108. Ekenstam, E. and Callen, J. (1984) Cutaneous

leukocytoclastic vasculitis: clinical and laboratory features of 82 patients seen in private practice. *Arch. Dermatol.*, **120**, 484–9.

109. Gilliam, J. N. and Smiley, J. D. (1976) Cutaneous necrotizing vasculitis and related disorders. *Ann. Allergy*, **37**, 328–39.

110. Gibson, L. E., Su, W. P. D. (1990) Cutaneous vasculitis. *Rheum. Dis. Clin. N. Am.*, **16**, 309–24.

111. Haber, M. M., Marboe, C. C. and Fenoglio, J. J. (1990) Vasculitis in drug reactions and serum sickness, in *Systemic Vasculitides*, (eds A. Churg and J. Churg), Igaku-Shoin, New York, pp. 305–13.

112. Calabrese, L. H., Michel, B. A., Bloch, D. A. *et al.* (1990) The American College of Rheumatology 1990 criteria for the classification of hypersensitivity vasculitis. *Arth. Rheum.*, **33**, 1108–13.

113. Grishman, E. and Spiera, H. (1990) Vasculitis in connective tissue disease, including hypocomplementemic vasculitis, in *Systemic Vasculitides*, (eds A. Churg and J. Churg), Igaku-Shoin, New York, pp. 273–92.

114. White, R. H. R. (1990) Henoch–Schönlein purpura, in *Systemic Vasculitides*, (eds A. Churg and J. Churg), Igaku-Shoin, New York, pp. 203–17.

115. Borges, W. H. (1972) Anaphylactoid purpura. *Med. Clin. N. Am.*, **56**, 201–6.

116. Meadow, S. R., Glasgow, E. F., White, R. H. R. *et al.* (1972) Schönlein-Henoch nephritis. *Q. J. Med.*, **163**, 241–58.

117. Allen, D. M., Diamond, L. K. and Howell, D. A. (1960) Anaphylactoid purpura in children (Schönlein–Henoch syndrome): review with a follow-up of the renal complications. *Am. J. of Dis. of Children*, **99**, 147–68.

118. Austin, H. A., Balow, J. E. (1983) Henoch–Schönlein nephritis: prognostic features and the challenge of therapy. *Am. J. Kidney Dis.*, **5**, 512–20.

119. Ansell, B. M. (1970) Henoch–Schönlein purpura with particular reference to the prognosis of the renal lesion. *Br. J. Dermatol.*, **82**, 211–5.

120. Meadow, S. R. (1978) The prognosis of Henoch–Schöenlein nephritis. *Clin. Nephrol.*, **9**, 87–90.

121. Koskimies, O., Mir, S., Rapola, J. *et al.* (1981) Henoch–Schönlein nephritis: long-term prognosis of unselected patients. *Arch. Dis. Children*, **56**, 482–4.

122. Counahan, R. , Winterborn, M. H., White, R.

H. R. *et al.* (1977) Prognosis of Henoch–Schönlein nephritis in children. *Br. Med. J.*, **2**, 11–4.

123. Lee, H. S., Koh, H. I., Kim, M. J. *et al.* (1986) Henoch–Schönlein nephritis in adults: a clinical and morphological study. *Clin. Nephrol.*, **26**, 125–30.

124. Fogazzi, G. B., Pasquali, S., Moriggi, M. *et al.* (1989) Long-term outcome of Schönlein–Henoch nephritis in the adult. *Clin. Nephrol.*, **31**, 60–6.

125. Ballard, H. S., Eisinger, R. P. and Gallo, G. (1970) Renal manifestations of the Henoch–Schöenlein syndrome in adults. *Am. J. Med.*, **49**, 328–35.

126. Kauffmann, R. H. and Houwert, D. A. (1981) Plasmapheresis in a rapidly progressive Henoch-Schönlein glomerulonephritis and the effect on circulating IgA immune complexes. *Clin. Nephrol.*, **16**, 155–60.

127. Ilan, Y. and Naparstek, Y. (1991) Schönlein-Henoch syndrome in adults and children. *Sem. Arth. Rheum.*, **21**, 103–9.

128. Cream, J. J., Gumpel, J. M. and Peachy, R. D. G. (1970) Schönlein–Henoch purpura in the adult: a study of 77 adults with anaphylactoid or Schönlein–Henoch purpura. *Q. J. Med.*, **156**, 461–84.

129. Faull, R. J., Woodroffe, A. J., Aarons, I. *et al.* (1987) Adult Henoch–Schönlein nephritis. *Aust. NZ J. Med.*, **17**, 396–401.

130. Lie, J. T. (1991) Takayasu's arteritis, in *Systemic Vasculitides*, (eds A. Churg and J. Churg), Igaku-Schoin, New York, pp. 159–79.

131. Fraga, A. and Lavalle, C. (1980) Takayasu's arteritis. *Clin. Rheum. Dis.*, **6**, 405–12.

132. Lupi-Herrera, E., Sanchez-Torres, G., Marcushamer, J. *et al.* (1977) Takayasu's arteritis: clinical study of 107 cases. *Am. Heart J.*, **93**, 94–103.

133. Nakao, K., Ikeda, M., Kimata S-I. *et al.* (1967) Takayasu's arteritis: clinical report of eighty-four cases and immunological studies of seven cases. *Circulation*, **35**, 1141–55.

134. Hall, S. and Buchbinder, R. (1990) Takayasu's arteritis. *Rheum. Dis. Clin. N. Am.*, **16**, 411–22.

135. Hall, S., Barr, W., Lie, J. T. *et al.* (1985) Takayasu arteritis: a study of 32 North American patients. *Medicine*, **64**, 89–99.

136. Sise, M. J., Counihan, C. M., Shackford, S. R. *et al.* (1988) The clinical spectrum of Takayasu's arteritis. *Surgery*, **104**, 905–10.

137. Lande, A. and Rossi, P. (1975) The value of total aortography in the diagnosis of

Takayasu's arteritis. *Radiology*, **114**, 287–97.

138. Shelhamer, J. H., Volkman, D. J., Parrillo, J. E. *et al.* (1985) Takayasu's arteritis and its therapy. *Ann. Intern. Med.*, **103**, 121–6.

139. Ishikawa, K. (1978) Natural history and classification of occlusive thromboaortopathy (Takayasu's disease). *Circulation*, **57**, 27–35.

140. Fraga, A., Mintz, G., Valle, L. *et al.* (1972) Takayasu's arteritis: frequency of systemic manifestations (study of 22 patients) and favorable response to maintenance steroid therapy with adrenocorticosteroids (12 patients). *Arth. Rheum.*, **15**, 617–24.

141. Subramanyan, R., Joy, J. and Balakrishnan, K. G. (1989) Natural history of aortoarteritis (Takayasu's disease). *Circulation*, **80**, 429–37.

142. Ishikawa, K. (1991) Effects of prednisolone therapy on arterial angiographic features in Takayasu's disease. *Am. J. Cardiol.*, **68**, 410–13.

143. Ishikawa, K. and Yonekawa, Y. (1987) Regression of carotid stenoses after corticosteroid therapy in occlusive thromboaortopathy (Takayasu's disease). *Stroke*, **18**, 677–9.

144. Ishikawa, K. (1988) Diagnostic approach and proposed criteria for the clinical diagnosis of Takayasu's arteriopathy. *J. Am. Coll. Cardiol.*, **12**, 964–72.

145. Tanigawa, K., Eguchi, K., Kitamura, Y. *et al.* (1992) Magnetic resonance imaging detection of aortic and pulmonary artery wall thickening in the acute stage of Takayasu arteritis: improvement of clinical and radiographic findings after steroid therapy. *Arth. Rheum.*, **35**, 476–80.

146. Miller, D. L., Reinig, J. W. and Volkman, D. J. (1986) Vascular imaging with MRI: inadequacy in Takayasu's arteritis compared with angiography. *Am. J. Roentgenol.*, **146**, 949–54.

147. Oneson, S. R., Lewin, J. S. and Smith, A. S. (1992) MR angiography of Takayasu's arteritis. *J. Computed Assisted Tomography*, **16**, 478–80.

148. Wong, V. C. W., Wang, R. Y. C. and Tse, T. F. (1983) Pregnancy and Takayasu's arteritis. *Am. J. Med.*, **75**, 597–601.

149. Ishikawa, K. and Matsura, S. (1982) Occlusive thromboaortopathy (Takayasu's disease) and pregnancy. *Am. J. Cardiol.*, **50**, 1293–1300.

150. Ishikawa, K. (1981) Survival and morbidity after diagnosis of occlusive thromboaortopathy (Takayasu's disease). *Am. J. Cardiol.*, **47**, 1026–32.

151. Mevorach, D., Leiboewitz, G., Brezis, M. *et al.* (1992) Induction of remission in a patient with Takayasu's arteritis by low dose pulses of methotrexate. *Ann. Rheum. Dis.*, **51**, 904–5.

152. Liang, G. C., Nemickas, R. and Madayag, M. (1989) Multiple percutaneous transluminal angioplasties and low dose methotrexate for Takayasu's arteritis. *J. Rheumatol.*, **16**, 1370–3.

153. Hoffman, G. S., Leavitt, R. Y., Kerr, G. S. *et al.* (1991) Treatment of Takayasu's arteritis (TA) with methotrexate (MTX). *Arth. Rheum.*, **34S**, A49.

154. Buckley, A., Southwood, T., Culham, G. *et al.* (1991) The role of ultrasound in evaluation of Takayasu's arteritis. *J. Rheumatol.*, **18**, 1073–80.

155. Maeda, H., Handa, N., Matsumoto, M. *et al.* (1991) Carotid lesions detected by B-mode ultrasonography in Takayasu's arteritis: 'macaroni sign' as an indicator of the disease. *Ultrasound Med. Biol.*, **17**, 695–701.

156. Giordano, J. M., Leavitt, R. Y., Hoffman, G. *et al.* (1991) Experience with surgical treatment of Takayasu's disease. *Surgery*, **109**, 252–8.

157. Weaver, F. A., Yellin, A. E., Campen, D. H. *et al.* (1990) Surgical procedures in the management of Takayasu's arteritis. *J. Vascular Surgery*, **12**, 429–39.

158. Park, J. H., Han, M. C., Kim, S. H. *et al.* (1989) Takayasu arteritis: angiographic findings and results of angioplasty. *Am. J. Radiol.*, **153**, 1069–74.

159. Cravioto, H. and Feigin, I. (1959) Noninfectious granulomatous angiitis with a predilection for the nervous system. *Neurology*, **9**, 599–609.

160. Hughes, J. T. and Brownell, B. (1966) Granulomatous giant-celled angiitis of the central nervous system. *Neurology*, **16**, 293–8.

161. Valvanis, A., Friede, R., Schubiger, O. *et al.* (1979) Cerebral granulomatous angiitis simulating brain tumor. *J. Computer Assisted Tomography*, **3**, 536–8.

162. Budzilovich, G. N., Feigin, I. and Siegal, H. (1963) Granulomatous angiitis of the nervous system. *Arch. Pathol.*, **76**, 250–6.

163. Calabrese, L. H. and Mallek, J. A. (1987) Primary angiitis of the central nervous system: report of 8 new cases, review of the literature and proposal for diagnostic criteria. *Medicine*, **67**, 20–39.

164. Sigal, L. H. (1993) Cerebral Vasculitis, in *Arthritis and Allied Conditions*, 12th edn, (eds

D. J. McCarty and W. J. Koopman), Lea and Febiger, Philadelphia, pp. 1131–42.

165. Moore, P. M. (1989) Diagnosis and management of isolated angiitis of the central nervous system. *Neurology*, **39**, 167–73.

166. Koo, E. H. and Massey, E. W. (1988) Granulomatous angiitis of the central nervous system: protean manifestations and response to treatment. *J. Neurol.*, Neurosurgery and Psychiatry, **51**, 1126–33.

167. Cupps, T. R., Moore, P. M. and Fauci, A. S. (1983) Isolated angiitis of the central nervous system: prospective diagnostic and therapeutic experience. *Am. J. Med.*, **74**, 97–105.

168. Sigal, L. H. (1987) The neurologic presentation of vasculitic and rheumatologic syndromes: a review. *Medicine*, **66**, 157–80.

169. Lie, J. T. (1991) Angiitis of the central nervous system. *Curr. Opin. Rheumatol.*, **3**, 36–45.

170. Feigin, I., Ewald, E. A. and Silverstein, A. (1991) Primary (granulomatous) vasculitis of the central nervous system, in *Systemic Vasculitides*, (eds A. Churg and J. Churg), Igaku-Shoin, New York, pp. 133–41.

171. Ewald, E. A., Arsen, A., Albin, R. *et al.* (1988) Magnetic resonance imaging (MRI) abnormalities in isolated angiopathy of the central nervous system (IACNS). *Arth. Rheum.*, **31**, 42N.

172. Vanderzant, C., Bromberg, M., MacGuire, A. *et al.* (1988) Isolated small vessel angiitis of the central nervous system. *Arch. Neurol.*, **45**, 683–7.

173. Ferris, E. J. and Levine, H. L. (1973) Cerebral arteritis: classification. *Radiology*, **109**, 327–41.

174. Garner, B. F., Burns, P., Bunning, R. D. *et al.* (1990) Acute blood pressure elevation can mimic arteriographic appearance of cerebral vasculitis (a postpartum case with relative hypertension). *J. Rheumatol.*, **17**, 93–7.

175. Stein, R. L., Martino, C. R., Weinert, D. M. *et al.* (1987) Cerebral angiography as a guide for therapy in isolated central nervous system vasculitis. *J. Am. Med. Assoc.*, **257**, 2193–5.

176. Griffin, J., Price, D. L., Davis, L. *et al.* (1973) Granulomatous angiitis of the central nervous system with aneurysms on multiple cerebral arteries. *Trans. Am. Neurolog. Assoc.*, **98**, 145–8.

177. Sigal, L. H. (1989) Isolated CNS angiitis. *Neurology*, **39**, 1645.

178. Cogan, D. G. (1945) Syndrome of non-syphilitic interstitial keratitis and vestibulo-auditory symptoms. *Arch. Ophthalmol.*, **33**, 144–9.

179. Haynes, B. F., Kaiser-Kupfer, M. I., Mason, P. *et al.* (1980) Cogan syndrome: studies in thirteen patients, long-term follow-up, and a review of the literature. *Medicine*, **59**, 426–41.

180. Vollertsen, R. S., McDonald, T. J., Younge, B. R. *et al.* (1986) Cogan's syndrome: 18 cases and a review of the literature. *Mayo Clin. Proc.*, **61**, 344–61.

181. McCallum, R. M. (1992) Cogan's syndrome: clinical features and outcomes. *Arth. Rheum.*, **35**, (Supp 9), S51.

182. McCallum, R. M. and Haynes, B. F. (1993) Cogan's syndrome, in *Ocular Infection and Immunity*, (eds J. S. Pepose, G. N. Holland and K. R. Wilhelmus), Mosby-Year Book, Philadelphia, (in publication).

183. Allen, N. B., Cox, C. C., Cobo, M. *et al.* (1990) Use of immunosuppressive agents in the treatment of severe ocular and vascular manifestations of Cogan's syndrome. *Am. J. Med.*, **88**, 296–301.

184. Haynes, B. F., Pikus, A., Kaiser-Kupfer, M. *et al.* (1981) Successful treatment of sudden hearing loss in Cogan's syndrome with corticosteroids. *Arth. Rheum.*, **24**, 501–3.

185. McCallum, R. M. (1993) Cogan's syndrome, in *Current Ocular Therapy*, 4th edn, (eds F. T. Franunfelder and R. Hampton), W. B. Saunders, Philadelphia, (in publication).

186. Haynes, B. F. (1992) Cogan's syndrome, in *Current Therapy in Allergy, Immunology, and Rheumatology*, 4th ed, (eds L. M. Lichtenstein and A. S. Fauci), Mosby-Year Book/B. C. Decker, St. Louis, pp. 228–30.

187. Bielory, L., Conti, J. and Frohman, L. (1990) Cogan's syndrome. *J. Allergy and Clin. Immunol.*, **85**, 808–15.

SECONDARY VASCULITIS

9

R. A. Watts and D. G. I. Scott

INTRODUCTION

Vasculitis may be a primary event (e.g. polyarteritis nodosa) or secondary to established autoimmune rheumatic disease (e.g. rheumatoid arthritis (RA)), malignancy or to other exogenous antigens including drugs and infection. The primary vasculitides and vasculitis secondary to autoimmune conditions are described elsewhere (Chapter 8 and others). This chapter concentrates on vasculitis occurring secondary to infection, malignancy and drugs, together with conditions which simulate vasculitis.

CLASSIFICATION

The classification of vasculitis is difficult: there is much clinical overlap between the different vasculitis syndromes and often the cause of vasculitis is unknown. Even known etiological agents may be associated with several different clinical syndromes. Infection with hepatitis B virus has been associated with small vessel vasculitis[1,2] cryoglobulinemia with or without vasculitis[3] glomerulonephritis[4] and polyarteritis nodosa[5]. A classification based on the size of the predominant vessel involved and the type of inflammatory change seems the most logical (Table 9.1). This classification is developed from the schemes proposed by Zeek[6], Alarcón-Sergovia[7] and Lie[8]. The strong association between ANCA and vasculitis has led to some confusion about disease definition and classification. This is especially true of polyarteritis nodosa, described in Chapter 8, which can be defined as classical or microscopic PAN. If we confine classical PAN to those patients with pure medium vessel disease without glomerulonephritis, this disease is rare and not usually associated with ANCA. The clinical consequences are major organ infarction and hemorrhage. This leaves three diseases characterized by medium artery and small vessel involvement. Microscopic PAN is more accurately defined as microscopic polyangiitis to recognize the involvement of small vessels and together with Wegener's granulomatosis and Churg–Strauss syndrome have the closest association with ANCA and the highest incidence of severe glomerulonephritis.

This classification also reflects therapeutic strategies (Table 9.2). Diseases with predominant medium artery involvement, especially those associated with ANCA, respond best to immunosuppression (usually cyclophosphamide and corticosteroids) while the small vessel vasculitides can often be managed conservatively. Large vessel disease can be controlled with corticosteroids alone. Pure small vessel vasculitis has a good prognosis, while medium-sized artery involvement is associated with significant mortality (of up to 25% at 2 years[9]).

The systemic vasculitides are generally considered to be uncommon, but recent studies have suggested that the incidence is increasing which may be attributable to increased

Connective Tissue Diseases. Edited by Jill J. F. Belch and Robert B. Zurier. Published in 1995 by Chapman & Hall, London. ISBN 0 412 48620 2

Table 9.1   Classification of vasculitis

Vessel involved	Primary	Secondary
Large arteries	Giant cell arteritis	Aortitis associated with RA
	Takayasu's arteritis	Infection (syphilis)
Medium arteries	Classical PAN	Infection (e.g. hepatitis B)
	Kawasaki disease	
Small vessels and medium arteries	Wegener's granulomatosis*	Vasculitis 2° to RA, SLE,
	Churg–Strauss syndrome*	Sjögren's syndrome
	Microscopic polyangiitis*	Drugs
		Infection (HIV)
Small vessels (leucocytoclastic)	Henoch–Schönlein purpura	Drugs
	Essential mixed cryoglobulinemia	Infection

* Diseases commonly associated with ANCA (anti-myeloperoxidase and anti-proteinase 3 antibodies), a significant risk of renal involvement and which are most responsive to cyclophosphamide.

Table 9.2   Relationship between vessel size and treatment

Vessel involved	Corticosteroids alone	Cyclophosphamide ± corticosteroids	Others
Large arteries	+++	–	+
Medium arteries	+	++	++*
Small vessels and medium arteries	+	+++	–
Small vessels	+	–	++

+++ Good response.
++ Moderate response
+   Some response.
–   No response.
* Includes plasmapheresis, anti-viral therapy for hepatitis B associated vasculitis, intravenous immunoglobulin for Kawasaki disease.

diagnostic awareness. In Leicester, UK, the incidence of Wegener's granulomatosis (and microscopic polyangiitis) over two decades increased four-fold to 6.1/million/year following introduction of the ANCA test[10]. In Norfolk, UK, we have seen approximately 120 patients with systemic vasculitis, over the 5-year period 1988–93, suggesting an annual incidence of Wegener's granulomatosis of 7/million/year and of systemic vasculitis associated with RA 11/million/year. Vasculitis associated with infection was rare, but comprised one patient with small vessel vasculitis associated with chlamydia and another with herpes zoster. A case of aortitis was associated with a pneumococcal mycotic aneurysm. There were two cases of vasculitis associated with malignancy (nasopharyngeal carcinoma, chronic lymphatic leukemia) and two with cryoglobulinemic vasculitis. Data associating vasculitis with drugs was unavailable from this study. Thus in our experience secondary causes of vasculitis (excepting RA and systemic lupus erythematosus (SLE)) are rare.

ANCA AND SECONDARY VASCULITIS

A positive ANCA is most commonly associated with primary vasculitis. As documented in Chapter 8, two main staining patterns have

Table 9.3 ANCAs in diseases other than systemic vasculitis

1. Infection:	HIV, mycobacterial infections, severe pneumonia, bacterial endocarditis, cystic fibrosis with secondary infection, sepsis
2. Chronic:	rheumatoid arthritis, inflammatory bowel disease, Sweet's syndrome, eosinophilia-myalgia syndrome, Goodpasture's syndrome
3. Neoplasms:	atrial myxoma, small cell lung cancer, hypernephroma, non-Hodgkin's lymphoma, myelodysplasia, colon carcinoma

From [16].

Table 9.4 Infection and vasculitis

Vessel involved		*Infection*
Large arteries	Bacterial:	*Staphylococcus, Salmonella, Mycobacteria, Streptococcus*
	Spirochaetal:	*Treponema pallidum*
	Fungal:	*Coccidiodomycosis*
Medium arteries	Bacterial:	Group A *Streptococcus* (childhood PAN) *Mycobacteria*
	Viral:	hepatitis B, C, HIV, parvovirus
Small vessels and medium arteries	Bacterial:	*Streptococcus*
	Viral:	hepatitis B, C, HIV, CMV
Small vessels (leucocytoclastic)	Bacterial:	*Streptococcus, Staphylococcus, Salmonella, Yersinia, Mycobacteria, Neisseria*
	Viral:	HIV, CMV, herpes zoster, parvo B19
	Bacterial:	Rickettsiae

been observed using indirect immunofluorescence (IIF): cytoplasmic (cANCA) and perinuclear (pANCA). A third pattern xANCA (atypical) is seen in some non-vasculitic diseases, such as inflammatory bowel disease.

cANCA is strongly associated with Wegener's granulomatosis and less frequently with microscopic polyangiitis and Churg–Strauss syndrome. The antigenic specificity is in most cases proteinase-3. cANCA have been reported in infective disorders such as HIV[11], endocarditis and pneumonia[12]. They have also been described in patients with monoclonal gammopathy[13] and malignancy[14] without evidence of vasculitis, but the antigen specificity in these cases has not been defined.

pANCA are less specific. They are most commonly found in microscopic polyangiitis and Churg–Strauss syndrome. The most important target antigen for pANCA is myeloperoxidase. pANCA has been reported in patients with RA, particularly in those with extra-articular manifestations, vasculitis or Felty's syndrome[15]. This relationship has not been confirmed by other groups[16], and the antigen specificity of the pANCA may not be myeloperoxidase. In some studies the ANCA specificity has been shown to be anti-lactoferrin.

ANCA has also been described in a number of other diseases (Table 9.3). These include a wide variety of infections, other chronic inflammatory diseases and malignancy. The specificity of the ANCA in these non-vasculitic diseases is not known. ANCA has

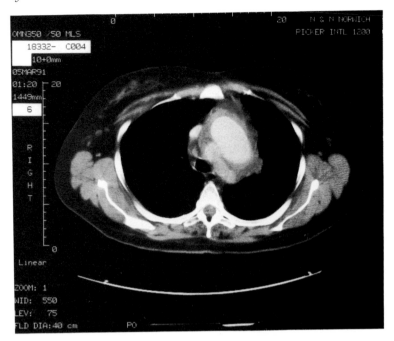

Fig. 9.1 Thoracic CT scan showing an aneurysm of the descending aorta. *Pneumococcus pneumoniae* was cultured from the resected vessel. (From Chakravarty *et al.* (1992), with permission.)

also been described in hydrallazine-induced glomerulonephritis and more recently pro-pylthiouracil induced vasculitis[17]. In the later report, 6 patients were described. The specificities of the ANCA were: myeloperoxi-dase[3,5], proteinase-3 and human neutrophil elastase[6].

It is important to recognize that although vasculitis can occur in association with infection or malignancy as can ANCA, the relationship between ANCA, the vasculitis and the infection/malignancy is not at all clear. The presence of ANCA does not necessarily indicate the presence of vasculitis or vice versa.

INFECTION-RELATED VASCULITIS

Many cases of vasculitis are considered to have an infectious cause, although frequently a causal relationship has not been established. A wide variety of organisms have been implicated (Table 9.4). Two mechanisms for infection related vasculitis have been proposed:

first, direct microbial toxicity either by endothelial invasion or the effect of microbial toxins on endothelium; secondly, immune-mediated by either humoral (immune complex) or cellular responses[18].

BACTERIAL INFECTIONS

Direct endothelial invasion by pyogenic organisms (*Staphylococcus* and *Streptococcus*) is a well-documented cause of vasculitis. More recently vasculitis has been described in association with unusual infections including *Mycobacterium fortuitum*[19] and *Salmonella* [20], which probably reflects the changing pattern of infections since the introduction of antibiotics.

The vascular reaction to direct infection depends on the organism and the site of infection. In large arteries, the infection leads to an erosive arteritis with mycotic aneurysm formation (Figure 9.1). In small arteries and arterioles, it manifests as a necrotizing vasculitis or thrombosis. In around 60% of cases there is a predisposing condition of which the most common is diabetes mellitus[20]. Infection often occurs at a site of pre-existing vascular damage by atherosclerosis or at a site of previous surgery[20].

Neisseria gonorrhoeae and *N. meningitides* may directly infect vascular endothelium, causing maculopapular or purpuric skin lesions. Biopsies of early lesions show a small vessel vasculitis with mononuclear cells, neutrophils, leucocytoclasis, necrosis and neisserial organisms[21,22].

Group A streptococcal infection has been associated with development of polyarteritis nodosa in childhood[22], but not observed in adults. Vasculitis is a rare (<1%) feature of adult rheumatic fever and post-streptococcal reactive arthritis[23].

SPIROCHETAL INFECTION

Treponema pallidum (syphilis, Table 9.1) is well recognized as a cause of aortitis, with aneurysm formation and development of aortic incompetence. The primary histological changes are in the vasa vasorum with endarteritis and perivascular infiltration with lymphocytes and plasma cells. Infection occurs early in the disease and organisms lie dormant in the aortic wall. Spirochetes can, however, only rarely be detected in tissue. Symptomatic aortic disease occurs as a feature of tertiary disease. Diagnosis is based on the radiographic appearances and serological tests.

Lyme disease is caused by infection with the spirochete *Borrelia burgdorferi*. Features of Lyme disease include polyarthritis, typical skin rash (erythema chronicum migrans), neurological (meningitis, encephalitis, radiculopathy) and cardiac conduction defects. A mild vasculitis may occur as part of the disseminated stage of infection[24] but major vasculitis is uncommon. Treponemes may be demonstrated in infected tissue.

RICKETTSIAL INFECTIONS

Vascular lesions are a prominent feature of some rickettsial infections, particularly Rocky Mountain spotted fever, epidemic typhus and scrub typus. In humans the organisms are usually found in vascular endothelium and in some circumstances vascular smooth muscle. The pathology of the vascular lesion of *Rickettsia rickettsii* infection (Rocky Mountain spotted fever) follows a characteristic pattern. In the early stages, endothelial cell swelling is seen in association with intracellular rickettsiae. Later in the disease vasculitis with increased vascular permeability, hemorrhage and occasionally thrombosis develops with deposition of immunoglobulin and complement[25–27] suggesting an immune mediated mechanism.

FUNGAL INFECTIONS

Fungal infections may cause vasculitis by direct spread into the vessel wall with formation of a mycotic aneurysm. This usually occurs in patients who are already severely immunocompromized from other diseases. Fungi such as *Coccidioides immitis* may also cause a localized CNS vasculitis, presenting abruptly with stroke-like lesions[28]. These patients have a high mortality (70%) and require aggressive anti-fungal therapy.

MYCOBACTERIAL INFECTION

Blood vessels of any size may be involved in tuberculous infection, with veins being more vulnerable than arteries. The usual clinical lesion being erythema nodosum. Histologically, tuberculous vasculitis of large and small arteries appears as a granulomatous panarteritis or thrombophlebitis. Acid-fast bacilli may be demonstrated in or adjacent to the vessel wall.

The vascular lesions of *M. leprae* infection are focal in distribution and involve arteries and veins with equal frequency. The most common site is invasion of small vessels, e.g. erythema nodosum leprosum or the vasa vasorum of large vessels. The clinical consequence of vasculitis is rarely significant.

VIRAL INFECTIONS

Hepatitis B virus (HBV) is recognized as a cause of a systemic vasculitis which may be histologically indistinguishable from polyarteritis nodosa. The frequency of HBV infection in PAN varies greatly between different centres. This probably reflects the incidence of HBV in the indigenous population. The incidence of HBV in PAN ranges from very rare to 100% but appears to be declining especially in Europe. We have not seen a case of HBV associated vasculitis in the last 10 years.

In patients with HBV infection hepatitis B surface antigen has been demonstrated in immune complexes and in vascular lesions by immunofluorescence[5] and Christian has suggested that vasculitis (clinical or subclinical) may be a feature of virtually all patients with HBV infections[29].

Quint *et al.* explored the role of hepatitis C virus (HCV) in 35 patients with polyarteritis nodosa[30]. They stressed that the prevalence of HCV in PAN is similar to that found in HCV chronic hepatitis and that sera positive for HCV were also positive for HBV, thus no conclusion could be drawn about the relationship between HCV and vasculitis. No data as yet exists regarding hepatitis D and E virus infection and vasculitis.

The hepatitis viruses have been associated with other types of vasculitis. Cryoglobulinemia (see below) is associated with small vessel vasculitis. Hepatitis viruses A, B and C have all been associated with mixed cryoglobulinemia, with reports that 50% of cases of mixed cryoglobulinemia are associated with hepatitis B or C infection[31]. Hepatitis B has also been associated with urticarial vasculitis (below).

Human immunodeficiency virus (HIV) has been associated with almost the entire clinical spectrum of vasculitis[18].

Polyarteritis nodosa has been described in at least 16 patients with HIV infection. The status of HIV infection spanned the whole spectrum from asymptomatic to advanced disease with opportunistic infections. The predominant organs involved were nerve and muscle. Presentation is with a peripheral neuropathy or digital ischemia. Renal and testicular abnormalities have not so far been reported[32]. The majority of cases reported have been negative for hepatitis B surface antigen[32]. ANCA has been reported in HIV infection[11].

Gheradi and colleagues studied muscle, nerve and skin biopsy specimens from 148 symptomatic HIV infected patients. They found inflammatory vascular disease in 34 cases. Using the ACR criteria for classification of vasculitis, 11 patients had a distinct form of vasculitis including: PAN(4), Henoch–Schönlein purpura(1) and drug-induced hypersensitivity vasculitis(6), 23 were unclassified. One patient had HBV surface antigenemia, 2 had cryoglobulinemia and 2 were co-infected with human T-lymphotropic virus type 1. Cytomegalovirus (CMV) inclusion bodies and antigens were detected in endothelial cells from 1 patient. HIV antigens and genome were detected in the perivascular cells of 2 patients with a necrotizing arteritis[32]. Thus a wide range of inflammatory vascular disease occurs in HIV, and may result from exposure to infectious agents and drugs as well as to HIV itself.

A solitary case of Churg–Strauss syndrome has been described in association with HIV[33]. The patient had asthma, rhinitis, eosinophilia (3.1×10^9/l) and a purpuric skin eruption. Lung biopsy showed granulomas.

Small vessel vasculitis has been associated with HIV infection[18,32], in some cases there has been evidence of another viral infection, such as CMV, and the possibility of drug-induced vasculitis in these patients needs to be considered[32].

Primary vasculitis of the central nervous system has also been associated with HIV in 6

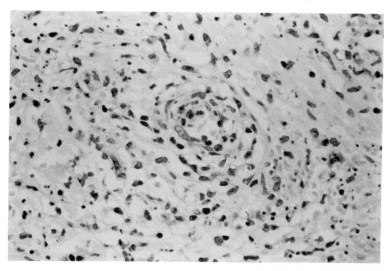

Fig. 9.2 Skin biopsy from a patient with herpes zoster infection and vasculitis. There is a perivascular leucocyte infiltrate with nuclear debris, intramural leucocytes and extravasation of erythrocytes. Hematoxylin and Dosin stain, ×100. (Courtesy of Dr R. Y. Ball.)

cases[18]. No other infectious cause for cerebral vasculitis has been found in these cases.

Lymphomatoid granulomatosis has been reported in at least 6 cases of HIV infection and this association has led to the suggestion that HIV-induced immune dysregulation can lead to uncontrolled lymphoproliferation of T-cell lineages with an angiocentric disposition[18].

Wegener's granulomatosis, Takayasu's arteritis and giant cell arteritis have not so far been associated with HIV infection.

Other viral infections associated with vasculitis include *Parvovirus B19*, *herpes zoster* (Figure 9.2), CMV, Epstein–Barr virus, hantavirus and rubella[34,35]. The incidence of vasculitis in these infections is unknown.

Several mechanisms have been proposed for viral-induced vasculitis. These include immune complex deposition and direct viral infection leading to necrosis of endothelial cells. A well-studied example of the latter is equine viral arteritis, which is associated with a fulminant systemic vasculitis[36]. A similar process may occur with CMV infection in humans, where typical viral inclusion bodies

are seen in vascular endothelium[37]. Viral infection of endothelial cells may also lead to a cell mediated response. This has been suggested in experimental border disease of sheep[38], but no evidence exists for this mechanism in humans.

OTHER INFECTIONS

Vasculitis has only rarely been associated with parasitic infection. Churg–Strauss syndrome has been associated in a single patient with *Ascaris lumbricoides* infection[39]. The infection was confined to the biliary tree. Following antibiotics and immunosuppression the vasculitic illness settled.

Despite the extensive literature relating infection to vasculitis, the direct relationship between specific organisms and vascular damage is often unclear. It is likely that new methods of diagnosis (e.g. *in situ* hybridization, polymerase chain reaction) will lead to a better understanding of the role of infection in vasculitic diseases.

Treatment of vasculitis associated with infection is that of the infection. PAN associated with hepatitis B responds to antiviral therapy with α-interferon combined with plasma exchange[40]. Plasma exchange may be required for severe disease.

KAWASAKI DISEASE

Kawasaki disease is an acute vasculitis of unknown etiology which primarily affects infants and young children. The disease occurs in both endemic and epidemic forms worldwide. The clinical features are described in Chapter 12.

The occurrence of epidemic Kawasaki disease has lead to the notion that the condition is caused by an infectious agent. *Streptococcal,* sp., *Propionibacterium acnes, Rickettsia* sp., Epstein–Barr virus, and retroviruses have all been proposed as causative agents for Kawasaki disease, but none have been confirmed[41].

Table 9.5 Immunoregulatory abnormalities during acute Kawasaki disease

Increased percentage of CD4$^+$ activated T-cells
Selective expansion of V$_\beta$2$^+$ and V$_\beta$8$^+$ T-cells
Decreased percentage of CD8$^+$ T-cells
Increased levels of soluble CD25, CD4, CD8
Polyclonal B-cell activation
Antibodies against endothelial cell antigens
Increased IL-1, IL-6, IFN-γ, TNF-α production

From [43].

Acute Kawasaki disease is associated with marked immune activation (Table 9.5). There is polyclonal B-cell activation with increased numbers of activated CD4$^+$ T-cells and monocytes, which is accompanied by elevated levels of interleukin-1 (IL-1), tumor necrosis factor alpha and interferon gamma and IL-6. There is histological evidence of vascular endothelial cell activation and necrosis, with infiltration of mononuclear cells and neutrophils into the media, and adventitia of arteries and venules. The production of pro-inflammatory cytokines

(IL-1, TNF-α) may be prothrombotic induce endothelial leukocyte adhesion molecules. Such activation of T-cells and monocytes is a feature of bacterial superantigens. Superantigens are able to activate T-cells by binding directly to the β region of the T-cell receptor. This results in selective expansion of β T-cell populations. Abe and colleagues have demonstrated that there is a bias in the T-cell repertoire of patients with acute Kawasaki disease[42], which returns to normal during convalescence. This supports the idea that Kawasaki disease is caused by a superantigen, which might be derived from Streptococci. Antibodies against streptococcal pyrogenic exotoxin A (which can act as a super-antigen) are present in serum from patients with Kawasaki disease. Leung and colleagues have suggested that streptococcal exotoxins or exotoxins with a structural homology to them may be involved in the pathogenesis of Kawasaki disease[43].

VASCULITIS AND MALIGNANCY

Neoplasia has been associated with a variety of vasculitic syndromes. Curth has described six criteria for cutaneous paraneoplastic syndromes:

1. both conditions start at about the same time;
2. both follow a parallel course;
3. consistent relation between a specific tumor and the concurrent paraneoplastic syndrome;
4. rarity;
5. unexpected frequency of association; and
6. heredity[44].

Only a few vasculitic syndromes meet these criteria.

VASCULITIS OF MEDIUM AND SMALL ARTERIES

The best-known association between malignancy and vasculitis is that between hairy cell leukemia and systemic necrotizing vasculitis especially PAN. Hairy cell leukemia is a rare malignancy of mononuclear cells which typically presents with progressive pancytopenia and splenomegaly with circulating hairy cells. Since the first description at least 22 cases have been described[45,46]. In 17 out of 22 cases the diagnosis of hairy cell leukemia was made before the vasculitis and in at least 8 this was more than a year before the onset of vasculitis. Splenectomy was performed in 14 cases before the diagnosis of vasculitis. Sixteen patients developed PAN diagnosed on clinical, radiological and histological criteria, while 5 patients had cutaneous vasculitis and 1 a granulomatous vasculitis. The patients with cutaneous vasculitis had palpable purpura but no other organ involvement. The clinical manifestations of hairy cell leukemia associated PAN are similar to those seen with classical PAN. Arteriography shows characteristic aneurysm formation. Histology shows acute and chronic inflammation of medium-sized arteries. In 5 patients with systemic disease non-giant cell temporal arteritis was present. Arthritis and arthralgias were present in both groups. In 3 patients hairy cells were demonstrated in the vessel wall cellular infiltrate.

Several theories have been proposed to account for the occurrence of vascular injury in hairy cell leukemia. The hairy cell is of B-cell origin and is therefore able to produce immunoglobulins. These could form immune complexes and be deposited[47], alternatively the immunoglobulin may be able to bind to endothelial cell antigens and provoke vascular injury. This is not supported in patients where circulating immune complexes, cryoglobulins and hypocomplementemia are rarely seen. Posnett and colleagues demonstrated an epitope on hairy cells that is also present on endothelial cells[48].

Vasculitis is rarely the cause of death, the majority of patients have died of a complication of leukemia, infection or bleeding due to thrombocytopenia or impaired coagulation.

Other lymphoproliferative malignancies rarely associated with PAN include lymphatic leukemia[49] and monocytic leukemia[50]. Cutaneous necrotizing arteritis without systemic involvement has been associated with lymphosarcoma, Hodgkin's lymphoma and multiple myeloma[51,52].

Sanchez-Guerro reported two cases of medium-sized arteritis of the bowel, one in association with a ductal adenocarcinoma of the breast and the second in a patient with myelofibrosis[53].

Churg–Strauss syndrome has been associated with malignant melanoma in one patient[54], and with a non-Hodgkin's lymphoplasmacytoid B-cell lymphoma in a further patient[55]. Single case reports involving Wegener's granulomatosis and papillary adenocarcinoma of thyroid and hepatocellular carcinoma have been described[56].

Cerebral granulomatous angiitis is an uncommon condition which has been described in six cases of Hodgkin's disease and one each of chronic myeloid leukemia and primary cerebral lymphoma[57,58]. In these cases the temporal relationship was variable, with vasculitis developing 18 months before or up to 3 years after discovery of the malignancy.

LARGE VESSEL VASCULITIS

Giant cell arteritis and Takayasu's disease do not appear to be associated with malignancy. A recent controlled study looking at any possible association between malignancy and polymyalgia rheumatica/temporal arteritis concluded that there was no evidence to support a paraneoplastic mechanism[59]. However, non-giant cell vasculitis of the temporal arteries has been reported in association with hairy cell leukemia[45,60,61,62], malignant histiocytosis[63] and follicular small cleaved cell lymphoma[64]. In the latter case malignant cells were demonstrated in the perivascular infiltrate around the temporal artery.

SMALL VESSEL VASCULITIS

Vasculitis of small vessels has been described in association with lympho-proliferative disorders and less frequently with solid tumors. One series described six patients with myelo-proliferative disorders and cutaneous leuco-cytoclastic vasculitis[65]. Clinically, the lesions were described as maculopapular rash, palpable purpura or erythema multiforme with urticaria. In 4 cases the skin eruptions preceded the malignancy by 1–17 months (mean 6 months). There was no clear relation between the clinical course of the vasculitis and the underlying malignancy. Five patients died as a consequence of their malignancy. Autopsy in 4 cases showed no evidence of cutaneous or visceral vasculitis. Other myeloproliferative diseases associated with small vessel vasculitis include 3 patients with T-cell lymphomas[53,66,67] and in a single patient with Wiskott–Aldrich syndrome[68]. Hodgkin's disease has been described in 8 cases[69]. In 6 patients vasculitis preceded diagnosis of Hodgkin's disease. Vessel wall infiltration by lymphocytes or Reed–Sternberg cells was not seen.

More recently, Sanchez-Geurro described 11 patients with malignancy occurring in a series of 222 patients with vasculitis[53]. Two patients had myeloproliferative neoplasia (thrombocytosis, myelofibrosis), 3 lympho-proliferative disease (non-Hodgkin's lymphoma(2), T-cell lymphoma(1)), 4 carcinoma (below), and 2 with leukemia (myeloblastic leukemia, chronic granulocytic leukemia). In 9 patients vasculitis was confined to the skin, and showed histological evidence of leucocytoclastic vasculitis. In two patients with bowel involvement, the vasculitis involved medium-sized arteries. In 8 patients vasculitis followed the malignancy with a time interval of 1 month to 17 years (mean 5.5 years), in 2 cases both disease processes developed contemporaneously and in the remaining vasculitis preceded the malignancy. An interesting feature of this series was the occurrence of four solid tumors (2 breast, 1 vocal cord and 1 esophagus).

Vasculitis associated with a solid tumor is uncommon and restricted to single case reports (Table 9.6). In our own series of 120 patients with vasculitis, two had an associated tumor (laryngeal adenocarcinoma, chronic lymphatic leukemia).

Vasculitis may precede the diagnosis of malignancy, and the investigation of small vessel vasculitis should include a search for malignant disease.

It is also important to recognize that malignancy may occur as a consequence of treatment of systemic vasculitis with immunosuppressive drugs, especially cyclophosphamide and azathioprine. Cyclophosphamide is particularly associated with bladder tumors and the risk may be related to the total dose administered. Pulse cyclophosphamide regimen appear to be less toxic than continuous oral therapy. Oral cyclophosphamide has also been associated with an increased incidence of skin cancers and non-Hodgkin's lymphomas[79].

VASCULITIS MIMICKING MALIGNANCY

Large masses of vasculitic tissue associated with constitutional symptoms can be misdiagnosed as a malignancy. Giant cell arteritis of the breast may present with a breast mass and be mistaken for carcinoma[80]. The differentiation between lymphoma and Wegener's granulomatosis of the upper airway can be difficult[81].

CRYOGLOBULINEMIC VASCULITIS

Cryoglobulins are plasma proteins which reversibly precipitate or gel in the cold, and were first described by Wintrobe and Benell in 1933[82]. Waldenström initially reported that cryoglobulins contained immunoglobulin[83] and in 1962 Lospalluto *et al.* observed that cryoglobulins may contain more than one immunoglobulin and that rheumatoid factor

Table 9.6 Small vessel vasculitis and solid malignancy

Reference	Case	Age	Sex	Neoplasm	Type of vasculitis	Temporal relationship vasculitis to neoplasm
[71]	1	52	M	Colon adenocarcinoma	Leucocytoclastic	3 months before
[72]	1	NA	NA	Renal cell carcinoma	Leucocytoclastic	NA
[73]	1	60	M	Prostate adenocarcinoma	HSP	NA
[74]	1	63	M	Squamous cell Ca bronchus	HSP	1 year before
	2	73	M	Squamous cell Ca bronchus	HSP	3 months before
[75]	1	57	M	Squamous cell Ca bronchus	Leucocytoclastic	3 years
[76]	1	59	M	Squamous cell Ca bronchus	HSP	3 months
[77]	1	69	F	Colon adenocarcinoma	UV	NA
[53]	1	79	M	Squamous cell Ca esophagus	Leucocytoclastic	0
[76]	1	32	M	Phaeochromocyta	Leucocytoclastic	18 months
[70]	1	75	F	Renal cell carcinoma	Leucocytoclastic	3 weeks
	2	77	F	Renal cell carcinoma	Leucocytoclastic	5 months

NA = not available.
HSP = Henoch–Schönlein vasculitis.

activity may be present in the cryoprecipitate[84]. Cryoglobulins have been classified into three types on the basis of the type of immunoglobulin contained within the cryoprecipitate[85]. Type I cryoglobulinemia contains only a monoclonal immunoglobulin (usually IgM), whereas types II and III are mixed cryoglobulinemias containing more than one class of immunoglobulin. In type II cryoglobulinemia there is a polyclonal component (usually IgG) and a monoclonal component (IgMκ with anti-globulin activity). Type III cryoglobulinemia contains a mixture of two types of polyclonal immunoglobulin, one of which has rheumatoid factor activity.

Cryoglobulins can be found in association with a wide variety of clinical conditions including myeloma, macroglobulinemia, chronic infections and inflammatory disorders. Type I cryoglobulins are seen in patients with lymphoproliferative disorders, especially Waldenström's macroglobulinemia and multiple myeloma, while Type III cryoglobulins are found in patients with autoimmune disorders and infections (e.g. hepatitis A, B, C or chronic inflammatory conditions. Type II and III cryoglobulinemia may occur in the absence of underlying

disease ('essential mixed cryoglobulinemia'), first described by Meltzer *et al.* in 1966[86].

The clinical features associated with cryoglobulinemia are shown in Table 9.7. Vascular purpura is more common in types II and III, while skin necrosis, necrotic purpura and severe Raynaud's phenomenon are features of type I cryoglobulinemia.

Arthralgias were a component of the syndrome reported by Meltzer *et al.*[86].

Arthralgias are a common feature of essential mixed cryoglobulinemia and frank arthritis even with erosions can occur[87]. Renal involvement ranges from isolated proteinuria with microscopic hematuria to an acute nephritic syndrome. Histology shows a mesangiocapillary glomerulonephritis with prominent monocytic infiltration with active vasculitis of small- and medium-sized vessels seen in about one-third of patients[88]. Renal disease is an important cause of morbidity with 17% of patients becoming dialysis dependent[89] and mortality up to 62%[90].

The demonstration of cryoglobulins requires that the blood be kept at 37°C until analysis. The amount of cryoglobulins may exceed 1 g/l. There is evidence of activation of the classical pathway of complement with

Table 9.7   Clinical features of cryoglobulinemia

	Type I*	Type II*	Type III*	Types II + III†	Type II‡
Cutaneous					
Vascular purpura	15	60	70	100	94
Distal necrosis	40	20	0	–	–
Urticaria	15	0	10	–	–
Livedo	1	0	14	–	–
Leg ulcers	8	0	4	30	–
Raynaud's	40	40	60	25	70
Acrocyanosis	15	15	2	–	–
Articular	5	20	28	72.5	54
Renal	25	35	12	55	54
Neurological	15	5	25	20	44
Hemorrhage	20	5	0	–	–
Arterial thrombosis	5	0	0	–	–

* From [85].
† From [91].
‡ From [90].
(All expressed as %)

greatly reduced levels of C4 but only moderately reduced levels of C3[90]. A normochromic normocytic anemia, with a mild leucocytosis and eosinophilia, may be present. Measurement of the acute phase response (CRP, ESR, PV) should be performed on blood separated at 37°C. Cryoprecipitation may reduce these indices. Cryoglobulin levels do not correlate well with disease activity or act as an index of renal involvement. However, monitoring levels is useful in predicting relapse as symptoms recur if levels return to those seen at presentation.

Because cryoglobulins precipitate in the cold they deposit in the extremities causing a local inflammatory response (vasculitis) and they can be recognized by immunofluorescence. The site of deposition is most commonly the skin and gomerular capillaries (plates 6–8). They can also deposit in small arteries and arterioles and may be widespread involving muscle, fat, liver, kidney, gut, spleen and lungs.

The pathogenesis of the vasculitis in cryoglobulinemia is poorly understood. A murine model has been described in which monoclonal IgG with rheumatoid factor activity is injected into experimental animals. Within 5–10 days severe glomerulonephritis and leucocytoclastic vasculitis develop[92]. A specific monoclonal IgG anti-idiotypic antibody can prevent cryoprecipitation and so inhibit cutaneous vasculitis and glomerulonephritis.

Treatment of cryoglobulinemia is by plasma exchange, which can control acute disease with resolution of cutaneous and joint symptoms, retinal vasculitis, acute pulmonary hemorrhage and acute glomerulonephritis[90]. Plasma exchange may work by reducing immune complex induced inflammation and also reduction of immune complex load may improve the ability of the reticuloendothelial system to clear immune complexes.

The effect of plasma exchange is usually transient and additional immunosuppressive therapy with corticosteroids and cytotoxic drugs, such as azathioprine, cyclophosphamide and chlorambucil, is required to control the disease. No controlled trials of these regimen have been performed. It is also important to treat any underlying disease, especially infection.

DRUG-INDUCED VASCULITIS AND SERUM SICKNESS

The definition of a drug-induced vasculitis is often empirical. Ideally, there should be an appropriate history of drug administration, biopsy of affected organs and positive rechallenge. In many cases the diagnosis is made on the basis of a suggestive history and a purpuric skin rash. Biopsy is often not performed and rechallenge may be unethical because of the risks of inducing generalized disease.

Most cases of drug-induced vasculitis involve small vessels with a hypersensitivity type of reaction. Very few cases of drug-induced vasculitis have been reported in association with medium or large vessel vasculitis.

DRUG-INDUCED HYPERSENSITIVITY (SMALL VESSEL) VASCULITIS

Drug-induced vasculitis is generally considered to be immunologically mediated. Serum from patients with vasculitis has been shown to contain increased levels of circulating immune complexes, and decreased levels of complement. Immunoglobulin deposition in vessel walls has been documented. These changes suggest a type III immune response similar to that seen in the Arthus reaction and serum sickness. These immunological changes are not constant and many cases show little if any immunological disturbance.

The commonest histological appearance of small vessel involvement is a leucocytoclastic vasculitis. This is thought to represent the response to immune complex deposition and hypersensitivity. Surprisingly, a recent review suggests that leucocytoclastic vasculitis is less common than a mononuclear vasculitis[93].

Similarly, Mullich studied 30 patients with drug-induced vasculitis and found a mononuclear vasculitis without evidence of fibrinoid change or leucocytoclasis[94].

The frequency of drug-induced hypersensitivity vasculitis is unknown but may account for 10–20% of cases with dermal vasculitis. These figures are probably an underestimate, since many cases are mild and self-limiting following drug withdrawal, and hence are not reported.

The clinical presentation of drug-induced vasculitis is indistinguishable from other hypersensitivity vasculitides. The most common skin lesion is 'palpable purpura', which occurs in at least 50% of cases, with urticarial lesions occurring in 10% of cases. The eruption is symmetrical and often affects the extremities (Figure 9.3). The lesions are usually all of the same age and disappear within several weeks of drug withdrawal. They may scar or leave hemosiderosis.

Involvement of extra-cutaneous sites is uncommon. However, one series reported 50–60% of cases with extra-cutaneous involvement but this is probably an overestimate reflecting the specialist referral of more severe cases[94]. There are no major reviews of unselected cases, so much of the following discussion is based on Mullich's work. The systemic nature of his patients is exemplified by the frequency of constitutional illness with malaise and fever in 90%[94].

Renal involvement occurs in 60% of patients with disseminated disease. In most cases, this is mild with microscopic hematuria and proteinuria. Progression to renal failure is uncommon. Biopsy typically shows a glomerulonephritis, either focal or segmental, but only occasionally associated with fibrinoid necrosis.

Most patients develop arthralgia, but arthritis is not uncommon. Knees, elbows, wrists and ankles are the most commonly involved joints, usually in an asymmetric oligoarticular pattern. Synovial biopsy shows inflammatory changes with no specific features[95].

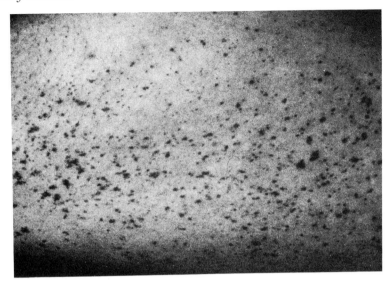

Fig. 9.3 Drug-induced vasculitis (sulphonamide).

Myalgias also occur and muscle biopsy is either normal or shows a small vessel vasculitis[96].

Pulmonary involvement is uncommon but may present with hemoptysis, pulmonary infiltrates on X-ray, pleuritic pain and dry cough. Cardiac disease is more common being found in 13 out of 30 cases reported by Mullich *et al.*, with either a myocarditis or a coronary vasculitis. Such involvement was associated with a high mortality[94].

Hepatic involvement occurs in around 50% of cases and is frequently asymptomatic: the only abnormalities being raised liver enzymes. Biopsy findings include hepatic necrosis, portal inflammatory infiltrate and epithelioid granulomas.

Drug-induced vasculitis affecting the nervous system is uncommon, but has been particularly associated with substance abuse (below). Mononeuritis multiplex and/or focal seizures occur, the latter has been reported occurring after Allopurinol[97].

Other laboratory findings are usually non-specific with leucocytosis and an acute phase response with elevation of ESR and CRP. These findings occur also in other forms of vasculitis. An eosinophilia is suggestive of a drug etiology but is also a typical feature of the Churg–Strauss syndrome. Hypocomplementemia is an inconsistent, non-specific finding which may also occur in other types of small vessel vasculitis. The role of ANCA in drug-induced vasculitis is unclear. Six patients with vasculitis induced by propylthiouracil were found to be ANCA positive[17]. The specificities were overlapping including 5 against proteinase-3, 3 against myeloperoxidase and 6 against human neutrophil elastase. ANCA titers fell on withdrawl of the drug.

Drugs which have been associated with hypersensitivity vasculitis are listed in Table 9.8. Many are single case reports and do not satisfy the criteria for a drug reaction (above).

The therapy of drug-induced hypersensitivity is unclear. The majority of cases respond to simple withdrawal of the inducing drug. Reported cases reflect the severe end of the disease spectrum and therapies thus have included corticosteroids, plasmapharesis and cyclophosphamide. Disseminated disease is more likely to require aggressive therapy than vasculitis confined to the skin.

Table 9.8 Drugs associated with hypersensitivity vasculitis

Acetylsalicylic acid	Isotretinoin
Alclocofenac	Levamisole
Allopurinol	Maprotiline
Ampicillin	Mefenamic acid
Atenolol	Melphalan
Bromide	Metformin
Busulphan	Methamphetamine
Captopril	Methotrexate
Carbamazepine	Methylthiouracil
Cefoxitin	Naproxen
Chloramphenicol	Nifedipine
Chlorothiazide	Oxyphenbutazone
Chlorpropamide	Penicillamine
Chlorthalidone	Penicillin
Cimetidine	Phenacetin
Ciprofloxacin	Phenothiazines
Colchicine	Phenylbutazone
Cotrimoxazole	Piroxicam
Dextran	Potassium iodide
Diazepam	Procainamide
Diclofenac	Propylthiouracil
Dihydan	Quinidine
Diltiazem	Rifampicin
Diphenhydramine	Sodium cromoglycate
Erythromycin	Spironolactone
Fenbufen	Streptokinase
Frusemide	Sulfasalazine
Griseofulvin	Sulfonamides
Hematoporphyrin	Terbutaline
Hydralazine	Tetracycline
Ibuprofen	Troxidone
Indium 113m	Tryptophan
Indomethacin	Vaccines
Iproniazid	Vitamins
Isoniazid	

From [98].

MEDIUM AND LARGE VESSEL DRUG-INDUCED VASCULITIS

Prior to Zeek's classification of vasculitis, drugs were considered to be a cause of PAN. Subsequently, most cases have been classified as hypersensitivity vasculitis and not PAN. A necrotizing vasculitis with the histological features of PAN has occasionally been reported in association with drugs, e.g. hydrallazine, penicillamine and fenoprofen[98].

Churg–Strauss syndrome has occasionally been reported in association with drugs. However, in most cases the evidence is circumstantial because of the absence of positive histology showing granulomas. Furthermore eosinophilia is itself a feature of drug reactions. A single case of drug-induced Wegener's granulomatosis has been reported in association with isotretinoin[99].

Acute necrotizing temporal arteritis developed in a cardiac allograft recipient who received OKT 3, a murine anti-CD3 monoclonal antibody for treatment of refractory rejection. The patient developed temporal headaches, arthralgia, myalgia with tender, pulsatile temporal arteries and a raised ESR. Biopsy of the temporal artery showed fibrinoid necrosis of the arterial wall with deposition of murine IgG[100].

Vaccines and hyposensitization therapy for allergy have been reported to cause a PAN-like illness. PAN with eosinophilia developed in 6 patients receiving hyposensitization therapy for asthma[101].

Vasculitis has been described following influenza vaccination. In 10 out of 13 cases there were systemic features with kidney and lung being the most common non-cutaneous organs involved. The interval between immunization and onset of vasculitis was 2–20 days with a mean of 9 days. One case was fatal and post-mortem examination confirmed a diagnosis of PAN[102].

Erythema nodosum and Takayasu's arteritis have been reported in a single case after immunization with plasma derived hepatitis B vaccine[103].

SUBSTANCE ABUSE RELATED VASCULITIS

Widespread use of illicit substances has resulted in an increased recognition of their complications. Vasculitis is one complication and appears to be restricted to the central nervous system. Amphetamine[104], cocaine [105], heroin[106], phenylpropylamine[107], ephedrine[108] and pseudoephedrine[109] have all been reported as causing a cerebral vasculitis.

The typical presentation is with neurological symptoms developing rapidly within minutes or hours of drug use. Headache is often the initial feature but encephalopathy may supervene quickly. Focal signs may develop but fits are uncommon.

Computerized tomography and magnetic resonance imaging reveal intracerebral hematoma, subarachnoid hemorrhage or cerebral infarction. Cerebral arteriography characteristically demonstrates segmental regions of stenosis and dilatation often described as 'beading' or 'sausage-like', with non-specific, small vessel occlusions. These changes may resolve.

Until recently, vasculitis was diagnosed only at post-mortem. Several cases have recently been diagnosed by brain biopsy[110,111]. Vasculitis predominantly affects small vessels with a lymphocytic infiltrate; giant cells and granulomas are not present. Attribution of these changes to a single agent is in many cases difficult as chronic use and multiple drug use are common, and purity questionable. Many abused substances are vasospastic and it has been suggested that vasospasm may damage endothelium with release of autoantigen[111], and the development of vasculitis.

The clinical course depending on severity is for resolution following stopping substance abuse. The role of immunosuppressive agents, such as corticosteroids or cyclophosphamide, is uncertain, with reports of both success and failure[110,111].

SERUM SICKNESS

Serum sickness is an immune complex mediated phenomenon occurring after repeated administration of heterologous proteins. The immunological mechanisms were extensively investigated in the 1950s[112]. In acute 'one-shot' serum sickness a single large dose of bovine serum albumin injected into a rabbit results in an acute disease characterized by nephritis, arthritis and vasculitis. The lesions develop when soluble complexes of antigen and antibody form in conditions of excess antigen, and heal when after antigen clearance, free antibody appears in the serum. Chronic experimental serum sickness can be induced by repeated administrations of foreign protein, so that immune complexes are present in the serum for much longer periods of time. These animals develop chronic glomerulonephritis but not a vasculitis. The development of glomerulonephritis depends on the balance between antigen and antibody; those animals which produce only small amounts of antibody and form soluble complexes when antigen is given in antigen excess develop chronic glomerulonephritis. Immunoglobulin and complement are detectable in a granular pattern along the glomerular basement membrane.

Hyperimmune heterologous sera are no longer in use; however, antilymphocyte or antithymocyte globulins are still used in the treatment of autoimmune disease or allograft rejection. Bielory *et al.* prospectively analysed 35 patients who received equine antithymocyte globulins for bone marrow failure[113]. Serum sickness occurred 5–7 days after starting antithymocyte therapy with development of fever, malaise, headache, arthralgias and skin rash. Urinary abnormalities (hematuria, proteinuria and hemoglobulinuria) occurred in 50% of patients. Skin biopsy showed a perivascular infiltrate of lymphocytes and monocytes with edema. Leucocytoclasis was uncommon and fibrinoid necrosis was not seen. Serum complement levels were decreased and immune complex levels raised. The course was benign with resolution in 1–2 weeks.

The development of monoclonal antibody (MAb) technology has resulted in the therapeutic use of mouse or rat MAbs in the treatment of allograft rejection and autoimmune disease. Use of rodent MAbs invariably results in an antiglobulin response with detectable levels of human anti-rodent antibodies[114]. Development of an antiglobulin response has not prevented repeated courses of therapy; however, they may be less effective and potentially may result in serum sickness or an anaphylactic reaction[115]. Significant serum sickness reaction seems to be infrequent, occurring in 3% of patients retreated with OKT3 (an anti-CD3 MAb) for recurrent allograft rejection[116,117]. Chimeric (human constant region with rodent variable region) or humanized (human constant and variable framework regions with rodent complementarity determining regions) MAbs are less immunogenic than rodent MAbs. Their use should reduce the antiglobulin response although it is still possible for an anti-idiotypic or antiallotypic response to develop. Studies using the humanized MAb CAMPATH-IH suggest that it is less immunogenic than its rodent counterpart CAMPATH-IG[114,118], thus making repeated courses of therapy safer.

Serum sickness may also occur after administration of intravenous or intracardiac streptokinase[119] and anisoylated plaminogen streptokinase activator complex (AP-SAC)[120] in the treatment of myocardial infarction. IgG and IgE anti-streptokinase antibody concentrations are raised in patients with serum sickness following streptokinase therapy. Bucknall *et al.* reported serum sickness occurring in 6 out of 253 patients treated with APSAC for myocardial infarction. All 6 patients developed a purpuric rash on the lower extremities associated with an arthritis in 5 patients and proteinuria/hematuria in 2 patients. The skin lesions resolved over 3 weeks without specific therapy. In 2 patients skin biopsy showed a lymphocytic vasculitis[120].

A serum sickness-like illness can also occur following certain non-protein drugs, such as penicillin, sulphonamides, thiouracil and hydantoin, presumably following hapten formation.

HYPOCOMPLEMENTEMIC URTICARIAL VASCULITIS

Hypocomplementemic urticarial vasculitis syndrome (HUVS) is an uncommon vasculitic syndrome initially described as a triad of hypocomplementemia, cutaneous vasculitis and arthritis[121,122]. The rash clinically resembles urticaria; however, on biopsy there is evidence of a leucocytoclastic vasculitis with involvement of post-capillary venules. The skin lesions present as recurrent episodes of an urticarial-like rash which burns and is painful rather than itchy. They may resolve with purpura or hyperpigmentation[123]. Patients may have associated angioderma, arthralgias, arthritis, abdominal pain, chest pain, fever, renal disease (proteinuria, hematuria, impairment of function), episcleritis and uveitis.

Hypocomplementemia was initially thought to be a typical feature of all urticarial vasculitis syndromes. However, some patients have persistently normal complement levels[123,124]. Mehregan *et al.* studied 72 patients with urticarial vasculitis diagnosed on skin biopsy. One-third (23 out of 72) had hypocomplementemia. Patients with hypocomplementemia were more likely to have systemic symptoms, such as arthralgias, abdominal pain and chronic obstructive airways disease[124].

Urticarial vasculitis has been associated with SLE[125] and may be an early presentation of the disease[126]. In the Mehregan study, 11% of patients with urticarial vasculitis met the ACR criteria for the diagnosis of SLE. Hypocomplementemia or biopsy findings were not reliable predictors of SLE[124]. Other associations of urticarial vasculitis include hepatitis B, infectious mononucleosis, IgA multiple myeloma, IgM gammopathy (Schnitzler's syndrome), serum sickness and exposure to ultraviolet light and drugs[127–130].

Histologically, urticarial vasculitis is differentiated from uncomplicated urticaria by the presence of swelling of endothelial cells damage, fibrinoid necrosis, leucocytoclasis and dermal hemorrhage. In patients with hypocomplementemia there may be in addition an interstitial neutrophilic dermal infiltrate with immunoglobulin and complement deposition in the blood vessels and dermal basement membrane.

The pathogenesis of urticarial vasculitis is believed to be a type III hypersensitivity reaction, similar to other types of leucocytoclastic vasculitis[131]. Circulating immune complexes have been reported in up to 75% of patients with urticarial vasculitis[127]. Alternatively, the disease may result from an intrinsic abnormality of the complement system, e.g. HUVS[122]. Serum levels of early components of the complement pathways are low, in particular, C4, C2 and C3, while later components are normal. This pattern is typical of activation of the classical complement pathway.

In serum from patients with hypocomplementemia there is an IgG precipitin which binds to ClQ through its Fc portion[132]. Autoantibodies to ClQ in patients with HUVS are similar to Cl-binding autoantibodies found in SLE[133], suggesting that both bind to the same collagen-like region epitopes of ClQ. Thus patients with HUVS and SLE have some immunological similarities.

The treatment of HUVS is uncertain. Antihistamines are not always successful in clearing skin lesions[124,134], suggesting that the urticaria is not simply caused by most cell degranulation and histamine release. Nonsteroidal anti-inflammatory drugs (in particular Indomethacin) have also been used successfully[135]. Oral corticosteroids and antimalarials may be useful.

BEHÇET'S DISEASE

Behçet's disease is a chronic relapsing inflammatory vascular process. The characteristic feature is the triad of recurrent orogenital

Table 9.9 International study group criteria for diagnosis of Behçet's disease (1990)

Diagnosis requires recurrent aphthous stomatitis*
  plus two of the following:
Genital aphthae
  Aphthous ulcer or scarring
Eye lesions
  Anterior or posterior uveitis
  Cells in vitreous humor on slit-lamp
    examination
  Retinal vasculitis observed by ophthalmologist
Skin lesions
  Erythema nodosum
  Pseudo folliculitis
  Papulopustular lesions
  Acneiform nodules (absence of steroid
    treatment in post-adolescent patient)
Positive pathergy test results[†]
  Read by physician at 24–48 hours

---

* Three times in one year. Diagnosis excludes other clinical syndromes (e.g. inflammatory bowel disease, relapsing polychondritis, infections and sarcoidosis).
† Method: subcutaneous injection of small volume sterile normal saline. Test results less commonly positive in USA and UK than in the Mediterranean and Japan.
(From [137]

ulceration and uveitis. The first modern description was by Behçet in 1937, but the disease has been known since the time of Hippocrates[136].

The major clinical feature of Behçet's disease is recurrent oral and genital aphthous ulceration. These ulcers are often painful. Uveitis is the third component of the classical triad. Cutaneous lesions include thrombophlebitis, erythema nodosum and acneiform nodules. Systemic manifestations include vasculitis, polyarthritis, central nervous system, pulmonary and gastrointestinal involvement. Because of the variable multisystem nature of the disease, diagnostic criteria have been proposed (Table 9.9).

Behçet's disease occurs more commonly in Japan and the Mediterranean than in Europe or North America. The disease occurs most commonly in adults aged 18–40 years with a 2:1 male preponderance. It can occur rarely in childhood (Chapter 12). The course of the

Table 9.10   Vascular involvement in Behçet's disease

	Koc series	Literature review
Patients	38	728
Venous		
Occlusions of upper and lower limb	–	221 (30.4%)
Subcutaneous thrombophlebitis	18 (47.3%)	205 (28.2%)
Superior vena cava	6 (15.8%)	122 (16.7%)
Inferior vena cava	6 (15.8%)	93 (12.8%)
Cerebral sinus	3 (7.9%)	30 (4.0%)
Budd Chiari	2 (5.2%)	17 (2.3%)
Subclavian	2 (5.2%)	8 (1.1%)
Iliac vein	–	7 (1.0%)

From [139].

disease is more severe among Japanese and Eastern Mediterraneans who have more severe uveitis. Among this group of patients there is an association with HLA-B5 and its subtype B51.

VASCULAR INVOLVEMENT IN BEHÇET'S DISEASE

Vascular involvement in Behçet's disease, although not a diagnostic feature, occurs in up to 35% of patients[138]. The spectrum of vascular involvement has recently been described by Koc *et al.* together with an extensive literature review[139]. He studied a series of 137 consecutive Turkish patients with Behçet's disease, of whom 38 had vascular involvement (Table 9.10). Venous involvement was more common (33 patients) than arterial disease, in particular deep venous thrombosis of the extremities, trunk and intracranial sinuses are common and may be accompanied by superficial thrombophlebitis. Arterial involvement is less common, with the most frequently involved arteries being the aorta and pulmonary arteries. Aneurysm formation occurs more commonly than occlusions and can occur in any large or medium artery. Rupture of large artery aneurysms is a major cause of death in patients with Behçet's disease.

Small vessel vasculitis is common in Behçet's disease[138]. Vascular necrosis together with a lymphocytic infiltrate have been found in all organs involved in the disease process.

There are no specific laboratory abnormalities in Behçet's disease. The cutaneous pathergy test can be elicited in 25–75% of patients from Japan and Turkey. No specific microorganisms have been consistently isolated from patients with Behçet's disease, but streptococcal antigens may have a role[140].

Suzuki and colleagues have demonstrated an increased percentage of circulatory gamma-delta T-cells in Behçet's disease patients[141].

There are no good controlled trials of treatment of Behçet's disease. Mild to moderately severe disease can be treated with anti-inflammatory drugs and either local or systemic corticosteroids. More severe disease requires immunosuppression with cyclophosphamide, cyclosporin A, azathioprine, methotrexate. Vascular thrombosis may be treated with low-dose aspirin or anticoagulation.

TRANSPLANT VASCULITIS

Transplant vasculitis occurs in the setting of allograft rejection, and is classified depending on the time interval following transplantation. The clinical and immunological features are similar with all allografts, but the following discussion concentrates on renal transplantation.

Hyperacute rejection occurs during the first 24 hours after surgery but may become apparent during the operation itself[142]. The recipient has preformed donor-specific cytotoxic antibodies which react with HLA antigens on donor T- and B-lymphocytes. Proper cross-matching and avoidance of ABO incompatibility usually prevents this problem. There is rapid development of inflammation with thrombosis and necrosis of renal vessels. Severe ischemia ensues and the graft is lost.

Delayed hyperacute rejection occurs around 2 weeks after renal transplant but only under certain circumstances. It occurs in recipients of serologically HLA identical, mixed lymphocyte culture non-stimulatory living-related grafts. The graft functions satisfactorily, but suddenly becomes tender, swollen and function rapidly deteriorates. The rejection is characterized by aggressive vascular lesions with fibrinoid necrosis, interstitial hemorrhage, thrombosis and cortical necrosis. The pathogenesis is unknown but is believed to be antibodies against vascular endothelial cell antigens which cross-react with monocyte antigens.

Treatment of hyperacute and delayed hyperacute rejection is generally unsuccessful with little response to conventional immunosuppression.

Acute cellular rejection is the most common form of rejection and is seen in the first year after transplantation but can occur in the first month[143]. Presentation is with low grade fever, diminishing urine output, increasing serum creatinine and a swollen, tender allograft. The characteristic histological feature of acute cellular rejection is an interstitial infiltrate comprised of T- and B-lymphocytes, macrophages, monocytes, neutrophils and natural killer cells. These infiltrates develop initially in the perivascular areas and then in

Table 9.11 Vasculitis mimicks

1. Systemic multisystem disease		
Tumors:	Metastatic carcinoma	*
	Lymphoproliferative	*
	Paraneoplastic	*
	Atrial myxoma	*
Infection:	Neisseria	*
	Rickettsiae	*
	Borrelia	*
	Endocarditis	*
Sweet's syndrome		
2. Occlusive vasculopathy		
Embolic	Cholesterol	
	Mycotic aneurysm	*
	Atrial myxoma	*
	Endocarditis	*
Anti-phospholipid antibody syndrome		
Ergotism		
Radiation		
Degos		
3. Aneurysms	Pseudoxanthoma elasticus	
	Neurofibromatosis	
	Mycotic	
	Myxomas	
	Radiation	

* These conditions can mimic a multisystem disease or emboli and can, in addition, be associated with a true vasculitis.

the interstitium. If untreated there is vascular necrosis and lumenal narrowing. The graft sensitizes the recipient, such that circulating antibodies against the graft appear. These may be cytotoxic or complement activating.

Treatment of acute cellular rejection is with methylprednisolone, cyclosporin and azathioprine. Monoclonal anti-T-cell antibodies (e.g. OKT3, CAMPATH-IG) have been shown to be effective at reversing acute cellular rejection.

Chronic rejection develops weeks to years after transplantation, with a slow deterioration of graft function. There is intimal thickening with preservation of the media and elastic laminae[144]. Lumenal narrowing results in tissue atrophy and infarction. There is little evidence of active inflammation. Treatment is conservative, aggressive immunosuppression is avoided and treatment is aimed at preservation of graft function.

VASCULITIS MIMICKS

The clinical manifestations of systemic vasculitis are protean. Different vasculitis syndromes are recognized on the basis of a combination of clinical, histological and laboratory features (Table 9.1). Systemic vasculitis may, however, be mimicked by a variety of non-vasculitic diseases (Table 9.11). In general, these vasculitis mimicks present with a systemic multiorgan illness or with a non-inflammatory vascular disease or both.

Biopsy of involved organs is important and will identify non-inflammatory emboli or thrombosis. It is important to remember that aneurysm formation, although a typical feature of PAN, also occurs in a number of other conditions including bacterial endocarditis and cardiac myxoma. A good history and appropriate investigations (e.g. blood cultures and echocardiography) should help define these vasculitis mimicks.

CHOLESTEROL ATHEROEMBOLISM

Although described over a century ago, clinically significant disease-mimicking systemic vasculitis is extremely uncommon. Minor vascular abnormalities due to spontaneous atheroembolism has been observed in 3% of unselected post-mortem examinations and in up to 30% of patients undergoing aortic surgery or arteriography[145,146]. Cholesterol embolization mimicking systemic vasculitis was reviewed by Cappiello and colleagues[147]. This review suggests that multiple cholesterol emboli produce a spectrum of clinical signs and symptoms depending on their size, number, site of origin and ultimate organ enlodgement. Multisystem involvement can mimic a necrotizing vasculitis, cryoglobulinemia, macroglobulinemia,

Table 9.12 Laboratory abnormalities in cholesterol embolism

Abnormalities	Frequency (%)
Leucocytosis	40
Eosinophilia	80
Hypocomplementemia	73
Thrombocytopenia	85
Raised ESR	80
Elevated muscle enzymes	10
Hyperamylasemia	43
Uremia	90
Abnormal urinalysis	20
Disseminated intravascular coagulation	50

Adapted from [147].

or emboli of cardiac origin. Cutaneous lesions include livedo reticularis and digital infarction. Other common systemic features include fever, weight loss, renal impairment, neurological changes and abdominal pain (Table 9.12)[147]; they are usually non-specific but are similar to those seen in systemic vasculitis. Eosinophilia is common and may lead to confusion with Churg–Strauss syndrome.

Biopsy of clinically involved sites is diagnostic, showing cholesterol crystals in small arteries and capillaries. The diagnosis should be considered in older patients with an aneurysm and/or peripheral vascular disease or following catheterization.

Treatment is unsatisfactory; low molecular weight dextrose, antiplatelet drugs, vasodilator drugs and corticosteroids are generally ineffective[147].

CARDIAC MYXOMA

Cardiac myxomas are rare benign tumors most commonly found in the left atrium (90% of cases). Constitutional symptoms and systemic embolization may lead to a mistaken diagnosis of vasculitis[148–150].

Constitutional features seen in 90% include: fever, weight loss, Raynaud's phenomenon, clubbing, raised erythrocyte sedimentation rate and, elevated acute phase proteins and serum immunoglobulin levels.

Systemic embolization occurs in approximately 40% of cases. Emboli may be the first manifestation of disease and their size varies greatly; the biggest are able to occlude the aortic bifurcation. Microemboli from cardiac myxoma may remain viable, and so are capable of invading the vessel wall and destroying the internal elastic lamina, and media, resulting in aneurysm formation which mimicks PAN[151].

Small vessel vasculitis in muscle has been reported in a patient with a cardiac myxoma[150], suggesting that myxoma is not always a mimic. ANCA has also been described in patients with atrial myxoma[16].

Cardiac myxomas are readily diagnosed by echocardiography[149], an investigation which should be performed in all cases of suspected vasculitis.

Treatment is by surgical excision of the primary tumor. Embolized myxomas should also be excised if possible, as they are autonomous and can continue to grow after resection of the primary tumor.

ANTIPHOSPHOLIPID ANTIBODY SYNDROME

Vasculitis is not a feature of the antiphospholipid antibody syndrome[152], but the occurrence of widespread occlusive vascular lesions may mimick vasculitis. The presence of these autoantibodies have been associated with recurrent arterial and venous thrombosis, fetal loss and thrombocytopenia[153] [Table 9.13]. The most common manifestations are stroke and deep venous thrombosis, but many other sites have been described[154]. A devastating multisystem non-inflammatory vasculopathy may rarely occur. The pathology is unimpressive with occlusions of capillaries and small arterioles(155,156).

The widespread vascular occlusion of large

Table 9.13 Manifestations of antiphospholipid antibody syndrome

Major features

Arterial, thrombosis:	Stroke
	Transient ischemic attack
	Multi-infarct dementia
	Peripheral vascular disease
	Coronary artery
Venous thrombosis:	Deep veins of legs
	Hepatic vein
Fetal loss:	Recurrent abortion
Thrombocytopenia	

Minor clinical features
Chorea
Epilepsy
Optic neuritis
Transverse myelitis
Guillain–Barré syndrome
Migraine
Pulmonary hypotension
Libman–Sachs endocarditis
Livedo reticularis (Sneddon's syndrome)
Positive direct Coombs test

and small vessels occurring at different times mimicks vasculitis. The absence of a brisk acute phase response, or histological evidence of vasculitis together with the presence of antiphospholipid antibodies, should enable the diagnosis to be made.

Intra-alveolar hemorrhage can occur in the antiphospholipid antibody syndrome and can mimick pulmonary vasculitides, such as Wegener's granulomatosis[157].

KÖHLMEIER–DEGOS DISEASE

Köhlmeier–Degos disease (malignant atrophic papulosis) is a rare and lethal condition which involves skin, gut and the nervous system. The pathognomic skin lesions are circular, porcelain-white in color with a depressed centre 4–8 mm in diameter, with a slightly elevated erythematous margin. The arterial lesion is luminal stenosis or occlusion due to intimal proliferations and consequent thrombosis[158]. Presentation is usually with acute abdominal pain (in association with the skin lesion), leading to bowel perforation and peritonitis, which may be fatal.

The multisystem nature of Köhlmeier–Degos disease mimicks a vasculitis; however, the vascular lesions are due to an obliterative intimal proliferation rather than a vasculitic process. The distinction can be made on biopsy.

ACUTE FEBRILE NEUTROPHILIC DERMATOSIS (SWEET'S SYNDROME)

Sweet described a syndrome occurring in young women comprising a quartet of major features: fever, painful red skin plaques, leucocytosis and a dermal infiltrate with neutrophils[159]. Other systemic manifestations include arthritis, inflammatory bowel disease, paraproteinemia and ocular signs. Sweet's syndrome is associated with myelodyplasia and leukemia. The systemic features and skin lesions may lead to consideration of a diagnosis of vasculitis. Sweet's syndrome is usually diagnosed by skin biopsy, which shows an intense infiltration of neutrophils into the dermis, without any evidence of vasculitis. Treatment is with steroids or other immunosuppressive agents.

RADIATION VASCULOPATHY

Radiation has been known to cause vascular injury since 1893[160], only 3 years after the discovery of X-rays by Röntgen. Vascular injury after radiation can be classified as either acute (occurring within hours of irradiation) or chronic (developing months to years after irradiation). Acute changes include hemorrhage and an 'acute cardiovascular syndrome' characterized by progressive hypotension, shock and death. These phenomena occur after high doses of total body irradiation.

Three types of chronic vascular lesion are recognized:

1. internal injury and mural thrombosis occurring within 5 years;

2. progressive sclerosis of arterioles and arteries occurring within 10 years and which can lead to lumenal occlusion; and

3. accelerated atherosclerosis with a latency of approximately 20 years[161,162].

The endothelial cell is the most radiation sensitive part of the vascular system. Following irradiation endothelial cells fail to replicate and endothelium is not adequately renewed. The basement membrane becomes exposed, on to which platelets come into contact and thrombotic mechanisms are activated, with consequent thrombosis and atherosclerosis. The resulting reduction in perfusion causes organ ischemia and necrosis. These changes affect vessels of all sizes, although lesions of large vessels are often difficult to distinguish from 'idiopathic' atherosclerosis.

Clinically, the manifestations depend on the organs included within the field of therapy and the dose and type of radiation used. The features include arterial stenosis and occlusion, arterial rupture and aneurysm formation[163,164]. Arteriographic changes may be similar to those seen in atherosclerosis. Radiation vasculopathy can be distinguished from systemic vasculitis by the history of cancer therapy, irradiation to the ischemic vascular bed and lack of an acute phase inflammatory response.

CHRONIC ERGOTISM

Epidemic ergotism occurs after consumption of grain contaminated with ergot (*Claviceps purpurea*). During and since the Middle Ages, epidemics have been described in which painful gangrene of the peripheries occurred with loss of the extremities.

Chronic ergotism may also follow the consumption of large amounts of ergotamine tartrate which is sometimes used for migraine headaches. Patients may develop peripheral, carotid, coronary and visceral ischemia. The angiographic appearances may simulate vasculitis with irregular, long and short segmental stenoses, but without histological evidence of vasculitis. Diagnosis depends on the history of ergot ingestion. The lesions may not be fully reversible on withdrawal of ergot[164].

REFERENCES

1. Gover, R. G., Sausker, W. F., Kohler, P. F., *et al.* (1978) Small vessel vasculitis caused by hepatitis B virus immune complexes. *J. Allergy. and Clin. Immunol.*, **62**, 222–8.

2. Neumann, H. A. M., Berretty, P. J. M. and Reinders-Folmer, S. C. C. (1981) Hepatitis B surface antigen deposition in the blood vessels of urticarial lesions in acute hepatitis B. *Br. J. Dermatol.*, **104**, 383–8.

3. Levo, Y., Gorevic, P. D., Kassab, H. J. *et al.* (1977) Association between hepatitis B virus and essential mixed cryoglobulinaemia. *N. Eng. J. Med.*, **296**, 1501–4.

4. Combes, B., Stastny, P., Shorez, J. *et al.* (1971) Glomerulonephritis with deposition of Australia antigen-antibody complexes in glomerular basement membrane. *Lancet*, **11**, 234–7.

5. Gocke, D. J., Hsu, K., Morgan, C. *et al.* (1970) Association between polyarteritis and Australia antigen. *Lancet*, **11**, 1149–53.

6. Zeek, P. M. (1953) Periarteritis nodosa and other forms of necrotizing angiitis. *N. Eng. J. Med.*, **248**, 764–72.

7. Alarcon-Sergovia, D. and Brown, A. L. (1964) Classification and aetiologic aspects of necrotizing angitides. *Mayo Clin. Proc.*, **39**, 205–22.

8. Lie, J. T. (1988) Classification and immunodiagnosis of vasculitis – a new resolution or promises unfilled? *J. Rheumatol.*, **15**, 5.

9. Adu, D. (1993) Polyarteritis, Wegener's granulomatosis and Churg–Strauss syndrome, in *Oxford Textbook of Rheumatology*, (eds P. Maddison, D. Isenberg, P. Woo *et al.*) Oxford.

10. Andrews, M., Edmunds, M., Campbell, A. *et al.* (1990) Systemic vasculitis in the 1980's – is there an increasing incidence of Wegener's granulomatosis and microscopic polyarteritis? *J. R. Coll. Physicians*, **24**, 284–8.

11. Klaasen, R. J., Goldschmeding, R., Dolman, K. M. *et al.* (1992) Anti-neutrophil cytoplasmic antibodies in symptomatic HIV infection. *Clin. Exp. Immunol.*, **87**, 24–30.

12. Efthimiou, J., Spickett, G., Lane, D. *et al.* (1991) Anti-neutrophil cytoplasmic antibodies, cystic fibrosis and infection. *Lancet*, **337**, 1037–8.

13. Esnault, V. C. M., Jayne, D. R. W., Keoghan, M. T. *et al.* (1990) Anti-neutrophil antibodies in patients with monoclonal gammopathies. *Clin. Lab. Immunol.*, **32**, 153–9.

14. Davenport, A. (1991) 'False positive' perinuclear and cytoplasmic anti-neutrophil cytoplasmic antibodies results leading to a misdiagnosis of Wegener's granulomatosis and/or microscopic polyarteritis. *Clin. Nephrol.*, **37**, 124–30.

15. Juby, C., Johnston, C., Davis, P. *et al.* (1992) Anti-nuclear and anti-neutrophil cytoplasmic antibodies (ANCA) in the series of patients with Felty's syndrome. *Br. J. Rheumatol.*, **31**, 185–8.

16. Peter, H. H., Mertzger, D., Rump, A. *et al.* (1993) ANCA in diseases other than systemic vasculitis. *Clin. Exp. Immunol.*, **93** (Suppl 1), 12–14.

17. Dolman, K. M., Gans, R. O. B., Verraat, T. J. *et al.* (1993) Vasculitis and anti-neutrophil cytoplasmic autoantibodies associated with propylthiouracil therapy. *Lancet*, **342**, 651–2.

18. Calabrese, L. H. (1991) Vasculitis and infection with the human immuno-deficiency virus. *Rheum. Dis. Clin. North. Am.*, **17**, 131–47.

19. Schlossberg, D. and Aaron, T. (1991) Aortitis caused by *Mycobacterium fortuitum*. *Arch. Intern. Med.*, **152**, 1010–11.

20. Oskoui, R., David, W. A. and Gomes, M. D. (1993) *Salmonella* aortitis. *Arch. Intern. Med.*, **153**, 517–25.

21. Sotto, M. N., Langer, B., Hoshino-Shimizu, S. *et al.* (1976) Pathogenesis of cutaneous lesions in acute meningococcaemia in humans: light, immunofluorescence, and elective microscopic studies in humans. *J. Infect. Dis.*, **133**, 506–14.

22. Fink, C. W. (1991) The role of the streptococcus in post-streptococcal reactive arthritis and childhood polyarteritis nodosa. *J. Rheumatol.* **18** (Suppl), 14–20.

23. Deighton, C. (1993) Beta haemolytic streptococci and reactive arthritis in adults. *Ann. Rheum. Dis.*, **52**, 475–82.

24. Steer, A. C. (1989) Lyme disease. *N. Eng. J. Med.*, **321**, 586–96.

25. Walker, D. H. and Mattern, W. D. (1980)

Rickettsial vasculitis. *Am. Heart J.*, **100**, 896–900.

26. Torres, J., Humphrey, E. and Bisns, A. L. (1973) Rocky Mountain spotted fever in the mid south. *Arch. Intern. Med.*, **132**, 340–7.

27. Woodward, T. E., Petersen, C. E., Oster, C. N. *et al.* (1976) Prompt confirmation of Rocky Mountain spotted fever: identification of Rickettsiae in skin tissue. *J. Infect. Dis.*, **134**, 297–301.

28. Williams, P. L., Johnson, R., Pappagionis, D. *et al.* (1992) Vasculitic and encephalitic complications associated with *coccidioidis immitis* infection of the central nervous system. *Clin. Infect. Dis.*, **14**, 673–82.

29. Christian, C. L. (1991) Hepatitis B virus (HBV) and systemic vasculitis. *Clin. Exp. Rheumatol.*, **9**, 1–2.

30. Quint, L., Deny, P., Guillevin, L. *et al.* (1991) Hepatitis C virus in patients with polyarteritis nodosa. Prevalence of 38 patients. *Clin. Exp. Rheumatol.*, **9**, 253–7.

31. Abel, G., Zhang, Q-X. and Agnello, V. (1993) Hepatitis C virus infection in type II mixed cryoglobulinaemia. *Arth. Rheum.*, **30**, 1341–9.

32. Gheradi, R., Belec, L., Mhiri, C. *et al.* (1993) The spectrum of vasculitis in human immunodeficiency virus infected patients. *Arth. Rheum.*, **36**, 1164–74.

33. Cooper, L. M. and Patterson, J. A. K. (1989) Allergic granulomatosis and angiitis of Churg–Strauss: case report in a patient with antibodies to human immunodeficiency virus and hepatitis B virus. *J. Dermatol.*, **28**, 597–8.

34. Corman, L. C. and Dolson, D. J. (1992) Polyarteritis nodosa and parvovirus B 19 infection. *Lancet*, **339**, 491.

35. Pesther, J. U. S., Thurlow, J., Palferman, T. *et al.* (1993) Acute hantavirus infection presenting as hypersensitivity vasculitis with arthropathy. *J. Infect.*, **26**, 75–7.

36. Hensen, J. B. and Crawford, T. B. (1974) The pathogenesis of virus-induced arterial disease – Aleutian disease and equine viral arthritis. *Adv. Cardiol.*, **13**, 183–91.

37. Tatum, E. T., Sun, P. C. and Cohn, U. L. (1989) Cytomegalovirus vasculitis and colon perforation in a patient with acquired immuno-deficiency syndrome. *Pathology*, **21**, 235–8.

38. Zakarain, B., Barlow, R. M. and Rennie, J. C. (1976) Periarteritis in experimental border disease of sheep. *J. Comp. Pathol.*, **86**, 477–87.

39. Chauhan, A., Scott, D. G. I., Neuberger, J. *et al.* (1990) Churg–Strauss vasculitis and ascaris infection. *Ann. Rheum. Dis.*, **49**, 320–2.

40. Chote, F., Guillevin, L. and Saubaget, F. (1993) Treatment of polyarteritis nodosa related to Hepatitis B virus with alpha interon and plasma exchange. Results in 6 patients. *Arth. Rheum.*, **36** (Suppl1), 596.

41. Gibb, D. (1991) Kawasaki disease: a disorder looking for an organism? *Paediatri. Perinat. Epidemiol.*, **5**, 123–32.

42. Abe, J., Kotzin, B. L., Jujoh, K. *et al.* (1992) Selective expansion of T cells expressing T-cell receptor variable regions UB2, UB8 in Kawasaki disease. *Proc. Nat. Acad. Sci. USA*, **89**, 4066–70.

43. Leung, D. Y. M. (1993) Kawasaki disease. *Curr. Opin. Rheumatol.*, **5**, 41–7.

44. Curth, H. O. (1976) Skin lesions and internal carcinoma, in *Cancer of the Skin*, (eds R. Adrade, S. L. Crumpert, G. L. Popkin *et al.*), Philadelphia, Saunders, pp. 1308–43.

45. Hughes, G. R. V., Elkon, K. B., Spiller, R. *et al.* (1979) Polyarteritis nodosa and hairy cell leukaemia. *Lancet*, **317**, 280–2.

46. Gabriel, S. E., Conn, D. L., Phyliky, R. L., *et al.* (1986) Vasculitis in hairy cell leukaemia: review of literature and consideration of possible pathogenic mechanisms. *J. Rheumatol.*, **13**, 1167–72.

47. Golde, D. W., Stevens, R. H., Quan, S. G. *et al.* (1977) Immunoglobulin synthesis in hairy cell leukaemia. *Br. J. Haematol.*, **35**, 359–65.

48. Posnett, D. N., Marloe, C. C. and Knowles, D. M. (1984) A membrane antigen (HCI) selectively present on hairy cells, leukaemia cells, endothelial cells, and epidermal basal cells. *J. Immunol.*, **132**, 2700–2.

49. Gerber, M. A., Brodin, A., Steinberg, A. D. *et al.* Periarteritis nodosa, Australia antigen and lymphatic leukaemia. *N. Eng. J. Med.*, **286**, 14–17.

50. Leung, A. C. T., McLay, A. and Boulton-Jones, J. M. (1986) Polyarteritis nodosa and monocyte leukaemia. *Postgrad. Med. J.*, **62**, 35–7.

51. Greer, J. M., Longley, S., Edwards, N. L. *et al.* (1988) Vasculitis associated with malignancy. *Medicine* (Baltimore), **67**, 220–30.

52. Sams, W. M., Harville, D. D. and Winkelmann, R. K. (1988) Necrotizing vasculitis associated with lethal reticulo endothelial disease. *Br. J. Dermatol.*, **80**, 555–60.

53. Sanchez-Guerro, J., Guteirrez-Urevia, S.,

Vidaller, A. *et al.* (1990) Vasculitis as a para-neoplastic syndrome. Report of 11 cases and review of the literature. *J. Rheumatol.*, **17**, 1458–62.

54. Cupps, T. R. and Fauci, A. S. (1982) Neoplasm and systemic vasculitis: a case report. *Arth. Rheum.*, **25**, 475–7.

55. Calonje, J. E. and Gleaves, M. W. (1993) Cutaneous extravascular necrotizing granu-loma (Churg–Strauss syndrome) as a par neoplastic manifestation of non-Hodgkin's B-cell lymphoma. *J. R. Soc. Med.*, **86**, 549–50.

56. Araki, R., Shimi, T., Goto, H. *et al.* (1992) Wegener's granulomatosis with papillary ad-enocarcinoma of the thyroid. *Intern. Med.*, **31**, 1065–8.

57. Greco, F. A., Kolins, J., Rajjoub, R. K. *et al.* (1976) Hodgkins disease and granulomatous angiitis of the central nervous system. *Cancer*, **38**, 2027–32.

58. Boreinstein, D., Costa, M., Jannotta, F. *et al.* (1988) Localised isolated angiitis of the central nervous system associated with primary intracerebral lymphoma. *Cancer*, **62**, 375–80.

59. Haga, H-J., Eide, G. E., Johanssen, A. *et al.* (1993) Cancer in association with polymyalgia rheumatica and temporal arteritis. *J. Rheu-matol.*, **20**, 1335–9.

60. Elkon, K. B., Hughes, G. R. V., Catovsky, D. *et al.* (1979) Hairy cell leukaemia with polyar-teritis nodosa. *Lancet*, **317**, 280–2.

61. Behn, A. and Sykes, H. (1982) Polyarteritis nodosa and hairy cell leukaemia. *Rheumatol. Rehab.*, **21**, 164–6.

62. Krol, T., Robinson, J., Beketis, L. *et al.* (1983) Hairy cell leukaemia and a fatal periarteritis nodosa-like syndrome. *Arch. Pathol. Lab. Med.*, **107**, 583–5.

63. Hammoudeh, M. and Kahn, M. A. (1982) Cranial arteritis as the initial manifestation of malignant histiocytosis. *J. Rheumatol.*, **9**, 445–7.

64. Webster, E., Corman, L. C., Braylan, R. C. (1986) Syndrome of temporal arteritis with perivascular infiltration by malignant cells in a patient with follicular small cell lymphoma. *J. Rheumatol.*, **13**, 1163–6.

65. Longley, S., Caldwell, J. R. and Panush, R. S. (1986) Paraneoplastic vasculitis: unique syn-drome of cutaneous angiitis and arthritis associated with myeloproliferative disorders. *Am. J. Med.*, **80**, 1027–30.

66. O'Shea, J. J., Jaffe, E. S., Lane, H. C. *et al.* (1987) Peripheral T cell lymphoma presenting as hypereosinophilia with vasculitis. *Am. J. Med.*, **82**, 539–45.

67. Delmar, A., Audoin, J. and Rio, B. (1988) Peripheral T cell lymphoma presenting as hypereosinophilia. *Am. J. Med.*, **85**, 565–6.

68. Watson, R. D., Gershwin, M. E., Smithwick, E. *et al.* (1985) Cutaneous T cell lymphoma and leucocytoclastic vasculitis in a long term survivor of the Wiskott–Aldrich syndrome. *Ann. Allergy*, **55**, 654–7.

69. Cransac, M., Vidal, E., Liozon, E. *et al.* (1993) Hodgkins disease revealed by cutaneous vas-culitis: two cases. *Am. J. Med.*, **90**, 53–55.

70. Lacour, J-P., Castanet, J., Perrin, C. *et al.* (1993) Cutaneous leucocytoclastic vasculitis and renal cancer: two cases. *Am. J. Med.*, **94**, 104–8.

71. Callen, J. P. (1987) Cutaneous leucocytoclastic vasculitis in a patient with adenocarcinoma of the colon. *J. Rheumatol.*, **14**, 386–9.

72. Hoag, G. N. (1987) Renal cell carcinoma and vasculitis: a report of 2 cases. *J. Surg. Oncol.*, **35**, 35–8.

73. Garcias, V. A. and Herr, H. (1982) Henoch–Schönlein purpura associated with cancer of prostate. *Urology*, **6**, 155–8.

74. Cairns, S. A., Mallick, N. P., Lawler, W. *et al.* (1978) Squamous cell carcinoma of bronchus presenting with Henoch–Schönlein purpura. *Br. Med. J.*, **2**, 474.

75. Mitchell, D. M. and Hoffbrand, B. I. (1979) Relapse of Henoch–Schönlein disease associ-ated with lung cancer. *J. R. Soc. Med.*, **72**, 614–5.

76. Maurice, T. R. (1978) Carcinoma of bronchus presenting with Henoch-Schönlein purpura. *Br. Med. J.*, **2**, 831.

77. Lewis, J. E. (1990) Urticarial vasculitis occur-ring in association with visceral malignancy. *Acta Dem. Venerol.*, **70**, 345–7.

78. Kulp-Shorten, L., Rhodes, R. H., Peterson, H. *et al.* (1990) Cutaneous vasculitis associated with phaechromocytoma. *Arth. Rheum.*, **33**, 1852–6.

79. Kinlen, L. J. (1985) Incidence of cancer in rheumatoid arthritis and other disorders after immunosuppression. *Am. J. Med.*, **78**, 44–9.

80. Cook, D. J., Bensen, W. G., Carroll, J. J. *et al.* (1988) Giant cell arteritis of the breast. *Can. Med. Assoc. J.*, **139**, 513–5.

81. Noorduyn, L. A., Torenbeck, R., van de Valk, P. *et al.* (1991) Sinonasal non-Hodgkin's lymphomas and Wegener's granulomatosis: a

clinico-pathological study. *Virchow's Arch.* (A), **418**, 235–40.

82. Wintrobe, M. M. and Beuell, M. V. (1933) Hypoproteinaemia associated with multiple myeloma. *Bull. Johns Hopkins Hosp.*, **52**, 156–65.

83. Waldenström, J. (1943) Kliniska metoder for pavisande av hyper-proteinami och deras praktiska varde for diagnostiken. *Nord. Med.*, **20**, 2288–95.

84. Lospalutto, J., Dorvand, B., Miller, W. *et al.* (1962) Cryoglobulinaemia based on interaction between a gamma macroglobulin and 7S gamma globulins. *Am. J. Med.*, **32**, 142–7.

85. Brouet, J. C., Clawvel, J. P., Danon, F. *et al.* (1957) Biological and clinical significance of cryoglobulins. *Am. J. Med.*, **57**, 775–86.

86. Meltzer, M., Franklin, E. C., Elias, K. *et al.* (1966) Cryoglobulinaemia – a clinical and laboratory study. *Am. J. Med.*, **40**, 837–56.

87. Weinberger, A., Berliner, A., Russo, I. *et al.* (1985) X-ray findings of peripheral joints in essential cryoglobulinaemia. *Israeli J. Med. Sci.*, **21**, 529–31.

88. D'amico, G., Colasanti, G., Ferrario, F. *et al.* (1989) Renal involvement in essential mixed cryoglobulinaemia. *Kidney International*, **35**, 1004–14.

89. Cordonnier, D., Vialtel, P., Renversez, J. *et al.* (1985) Renal disease in 18 patients with mixed type II IgM-Igb cryoglobulinaemia. *Adv. Nephrol.*, **12**, 177–204.

90. Frankel, A. H., Singer, D. R., Winnearls, C. G. *et al.* (1992) Type II essential mixed cryoglobulinaemia; presentation, treatment and outcome in 13 patients. *Q. J. Med.*, **82**, 101–24.

91. Gorevic, P. D., Kassab, H. J., Levo, Y. *et al.* (1980) Mixed cryoglobulinaemia: clinical aspects and long term follow up of 40 patients. *Am. J. Med.*, **69**, 287–307.

92. Spertini, F., Donati, Y., Welle, I. *et al.* (1989) Prevention of murine cryoglobulinaemia and associated pathology by monoclonal anti-idiotype antibody. *J. Immunol.*, **143**, 2508–13.

93. Churg, J. and Churg, A. (1989) Idiopathic and secondary vasculitis: a review. *Mod. Pathol.*, **2**, 144–60.

94. Mullich, F. G., Mcallister, H. A., Wagner, B. M. *et al.* (1977) Drug related vasculitis. *Hum. Pathol.*, **10**, 313–25.

95. Mordes, J. P., Johnson, M. W. and Soter, H. A. (1980) Possible Naproxen associated vasculitis. *Arch. Int. Med.*, **145**, 985.

96. Rosenberg, J. M., Edlow, D. E. and Sneider, R. (1978) Liver disease and vasculitis in a patient taking Cromolyn. *Arch. Int. Med.*, **138**, 989–9.

97. Weiss, E. B., Forman, P. and Rosenthal, I. M. (1978) Allopurinol induced arteritis in HGPRT ase deficiency. *Arch. Int. Med.*, **138**, 1743–4.

98. Dubost, J-J., Souteyrand, P. and Sauvezie, B. (1991) Drug induced vasculitis. *Bailliere; Clin. Rheumatol.*, **5**, 119–138.

99. Epstein, E. H., McNutt, N. S., Beallo, R., *et al.* (1987) Severe vasculitis during isotretinoin therapy. *Arch. Dermatol.*, **123**, 1123–5.

100. Hammond, E. H., Watson, F. S., Bristow, M. R. *et al.* (1990) Fibrinoid necrosis of a temporal artery complicating the treatment of retractory cardiac alograft rejection with murine mono-clonal CD3 antibody (OKT3). *J. Heart Transplant*, **9**, 236–8.

101. Phanuphak, P. and Kohler, P. F. (1980) Onset of polyarteritis nodosa during allergic hyposensitization treatment. *Am. J. Med.*, **68**, 479–85.

102. Mader, R., Navendran, A., Lewtas, J. *et al.* (1993) Systemic vasculitis following influenza vaccination – report of 3 cases and literature review. *J. Rheumatol.*, **20**, 1429–1431.

103. Castresana-Isla, C., Herrera-Martinez, G. and Vega-Moline, J. (1993) Erythema nodosum and Takayasu's arteritis after immunization with plasma derived hepatitis B vaccine. *J. Rheumatol.*, **20**, 1417–18.

104. Citron, B. P., Halpern, M., McCarron, M. *et al.* (1970) Necrotizing angiitis associated with drug abuse. *N. Eng. J. Med.*, 1003–11.

105. Kaye, B. R. and Fainstat, M. (1987) Cerebral vasaculitis associated with cocaine abuse. *JAMA*, **258**, 2104–6.

106. King, J., Richards, M. and Tress, B. (1978) Cerebral arteritis associated with heroin abuse. *Med. J. Aust.*, **2**, 444–5.

107. Fallis, R. J. and Fisher, M. (1985) Cerebral vasculitis and haemorrhage associated with phenylpropanolamine. *Neurology*, **35**, 455–7.

108. Wootes, M. R., Khangure, M. S. and Murphy, M. J. (1983) Intracranial haemorrhage and vasculitis related to ephedrine abusage. *Ann. Neurol.*, **13**, 337–40.

109. Loizou, L. A., Hamilton, J. G. and Tsementzio, S. A. (1982) Intracranial haemorrhage in association with pseudoephedrine overdosage. *J. Neurol. Neurosurg. Neuropsych.*, **45**, 471–2.

110. Fredericks, R. K., Leftkovitz, D. S., Challs, U.

R. *et al.* (1991) Cerebral vasculitis associated with cocaine abuse. *Stroke*, **22**, 1437–9.

111. Krendal, D. A., Ditter, S. M., Frankel, M. R. *et al.* (1990) Biopsy proven cerebral vasculitis associated with cocaine abuse. *Neurology*, **40**, 1092–4.

112. Dixon, F. J. (1963) The role of antigen-antibody complexes in disease. *Harvey Lecture*, **58**, 21–52.

113. Bielory, L., Gascon, P., Lawley, T. J. *et al.* (1988) Human serum sickness: a prospective analysis of 35 patients treated with equine anti-thymocyte globulins for bone marrow failure. *Medicine*, **67**, 40–57.

114. Isaacs, J. D. (1990) The antiglobulin response to therapeutic antibodies. *Semin. Immunol.*, **2**, 449–56.

115. Watts, R. A. and Isaacs, J. D. (1992) Immuno-therapy of rheumatoid arthritis. *Ann. Rheum. Dis.*, **51**, 577–9.

116. Cosimi, A. B. (1978) Clinical development of orthoclone OKT3. *Transplant Proc.*, **19** (Supp 11), 7–16.

117. O'Connell, J. B., Rebund, D. G., Gay, W. A. *et al.* (1989) Efficacy of OKT3 retreatment for refractory cardiac allograft rejection. *Transplantation*, **47**, 788–92.

118. Isaacs, J. D., Watts, R. A., Hazleman, B. L. *et al.* (1992) Humanized monoclonal antibody therapy for rheumatoid arthritis. *Lancet*, **340**, 748–52.

119. Davidson, J. R., Bush, B. K., Grogon, E. W. *et al.* (1988) Immunology of a serum sickness/vasculitis reaction secondary to streptokinase used for acute myocardial infarction. *Clin. Exp. Rheum.*, **6**, 381–4.

120. Bucknall, C., Darley, C., Flax, J. *et al.* (1988) Vasculitis complicating treatment with intravenous anisoylated plasminogen streptokinase activator complex in acute myocardial infarction. *Br. Heart J.*, **59**, 9–11.

121. McDuffie, F. C., Sams, W. M., Maldonado, J. E. *et al.* Hypocomplementaemia with cutaneous vasculitis and arthritis. Possible immune complex syndrome. *Mayo Clin. Proc.*, **48**, 340–8.

122. Sissons, J. C. P., Williams, D. G., Peters, D. K. *et al.* (1974) Skin lesions, angioderma and hypocomplementaemia. *Lancet*, **2**, 1350–2.

123. Sanchez, N. P., Winkelmann, R. K., Schroeter, A. L. *et al.* (1982) The clinical and histopathologic spectrums of urticarial vasculitis: study of 40 cases. *J. Am. Acad. Dermatol.*, **7**, 599–605.

124. Mehregan, D. R., Hall, M. J. and Gibson, C. E. (1992) Urticarial vasculitis: a histopathological and clinical review of 72 cases. *J. Am. Acad. Dermatol.*, **26**, 441–8.

125. O'Loughlin, S., Schroeter, A. L. and Jordan, R. E. (1978) Chronic urticaria-like lesions in SLE. *Arch. Dermatol.*, **114**, 879–83.

126. Matarredona, J., Sendagorta, E., Rocamon, A. *et al.* (1986) Systemic lupus erythematosus appearing as urticarial vasculitis. *Int. J. Dermatol.*, **25**, 446–8.

127. Berg, R. E., Kantor, G. R. and Bergfeld, W. F. (1988) Urticarial vasculitis. *Int. J. Dermatol.*, **27**, 468–72.

128. Gammon, W. R. (1985) Urticarial vasculitis. *Dermatol. Clin.*, **3**, 97–105.

129. Borrodon, L., Rybojad, M., Puissant, A. *et al.* (1990) Urticarial vasculitis associated with monoclonal IgM gammopathy: Schnitzler's syndrome. *Br. J. Dermatol.*, **123**, 113–8.

130. Highet, A. S. (1980) Urticarial vasculitis and IgA myeloma. *Br. J. Dermatol.*, **102**, 355–7.

131. Jones, R. R., Bhogal, B., Dash, A. *et al.* (1985) Urticaria and vasculitis: a continuum of histological and immunopathological changes. *Br. J. Dermatol.*, **108**, 695–703.

132. Marder, R. J., Rent, R., Choi, E. Y. C. *et al.* (1976) C1q deficiency associated with urticarial lesions and cutaneous vasculitis. *Am. J. Med.*, **61**, 560–5.

133. Wisneski, J. J. and Jones, S. M. (1992) Comparison of autoantibodies to the collagen-like region of C1q in hypocomplementemic vasculitis syndrome and systemic lupus erythematosus. *J. Immunol.*, **148**, 1396–403.

134. Asherson, R. A. and Sontheimer, R. (1991) Urticarial vasculitis and syndromes in association with connective tissue diseases. *Ann. Rheum. Dis.*, **50**, 743–4.

135. Millns, J. L., Randle, H. W., Solley, G. O. *et al.* (1980) The therapeutic response of urticarial vasculitis to indomethacin. *J. Am. Acad. Dermatol.*, **3**, 349–50.

136. Behçet, H. (1940) Some observations on the clinical picture of the so-called triple symptom complex. *Dermatologica*, **81**, 73–8.

137. International study group of Behçet's disease. (1990) *Lancet*, **335**, 1078–80.

138. Lie, J. T. (1992) Vascular involvement in Behçet's disease: arterial and venous and vessels of all sizes. *J. Rheumatol.*, **19**, 341–3.

139. Koc, Y., Gullu, J., Akpek, G. *et al.* (1992) Vascular involvement in Behcet's disease. *J. Rheumatol.*, **19**, 402–10.

140. The Behçet's disease research committee at Japan (1989) Skin hypersensitivity to streptococcal antigens and the induction of systemic symptoms by the antigens in Behçet's disease. *J. Rheumatol.*, **15**, 506–11.

141. Suzuki, Y., Hoshi, K., Matsula, T. *et al.* (1992) Increased peripheral blood gamma-delta T cells and natural killer cells in Behçet's disease. *J. Rheumatol.*, **19**, 588–92.

142. Busch, G. J., Garovaz, M. R. and Tilney, N. C. (1979) Variant forms of arteritis in human renal allografts. *Transplant Proc.*, **11**, 100–3.

143. Busch, G. J., Galvanek, E. G. and Reynolds, E. S. (1971) Human renal allografts. Analysis of lesions in long term survivors. *Hum. Pathol.*, **2**, 253–98.

144. Kincaid-Smith, P. (1967) Histological diagnosis of rejections of renal allografts in man. *Lancet*, **2**, 849–52.

145. Lie, J. T. (1992) Cholesterol atheromatous embolism: the great masquerader revisited. *Pathol. Annu.*, **27**, 17–50.

146. Ramirez, G., O'Neill, W. M., Lambert, R. *et al.* (1978) Cholesterol embolization. A complication of angiography. *Arch. Intern. Med.*, **138**, 1430–2.

147. Cappiello, R. A., Espinoza, L. R., Adelman, H. *et al.* (1989) Cholesterol embolism: A pseudovasculitic syndrome. *Semin. Arth. Rheum.* **18**, 240–6.

148. Leonhardt, E. T. G. and Kullenberg, K. P. G. (1977) Bilateral myxomas with multiple arterial aneurysms: a syndrome mimicking poly-arteritis nodosa. *Am. J. Med.*, **62**, 792–4.

149. Buchanan, R. R. C., Cairns, J. C., Knagg, S. *et al.* (1979) Left atrial myxoma mimicking vasculitis; echocardiographic diagnosis. *Can. Med. Assoc. J.*, **120**, 1540–2.

150. Boussen, K., Mualla, M., Blondeau, P. *et al.* (1991) Embolisation of cardiac myxoma masquerading as polyarteritis nodosa. *J. Rheumatol.*, **18**, 283–5.

151. Price, D. L., Harris, J. L., Nes, P. F. J. *et al.* (1970) Cardiac myxoma: a clinicopathologic and angiographic study. *Arch. Neurol.*, **23**, 558–67.

152. Lie, J. T. (1989) Vasculopathy in the antiphospholipid antibody syndrome: thrombosis or vasculitis or both. *J. Rheumatol.*, **16**, 713–15.

153. Harris, E. N., Gharavi, A. E. and Hughes, G. R. V. (1985) Antiphospholipid antibodies. *Clinic. Rheum. Dis.*, **11**, 591–609.

154. Mackworth-Young, C. G., Loizou, S. and Walport, M. J. (1989) Antiphospholipid antibodies and disease. *Q. J. Med.*, **72**, 767–77.

155. Greisman, S. G., Thayaparan, R. S., Godwin, T. A. *et al.* (1991) Occlusive vasculopathy in systemic lupus erythematosus; association with anticardiolipin antibody. *Arch. Intern. Med.*, **III**, 389–92.

156. Smith, K. J., Skelton, H. G., James, W. D. *et al.* (1990) Cutaneous histopathologic findings in 'antiphospholipid syndrome'. *Arch. Dermatol.*, **126**, 1176–83.

157. Travis, W. D., Carpenter, H. A. and Lie, J. T. (1989) Capillaritis and pulmonary haemorrhage in Wegener's granulomatosis. *Am. J. Surg. Pathol.*, **13**, 78–9.

158. Magnat, G., Kerven, K. S. and Gabriel, D. A. (1989) The clinical manifestation of Degos' syndrome. *Arch. Pathol. Lab. Med.*, **113**, 354–62.

159. Sweet, R. D. (1964) An acute febrile neutrophilic dermatosis. *Br. J. Dermatol.*, **76**, 349–56.

160. Gassman, A. (1899) Zur histologie der Roentgenuclere. *Fortschr Geb Rontgent Nuklearmed Ergonzungsband*, **2**, 199–207.

161. Fonkalstud, R. A., Sanchez, R., Zerubavel, R. *et al.* (1977) Serial changes in arterial structure following radiation therapy. *Surg. Gunecol. Oncol.*, **145**, 395–430.

162. Butler, M. J., Lane, R. S. and Webster, J. H. H. (1980) Irradiation injury to large arteries. *Br. J. Surg.*, **67**, 341–3.

163. McCready, R. A., Hyde, G. L., Bivins, B. A. *et al.* (1983) Radiation induced arterial injuries. *Surgery*, **93**, 306–12.

164. Magee, R. (1991) Saint Anthony's fire revisited: vascular problems associated with migraine medication. *Med. J. Aust.*, **154**, 145–9.

POLYMYALGIA RHEUMATICA AND GIANT CELL ARTERITIS

10

J. K. Rao and N. B. Allen

INTRODUCTION

Temporal arteritis and polymyalgia rheumatica are two rheumatologic conditions frequently seen in older individuals. Temporal arteritis (TA) is a systemic granulomatous vasculitis that predominantly affects large- and medium-sized blood vessels and generally involves the cranial branches of the aorta. This disease, most often seen in patients over 50 years of age, is an important preventable cause of blindness. However, it has long been recognized that temporal arteritis is a disease with protean manifestations, and extracranial presentations are not uncommon. Common synonyms for temporal arteritis include cranial arteritis, Horton's disease, granulomatous arteritis, and giant cell arteritis. One of these diagnostic terms, giant cell arteritis, also describes the characteristic pathologic lesion of Takayasu's arteritis, a granulomatous vasculitis of large blood vessels which occurs predominantly in young women. For the purposes of this chapter, the term 'temporal arteritis' will be used to denote a granulomatous vasculitis that affects older individuals.

Classically considered as related ends of a clinical spectrum, some patients with polymyalgia rheumatica (PMR) may later develop symptoms of temporal arteritis. The exact relationship between these two diseases is not entirely clear because usually only patients with symptoms of ocular ischemia will undergo a temporal artery biopsy. In addition, patients with temporal arteritis may initially present with PMR-like symptoms. As a defined pathologic lesion does not exist for polymyalgia rheumatica, the diagnosis is usually made on the basis of clinical and laboratory evidence. This disease is characterized by aching and proximal muscle stiffness lasting longer than four weeks in association with an elevated erythrocyte sedimentation rate, and a prompt response to low-dose corticosteroids. Recent clinical studies have shown that a low-grade axial synovitis, rather than actual muscle inflammation, may be the primary cause of these symptoms. Because some patients experience progressive peripheral synovitis, certain authors believe that polymyalgia rheumatica may be a harbinger of rheumatoid arthritis or systemic lupus erythematosus of the elderly.

Our understanding of temporal arteritis and polymyalgia rheumatica, in terms of epidemiology, classification, clinical presentation, pathophysiology and treatment continues to improve with data from multiple clinical studies and reports. Both diseases should be considered in the differential diagnosis of older patients with an elevated erythrocyte sedimentation rate of unknown etiology. In this chapter, clinical aspects, as

Connective Tissue Diseases. Edited by Jill J. F. Belch and Robert B. Zurier. Published in 1995 by Chapman & Hall, London. ISBN 0 412 48620 2

well as the management of both diseases, are discussed in detail.

HISTORICAL PERSPECTIVE

While ancient hieroglyphics found on the tomb of Pa-Aton-Em-Heb (1350 BC, the 18th dynasty) may represent the earliest pictorial description of temporal arteritis, the writings of Ala Ibn Isa (AD 1000) first documented the relationship between inflamed temporal muscles and visual loss[1,2]. In 1890, Hutchinson reported the disease in the medical literature by describing an octogenarian whose inflamed, tender and subsequently pulseless temporal arteries prevented him from wearing a hat[3]. Horton and colleagues found granulomatous inflammation on temporal artery biopsies in two patients with symptoms of headaches, tender scalp and painful nodules of the temporal artery[4]. At the time of this initial publication, Horton was reluctant to attach a specific name to this interesting syndrome of 'localized periarteritis'. In a separate publication, Horton and colleagues discussed the clinical manifestations of this disease in a series of seven patients, concluding that symptoms of headache, anorexia, fevers, malaise, night sweats and weight loss were common[5]. Because all patients recovered without loss of sight, this syndrome was originally thought to be a benign and self-limited disease[5,6].

However, Jennings noted the systemic and relapsing nature of temporal arteritis, first documenting blindness as a disease complication, an outcome separately confirmed by Cooke[7,8]. In 1941, Gilmour coined the term 'giant cell arteritis' to describe the pathologic lesion found on the temporal artery biopsies[9]. With the discovery of corticosteroids, Birkhead demonstrated that this therapy was effective in decreasing the incidence of bilateral blindness in patients from 17 to 9%[10]. In this study, patients with pre-therapy blindness did not recover their visual acuity[10].

Thus, because of the documented risk of blindness with this disease, temporal arteritis is now commonly considered a medical emergency.

Like temporal arteritis, early pictorial descriptions of polymyalgia rheumatica exist in the paintings of the Dutch masters of the fifteenth century[2]. In 1888, Bruce, a Scottish physician, made the first report in the medical literature in describing five elderly patients with severe muscular pains that spontaneously resolved over one to two years[11]. The disease was named 'senile rheumatic gout' to make the distinction from acute rheumatism and gout[11]. In the 1940s and 1950s, this syndrome was denoted by several names, including periarthrosis humeroscapularis, peri-extra-articular rheumatism, myalgic syndrome of the elderly with systemic reaction, anarthritic rheumatoid disease, polymyalgia arteritica and rhizomelic inflammatory rheumatism of the aged[12,13]. Whether this symptom complex represented a separate rheumatic disease remained a point of controversy in the medical literature for several years.

This affliction of myalgias with constitutional symptoms was finally given its name, 'polymyalgia rheumatica' by Barber[14]. Barber also noted that patients with this disease were often thought to suffer from a psychoneurosis until an erythrocyte sedimentation rate was checked, thus confirming an association first documented in 1945[1,14]. Paulley described a connection between polymyalgia rheumatica and temporal arteritis in 1956; however, the exact nature of this relationship still remains the subject of debate[15]. Estimates of the incidence of temporal arteritis in patients with PMR range from 15–78%, likely reflecting differences in diagnostic criteria for both diseases[13,16]. In addition, as 'blind' biopsies are usually not clinically indicated or feasible, the true rate of 'occult' arteritis is unknown in polymyalgia rheumatica as only the symptomatic patients typically undergo this procedure.

EPIDEMIOLOGY

Among the systemic vasculitides, temporal arteritis is one of the more common entities although, in actuality, it is a relatively rare disease. A complete understanding of the epidemiology and patient outcome has been hampered by the low incidence of disease, different classification schemes and overlapping presentations with other forms of vasculitis and with polymyalgia rheumatica. Conversely, the true incidence of polymyalgia rheumatica is also not well understood. In many studies, patients with PMR are often classified with temporal arteritis as both diseases can have similar features initially. Retrospective case series data have broadened our knowledge of both diseases and raised interesting hypotheses for further studies in disease classification, causative factors and patient outcome.

Our best understanding of the incidence and prevalence of temporal arteritis comes from epidemiologic studies carried out in Olmsted County, Minnesota, from 1950–85. In Olmsted County, the estimated overall incidence rate in persons older than 50 years of age was 17.0 cases/100 000/year, and the age- and sex-adjusted prevalence was 223/100 000[17]. In Denmark, from 1982–5, the overall incidence and prevalence of temporal arteritis was estimated to be 76.6/100 000/year and 37.8/100 000, respectively, in persons aged 50 years or older[18]. Both series appear to show a higher incidence rate for persons of Northern European descent living in the northern hemisphere than is observed in studies from other regions of the world. Lower incidence rates of 1.58/100 000 and 6/100 000 in persons over the age of 50 in Shelby County, Tennessee, and Lugo, Spain, respectively, appear to reflect this notion [19,20]. It is important to note, however, that cases of temporal arteritis have been documented in Blacks, Hispanics and Orientals[21–24]. Interestingly, these patients had similar symptoms to those of White patients, but were frequently biopsied at a more advanced stage of disease when jaw claudication or visual loss had occurred[21]. Thus, it is important to consider this diagnosis in patients with compatible symptoms, regardless of ethnic background.

A 3 to 5 times higher incidence rate for females than for males is demonstrated in several studies, and the incidence increases with each decade as individuals reach 80+ years of age[17,18,25]. In one study, there was an increased incidence of temporal artery biopsies in women, indicating a possible detection bias[17,26]. Various potential risk factors for disease, including age, sex, socioeconomic factors, smoking, Quetelet index (body mass index) and comorbid illness have been examined, and only smoking was associated with a significant risk[26]. An increased risk of disease was also noted with atherosclerotic disease in general, but because the study had limited statistical power, further studies are needed to determine if these elevated risks are truly significant. Interestingly, although the disease affects the vascular system, several studies have shown no difference in the long-term survival of these patients[25,27,28].

Polymyalgia rheumatica is more common than temporal arteritis, but these two diseases are sometimes seen simultaneously, thus confusing the true estimates of the former. Estimates of the incidence and prevalence of this disease come from the data of several retrospective case series. In Olmsted County, Minnesota, from 1970–9, the calculated overall average incidence rate was 53.7/100 000/year for persons aged 50 years or older and 11.1/100 000 for the total population[29]. The prevalence was estimated to be 442/100 000/year, including the active cases as well as those cases in remission[29]. Incidence rates in persons 50 years or older residing in other regions of the world range from 68.3/100 000/year in Ribe County, Denmark (1982–5) to 12.7/100 000/year in Reggio Emilio, Italy [18,30,31]. Polymyalgia rheumatica rarely affects persons less than 40 years old, and the median age at disease onset is approximately 70 years of age[32]. Several studies document a 1.5 to 2 times higher incidence rate for females than for males, which is present in each decade of life[29,33]. Finally, like temporal arteritis, PMR has been observed in patients of non-Caucasian backgrounds[34]. Long considered a self-limited and benign disease, polymyalgia rheumatica has no significant effect on patient survival[29,35].

ETIOLOGY/PATHOGENESIS

Researchers continue to search for a cause of both temporal arteritis and polymyalgia rheumatica. Environmental and genetic factors are frequently implicated as important factors in disease expression. With several epidemiologic studies showing a higher incidence of temporal arteritis for inhabitants of the northern latitudes compared to the southern latitudes, the importance of environmental factors, such sunlight exposure, becomes an attractive theory[17–19]. Those who believe in the 'actinic hypothesis' speculate that solar radiation plays a role in the alteration or degeneration of the elastic lamina, resulting in inflammation of the temporal artery[36]. However, if this theory were true, a higher incidence of disease in the southern latitudes as well as a seasonal variation of rates would be expected[36]. It has also been speculated that differences in the indigenous populations of birds and infectious agents in various regions of the world may play an important role in determining who develops this disease. However, the search for a causative factor has been unsuccessful thus far.

Temporal arteritis has been reported to occur in married couples, siblings and twins[37,38]. While conjugal cases of temporal arteritis imply the importance of environmental factors, the familial cases demonstrate that genetic factors may also play a significant role. Several reports address the role of genetic factors, and show an association between the HLA-DR4 haplotype and temporal arteritis[38,39]. Further studies on affected sibling pairs is expected to reveal insights into the role of genetic factors in disease expression. While Caucasians have a higher expression of HLA-DR4, it is important to note that temporal arteritis has occurred in patients of other ethnic origins with a lower expression of this HLA haplotype[34].

Like temporal arteritis, a seasonal trend in incidence has not been observed in polymyalgia rheumatica[29]. Genetic factors are commonly thought to have a significant role as the disease largely affects females, and familial cases have also been reported in the literature. The frequent association of the HLA-DR4 haplotype with polymyalgia rheumatica is also supportive of this relationship, which may be stronger than that between temporal arteritis and HLA-DR4[39]. There appears to be a predilection for the Caucasian race, which is supported by the lower rates of disease in Blacks in whom HLA-DR4 is less common[34]. Studies performed in Reggio, Italy, show a lower rate of HLA-DR4 positivity in association with a lower incidence of disease[30]. The contribution of genetic factors is also reinforced by the higher incidence rates in females.

Cellular and humoral immunity have been implicated as possible pathogenic factors in both diseases, and their ultimate role has yet to be determined. Circulating lymphoblasts and altered cytotoxic/suppressor T-cell ratios have been observed in polymyalgia rheumatica[32,40]. Immune deposits have been found in the arterial walls of temporal artery biopsies, and circulating immune complexes have been found in the peripheral blood of some patients[41,42]. In a recent study of patients with polymyalgia rheumatica and temporal arteritis prior to treatment, it was found that these patients had elevated circulating interleukin-6 compared to normal controls[43]. These levels normalized after prolonged corticosteroid therapy, and may represent a method to monitor efficacy of treatment.

Antiphospholipid antibodies and factor VIII von Willebrand factor antigen (VWF) have been demonstrated in both diseases, leading to some interesting theories of the pathogenic role of these factors. It has been speculated that antiphospholipid antibodies may induce thrombotic events to occur, resulting in ischemic optic neuropathy and other severe vascular complications[44,45]. In studies of VWF, it was found that the levels were the highest in patients with temporal arteritis, with a correlation between titers and disease activity, while patients with both diseases had intermediate levels and those with PMR alone had the lowest levels[46]. Because VWF is produced in endothelial cells and can be seen early in the disease process, its presence in patients with polymyalgia rheumatica may be indicative of impending temporal arteritis. As our knowledge of cellular and humoral immunity continues to grow, the understanding of the role of these factors in temporal arteritis and polymyalgia rheumatica will improve.

CLINICAL PRESENTATION

Temporal arteritis may present abruptly or insidiously, and it is the latter presentation which can lead to a delay in diagnosis. While headaches and sudden blindness are the classical symptoms associated with this disease, vague constitutional symptoms, such as fever, weakness, anorexia, malaise, myalgias and fatigue, may be the earliest manifestations[8,47]. Approximately 10–15% will initially present with fever of unknown origin as a primary symptom[48–50]. The fevers may be low grade or occasionally high as 104°F with associated night sweats in some[6,8,51]. Others may exhibit depression, confusion or psychosis, which is often incorrectly attributed to dementia or the aging process-[15,52,53]. In two retrospective studies of patients with biopsy-proven temporal arteritis, nearly 40% of individuals presented with

Table 10.1   Symptoms of temporal arteritis

Constitutional: fevers, anorexia, weight loss, fatigue, malaise
HEENT*: headache (occipital, frontal, temples), jaw claudication, tongue claudication, visual disturbance (diplopia, amaurosis fugax, blindness), dysphagia, throat pain, hearing loss, tinnitus
Peripheral vascular: extremity claudication, decreased pulses, Raynaud's phenomenon
Cardiopulmonary: congestive heart failure, myocardial infarction and arrhythmias, myocarditis, pericarditis, angina
Gastrointestinal/renal: bowel infarction, hepatitis, gastrointestinal bleeding, hematuria
Musculoskeletal: arthralgias, myalgias, morning stiffness
Neurologic: transient ischemic attacks (carotid, vertebrobasilar), stroke, cranial neuropathy, peripheral neuropathy, mononeuropathy, seizure, vertigo
Psychiatric: organic/affective disorder, dementia, visual hallucinations, confusion

HEENT: head, eyes, ears, nose, throat.

'masked' or unusual symptoms of temporal arteritis[48,54]. Approximately 50% of patients with temporal arteritis will have symptoms of polymyalgia rheumatica[25,55]. These symptoms of myalgias and arthralgias may actually mask 'occult' temporal arteritis, and may ultimately cause a delay in the diagnosis until a visual or vascular obliterative event has occurred. Thus, it is important to consider this diagnosis when evaluating elderly patients who have symptoms of fever, fatigue or weight loss of indeterminate etiology.

The general pattern of involvement in this disease includes large- and medium-sized arteries, and symptoms are usually referable to the involved branches of the internal and external carotid artery (Table 10.1). The ophthalmic and posterior ciliary branches of the internal carotid artery are commonly affected, but the superficial temporal, maxillary, lingual, occipital and facial branches of the external carotid artery can also be involved[47]. Widespread arterial inflammation of the aortic arch, coronary arteries, mesenteric and renal circulation has also been reported in this disease[47,56–58]. As the arteries become inflamed, there is gradual occlusion and loss of the pulse.

Headaches are a typical complaint, and may be localized to the region of the superficial temporal arteries or generalized, resembling a tension headache. While 77% had headache as a clinical manifestation in the Olmsted County study, this symptom is considered a relatively nonspecific finding[17]. Descriptions of the headaches range from sharp and lancinating to a dull, continuous pain that radiates to the neck, occiput, face and/or jaw. Scalp tenderness can also be a prominent feature, and some individuals experience difficulty when wearing a hat, combing their hair or laying upon a pillow. This symptom, which is secondary to involvement of the superficial temporal and occipital arteries, may cause a sleep disturbance in these patients[8,53].

Jaw claudication, like headache and scalp tenderness, has historically been considered a pathognomonic sign of temporal arteritis, and has been observed in approximately 50% of cases[17,47]. However, patients with other diseases, such as Wegener's granulomatosis, classic polyarteritis nodosa and systemic amyloidosis, can have this same complaint[59,60]. Jaw claudication results from facial and maxillary artery involvement, which induces ischemia to the muscles of mastication. Patients will often complain of pain when chewing foods of a firm consistency, particularly meat. Involvement of the occipital and lingual arteries can manifest as retroauricular pain and a loss of taste sensation, respectively[6]. A chronic sore throat, dysphagia and tongue claudication have also been described and, rarely, this disease can result in glossitis and tongue necrosis[61–63]. Any of these symptoms can contribute to weight loss in patients.

According to several series, some degree of permanent or temporary visual loss occurs in approximately 15% of individuals, and these rates are in sharp contrast to earlier series which showed an incidence of visual impairment before treatment approaching nearly 40%[10,17,25,64,65]. True blindness occurs in 1% of patients, although this complication is expected to continue to decrease with better awareness of the disease. Sudden visual loss, either partial or complete, is a consequence of narrowing or occlusion of the ophthalmic or posterior ciliary arteries. Once this catastrophic event occurs, it is irreversible, even with corticosteroid therapy[10]. Blindness, which can be unilateral or bilateral, may be preceded by transient symptoms of visual blurring, diplopia or amaurosis fugax. Patients who develop blindness will often have had 2–5 months of non-visual symptoms, such as arthralgias or headaches, prior to this dreaded event[47,66].

The posterior ciliary artery is most commonly affected by the disease, followed by involvement of the ophthalmic and retinal arteries[64]. Another under-reported manifestation is the ocular ischemic syndrome, caused by a decreased perfusion to the optic nerve or retina[67]. Symptoms of this steroid-responsive event include corneal edema and uveitis in addition to visual loss[67]. Thus, temporal arteritis can have other visual symptoms, such as uveitis, amaurosis fugax or diplopia, and it is important to recognize these premonitory signs of temporal arteritis before blindness occurs. In Birkhead's study, improvement of pre-therapy visual symptoms, short of blindness, occurred in only 43% with treatment[10].

Arteritis of the large vessels, causing claudication of the extremities and Raynaud's phenomenon, occurs in approximately 10% of patients[57,68,69]. Clinical improvement of claudication and a gradual return of pulses occurs with steroid therapy in the majority of patients[68]. Cardiac manifestations of the disease include congestive heart failure, granulomatous myocarditis and pericarditis[63,70]. A few reports of patients with vasculitis of the coronary arteries, aortic aneurysms and aortitis in association with temporal arteritis are in the literature[58]. Some of these entities can be easily missed without a high index of suspicion and often have a fatal outcome if untreated. Thus, every patient with suspected or proven temporal arteritis should be examined carefully for the presence of large vessel disease.

Pulmonary involvement has been demonstrated in temporal arteritis. Respiratory symptoms have been a presenting symptom in approximately 4% of individuals[71]. Chronic hoarseness and a nonproductive cough are problems experienced by some individuals[71]. A sore throat that involves the entire anterior portion of the neck in addition to the oropharynx is also not uncommon. Other more serious manifestations can include pleural effusions, pulmonary nodules, interstitial pulmonary edema as well as pulmonary artery vasculitis[63,72,73]. Biopsies of the lung nodules may show necrosis and granulomatous inflammation involving the blood vessels and bronchioles[74]. This picture may be difficult to distinguish from limited Wegener's granulomatosis. Conversely, there have been reports of patients with Wegener's granulomatosis, who initially were thought to have temporal arteritis and even had vasculitis on temporal artery biopsy[75–77].

Renal involvement is not often described, likely because kidney biopsies are not generally performed in these patients. Microscopic hematuria and red cell casts have been demonstrated in some individuals with the disease, and biopsies have demonstrated focal glomerulonephritis, with or without crescents, or vasculitis involving the renal arterioles and small arteries[57,63,78,79]. These abnormalities typically resolve if treated promptly. Proteinuria and elevated serum creatinine has been described in those with more disseminated giant cell vasculitis. This clinical scenario can be difficult to differentiate from a systemic necrotizing vasculitis of medium-sized vessels.

Symptoms of nausea, fatigue and anorexia may result from liver inflammation[63]. Gastrointestinal hemorrhage and small bowel infarction have also been reported[80]. Dermatologic findings are usually limited to nodules and erythema overlying the involved artery. Other skin lesions, such as gangrene, purpura and ulcers, are unusual, but have been seen in a few patients[6,81]. Granulomatous vasculitis of the skin has been described in the literature, but is a rare phenomenon[81].

The neurologic findings can be diverse and include a sensorineural hearing loss, carpal tunnel syndrome, vertigo and stroke. Some individuals have presented with hearing loss or vertigo as an initial manifestation[61]. Classically thought to be strictly an extracranial process, autopsy studies have shown that intracranial vessels can also be affected by this disease[82,83]. Vasculitis of the vertebrobasilar system or the circle of Willis can cause hemorrhages or transient ischemic attacks [52,84]. Although an uncommon event, some patients may sustain an embolic cerebral infarction of the brain stem in association with temporal arteritis; this event is thought to be caused by thrombus formation around the site of inflammation of the vertebral arteries proximal to its penetration of the dura[56].

Synovitis has been detected in approximately 15% of patients with temporal arteritis, and many persons complain of diffuse arthralgias and myalgias[85]. The affected joints include the knees, shoulders and hips. Effusions, if present, are mildly inflammatory and transient. Temporal arteritis has occurred in patients with seropositive rheumatoid arthritis[85,86]. If symptoms of the former are vague and nonspecific, then jaw claudication or occipital headaches in these patients may be incorrectly attributed to the rheumatoid arthritis, leading to a delay in the ultimate diagnosis.

Like temporal arteritis, polymyalgia rheumatica may begin abruptly or insidiously, and fevers, anorexia and malaise are typical early symptoms. Frequently, severe morning stiffness that improves during the day is a prominent feature with a dramatic onset in many individuals[32]. Patients may actually remember the day that their symptoms began. A second major component of the syndrome includes severe pain and limitation of the proximal muscles. The physician may elicit a history of patient difficulty in going upstairs, arising from a chair and raising the arms over the head. These symptoms are initially due more to pain and stiffness than to true muscle weakness. The shoulders are most commonly affected followed by the proximal portions of the thighs, hip and neck[40]. Nearly 100% of patients have involvement of the proximal arm muscles, and there may be discomfort on minor movement, often along with a sleep disturbance[16,29]. In some cases, the symptoms are of such severity that a previously healthy and active individual can become bedridden. In these rare instances, disuse atrophy of the muscles can result. While patients with polymyalgia rheumatica often localize their symptoms to the muscles and muscular attachments, there may be actual involvement of the peripheral joints with synovitis and effusions[87,88]. Transient synovitis occurs in approximately 15–30%[33,89]. The knees and shoulders are typically affected and the synovitis usually resolves with low-dose corticosteroid therapy.

Inflammatory conditions, such as rheumatoid arthritis, Wegener's granulomatosis and systemic lupus erythematosus, deserve special mention as a polymyalgia rheumatica-like onset of these diseases in the elderly is now well recognized[32,90–92]. Systemic lupus erythematosus may manifest in older individuals as arthralgias, myalgias, fevers and weight loss. Patients who develop rheumatoid arthritis after 60 years of age often first have symptoms similar to polymyalgia rheumatica. Certain authors believe that seronegative rheumatoid arthritis of the elderly and polymyalgia rheumatica may be the same entity. Unlike younger patients with rheumatoid arthritis, there is a lower frequency of positive rheumatoid factor and a higher frequency of shoulder, wrist and knee involvement in this group[93]. However, like polymyalgia rheumatica, the outcome in these older patients is often favorable with symptoms controlled by low-dose corticosteroids without progression to joint deformity or radiographic erosions[93]. It is not uncommon for patients with both of these inflammatory conditions to be first diagnosed with polymyalgia rheumatica.

As previously stated, constitutional symptoms of fever, anorexia, malaise, night sweats and weight loss are common, but rash, oral ulcers or systemic symptoms of vascular involvement are rare without an associated vasculitis. Low-grade fevers of 100–101°F were observed in 13% of patients with polymyalgia rheumatica, while high spiking fevers with sweats may be indicative of associated temporal arteritis or a septic process[29,32]. As in the case of temporal arteritis, these nonspecific symptoms may predate the onset of the musculoskeletal symptoms by several weeks. Jaw claudication, visual symptoms and headaches can also occur with associated temporal arteritis, and patients should be examined carefully to detect these often subtle signs.

DIFFERENTIAL DIAGNOSIS

In patients with suspected temporal arteritis and polymyalgia rheumatica, a thoughtful approach is indicated as the differential diagnosis encompasses a wide range of diseases in which steroid treatment may actually be contraindicated. For this reason, empiric steroid therapy is discouraged without a thorough evaluation of the patient to rule out other etiologies that may present with similar symptoms (Table 10.2). The patient with visual symptoms or impending blindness remains the one exception to this rule, and corticosteroids should be initiated prior to or coinciding with obtaining a temporal artery biopsy or further evaluation.

Table 10.2 Differential diagnosis of temporal arteritis and polymyalgia rheumatica

Category	TA	Shared	PMR
Malignancy		Lymphoma Leukemia Multiple myeloma	Colon cancer Breast cancer Renal cell carcinoma
Infections		SBE Fungal infections Tuberculosis Viral syndromes	
Endocrinopathy		Hypothyroidism Hyperparathyroidism	
Connective tissue musculoskeletal	Takayasu's arteritis LCV PMR	Wegener's granulomatosis SLE Systemic vasculitis PAN Ankylosing spondylitis	GCA RA Fibromyalgia Polymyositis Osteoarthritis Pseudogout Sjögren's syndrome Scleroderma
Neurologic	Stroke TIA Brain tumor Atherosclerosis Trigeminal neuralgia Migraines Cluster headaches Internal carotid artery thrombosis	Depression	
HEENT	TMJ arthritis Carotidynia Sinusitis Dental pain Referred pain Nasopharyngeal tumor Retinal detachment Angle closure glaucoma Central retinal artery occlusion		

GCA: giant cell arteritis; HEENT: head, eyes, ears, nose, throat; LCV: leukocytoclastic vasculitis; PAN: polyarteritis nodosa; PMR: polymyalgia rheumatica; RA: rheumatoid arthritis; SBE: subacute bacterial endocarditis; SLE: systemic lupus erythematosus; TIA: transient ischemic attacks; TMJ: temporomandibular joint.

General categories to consider include malignancies, occult infections, other connective tissue diseases and endocrinopathies. Malignancies, such as lymphomas, multiple myeloma, leukemia and colon cancer, often occur in older individuals with weight loss and malaise. As in the evaluation of any systemic illness, occult infections, such as tuberculosis, brucellosis, subacute bacterial endocarditis, bacterial abscesses and viral syndromes, are included as diagnoses to exclude, particularly in those with fever of unknown origin as a prominent symptom. Other connective tissue diseases, such as Wegener's granulomatosis, polyarteritis nodoso (Chapter 8), Sjögren's syndrome (Chapter 5), and systemic lupus erythematosus (Chapter 2) can produce a constellation of symptoms reminiscent of temporal arteritis and polymyalgia rheumatica. Endocrinopathies, for example, hyperparathyroidism or hypothyroidism, represent another major category in the differential diagnosis. Thus, as one can see, the range of diagnostic possibilities in patients suspected to have either disease is quite broad.

The differential diagnosis of temporal arteritis can be defined further by the symptom complex exhibited by the patient. Increased intracranial pressure from brain tumors, migraines and cluster headaches are a few entities to contemplate in those with new onset headaches[56]. Scalp infections can result in scalp tenderness, and jaw claudication can be caused by temporomandibular joint dysfunction as well as other diseases, such as Wegener's granulomatosis and atherosclerosis[17,59,94]. In the patient with facial pain as a predominant feature, the diagnostic considerations include referred pain from the sinuses, skull or dental cavity in addition to otologic diseases, trigeminal neuralgia, nasopharyngeal tumor and carotidynia[47]. Retinal detachment, central retinal artery or vein occlusion, as well as angle-closure glaucoma and thrombosis of the internal carotid artery are other explanations for sudden visual loss[47]. As is evident, this short list includes some entities which would be exacerbated by steroid therapy.

Like temporal arteritis, the differential diagnosis of polymyalgia rheumatica is broad and includes many of the same entities with a few important additions. Osteoarthritis often affects this age group, but usually does not cause an elevation of the erythrocyte sedimentation rate. Pseudogout, or calcium pyrophosphate deposition disease, with shoulder, wrist and knee involvement as prominent features, is another syndrome that clinicians should consider in the differential diagnosis. Likewise, patients with fibromyalgia or depression may present with symptoms reminiscent of polymyalgia rheumatica without any associated laboratory abnormalities.

While inflammatory myopathies, such as polymyositis and dermatomyositis, can have associated severe myalgias, additional physical findings of muscle weakness as well as an elevated creatine phosphokinase are also evident. Finally, the clinician should consider the possibility of associated temporal arteritis, seronegative rheumatoid arthritis, systemic lupus erythematosus and Wegener's granulomatosis, which as previously stated, may have a polymyalgia rheumatica-like presentation. A directed history, physical examination and laboratory examination is clearly indicated as polymyalgia rheumatica remains a diagnosis of exclusion.

PHYSICAL EXAMINATION

Classic findings associated with superficial temporal artery involvement include a thickened, nodular, pulseless, tender and/or swollen artery. The nodules may be transient, and there may be associated overlying erythema of the skin overlying the artery. Occasionally, these findings of swelling and tenderness may be localized to the occipital arteries[95]. However, it is well recognized that patients may have biopsy proven temporal arteritis without any obvious abnormally on physical examination[17,96,97]. In these cases, clinical history and laboratory data may be more important. Scalp tenderness, if present, must be distinguished from pains in the muscles or muscular attachments[98]. Associated large vessel involvement is heralded by bruits, particularly of the subclavian and carotid arteries. On physical examination, palpation of the distal pulses may reveal an asymmetry with an associated auscultatory difference in blood pressure recordings. Bilateral blood pressure measurements should be performed on all individuals with suspected temporal arteritis.

Ischemia to cranial nerves III, IV and VI can result in oculomotor ophthalmoplegia as evidenced by diplopia or ptosis, and occurs in approximately 10% of individuals[64,67].

Visual field cuts and/or scotoma can be demonstrated in some patients. As blindness can occur one of three ways, depending upon the site involved, the funduscopic examination may or may not be abnormal. If the central retinal artery is affected, the funduscopic examination may be quite impressive with obliteration of the retinal vessels, a pale retina and a cherry-red spot in the macula[61]. A pale and swollen optic disc with hemorrhages in the adjacent retina is seen in ischemic optic neuropathy caused by posterior ciliary artery involvement[99]. Sometimes rouleaux formation can be seen in the blood vessels. Finally, the funduscopic examination can appear normal in ischemic retrobulbar optic neuritis even though loss of vision has occurred[65].

In contrast, the physical findings in polymyalgia rheumatica can be less impressive than in temporal arteritis. The physical examination in these patients is largely characterized by tender points and discomfort and stiffness upon movement of the shoulder girdle region and of the proximal muscles. If the symptoms are allowed to persist, subsequent muscle weakness may result from disuse atrophy. It is important to distinguish the 'give-way' weakness associated with muscular pain from true muscle weakness. Synovitis of the knees and sternoclavicular joints may be found on examination, and other commonly affected areas include the wrists, shoulders, ankles and metacarpophalangeal joints[29,40]. Effusions, if present, can have white cell counts ranging from 1300 to $20\,000 \times 10/ml$, predominantly consisting of polymorphonuclear leukocytes[33]. Some patients with wrist synovitis also develop carpal tunnel syndrome, which usually resolves with low-dose corticosteroid therapy and the use of wrist splints.

LABORATORY STUDIES

There is no specific diagnostic laboratory test for either disease entity. Nearly all patients with temporal arteritis or polymyalgia rheumatica have an erythrocyte sedimentation rate (ESR) greater than 50 mm/h, and this laboratory parameter is often used as a diagnostic tool as well as a measure of disease activity[6,25,29,47,100]. In the case of temporal arteritis, this percentage is derived from biopsy-proven cases and may actually represent an overestimation of this relationship. Temporal arteritis has been associated with an ESR less than 40 mm/h in some patients[95,101–103]. A low sedimentation rate does not appear to protect the patient from blindness, and overreliance on this laboratory parameter can lead to a delay in therapy and development of this complication. In one study, it was found that the sedimentation rate was not predictive of ocular complications from this disease[104]. Thus, a normal sedimentaion rate should not dissuade the clinician from considering this diagnosis.

With treatment, the ESR usually returns to normal. Because this laboratory parameter can be abnormal in many settings, other acute phase reactants such as C-reactive protein, fibrinogen and haptoglobin have been measured in these patients. In a study of patients with polymyalgia rheumatica or temporal arteritis, the C-reactive protein was not always elevated at the onset of disease[105]. Several studies show that the C-reactive protein normalized more rapidly and correlated with an improvement in patient's symptoms, but the ESR was more predictive of increases in disease activity[105–107]. Interleukin-6 levels may become helpful in monitoring disease activity in the future[43]. These studies show that the laboratory parameters, such as the acute phase reactants or ESR are an important adjunct in monitoring disease activity along with the patient's symptoms and clinical findings.

General laboratory testing may reveal a normocytic, normochromic anemia as well as thrombocytosis. The anemia usually responds to corticosteroid therapy. In some patients with temporal arteritis, elevated platelet counts are associated with thrombosis, causing ocular and cerebral ischemic complications[108]. Elevations in the serum transaminases and alkaline phosphatase are considered a characteristic finding in both diseases. Liver biopsies are often normal in these patients although a few cases of granulomatous hepatitis have been reported in the literature[47]. In one study, antimitochondrial antibodies were detected in patients with polymyalgia rheumatica, but did not correlate with biochemical, or hepatic dysfunction or other parameters of muscle inflammation[109]. Creatine kinase, an indicator of muscle damage, as well as electromyographic studies, are often normal in patients with polymyalgia rheumatica[13,16]. Steroid-responsive EMG abnormalities, such as spontaneous activity and abnormal motor unit recruitment, have been reported in association with polymyalgia rheumatica, but these are rare findings[110].

Other serologic parameters have been widely studied in both entities in order to find a disease marker and to predict outcome. Rheumatoid factor and anti-nuclear antibodies are generally normal in these patients. As previously stated, anti-phospholipid antibodies, and VWF have been associated with both diseases, and may play a role in the associated complications [44–46,111,112]. Antineutrophil cytoplasmic antibodies (ANCA), a serologic marker for Wegener's granulomatosis (Chapter 8), have also been demonstrated in a few patients with temporal arteritis[111,113]. In a consecutive series of 45 patients with biopsy-proven temporal arteritis, c-ANCA was present in 6% of the patients at the onset of their disease, and the titers became negative with treatment[113].

Some patients with temporal arteritis, particularly those with large vessel disease, may undergo arteriography. In a study of patients with large vessel involvement from the temporal arteritis, it was found that several features were suggestive of arteritis. These features were: areas of stenosis alternating

Table 10.3 Suggested laboratory tests for patients with possible polymyalgia rheumatica and/or temporal arteritis

---

Complete blood count (hematocrit, white blood cell count and differential, platelet count)
Serum chemistries (BUN, creatinine, liver function tests, total protein, albumin)
Urinalysis with microscopy
Thyroid function tests
Creatine phosphokinase
Serum protein electrophoresis
Erythrocyte sedimentation rate and/or C-reactive protein
Rheumatoid factor
Anti-nuclear antibody
Antineutrophil cytoplasmic antibody (suggested)
Lupus anti-coagulant, anti-phospholipid antibody (suggested)

---

with areas of normal caliber, smooth tapered occlusions of large arteries and lack of ulcerations[57]. Some of these features have been documented in other patients with large vessel disease[68,69]. Arteriography of the temporal artery is not considered a replacement for histologic confirmation, as arterial spasm can mimic areas of stenosis[114]. Likewise, dopplers can provide clues to areas of stenosis, but in one study had a false-positive rate of 43%[115]. These ancillary studies may be helpful in guiding, but not replacing temporal artery biopsies.

The laboratory testing, like the physical examination, should be thorough to rule out possible malignancy, infections, endocrinopathies or systemic vasculitis, and should be guided by the patient's clinical history and findings (Table 10.3). Thyroid function tests, creatine kinase, aldolase, urinalysis with microscopy, BUN, creatinine, serum electrophoresis, tuberculosis screen, testing of stools for occult blood and chest X-ray remain as a few additional basic laboratory tests to obtain in patients with suspected temporal arteritis or polymyalgia rheumatica. A blind search for malignancy is not cost effective or necessary.

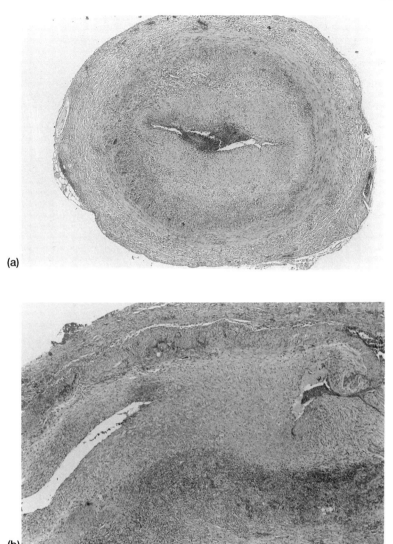

(a)

(b)

Fig. 10.1a, b   Cross-section and longitudinal section of temporal artery. Hematoxylin and eosin stain, ×40. Profound intimal proliferation causing occlusion of the lumen of the artery. Even at this low power, giant cells can be seen at the intima-media junction along with an inflammatory infiltrate.

PATHOLOGY

The diagnosis of temporal arteritis is made clinically with pathologic confirmation. Because the disease predominantly affects older individuals with potential contraindications to long-term corticosteroid therapy, it is important to obtain this information before making this commitment. Several studies address the necessity of obtaining a temporal artery biopsy. Symptom clusters for temporal arteritis were found to be highly specific, but the sensitivity in predicting positive biopsy results was only 17% in one analysis[116].

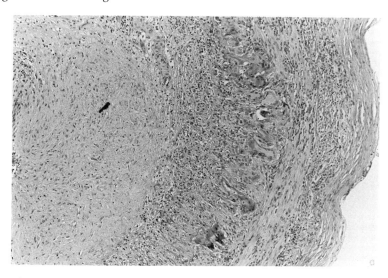

Fig. 10.2 Temporal artery. Hematoxylin and eosin stain, ×160. A series of giant cells at the intima-media junction with a predominantly mononuclear inflammatory infiltrate and intimal proliferation.

Similarly, another study found that 53% of patients with negative biopsies were misclassified by a symptom complex that included temporal artery tenderness with headache or visual changes in association with an elevated ESR[117]. While empiric corticosteroids seem to be an attractive and cost-effective alternative in the correct clinical setting, the biopsy becomes even more important when the patient's symptoms or the ESR fail to respond to therapy and the actual diagnosis in question.

The hallmark of the diagnosis of temporal arteritis is a biopsy that shows granulomatous inflammation, but this lesion is actually seen in less than 50% of positive biopsies[25,96]. Estimates of the sensitivity range from 65–97%[51,97,118]. A false-negative rate of approximately 5% for temporal artery biopsy has been documented in several studies [118,119]. There are three histological variants found on biopsy, but some features are common to all. Fragmentation of the internal elastic lamina, part of the normal aging process, and fibrous intimal proliferation, a major cause of stenosis and vessel occlusion, are seen in all three variants (Figure 10.1)[120]. In

the typical or granulomatous type, giant cells, either foreign body or Langerhans, can be found at the intima-media junction, sometimes seen to be ingesting bits of elastic lamina[121,122]. The number and location of these giant cells is highly variable (Figures 10.2 and 10.3). A mixed cellular infiltrate, consisting predominantly of chronic inflammatory cells (lymphocytes, monocytes, histiocytes), can be limited to the media or be seen transmurally. In the atypical or nongranulomatous type, an inflammatory infiltrate is still present and of the same composition as the granulomatous variety[96]. The third histological appearance has focal, scanty or no discernible inflammation, but consists predominantly of intimal fibrous proliferation[96]. Focal adventitial inflammation may be seen in early temporal arteritis, while intimal fibrosis and scarring is suggestive of healed temporal arteritis[6,25].

The artery on the more symptomatic side should be sampled. The biopsy is commonly performed as an outpatient procedure with local anesthesia[123]. Because this disease involves the temporal artery in a focal and segmental manner, with skip lesions found in

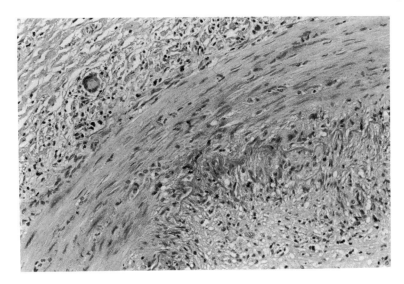

Fig. 10.3 Cross-section of temporal artery. Hematoxylin and eosin stain, ×400. Lone giant cell with predominantly mononuclear inflammatory infiltrate. Skip lesions are not uncommon, and giant cells can be easily missed if the sections are not thoroughly scanned by the pathologist.

28% of biopsies, at least 2–3 cm sample of the superficial temporal artery should be obtained with 3 mm sections performed[96,124]. Isolated frozen sections are not dependable to rule in or rule out this disease. All sections should be stained with elastic stain and hematoxylin-eosin stain and thoroughly scanned in order to localize any focal areas of vasculitis. If systemic amyloidosis is a consideration, then Congo red staining can be performed[125,126]. Direct immunofluorescence studies have shown deposition of IgG, IgM and IgA in biopsy specimens with active arteritis, although this is not routinely done[41,42].

A 'negative' biopsy in the setting of a high suspicion for the disease does not rule out the disease and should not preclude steroid therapy. One alternative might be to biopsy the contralateral side, and there is a minimal, but increased, risk of scalp necrosis with a second biopsy. Another approach might be to delay the second temporal artery biopsy until the patient fails to respond to steroid therapy. However, in studies of patients undergoing

temporal artery biopsy, 82% had a positive biopsy before steroid therapy with the percentage of positive results dropping to 60% after 1 week of steroid therapy and 10% thereafter[96,127]. Thus, with prolonged corticosteroid therapy, the probability of obtaining a positive biopsy decreases.

In patients with low likelihood of temporal arteritis, or with symptoms of polymyalgia rheumatica alone, an initial biopsy is unnecessary[128]. If the patient fails to respond to low-dose prednisone, then other diagnostic possibilities, such as temporal arteritis, malignancy or infection, become more important. The number of patients with temporal arteritis missed by this approach is not understood as the actual percentage of patients with polymyalgia rheumatica with 'silent' arteritis is not known. Estimates of 'occult arteritis' found on biopsy range from 10–40%, and as previously stated, the true relationship between the two diseases is unclear[16,25,55].

Muscle biopsies of patients with polymyalgia rheumatica are typically normal or show nonspecific type II changes. It is speculated that the symptoms of myalgias and stiffness is due to a low-grade axial synovitis, rather than actual muscle inflammation. Several studies have demonstrated the presence of synovial inflammation in these patients. Bone scans with increased uptake in the axial skeleton of patients with polymyalgia rheumatica had been noted as early as 1976[33,129,130]. A multicenter study, in which patients underwent a bone scan and tomography within two weeks of diagnosis, confirmed increased uptake in the shoulders, elbows and sternoclavicular joints[131]. Tomograms revealed erosions in the sternoclavicular joints in patients with long-standing symptoms[131]. An arthroscopic study of the shoulder joints of patients with polymyalgia rheumatica histologically demonstrated the presence of synovitis[132]. Light microscopy of synovial biopsy studies often show inflammatory changes with vascular congestion and mild proliferative changes of the synovial lining cells[12,129,132]. Microvascular changes and vesicular and granular debris in the synovial lining cells has been demonstrated on electron microscopy(12). These studies lend support to an immune basis for this disease although the complete mechanism has yet to be elucidated.

TREATMENT

Corticosteroids are the mainstay of treatment in both temporal arteritis and polymyalgia rheumatica. In the latter syndrome, a rapid response to low-dose corticosteroid therapy is considered as part of some diagnostic schemes[133]. Birkhead showed that this therapy was efficacious in preventing, but not reversing, blindness in 1957. In this study, 200–300 mg/day intramuscular cortisone, which is equivalent to 40–60 mg of prednisone, was used to treat these patients, with relapses occurring when the cortisone was tapered below 100 mg/day[10]. Because of the low incidence of temporal arteritis and the real

risk of blindness in this disease, a randomized, controlled trial of various steroid regimens has yet to be performed.

Patients with temporal arteritis are treated initially with divided dose oral prednisone equivalent of 40–60 mg/day. Those who are systemically ill are treated with a similar regimen of parental corticosteroids usually in the form of methylprednisolone. Patients will often show a dramatic response in symptoms and erythrocyte sedimentation rate within 48–72 hours after beginning treatment[47]. The corticosteroids are consolidated to single daily dose after 2–5 days, and are typically continued at this same dose for 2–4 weeks. At this time, there should be an improvement in symptoms and substantial decrease in ESR before the corticosteroids are tapered. The patient's symptoms and ESR should be followed carefully during this period.

After 2–6 weeks, the corticosteroids are gradually reduced in 5–10 mg decrements every 1–3 weeks to a total dose of 15 or 20 mg/day of prednisone. Any further tapering should be slower, perhaps by 2.5 mg decrements to 10 mg/day, and then by 1 to 2.5 decrements to a total dose of 5–7.5 mg/day of prednisone. The corticosteroids are tapered slowly in order to prevent relapses of the disease, which may occur in 30–50%[25,134].

Blindness has occurred in rare instances during this period of steroid tapering, and patients should be educated regarding the warning signs of disease reactivation. The duration of therapy varies on an individual basis, but most patients will require at least 1–2 years of treatment. In a recent study, the average duration of corticosteroid therapy for patients with temporal arteritis was nearly 6 years, and some may require treatment indefinitely[134,135]. Although initial alternate-day steroid therapy has been shown to be less effective than daily steroids, a change to this regimen after first controlling symptoms with daily-dose steroids may be an effective alternative as maintenance treatment [136,137].

While there are reports of successful treatment with nonsteroidal anti-inflammatory drugs alone, patients with polymyalgia rheumatica typically have a dramatic decrease in their symptoms with 10–20 mg/day of prednisone. Several studies demonstrate that this dosage will often successfully control the patient's symptoms[138–140]. It is well accepted that patients may need prolonged low-dose corticosteroid therapy for up to 2–3 years, but every attempt is made to taper to the lowest possible dose that will control the patient's symptoms and minimize associated side-effects. In an uncontrolled study, investigators showed that a regimen of 120 mg methylprednisolone intramuscularly every 3 weeks for 12 weeks with a gradual reduction to the lowest maintenance monthly dose of intramuscular methylprednisolone successfully controlled patients' symptoms without suppression of the pituitary-adrenal axis[141]. In general, the rate of relapse during corticosteroid taper approaches 50%, and some patients may experience a relapse even after 1 or 2 years of therapy[133,142]. One study addressed the issue of whether the initial corticosteroid dose played an important role in this rate and demonstrated a higher rate of relapse in patients treated initially with 'low-dose' regimens of 10 mg/day of prednisone than with higher doses of 20 mg/day[143].

The risks associated with chronic steroid therapy are well described and include osteoporosis, vertebral fractures, myopathy, hypertension, cataracts and hyperglycemia. In the elderly with multiple medical problems, these risks become even more important and can be associated with considerable morbidity. In a study of alternative steroid regimens, even those treated with a lower dose regimen of 10 mg/day of prednisone had a 25% risk of steroid-induced complications[138]. Patients should have careful follow-up of blood sugar and blood pressure while on steroid therapy. In addition, patients should be treated with 1–1.5 g of oral calcium supplementation as well as vitamin D therapy

400 IU/day in order to prevent bone loss. Additional measures, such as estrogens, etidronate or calcitonin, may be required in severe cases. A baseline bone densitometry measurement may be a useful tool to monitor bone mass during corticosteroid therapy. An aspirin (325 mg/day) may conceivably help prevent vascular occlusive events during the inflammatory phase of temporal arteritis, but no studies on the use of aspirin or low-dose anticoagulants in this disease exist to date.

There are few reports to date of patients treated with methotrexate, azathioprine or cyclophosphamide therapy, and usually these agents reserved for refractory cases or for steroid intolerance[98,144]. In some instances these agents are added in order to facilitate tapering of the corticosteroids. Large, randomized trials are needed to assess the efficacy of immunosuppressive agents in both diseases.

OUTCOME/SUMMARY

Several studies show that a diagnosis of temporal arteritis or polymyalgia rheumatica does not have a negative impact on the patient's long-term survival[27,29,134]. Most complications can be attributed to the prolonged therapy with corticosteroids, which is necessary in both entities. It is important to remember that blindness can occur, even while the patient is being treated with corticosteroids. The patient should be educated about the warning signs of visual loss, and when to seek medical attention.

In summary, temporal arteritis and polymyalgia rheumatica are two entities to consider in the older individual. Classically thought to be the ends of a clinical spectrum, the true relationship between these diseases as well as the etiology of either is not well understood. However, some common features are evident as both typically affect persons over 50 years of age, and are associated with an elevated ESR. In addition, patients with either entity have a dramatic response to corticosteroids, although the dosages required in temporal arteritis are higher than that needed to treat polymyalgia rheumatica. The diagnosis of temporal arteritis is made clinically with histologic confirmation, while polymyalgia rheumatica remains primarily a clinical diagnosis. If treated promptly, neither disease is associated with a negative impact on the long-term survival.

REFERENCES

1. Allen, N. B., Ferguson, B. J. and Farmer, J. C. (1987) Giant cell arteritis and polymyalgia rheumatica: review for the otolaryngologist. *Ann. Otol., Rhinol., Laryngol.*, **96**, 373.

2. Appelboom, T. and Eigem, A. V. (1990) How ancient is temporal arteritis? *J. Rheumatol.*, **17**, 929.

3. Hutchinson, J. (1890) Diseases of the arteries: on a peculiar form of thrombotic arteritis of the aged which is sometimes productive of gangrene. *Arch. Surg.*, **1**, 323.

4. Horton, B. T., Macgath, T. B. and Brown, G. E. (1934) Arteritis of the temporal vessels: a previously undescribed form. *Arch. Intern. Med.*, **53**, 400.

5. Horton, B. T. and Magath, T. B. (1937) Arteritis of the temporal vessels: report of seven cases. *Proc. of the Staff Meetings of the Mayo Clin.*, **12**, 548.

6. Hamilton, C. R., Shelley, W. M. and Tumulty, P. A. (1971) Giant cell arteritis: including temporal arteritis and polymyalgia rheumatica. *Medicine*, **50**(1), 1.

7. Jennings, G. H. (1938) Arteritis of the temporal vessels. *Lancet*, **1**, 424.

8. Cooke, W. T., Cloake, P. C. P., Govan, A. D. T. *et al.* (1946) Temporal arteritis: a generalized vascular disease. *Q. J. of Med.*, New Series, **15**, 47.

9. Gilmour, J. R. (1941) Giant cell chronic arteritis. *J. Path.*, **53**, 263.

10. Birkhead, N. C. and Wagener, H. P. (1957) Treatment of temporal arteritis with adrenal corticosteroids. *JAMA*, **163**(10), 821.

11. Bruce, W. (1888) Senile rheumatic gout. *Br. Med. J.*, **2**, 811.

12. Chou, C-T. and Schumacher, H. R. (1984) Clinical and pathologic studies of synovitis in polymyalgia rheumatica. *Arth. Rheum.*, **27**(10), 1107.

13. Hunder, G. G., Disney, T. F. and Ward, L. E. (1969) Polymyalgia rheumatica. *Mayo Clin. Proc.*, **44**, 849.

14. Barber, H. S. (1957) Myalgic syndrome with constitutional effects: polymyalgia rheumatica. *Ann. Rheum. Dis.*, **16**, 230.

15. Paulley, J. W. (1956) Anarthritic rheumatoid disease. *Lancet*, **2**, 946.

16. Chou, C-T. and Schumacher, H. R. (1983) Polymyalgia rheumatica. *Comprehen. Ther.*, **9**(9), 33.

17. Machado, E. B. V., Michet, C. J., Ballard, D. J. *et al.* (1988) Trends in incidence and clinical presentation of temporal arteritis in Olmstead County, Minnesota, 1950–1985. *Arth. Rheum.*, **31**(6), 745.

18. Boesen, P. and Sorenson, S. F. (1987) Giant cell arteritis, temporal arteritis, and polymyalgia rheumatica in a Danish county: a prospective investigation, 1982–1985. *Arth. Rheum.*, **30**(3), 294.

19. Smith, C. A., Fidler, W. J. and Pinals, R. S. (1983) The epidemiology of giant cell arteritis: report of a ten-year study in Shelby County, Tennessee. *Arth. Rheum.*, **26**(10), 1214.

20. Gonzalez-Gay, M. A., Alonso, M. D., Aguero, J. J. *et al.* (1992) Temporal arteritis in a northwest area of Spain: study of 57 biopsy proven patients. *J. Rheumatol.*, **19**(2), 277.

21. Love, D. C., Rapkin, J., Lesser, G. R. *et al.* (1986) Temporal arteritis in Blacks. *Ann. Intern. Med.*, **105**(3), 387.

22. Gonzalez, E. B., Varner, W. T., Lisse, J. R. *et al.* (1989) Giant cell arteritis in the Southern United States: an 11-year retrospective study from the Texas Gulf Coast. *Arch. Intern. Med.*, **149**, 1561.

23. Ballou, S. P., Khan, M. A. and Kushner, I. (1988) Giant-cell arteritis in a Black patient. *Ann. Intern. Med.*, **88**(2), 659.

24. Desai, M. C. and Vas, C. J. (1989) Temporal arteritis. The Indian scene. *J. Assoc. Physicians of India*, **37**(9), 609.

25. Huston, K. A., Hunder, G. G., Lie, J. T. *et al.* (1978) Temporal arteritis: A 25 year epidemiologic, clinical, and pathologic study. *Ann. Intern. Med.*, **88**, 162.

26. Machado, E. B. V., Gabriel, S. E., Beard, C. M. *et al.* (1989) A Population-based case-control study of temporal arteritis: evidence for an association between temporal arteritis and degenerative vascular disease? *Int. J. Epidemiol.*, **18**(4), 836.

27. Andersson, R., Malmvall, B-E. and

Bengtsson, B-A. (1986) Long term survival in giant cell arteritis including temporal arteritis and polymyalgia rheumatica. *Acta Med. Scand.*, **220**, 361.

28. Nordborg, E. and Bengtsson, B-A. (1989) Death rates and causes of death in 284 consecutive patients with giant cell arteritis confirmed by biopsy. *Br. Med. J.*, **299**, 549.

29. Chuang, T-Y., Hunder, G. G., Ilstrup, D. M. *et al.* (1982) Polymyalgia rheumatica: a 10 year epidemiologic and clinical study. *Ann. Intern. Med.*, **97**, 672.

30. Salvarani, C., Macchioni, P., Zizzi, F. *et al.* (1991) Epidemiologic and immunogenetic aspects of polymyalgia rheumatica and giant cell arteritis in Northern Italy. *Arth. Rheum.*, **34**(3), 351.

31. Franzen, P., Sutinen, S. and Knorring, J. V. (1992) Giant cell arteritis and polymyalgia rheumatica in a region of Finland: an epidemiologic, clinical, and pathologic study, 1984–1988. *J. Rheumatol.*, **19**(2), 273.

32. Cohen, M. D. and Ginsburg, W. W. (1990) Polymyalgia rheumatica. *Rheum. Dis. Clin. N. Am.*, **16**(2), 325.

33. Healey, L. A. (1984) Long-term follow-up of polymyalgia rheumatica: evidence for synovitis. *Sem. Arth. Rheum.*, **13**(4), 322.

34. Sanford, B. G. and Berney, S. N. (1977) Polymyalgia rheumatica and temporal arteritis in Blacks – clinical features and HLA typing. *J. Rheumatol.*, **4**(4), 435.

35. Levey, G. S., Carey, J. P. and Calabro, J. J. (1963) Polymyalgia rheumatica: a separate rheumatic entity? *Arth. Rheum.*, **6**(1), 75.

36. Hunder, G. G., Lie, J. T., Goronzy, J. *et al.* (1993) Pathogenesis of giant cell arteritis. *Arth. Rheum.*, **36**(6), 757.

37. Galetta, S. L., Raps, E. C., Wulc, A. E. *et al.* (1990) Conjugal temporal arteritis. *Neurology*, **40**, 1839.

38. Mathewson, J. A. and Hunder, G. G. (1986) Giant cell arteritis in two brothers. *J. Rheumatol.*, **13**(1), 190.

39. Richardson, J. E., Gladman, D. D., Fam, A. *et al.* (1987) HLA-DR4 in giant cell arteritis: association with polymyalgia rheumatica syndrome. *Arth. Rheum.*, **30**(11), 1293.

40. Espinoza, L. R., Silveira, L. H., Martinez-Osuna, P. *et al.* (1991) Epidemiology, diagnosis, and treatment of polymyalgia rheumatica. *Comprehen. Therapy*, **17**(6), 28.

41. Wells, K. K., Folberg, R., Goeken, J. A. *et al.* (1989) Temporal artery biopsies: correlation of light microscopy and immunofluorescence microscopy. *Ophthalmology*, **96**(7), 1058.

42. Chess, J., Albert, D. M., Bhan, A. K. *et al.* (1983) Serologic and immunopathologic findings in temporal arteritis. *Am. J. Ophthal.*, **96**, 283.

43. Roche, N., Weyand, C., Hunder, G. G. *et al.* (1992) Correlation between serum levels of interleukin 6 and TNF-alpha and the clinical course of giant cell arteritis and polymyalgia rheumatica. *Arth. Rheum.*, **35**(9 (Supp)), S164.

44. Espinoza, L. R., Jara, L. J., Silveira, L. H. *et al.* (1991) Anticardiolipin antibodies in polymyalgia rheumatica-giant cell arteritis: association with severe vascular complications. *Am. J. Med.*, **90**, 474.

45. Watts, M. T., Greaves, M., Rennie, I. G. *et al.* (1991) Antiphospholipid antibodies in the etiology of ischaemic optic neuropathy. *Eye*, **5**(part 1), 75.

46. Persellin, S. T., Daniels, T. M., Rings, L. J. *et al.* (1985) Factor VIII-von Willebrand Factor in giant cell arteritis and polymyalgia rheumatica. *Mayo Clin. Proc.*, **60**, 457.

47. Goodman, B. W. (1979) Temporal arteritis. *Am. J. Med.*, **67**, 839.

48. Wilke, W. S., Wysenbeek, A. J., Krall, P. L. *et al.* (1985) Masked presentation of giant-cell arteritis. *Cleveland Clin. Quart.*, **52**, 155.

49. Calima, K. T. and Hunder, G. G. (1981) Giant cell arteritis (temporal arteritis) presenting as fever of undetermined origin. *Arth. Rheum.*, **24**(11), 1414.

50. Ghose, M,. K., Shensa, S. and Lerner, P. I. (1976) Arteritis of the aged (giant cell arteritis) and fever of unexplained origin. *Am. J. Med.*, **60**, 429.

51. Malmvall, B-E. and Bengtsson, B-A. (1978) Giant cell arteritis. *Scand. J. Rheumatol.*, **7**, 154.

52. Neish, P. R. and Sergent, J. S. Giant cell arteritis: a case with unusual neurologic manifestations and a normal sedimentation rate. *Arch. Intern. Med.*, **151**, 378.

53. Hunder, G. G. (1983) Giant cell arteritis: a disease of the elderly. *Geriatrics*, **38**(3), 55.

54. Healey, L. A. and Wilske, K. R. (1980) Presentation of occult giant cell arteritis. *Arth. Rheum.*, **23**(6), 641.

55. Healey, L. A. and Wilske, K. R. (1984) Polymyalgia rheumatica and giant cell arteritis. *West. J. Med.*, **141**, 64.

56. Baumel, B. and Eisner, L. S. (1991) Diagnosis and treatment of headache in the elderly. *Med. Clin. N. Am.*, **75**(3), 661.

57. Klein, R. G., Hunder, G. G., Stanson, A. W. *et al.* (1975) Large artery involvement in giant cell (temporal) arteritis. *Ann. Intern. Med.*, **83**, 806.

58. Paulley, J. W. (1980) Coronary ischaemia and occlusion in giant cell (temporal) arteritis. *Acta Med. Scand.*, **208**, 257.

59. Gertz, M., Kyle, R., Griffing, W. *et al.* (1986) Jaw claudication in primary systemic amyloidosis. *Medicine*, **65**(3), 173.

60. Horton, B. T. (1962) Headache and intermittent claudication of the jaw in temporal arteritis. *Headache*, **2**, 29.

61. Hollenhorst, R. W., Brown, J. R., Wagener, H. P. *et al.* (1960) Neurological aspects of temporal arteritis. *Neurology*, **10**, 490.

62. Christensen, L. (1986) Ulceration and necrosis of the tongue due to giant cell arteritis. *Acta Med. Scand.*, **220**, 379.

63. Sonnenblick, M., Nesher, G. and Rosin, A. (1989) Nonclassical organ involvement in temporal arteritis. *Seminars in Arth. Rheum.*, **19**(3), 183.

64. Mehler, M. F. and Rabinowich, L. (1988) The clinical neuro-ophthalmologic spectrum of temporal arteritis. *Am. J. Med.*, **85**, 839.

65. Cohen, D. N. and Damaske, M. M. (1975) Temporal arteritis: a spectrum of ophthalmic complications. *Ann. Ophthal.*, August, 1045.

66. Lockshin, M. D. (1970) Diplopia as an early sign of temporal arteritis. *Arth. Rheum.*, **13**(4), 419.

67. Hamed, L. M., Guy, J. R., Moster, M. L. *et al.* (1992) Giant cell arteritis in the ocular ischaemic syndrome. *Am. J. Ophthal.*, **113**, 702.

68. Walz-Leblanc, B. A. E., Ameli, F. M. and Keystone, E. C. (1991) Giant cell arteritis presenting as limb claudication. Report and review of the literature. *J. Rheumatol.*, **18**(3), 470.

69. Ninet, J. P., Bachet, P., Dumontet, C. M. *et al.* (1990) Subclavian and axillary involvement in temporal arteritis and polymyalgia rheumatica. *Am. J. Med.*, **88**, 13.

70. Guillaume, M-P., Vachiery, F. and Cogan, E. (1991) Pericarditis: an unusual manifestation of giant cell arteritis. *Am. J. Med.*, **91**, 662.

71. Larson, T. S., Hall, S., Hepper, G. G. *et al.* (1984) Respiratory tract symptoms as a clue to giant cell arteritis. *Ann. Intern. Med.*, **101**, 594.

72. Romero, S., Vela, P., Padilla, I. *et al.* (1992) Pleural effusion as manifestation of temporal arteritis. *Thorax*, **47**, 398.

73. Ladanyi, M. and Fraser, R. S. (1987) Pulmonary involvement in giant cell arteritis. *Arch. Pathol. Lab. Med.*, **111**, 1178.

74. Bradley, J. D., Pinals, R. S., Blumenfeld, H. B. *et al.* (1984) Giant cell arteritis with pulmonary nodules. *Am. J. Med.*, **77**, 135.

75. Palaic, M., Yeadon, C., Moore, S. *et al.* (1991) Wegener's granulomatosis mimicking temporal arteritis. *Neurology*, **41**, 1694.

76. Small, P. and Brisson, M-L. (1991) Wegener's granulomatosis presenting as temporal arteritis. *Arth. Rheum.*, **34**(2), 220.

77. Nishino, H., Remee, R. D., Rubino, F. A. *et al.* (1993) Wegener's granulomatosis associated with vasculitis of the temporal artery: report of five cases. *Mayo Clin. Proc.*, **68**(115–121), 115.

78. Elling, H. and Kristensen, I. B. (1980) Fatal renal failure in polymyalgia rheumatica caused by disseminated giant cell arteritis. *Scand. J. Rheumatol.*, **9**, 206.

79. Truong, L., Kopelman, R. G., Williams, G. S. *et al.* (1985) Temporal arteritis and renal disease: case report and review of the literature. *Am. J. Med.*, **78**, 171.

80. Srigley, J. R. and Gardiner, G. W. (1980) Giant cell arteritis with small bowel infarction. *Am. J. Gastroenterol.*, **73**, 157.

81. Goldberg, J. W., Lee, M. L. and Sajjad, S. M. (1987) Giant cell arteritis of the skin simulating erythema nodosum. *Ann. Rheum. Dis.*, **46**, 706.

82. Russi, E., Aebi, M., Kraus-Ruppert, R. *et al.* (1979) Intracranial giant cell arteritis. *J. Neurol.*, **221**, 219.

83. Monteiro, M. L. R., Coppeto, J. R. and Greco, P. (1984) Giant cell arteritis of the posterior cerebral circulation presenting with ataxia and ophthalmoplegia. *Arch. Ophthal.*, **102**, 407.

84. Bogousslavsky, J., Deruaz, J. P. and Regli, F. (1985) Bilateral destruction of the internal carotid artery from giant cell arteritis and massive infarction limited to the vertebrobasilar area. *Euro. Neurol.*, **24**, 57.

85. Hall, S., Ginsberg, W. W., Vollertsen, R. S. *et al.* (1983) The coexistence of rheumatoid arthritis and giant cell arteritis. *J. Rheumatol.*, **10**, 995.

86. Broggini, M., Filardi, G. P., Volonte, S. *et al.* (1988) Temporal arteritis in seropositive rheumatoid arthritis with rheumatoid nodule. *Clin. Exp. Rheumatol.*, **6**, 141.

87. Fitzcharles, M-A. and Esdaile, J. M. (1990)

Atypical presentations of polymyalgia rheumatica. *Arth. Rheum.*, **33**(3), 403.

88. Al-Hussaini, A. S. and Swannell, A. J. (1985) Peripheral joint involvement in polymyalgia rheumatica: a clinical study of 56 cases. *Br. J. Rheumatol.*, **24**, 27.

89. Robbins, D. L. and White, R. H. (1988) Interrelationships between polymyalgia rheumatica and polyarthritis. *J. Rheumatol.*, **15**, 1323.

90. Healey, L. A. and Sheets, P. K. (1988) The relation of polymyalgia rheumatica to rheumatoid arthritis. *J. Rheumatol.*, **15**(5), 750.

91. Healey, L. A. (1992) Polymyalgia rheumatica and seronegative rheumatoid arthritis may be the same entity. *J. Rheumatol.*, **19**(2), 270.

92. Herrero-Beaumont, G., Armas, J. B., Amorim, R. *et al.* (1991) Limited forms of Wegener's granulomatosis presenting as polymyalgia rheumatica. *Br. J. Rheumatol.*, **30**, 382.

93. Deal, C. L., Meenan, R. F. Goldenberg, D. L. *et al.* (1985) The clinical features of elderly-onset rheumatoid arthritis. *Arth. Rheum.*, **28**(9), 987.

94. Venna, N., Goldman, R., Tilak, S. *et al.* (1986) Temporal arteritis-like presentation of carotid atherosclerosis. *Stroke*, **17**(2), 325.

95. Jundt, J. W. and Mock, D. (1991) Temporal arteritis with normal erythrocyte sedimentation rates presenting as occipital neuralgia. *Arth. Rheum.*, **34**(2), 217.

96. Lie, J. T. (1987) The Classification and diagnosis of vasculitis in large and medium-sized blood vessels. *Pathol. Ann.*, **22**(1), 125.

97. Fauchald, P., Rygvold, O. and Oystese, B. (1972) Temporal arteritis and polymyalgia rheumatica: clinical and biopsy findings. *Ann. Intern. Med.*, **77**, 845.

98. Hunder, G. G. (1990) Giant cell (temporal) arteritis. *Rheum. Dis. Clin. N. Am.*, **16**(2), 399.

99. Keltner, J. L. (1982) Giant cell arteritis: signs and symptoms. *Ophthalmalogy*, **89**(10), 1101.

100. Lauter, S. A., Reece, D. and Alvioli, L. V. (1985) Polymyalgia rheumatica. *Arch. Intern. Med.*, **145**, 1273.

101. Wong, R. L. and Korn, J. H. (1986) Temporal arteritis without an elevated erythrocyte sedimentation rate: a case report and review of the literature. *Am. J. Med.*, **80**, 959.

102. Wise, C. M., Agudelo, C. A., Chmelewski, W. L. *et al.* (1991) Temporal arteritis with low erythrocyte sedimentation rate: review of five cases. *Arth. Rheum.*, **34**(12), 1571.

103. Ellis, M. E. and Ralston, S. (1983) The ESR in

the diagnosis and management of polymyalgia rheumatica/giant cell arteritis syndrome. *Ann. Rheum. Dis.*, **42**, 168.

104. Jacobson, D. M. and Slamovits, T. L. (1987) Erythrocyte sedimentation rate and its relationship to hematocrit in giant cell arteritis. *Arch. Ophthal.*, **105**, 965.

105. Kyle, V., Cawston, T. E. and Hazleman, B. L. (1989) Erythrocyte sedimentation rate and C-reactive protein in the assessment of polymyalgia rheumatica/giant cell arteritis on presentation and during follow-up. *Ann. Rheum. Dis.*, **48**, 667.

106. Andersson, R., Malmvall, B-E. and Bengtsson, B-A. (1986) Acute phase reactants in the initial phase of giant cell arteritis. *Acta Med. Scand.*, **220**, 365.

107. Mallya, R. K., Hind, C. R. K., Berry, H. *et al.* (1985) Serum C-reactive protein in polymyalgia rheumatica: a prospective serial study. *Arth. Rheum.*, **28**(4), 383.

108. DeKeyser, J., DeKlippel, D. and Ebinger, G. (1991) Thrombocytosis and ischaemic complications in giant cell arteritis. *Br. Med. J.*, **303**(6806), 825.

109. Sattar, M. A., Cawley, M. I. D., Hamblin, T. J. *et al.* (1984) Polymyalgia rheumatica and antimitochondrial antibodies. *Ann. Rheum. Dis.*, **43**, 264.

110. Bromberg, M. B., Donofrio, P. D. and Segal, B. M. (1990) Steroid-responsive electromyographic abnormalities in polymyalgia rheumatica. *Muscle and Nerve*, **13**, 138.

111. McHugh, N. J., James, I. E. and Plant, G. T. (1990) Anticardiolipin and antineutrophil antibodies in giant cell arteritis. *J. Rheumatol.*, **17**, 916.

112. Olsson, A., Elling, P. and Elling, H. (1990) Serological and immunohistochemical determination of von Willebrand factor antigen in serum and biopsy specimens from patients with arteritis temporalis and polymyalgia rheumatica. *Clin. Exp. Rheumatol.*, **8**, 55.

113. Bosch, X., Font, J., Mirapei, E. *et al.* (1991) Antineutrophil cytoplasmic antibodies in giant cell arteritis. *J. Rheumatol.*, **18**(5), 787.

114. Horowitz, H. M., Pepe, P. F., Johnsrude, I. S. *et al.* (1977) Temporal arteriography and immunofluorescence as diagnostic tools in temporal arteritis. *J. Rheumatol.*, **4**(1), 76.

115. Barrier, J., Potel, G., Renaut-Hovasse, H. *et al.* (1982) The use of Doppler flow studies in the diagnosis of giant cell arteritis. *JAMA*, **248**(17), 2158.

116. Fernandez-Herlihy, L. (1988) Temporal arteritis: clinical aids to diagnosis. *J. Rheumatol.*, **15**(12), 1797.

117. Robb-Nicholson, C., Chang, R. W., Anderson, S. *et al.* (1988) Diagnostic value of the history and examination in giant cell arteritis: a clinical pathological study of 81 temporal artery biopsies. *J. Rheumatol.*, **15**(12), 1793.

118. Hall, S., Lie, J. T., Kurland, L. T. *et al.* (1983) The therapeutic impact of temporal artery biopsy. *Lancet*, **2**, 1217.

119. Hedges, T. R., Geiger, G. L. and Albert, D. M. (1983) The clinical value of negative temporal artery biopsy specimens. *Arch. Ophthal.*, **101**, 1251.

120. Meretoja, J. and Tarkkanen, A. (1975) Amyloid deposits of internal elastic lamina in temporal arteritis. *Ophthalmologica*, Basel, **170**, 337.

121. Kent, R. B. and Thomas, L. (1989) Temporal artery biopsy. *Am. Surgeon*, **56**(1), 16.

122. Nordborg, E., Bengtsson, B-A. and Nordborg, C. (1991) Temporal artery morphology and morphometry in giant cell arteritis. *APMIS*, **99**, 1013.

123. Stuart, R. (1989) Temporal artery biopsy in suspected temporal arteritis: a five year survey. *NZ Med. J.*, **102**(874), 431.

124. Klein, R. G., Campbell, R. J., Hunder, G. G. *et al.* (1976) Skip lesions in temporal arteritis. *Mayo Clin. Proc.*, **51**, 504.

125. Rao, J. K. and Allen, N. B. (1993) Primary systemic amyloidosis masquerading as giant cell arteritis. *Arth. Rheum.*, **36**(3), 422.

126. Taillan, B., Fuzibet, J-G., Vinti, H. *et al.* (1990) Amyloid deposits in temporal artery mimicking giant cell arteritis. *Clin. Rheumatol.*, **9**(2), 256.

127. Allison, M. C. and Gallagher, P. J. (1984) Temporal artery biopsy and corticosteroid treatment. *Ann. Rheum. Dis.*, **43**, 416.

128. Elliot, D. L., Watts, W. J. and Reuler, J. B. (1983) Management of suspected temporal arteritis: a decision analysis. *Med. Decision Making*, **3**(1), 63.

129. O'Duffy, J. D., Wahner, H. W. and Hunder, G. G. (1976) Joint imaging in polymyalgia rheumatica. *Mayo Clin. Proc.*, **51**, 519.

130. O'Duffy, J. D., Hunder, G. G. and Wahner, H. W. (1980) A follow-up of polymyalgia rheumatica: evidence of chronic axial synovitis. *J. Rheumatol.*, **7**(5), 685.

131. Paice, E. W., Wright, F. W. and Hill, A. G. S. (1985) Sternoclavicular erosions in polymyalgia rheumatica. *Ann. Rheum. Dis.*, **42**, 379.

132. Douglas, W. A. C., Martin, B. A. and Morris, J. H. (1983) Polymyalgia rheumatica: an arthroscopic study of the shoulder joint. *Ann. Rheum. Dis.*, **42**, 311.

133. Jones, J. G. and Hazleman, B. L. (1981) Prognosis and management of polymyalgia rheumatica. *Ann. Rheum. Dis.*, **40**, 1.

134. Andersson, R., Malmvall, B-E. and Bengtsson, B-A. (1986) Long-term corticosteroid treatment in giant cell arteritis. *Acta Med. Scand.*, **220**, 465.

135. Kyle, V. and Hazleman, B. L. (1990) Stopping steroids in polymyalgia rheumatica and giant cell arteritis. *Br. Med. J.*, **300**, 344.

136. Hunder, G. G., Sheps, S. G., Allen, G. L. *et al.* (1975) Daily and alternate-day corticosteroid regimens in the treatment of giant cell arteritis. *Ann. Intern. Med.*, **82**, 613.

137. Bengtsson, B-A. and Malmvall, B-E. (1981) An alternate-day corticosteroid regimen in maintenance therapy of giant cell arteritis. *Acta Med. Scand.*, **209**, 347.

138. Lundberg, I. and Hedfors, E. (1990) Restricted dose and duration of corticosteroid treatment in patients with polymyalgia rheumatica and temporal arteritis. *J. Rheumatol.*, **17**(10), 1340.

139. Delecoueillerie, G., Joly, P., DeLara, A. C. *et al.* (1988) Polymyalgia rheumatica and temporal arteritis: a retrospective analysis of prognosis features and different corticosteroid regimens (11 year survey of 210 patients). *Ann. Rheum. Dis.*, **47**, 733.

140. Behn, A. R., Perera, T. and Myles, A. B. (1983) Polymyalgia rheumatica and corticosteroids: how much for how long? *Ann. Rheum. Dis.*, **42**, 274.

141. Dasgupta, B., Fernandes, J. G. L. and Olliff, C. (1991) Treatment of polymyalgia rheumatica with intramuscular injections of depot methylprednisolone. *Ann. Rheum. Dis.*, **50**(12), 942.

142. Ayoub, W. T., Franklin, C. M. and Torretti, D. (1985) Polymyalgia rheumatica: duration of therapy and long-term outcome. *Am. J. Med.*, **79**, 309.

143. Kyle, V. and Hazleman, B. L. (1989) Treatment of polymyalgia rheumatica and giant cell arteritis. I. Steroid regimens in the first two months. *Ann. Rheum. Dis.*, **48**, 658.

144. De Silva, M. and Hazleman, B. L. (1986) Azathioprine in giant cell arteritis/polymyalgia rheumatica: a double-blind study. *Ann. Rheum. Dis.*, **45**, 136.

THE MOLECULAR BIOLOGY OF INHERITED DISORDERS OF CONNECTIVE TISSUE

11

A. Morgan and H. Bird

INTRODUCTION

Rapid advances in molecular biology over recent years have led to an improved understanding in the molecular basis of many human connective tissue disorders. The complexity of connective tissues and the importance of their macromolecular interactions has led to great conservation of some of their components at a molecular level. Recent advances in recombinant DNA technology including cloning, sequencing, restriction fragment cleavage and microinjection of the appropriate cell lines theoretically allows detailed analysis of any gene. The most time- and cost-effective method is to concentrate on possible candidate genes. When the candidate gene is unidentified, the use of restriction fragment length polymorphisms (RLFPs) may establish which structural protein gene carries the mutation. Such markers may detect linkage of a gene with the disorder, preferably in large families, and help analyse the type of inheritance. These techniques have been very successful in localizing the genes responsible for hemoglobinopathies, cystic fibrosis and Duchenne muscular dystrophy. In applying such techniques it is important to make a critical assessment of the phenotype through-out the family members to prevent apparent discordant segregation[1].

Many of the collagen genes have been extensively studied, not only to isolate the mutation, but also to try and determine the consequences at the molecular level. This is particularly the case for type I collagen and osteogenesis imperfecta. The creation of transgenic mice that carry specific mutations of type I collagen genes has helped to understand the structural consequence of relatively minor changes. However, it is still not clear how these molecular defects are translated into tissue abnormalities and into the clinical phenotype[2]. More information is certainly required on the complex intermolecular interactions that occur in connective tissues.

CONNECTIVE TISSUES

The majority of organs and tissues have specific parenchymal cells which are separated from the connective tissue by a basement membrane. Connective tissue consists of cells, fibers and ground substance. Two main types of fibers exist which include the collagenous fibers, collagen and reticulin, and those devoid of collagen, namely, microfibril and elastin fibers. The amorphous ground

Connective Tissue Diseases. Edited by Jill J. F. Belch and Robert B. Zurier. Published in 1995 by Chapman & Hall, London. ISBN 0 412 48620 2

Table 11.1   Composition of the different types of collagen

Collagen type	Chain composition	Gene(s)	Tissue distribution
I	$[\alpha 1(I)]_2\,\alpha 2(I)$	COL1A1 COL1A2	Abundant in skin, tendon, bone, most tissues except cartilage
II	$[\alpha 1(II)]_3$	COL2A1	Cartilage, vitreous humor, intravertebral disc
III	$[\alpha 1(III)]_3$	COL3A1	Most tissues notably skin, CV tissues, lung, stomach tissue, most organs, virtually absent in bone
IV	$[\alpha 1(IV)]_2\,\alpha 2(IV)$	COL4A1 COL4A2	Basal laminae
V	$[\alpha 1(V)]_2\,\alpha 2(V)_{\text{usually}}$ $[\alpha 1(V)]_3$ $[\alpha 3(V)]_3$ $\alpha 1(V)\,\alpha 2(V)\,\alpha 3(VI)$	COL5A1 COL5A2 COL5A3	Wide tissue distribution including tendons, blood vessels, bone, corneal stroma
VI	$[\alpha 1(VI)]_2\,\alpha 2(VI)$ $\alpha 1(VI)\,\alpha 2(VI)\,\alpha 3(VI)$	COL6A1 COL6A2 COL6A3	Wide tissue distribution in soft tissues, abundant in aorta, dermis
VII	$[\alpha 1(VII)]_3$	COL7A1	Anchoring fibrils at dermatoepidermal junction (stratified epithelium)
VIII	$[\alpha 1(VIII)]_3$	COL8A1	Endothelial cell matrix – most tissues
IX	$\alpha 1(IX)\,\alpha 2(IX)\,\alpha 3(IX)$	COL9A1 COL9A2 COL9A3	Cartilage
X	$[\alpha 1(X)]_3$	COL10A1	Hypertrophic zone cartilage
XI	$\alpha 1(XI)\,\alpha 2(XI)\,\alpha 3(XI)$	COL11A1 COL11A2 COL11A3	Cartilage

substance consists of many components, the best characterized of which are proteoglycans and glycoproteins which include fibronectin. The fibers and ground substance are metabolized by the constituent cells, some of which are tissue specific, such as chondrocytes and osteocytes. One of the major functions of connective tissue is mechanical support, but it also influences the differentiation and biosynthetic capabilities of many cells. Connective tissue also plays an important role in healing, and is involved in many inflammatory process[3,4]. This chapter will explain the biochemistry of some of the important connective tissue components with respect to the hereditary connective tissue diseases. It will then summarize the current molecular biological knowledge of some of these diseases.

COLLAGEN

Collagen is ubiquitous and constitutes up to one-third of the total body protein. It belongs to a family of at least 12 proteins, each having a characteristic tissue distribution and apparently unique biological function. It forms either fibers or network-like structures which largely define the size, shape and strength of most tissues[5]. The collagens, summarized in Table 11.1, have been broadly classified into three groups on the basis of their chemical structure.

Group I (types I, II, III, V and XI) have a continuous uninterrupted helical domain of approximately 300 mm and chains of approximately 95 000 kDa. These interstitial collagens are the best characterized and function as load bearing fibers. Group 2 molecules (types IV and VII) have helical domains interrupted by non-helical segments and chains larger than 95 000 kDa. Group 3 molecules (types VI, IX and X) have chains less than 95 000 kDa[3]. The last two groups, also known as non-fibrous collagens, do not form striated fibrils and are often located pericellularly. Their functions are more widespread in mediating cell membrane and matrix interactions[5].

GROUP I: INTERSTITIAL COLLAGENS (TYPES I, II, III, IV AND V AND XI)

These collagens form a major component of tendons, ligaments and joint capsules and are associated with a high-tensile strength. Type I collagen is the most abundant interstitial type and therefore the best characterized. It is associated with type III collagen in tissues that are extensible, e.g. arteries, skin and hollow organs. Type II, however, is found within cartilage and is able to withstand high compressive forces. Type V collagen has been identified as a minor component of most tissues. A number of roles have been suggested to explain its pericellular distribution, including the formation of an exocytoskeleton for connective tissue cells and possible roles in extra cellular matrix formation and differentiation. A similar role has been suggested for type XI collagen which is specifically located in cartilaginous tissues with type II collagen[3,5].

Collagen biosynthesis is very complex and is described in more detail below. Basically, three alpha chains of procollagen associate at their carboxy (C)-terminal ends and a small nucleus of a triple helix is formed which is propagated rapidly to the amino (N)-terminal end of the molecule. Correct folding of the triple helix is dependent on a repeating -Gly-X-Y-triplet. The precise nature of the component alpha chain varies with each type of collagen (Figure 11.1). The principle of nucleated growth extends to the extracellular matrix where the collagen monomers rapidly aggregate into fibrils once the C- and N-propeptides are cleaved. The structure of the triple helix and fibers are maintained by numerous covalent bonds.

Many mutations interfering with this process are known and are described according to the collagen type and clinical disease produced.

Collagen biosynthesis

To date at least 18 genes that encode the chains that are subunits of the various collagens are known. Certain functions and sequences of these genes are highly conserved throughout the animal kingdom, in particular the first four exons at the C-terminus and the areas encoding the triple helix. However, the introns may be quite diverse in size and sequence, constituting the majority of the collagen gene. There are up to 50 exons in the interstitial collagen genes and those coding the helix regions consist of multiples of 9 base pairs encoding the triplet sequence. Most exons contain 54 base pairs which may be the ancestral gene. The gene is firstly transcribed fully, and then the introns are spliced out. With additional processing messenger RNA is formed which migrates into the cytoplasm. Translation starts at the amino terminal end and the signal peptide of hydrophobic amino acid guides the polypeptide into the center of the rough endoplastic reticulum. The primary amino acid sequence consists of two terminal globular extensions known as the N- and C-propeptides and a central portion of approximately one thousand amino acids. The latter part consists of repeating tripeptide sequences of -Gly-X-Y-, where X is frequently proline and Y often hydroxyproline.

This primary sequence forms a left-handed minor helix which is subject to a number of enzymes acting simultaneously on this newly-formed chain. These post-translational modifications ensure the correct folding of the triple helix. The most important enzymes, hydroxylate proline and lysine, and require

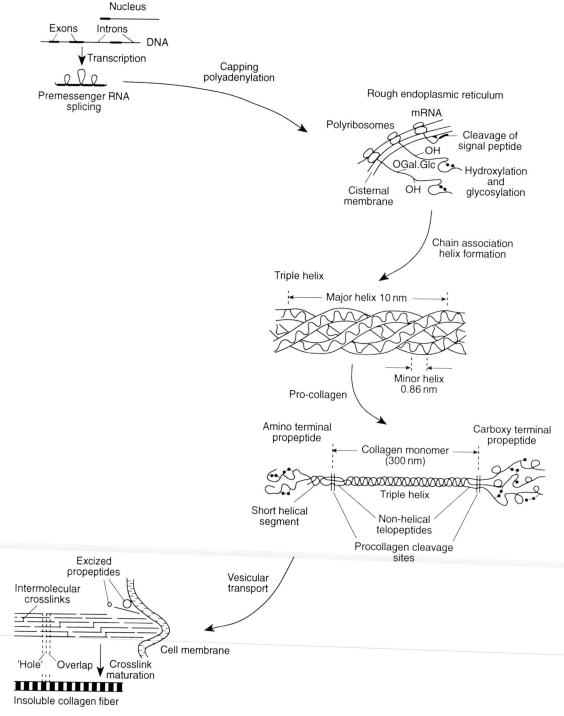

Fig. 11.1 Synthesis of interstitial collagen.

ferrous ions, 2-oxygluthrate, molecular oxygen and ascorbate as cofactors. Hydroxyproline is important for stability: its absence leads to increased lability at body temperatures and rapid degradation intracellularly. Hydroxylysine is important for the formation of stable cross-links, described later, and to the substrate for glycosylation. Two glycosyl transferase enzymes then add galactose and glucose to hydroxyl groups of hydrolysine. These sugars are the only sugars found in interstitial collagens and are assumed to regulate the packing of tropocollagen molecules into fibrils and fibers. Hydrophobic and electrostatic interactions between the carboxy-terminal ends of three pro-α chains then occur, which are stabilized by the formation of interchain disulphide bonds. This allows the correct alignment of the -Gly-X-Y- tripeptide units in the three chains providing a nucleus for triple helix formation. This is then rapidly propagated from the C- to the N-terminal. The chains come into contact at the glycine residues which occur every third amino acid resulting in the formation of a right-handed triple helix. This glycine periodicity is crucial as it is the smallest and only amino acid that can fit at the center of the helix. The triple helix is initially stabilized by hydrogen bonds between hydroxyproline residues of different chains. The formation of the triple helix prevents further enzymic modification to the primary structure. Therefore, anything that results in partial obstruction or inhibition of triple helix formation results in the over-modification of collagen. Once the triple helix has formed disulphide bonds stabilize the N-terminal peptides.

The pro-collagen is secreted via the golgi apparatus. Here further glycosylation occurs especially involving the arginine residues of the C-propeptide.

Once secreted the N- and C-terminal propeptides are cleaved by N- and C-procollagen proteinases respectively. This reduces the solubility about 2000 fold resulting in the monomers leaving solution and spontaneously polymerizing fibrils. The collagen monomers are aligned in a 'quarter staggered' array producing the characteristic cross striations, with a periodicity of 67 nm, visible under electron microscopy. Specific association is dependent on electrostatic and hydrophobic interaction and fibril formation on the principle of nucleated growth. This is a highly efficient mechanism for the assembly of large structures with defined architecture. Failure to remove the large C-propeptides results in the complete inhibition of fiber formation, whereas retention of the N-propeptide is associated with smaller, less well aligned fibers. Up to 40% of collagen is degraded intracellularly within minutes of synthesis. It has been suggested this may be a mechanism whereby the rate of collagen production may be altered. Fibril diameter grows in relation to the physical demands placed on the collagen in that tissue. Fibrils are stabilized by the formation of covalent cross links which are essential in the production of tensile strength. The final enzymic step involves lysyl oxidase whereby an aldehyde derivative of lysine or hydroxylysine is formed in a copper dependent process. The aldehyde groups are very reactive species and result in a sequence of reactions with the ultimate production of covalent cross-links. The exact sequence is dependent on the tissues and type of collagen.

In vivo, although fibril assembly is autonomous, it is likely to be influenced by other constituents of the extra-cellular matrix. Some fibres may also contain more than one type of collagen, in particular types I and III[3,5,6].

The complexity of collagen biosynthesis and the need for precise amino acid configurations in the formation of the triple helix and cross linking makes it vulnerable to a multitude of mutations. The best characterized are those of type I collagen and, in particular, for osteogenesis imperfecta. However, there is an increasing knowledge of other collagen mutations producing some rare and common conditions, such as aortic aneurysms and osteoarthritis[6]. Collagen mutations can result in clinical disease by a number of different mechanisms, but in general reduce the synthesis and secretion of normal procollagen monomers. When there is only a quantitative reduction in normal collagen the phenotype tends to be milder than when abnormal molecules are synthesized, when the mutation may be lethal. Mutations take a number of forms and include point substitutions, deletions and insertions which have either direct consequences at a structural level or result in aberrant splicing. Other mutations also alter the control of gene expression. Point mutations are relatively common and the phenotype is closely related to the site of the mutation.

Point mutations and deletions that disrupt the -Gly-X-Y- triplet sequence tend to increase the post-translational modification of chains on the amino terminal side of the mutation, due to delayed helix formation. Therefore, those near the carboxy terminal end of the triple helix tend to be lethal, whereas others at the amino terminal end are relatively mild. The presence of abnormal chains tends to impair the thermal stability and generally impairs the efficacy of secretion and proteolytic cleavage especially at the amino terminal propeptidase site. Although chain stability is primarily dependent on hydrogen bonding, charge interactions are also important. Even a small deletion may disrupt the normal charge interactions on formation of the triple helix and have consequences on fibrillogenesis. Abnormal molecules tend to be secreted less efficiently and once secreted they may be incorporated into fibrils with consequently more widespread interruption on matrix interactions. In bone, for example, abnormal molecules may be mineralized less efficiently than those containing normal collagen[7].

Type I collagen

This is the predominant collagen found in bones, tendons and dermis which is reflected in the clinical effects of its mutations. Mineralization only occurs in bones and it is not clear whether there is a specific three-dimensional orientation stabilized by different cross links in bone[5]. The best-characterized condition involving type I collagen is osteogenesis imperfecta, although mutations may also result in certain types of Ehlers–Danlos syndrome (EDS) particularly type VII. Some intermediate phenotypes have also been described with loose joint, blue sclerae and brittle bones[8]. More recently type I collagen mutations have been isolated in probands with osteopenia or osteoporosis[6].

Osteogenesis imperfecta

Osteogenesis imperfecta is characterized by bone fragility that becomes apparent early in life. Severe forms are lethal and death may occur *in utero*, whereas the milder forms have only mild bone deformities, impaired dentinogenesis and presenile hearing loss. Type I collagen constitutes 80% of the protein content of bone. However, considering the complexity and number of other minor proteins involved, it is somewhat surprising that over 90% of probands with osteogenesis imperfecta have mutations in type I collagen. More than 70 different mutations have been identified in the pro-α1(I) and pro-α2(I) chains of type I procollagen in unrelated patients with osteogenesis imperfecta. Some mutations reduce the synthesis whereas others result in structurally abnormal but partially functional chains[6].

The commonest mutations in osteogenesis imperfecta are single-base substitutions, particularly involving glycine residues. To date more than 40 have been described. The relation between their position and phenotypic effect, as described previously, is more closely worked out for the COL1A1 gene than for COL1A2. Many single exon deletions have been described and, with only one exception, those within the COL1A1 gene have been lethal or very severe with little apparent relationship to the exon site deleted. Similar deletions within the COL1A2 gene tend to be less severe, possibly due to contributing only one rather than two chains to the triple helix. The mildest forms of osteogenesis imperfecta tend to be the result of mutations that reduce the normal amount of type I procollagen produced. Relatively few mutations affecting gene expression, transcription and translation efficiency and molecular assembly have yet been identified. However, many deletions have been isolated that interfere with RNA splicing[2,6,7].

Ehlers–Danlos syndrome

In comparison to osteogenesis imperfecta, where clinical diversity reflects the nature of the type I collagen mutation, the phenotype in EDS is secondary to mutations in collagen genes, and abnormalities in processing enzymes and possible also other matrix components (Table 11.2). The best characterized to date are EDS types IV and VII with defects in type III collagen and N-propeptide cleavage of type I collagen respectively. Other types of EDS arise from abnormal function of one of three processing enzymes: lysyl oxidase, lysyl hydroxylase and procollagen peptidase. Fibronectin defects have been described in a number of families with EDS, described later. However, it is not clear whether this is the primary defect or arises secondary to the other matrix abnormalities.

Ehlers–Danlos syndrome type VII

In EDS, in particular type VII, rather than having predominant bony problems these patients have severe joint laxity with skin that is soft, silky and easily torn. EDS type VII was originally known as the arthromultiplex form, and three subtypes have now been defined on their molecular basis[19]. All three types have a defect in the processing of the N-propeptide of type I collagen. The persistence of this terminal extension completely disturbs fibril

Table 11.2 Biochemical defects in Ehlers–Danlos syndrome

Type	Defects noted/excluded
I	COL1A1, 1A2, 3A1 excluded[9]
	poor fibroblast proliferative activity[10]
II	COL1A1, 1A2, 3A1 excluded[11]
III	Some associated with type III collagen[12]
IV	COL3A1[12]
V	Lysyl oxidase[12]
VI	Lysyl hydroxylase[12]
VII	A. COL1A1: resistance to cleavage[13, 14, 15, 16, 17]
	B. COL1A2: procollagen N-proteinase
	C. Defect in procollagen N-proteinase[18]
VIII	Unknown
IX	Defect in copper metabolism impairing lysyl oxidase[12]
X	Fibronectin deficiency (1 family)[12]
	Cutis laxa lysyl oxidase

assembly and results in thin, highly distorted fibrils. They have a characteristic appearance under electron microscopy and are known as 'hieroglyphs'.

Type A results from mutations in the COL-1A1 gene which make the N-propeptide resistant to cleavage by the procollagen N-proteinase.

Type B is similar except the mutations occur in the COL1A2 gene. To date all the mutations characterized have been single base substitutions the majority in intron 6. These have resulted in a splicing defect with consequent deletion of sequences encoded by exon 6. This exon encodes the cleavage site for N-proteinase in both the pro-α1(I) and pro-α2(II) chains, and is also an important lysyl cross-linking site[13–17].

In type C the impaired processing of the N-propeptide occurs due to defects in the enzyme procollagen N-proteinase. This type is less well characterized partly related to the difficulty in assaying the membrane-bound enzyme[13]. This condition is very similar to dermatosparaxis, a recessively inherited connective tissue disorder of domesticated animals which results in fragile skin, joint laxity and premature death, usually from sepsis secondary to avulsion. Wertelecki first recorded this in humans in 1991[20], and recently two probands have been shown to have defective enzymic cleavage of the N-terminal propeptide[18].

Other type I collagen abnormalities

The possibility of type I collagen structural abnormalities in osteoporosis and osteopenia is starting to emerge. A woman with post-menopausal osteoporosis was found to have a single base substitution converting glycine to serine, in position 661 of the pro-α2(I) chain[21]. Two different mutations have been isolated in two patients with osteoporosis and joint hypermobility. One involved a single base substitution converting glycine to cystine at α-19 and the second due to an 11 base pair delation in the pro-α2(I) gene causing skipping of exon 9[22]. Less complete information is known about the presence of abnormal type I collagen in a patient with osteoporosis in association with ankylosing spondylitis[23] and a further patient with osteoporosis and idiopathic scoliosis[24]. Base insertions and deletions have been identified in patients with spondyloepiphyseal dysplasia.

Type II collagen

This is the major structural protein of cartilage and is also found in the vitreous gel of the eye. It consists of three identical chains, but compared to type I collagen there is a slower rate of chain association with consequently more extensive post-translational modification. In particular, there is increased glycosylation of hydroxylysine. The strength of cartilage is dependent on fibrils of type II collagen and it has, therefore, been suggested that many of the osteochondrodystrophies and other cartilage disorders may result from mutations in type II collagen. Single base substitutions have been identified in patients with Stickler

syndrome, achondrogenesis and primary generalized osteoarthritis associated with mild chondrodystrophies[7]. Phenotypic linkage of three families with osteoarthritis has been made with type II procollagen[25]. However, more recently patients with nodular generalized osteoarthritis were found to have no significant allelic differences at the locus of COL1A2 compared to controls. However, there was a slight tendency to have inherited COL1A1 alleles from their parents[26]. More work is clearly needed to see if certain subgroups and families with this common disease have a primary genetic defect.

Many more type II collagen genetic defects are likely to be found in the short-limbed dysmorphisms. However, the success will be dependent on the development of suitable protein assays from cultured chondrocytes. Cartilage cells are very difficult to culture with retention of their chondrocytic phenotype, as they usually revert to fibroblasts and then synthesise type I collagen. Even if such cultures can be isolated, there is likely to be a shortage of material as cartilage biopsies are difficult to justify.

Type II collagen abnormalities have been excluded to date as causative factors for achondroplasia and pseudoachondroplasia [8].

Type III collagen

Type III collagen is a major component of large arteries and is also found in association with type I collagen in soft tissues, especially in places where high compliance is necessary. It comprises 10–15% of collagen in adult skin and is also found in the walls of the gastrointestinal tract, uterus and lungs. The alpha chains are unique among fibrillar collagens in containing cystine residues within the helix. It has been postulated that they may give rise to additional stabilization through intermolecular bonding. The fibers are smaller when compared to type I collagen, which may be due to the retention of the amino terminal procollagen peptide for longer, thus giving rise to partial inhibition of fibril aggregation. The formation of type I and III cofibrils as seen on electron microscopy may be a relatively common occurrence[5].

The clinical manifestations of type III collagen defects are varied, but are characterized by arterial rupture and bruisability. The best documented is that of EDS type IV. This is one of the most severe subtypes, characterized by sudden rupture of large arteries, in particular, in the cerebral circulation and hollow organs of young adults. Widespread loose jointedness and hyperextensibility of the skin are uncommon, although there is an increased bruising tendency. A subset of EDS type III with lumbosacral striae, mitral valve prolapse and aortic rupture that resembles Marfan syndrome, as well as occasional patients with EDS type I, also have type III collagen defects documented[8]. Quantitative reductions in type III collagen have also been documented in scalp skin and superficial temporal arteries of patients with ruptured cerebral aneurysms [27]. Another family with a strong history of abdominal aortic aneurysms but no evidence of other genetic disease were found to have a single base substitution of arginine for glycine in type III procollagen[28]. Another family with aortic aneurysms that ruptured spontaneously was found to have easy bruisability, but no other characteristic features of EDS type IV. A single base mutation causing substitution of A for G_{+1} of intron 20 caused aberrant splicing of the transcribed RNA[29]. The possibility of phenotypic overlap and increased incidence of aneurysms in heterozygotes for EDS type IV needs to be assessed. Kontusaari *et al.* also suggested the potential role of DNA tests for mutations in the type III procollagen gene in the identification of individuals predisposed to developing aneurysms[29].

Ehlers–Danlos syndrome type IV

To date, at least 17 different mutations in the gene for type III procollagen have been characterized in probands for EDS type IV. These include single base substitutions that result in the substitution of glycine for amino acids with bulkier side chain mutations causing aberrant RNA splicing and partial gene deletions of varying sizes. The clinical picture appears to correlate poorly with the biochemical abnormality, although over-modification tends to occur the nearer to the C-terminal end of the protein. The amount of extracellular type III collagen is usually drastically decreased varying from 5–80% of normal[8].

More recently, a family has been described which secretes near normal amounts of apparently normal type III collagen and little is retained within the cells[30]. The small 27 base pair deletion within exon 37 presumably does not significantly impair helix formation in this case. Over-modification within the CB peptides may inhibit further processing by N-proteinase impairing normal fibril assembly. Another single base mutation results in the substitution of glycine for serine near the collagenase cleavage site making this product unusually sensitive to proteinases[31].

GROUP II COLLAGENS (TYPES IV AND VII)

This second group of collagens do not form striated fibers and are less well understood than the interstitial collagens.

Type IV collagen

Type IV collagen is found within the lamina densa of basement membranes. The molecular structure of the triple helix is not known with certainty, but unlike type I collagen these are 12 interrupted sequences where the triplet -Gly-X-Y- does not occur. These introduce a degree of flexibility into the molecule. A second major difference to other collagens is the incorporation of the large globular terminal dormants into the supramolecular structure. The collagen monomers are incorporated into the sheet-like structures resembling a two-dimensional chicken wire. This is stabilized via lysine derived cross-links and interchain disulphide bonds[3,5]. Mutations in the α5(IV) chain have been found in three families with X-linked Alport's syndrome[32].

Type VII collagen

Type VII collagen is thought to be associated with anchoring fibrils of the basement membrane. It is particularly important at the dermoepidermal junction and is also seen within the amnion[33]. It has been proposed that its main function is to enhance the adhesion of the basement membrane to the underlying connective tissue matrix. Its structure appears to consist of an unusually long triple helical domain with small terminal globular regions. A dramatic absence of type VII collagen has been found in the skin of patients with autosomal recessive dystrophic epidermolysis bullosa, which also lacks anchoring fibrils[29]. A structural mutation in type VII collagen has also been suggested. It is not known whether fibril disappearance is a secondary event. It is also possible that type IV abnormalities may contribute to other forms of epidermolysis bullosa localized to the lamina lucida[8].

GROUP III COLLAGENS TYPES (VI, IX, X, XII)

Type VI collagen

Type VI collagen is found in a wide variety of soft tissues accounting for up to 10% of total collagen. The structure has not been fully elucidated, but has two large globular domains and an uninterrupted triple helix. The triple helix monomers form dimers in antiparallel fashion which overlap and are held together by disulfide bonds in a supratwist[3]. These fibrils have occasionally been found perpendicular to the direction of collagen and elastin fibers. Further work is,

therefore, needed to determine their interactions with other matrix components[5].

Little is known about type VIII or endothelial cell collagen. Although it is produced in large amounts by endothelial cells in culture, it has not yet been identified within the extracellular matrix[3].

Types IX and X collagens

These are found in cartilage in addition to the predominant type II and XI collagens. Type IX collagen has a relatively short chain which lacks the classical 54 base pair repeat found in other collagens. It is found throughout the cartilage matrix and has a covalently bound glycosaminoglycan. The observation of covalent bonding between type IX and II collagens has led to suggestions that it may play a vital role in controlling fibril diameter of type II collagen and also in mediating proteoglycan interactions. Type X collagen has been isolated solely within zone 3 of the epiphysial growth plate. It is the only transient and developmentally regulated collagen isolated to date[3].

Type XII

Type XII collagen has been isolated in dense connective tissues alongside cross-striated type I collagen fibers, in a similar manner to the association between types II and IX collagens.

To date, no obvious diseases have been found in association with many types of collagens despite them forming substantial components of connective tissues. Many of the chondrodystrophies may be associated with type VI, IX and X collagen abnormalities and, similarly, many vascular abnormalities may be associated with type VI and VIII collagens.

MICROFIBRILLAR FIBER-SYSTEM

Microfibrillary fibers are composed of bundles of 10–12 nm slightly beaded microfibrils, that are widely distributed throughout the extra-cellular matrix of many tissues. These fibers are believed to form a scaffolding for elastin deposition and may be important in embryo-genesis. It has been postulated that they act as a structural protein system linking elastin to other matrix components. They may also be found in non-elastic tissues having a struc-tural role in their own right[34,35]. The molecular composition of the fibers is not clear but they appear to contain a number of structural glycoproteins, the best character-ized of which is fibrillin. The microfibrillary system has been noted to form a number of structures including lamellae, long rods and meshworks[36].

Fibrillin is a 350 kDa acidic glycoprotein that contains several repeated cystine-rich motifs, which are thought to participate in inter-molecular disulfide linkage[37]. Three motifs have been described. The commonest is type I which has some sequence homology with epidermal-growth-factor and forms an anti-parallel β-sheet conformation, the role of which is uncertain. Type II motif is analogous to the 8-cystine module seen in transforming growth factor-β banding protein[35].

The precise details of microfibrillary as-sembly and interactions with other com-ponents of the extracellular matrix remain to be elucidated.

The use of polyclonal and monoclonal anti-bodies have demonstrated the presence of microfibrillary fibers in skin, tendon, car-tilage, muscle, kidney, perichondrium, peri-osteum, blood vessels and the suspensory ligaments of the ocular lens[38]. Their pres-ence in the latter two tissues in particular led to the discovery of reduced amounts of fibril-lin in skin and fibroblast cultures of people with Marfan syndrome[36].

MARFAN SYNDROME

For over a decade, researchers had found the search for the molecular defect in Marfan syndrome frustratingly difficult. Much of the research centered around collagen. Some minor collagen abnormalities have been docu-mented, although recent candidate gene link-age studies have effectively excluded primary structural defects of the fibrillar collagens types I, II and III[39]. Elastin defects have also been suspected, due to the presence of fragmented elastic tissue in the tunica media of the aorta and skin of Marfan patients. Some biochemical studies indeed have shown increased urinary excretion of elastin metabolites. The possibility of linkage has, however, been excluded in several families. The absence of common restriction site polymorphisms have unfortu-nately prevented extensive studies[38].

Over-production of hyaluronic acid by cul-tured fibroblasts has been a consistent finding of unknown significance. The above bio-chemical abnormalities are now thought to be secondary to the basic defect or found in a minority of patients and are unable to explain the primary molecular abnormality in the majority of Marfan patients[8].

The marked unilateral decrease in fibrillin on the affected side of the unique patient with asymmetrical Marfan syndrome added further support to fibrillin being the basic molecular defect[40]. Further studies docu-mented consistent, relatively specific abnor-malities of the microfibrillary fibers in Marfan syndrome in contrast to other connective tissue disease and normal controls[38].

A different group of researchers chose the complementary pathway of searching for the defective gene and then looking for the gene product to try and elucidate the pathogenesis of Marfan syndrome. As suggested pre-viously, the early candidate genes were the fibrillar collagens, elastin and proteoglycans. Exclusion of these led to a large international collaborative study which using random link-age data managed to exclude 75% of the genome[41]. Shortly following this, linkage to three markers on chromosome it was found in five Finnish families, which was later con-firmed in British and American families with no evidence of locus heterogeneity[42].

In 1991, three separate reports confirmed the Marfan syndrome focus on chromosome 15 and the fibrillin gene were one and the same[43–45]. Since that time further studies have shown genetic linkage between ectopia lentis and the fibrillin gene on chromosome 15. Congenital contractual arachnodactyly is linked to a similar fibrillin gene on chromosome 5[46]. A third fibrillin gene has been identified on chromosome 17 and there will probably be an expanding gene family[47]. To date, a total of six fibrillin gene mutations have been characterized[47,48]. With the documentation of increasing numbers of mutations the genotypic-phenotypic relationships will become better understood. They may even overlap with some common conditions, such as aortic aneurysms, myopia and mitral valve prolapse[47]. The live biological significance of the mutations can only be speculated, although in a similar way to the collagens, they are likely to exert their effects by reduced synthesis and fibrillogenesis of fibrin. Alternatively, secretion and co-polymerization of mutant chain products with normal fibrillin may result in protein suicide. Characterization of the other glycoproteins present in the microfibrillary bundles may reveal further candidates for the defective gene products in Marfan syndrome[35,47].

ELASTIN

Elastin is present in virtually all soft tissues, especially where a high compliance and elastic recoil is necessary, e.g. the lungs and aorta. Elastin is synthesized by fibroblasts, smooth muscle cells, and, to a lesser extent, chondrocytes and endothelial cells. In comparison to collagen, elastin has a much greater percentage of hydrophobic amino acids, but also contains up to one-third glycose residues and 10–25% proline. On secretion, elastin becomes insoluble by the formation of desmosine and isodesmosine cross-links by lysyl oxidase. The newly formed elastin fibers are closely associated with the microfibrillary

fiber system, discussed later, which may regulate elastin deposition. There is a low turnover of mature elastin by elastases which are secreted by many cell types. In pathological conditions those released from neutrophil azurophil granules are the most important. Lack of the natural inhibitor $\alpha 1$ antitrypsin is an important factor in the pathogenesis of emphysema.

The random structure of elastin makes it relatively tolerant to amino acid mutations and no pathological defects in the primary structure have yet been described. However, a number of collagen abnormalities may also disrupt elastin structure, demonstrating the close physical interdependence particularly evident in the skin and aorta.

It has been suggested that changes in elastin may contribute to some of the heterogeneity of some collagen disorders. Elastin fragmentation occurs in pseudoxanthoma elasticum, although it may be secondary to an abnormal accumulation of glycosaminoglycans in the lesion. Elastin abnormalities have also been implicated in a number of other conditions, including Marfan syndrome, cutis laxa and Buschke–Ollendorff syndrome. Although the defect has not been fully localized in any of these[5].

GLYCOPROTEINS

The extracellular glycoproteins have important roles in controlling cellular behavior by regulating the local microenvironment. Two of their most important functions include cell adhesion and proving the optimal conditions for cell growth. The major extracellular glycoproteins, fibronectin, laminin and chondronectin, contain binding sites for proteoglycans and glycosaminoglycans[4].

Fibronectin is the best characterized and occurs in two isoforms. These arise through alternative splicing events of a single gene. Plasma fibronectin is a dimer which is synthesized primarily by the liver and possibly also by endothelial cells. Cellular fibronectin exists as dimers and multimers, which may be found on cell surfaces and also within the extracellular matrix. Fibronectin is a multifunctional binding protein that plays important roles in cellular adhesion and induction of mobility and differentiation of cells. It has high affinities for collagen, especially denatured fibrin and heparin. Fibronectin deposition and organization of other glycoproteins appears to initiate fibrillogenesis of the connective tissue matrix[4]. Fibronectin receptor expression is closely associated with fibronectin function and is reduced in a number of hereditary connective tissue diseases, including EDS, osteogenesis imperfecta and Marfan syndrome. Modest reductions in fibronectin receptor also occur in families of patients with EDS[49]. A paucity of fibronectin in the extracellular matrix *in vitro* has been described in EDS types I to VIII, which can be restored with co-cultivation of control fibroblasts[50]. Deregulation and alternative fibronectin splicing process have been found in skin fibroblasts from patients with EDS types III, IV and VII[51].

Laminin is closely associated with type IV collagen in the basal lamina of basement membranes implying an important role in epithelial cell adhesion.

Chondronectin is found in serum and in the interface between cells and the extracellular matrix of cartilage where it is thought to stimulate the attachment of chondrocytes to type II collagen[4].

PROTEOGLYCANS

Proteoglycans are a specialized family of glycoproteins which are found in most tissues but especially where the extracellular space is large and well developed, e.g. skin, cartilage and blood vessels. They consist of a protein core with up to 50 covalently linked glycosaminoglycan units. The high charge density of the long hydrophillic glycoaminoglycans make the proteoglycans very expanded molecules, resembling a 'bottle brush', which

excludes other macromolecules but returns permeability to small molecules. Proteoglycans either function as space-filling molecules important in maintaining hydration or are involved in matrix organization through molecular interactions.

The glycosaminoglycan side chains are highly anionic and unbranded containing repeating disaccharide units. These include heparin, heparan sulfate, dermatan sulfate, keratan sulfate, chondroitin sulfate and hyaluronic acid[4].

MECHANICAL PROPERTIES OF CONNECTIVE TISSUE

This is determined by the orientation of fibers and interactions occurring between the different types of collagen, elastin, glycoproteins and other matrix constituents. There are three important mechanical properties of connective tissues: elasticity, tensile strength and resilience.

Elasticity is the most important and is the ratio of stress (force applied) to strain (resulting change in shape) which is measured as Young's modulus (expressed in Newtons/m^2). A high Young's modulus indicates a high resistance to shape change for a given force, e.g. elastin $6 \times 10^5 \, \mathrm{Nm^{-2}}$ and collagen $8 \times 10^2 \, \mathrm{Nm^{-2}}$. Three phases can be identified, the early non-linear phase of initial high compliance is more apparent in tissues that resist tensile stress, e.g. tendons, ligaments and joint capsules. This is largely dependent on the structure of collagen fibers. The second linear phase is where molecular defects of connective tissues influence joint hypermobility and skin elasticity. This phase is dependent on collagen fiber diameter, orientation arrangement and cross-linking of fibers and interactions with other matrix components, particularly glycosaminoglycans. Finally, there is a non-linear rupture phase at high stress where disruption of collagen fibrils and breakage of cross-links occurs at the molecular level. The tensile strength of the 'breaking' strain which if exceeded the tissue will rupture. This is determined by the diameter and packing density of collagen fibers, cross-links and interactions with other matrix components.

Lastly, resilience is the efficiency of elastic recoil, i.e. the proportion of energy recovered when the tissue returns to the resting tension. The aorta, for example, with a high proportion of elastin has a resilience of greater than 90% compared to 75% in tendons[48].

EHLERS–DANLOS SYNDROME

This comprises a heterogenous group of inherited disorders involving particularly the skin, joints and blood vessels[52]. The term was first used by Poumeau-Delille[53] in 1934 though Tschernogobow (1892)[54], Ehlers (1901)[55] and Danlos (1908)[56] probably all described a variant of the same condition. Subsequently, Beighton's seminal monograph[57], based upon a thorough clinical examination of 100 patients[58], delineated the five main clinical variants of the EDS, separated on the grounds of either clinical features or patterns of inheritance.

The evidence of molecular genetics then allowed additional gene defects to be identified, characteristically linked to particular clinical features. As a result, six further variants were added to the classification, some of which (types 9 and 11) have now been withdrawn following their more rational reclassification alongside other medical conditions. A full clinical nosology was proposed at a workshop held during the 7th International Congress of Human Genetics, Berlin, in 1986[19] and a molecular nosology of hereditable disorders of connective tissue based on the specific abnormalities of collagen so far identified was published in 1992 in the *American Journal of Medical Genetics*[59]. With recent revolutionary developments in recombinant and DNA technology, it is likely that further varieties will be defined and that each of the fundamental molecular defects may ultimately be elucidated.

PATHOLOGY

The basic synthesis of collagen, its many types and their widespread distribution throughout different organs of the body are described above. It is likely most examples of EDS will be ascribed to a specific abnormality in the synthesis of collagen, but the extent to which this causes clinical symptoms may still vary. Simplistically, while the extent of the inheritance may vary from individual to individual, once faulty collagen has been formed only the extent to which this is subject to stress, e.g. the pressure of blood within vessels or external forces applied to the skin, will determine the extent of the clinical damage observed. Attention has been directed to sites where the integrity of collagen is important. Prolapse of the heart valves has been described but also disputed. The propensity to formation of herniae and varicose veins is recognized. The extent to which EDS might contribute to conditions as diverse as diverticulitis in the bowel, spontaneous pneumothorax and aneurysm formation in the cerebral circulation is barely explored. At present, aneurysm formation in large arteries remains the most common cause of sudden death.

CLINICAL PRESENTATION

The cardinal manifestations of EDS comprise:

- skin hyperextensibility with soft, velvety, doughy texture;
- dystrophic scarring;
- easy bruising;
- joint hypermobility;
- connective tissue fragility.

These features are found in varying degree in different clinical subdivisions of EDS. The 11 currently accepted variants (two types IX and XI no longer thought to be variants of EDS) are listed in Table 11.3 along with their clinical

Table 11.3   Clinical features of Ehlers–Danlos syndrome

Type I: gravis – autosomal dominant
Prominent skin hyperextensibility, fragility and easy bruisability; 'cigarette paper scars'; molluscoid pseudotumors (swellings in the skin) and subcutaneous spheroids (soft accumulations of tissue under the skin which cause soft, non-malignant lumps); large and small joint hypermobility; frequent varicose veins. Premature birth due to early rupture of membranes is common.

Type II: mitis – autosomal dominant
Skin is soft with easy bruisability but less hyperextensible and with less tendency to split and scar than gravis type. Joint hypermobility is less marked. Varicose veins and hernia may occur.

Type III: benign hypermobility – autosomal dominant
Skin is soft but hypertextensibility, splitting and scarring are limited. Joint hypermobility is generalized, affecting large and small joints; dislocation is common. Bruising tendency variable. Some patients in this category have defects similar to those causing EDS type IV and this group is also distinguished from the original type XI (benign familial articular hypermobility) which may lack the characteristic abnormality in collagen.

Type IV: ecchymotic or arterial: autosomal dominant/recessive
Skin is characteristically thin (translucent) with veins easily seen over trunk, arms, legs and abdomen. Skin is not usually hyperextensible. Minor trauma leads to extensive bruising (eccymosis). Joint mobility is usually normal aside from the small joints in the hands. Cardiovascular and gastrointestinal damage can occur (e.g. arterial rupture and intestinal perforation). Uterine rupture in pregnancy may occur, thus pregnancy should be approached with caution.

IV-A	Acrogeric type	AD (13005)
IV-B	Acrogeric type	AD (22535)
IV-C	Ecchymotic type	AD (13005)
VI	Ocular-scoliotic type	AR (22540)
VII	Arthrochalasis multiplex congenita	
	VII-A Structural defect of pro-cx 1(1)	AD (13006)
	VII-B Structural defect of pro-cx 2(1)	AD(13006)

Type V: X-linked – X-recessive
Some velvety, hyperextensible skin, hypermobile joints and scoliosis (curvature of the spine). Scarring usually less severe than type I. Marfanoid habitus. Some individuals have ocular fragility and keratoconus (excessive curvature and thinning of the cornea).

Type VII: arthrochalasis multiplex congenita – autosomal dominant/recessive
Soft skin with relatively normal scarring, marked joint hypermobility, marked hypotonia, congenital hip dislocation, short stature. Part of one or other of the collagen genes has been shown to be faulty in five different Type VII families. Genetic prenatal diagnosis can be offered to this particular subgroup of type VII.

Type VIII: periodontal – autosomal dominant
Prominent skin fragility with abnormal pigmented scars. Skin hyperextensibility is normal. Joint laxity may be present. Often there is generalized weakness (aesthenic habitus) and periodonitis.

Type IX: category currently unallocated
Originally used to denote X-linked cutis laxa which is no longer regarded as EDS.

Type X: fibronectin platelet defect – uncertain
Soft, mildly extensible skin, mild joint hypermobility, bruising.

Type XI: category currently unallocated
This was originally used to describe patients with benign familial articular hyperlaxity, a condition no longer thought to be a variant of EDS because of a failure to demonstrate the classical chemical changes.

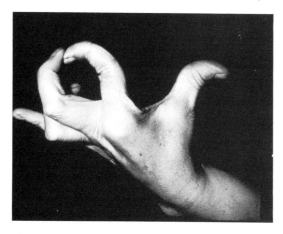

Fig. 11.2　Ehlers–Danlos syndrome. Hyperlaxity of the hands can be extreme.

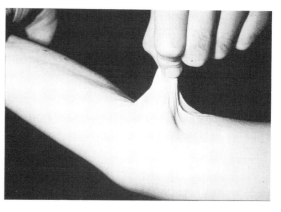

Fig. 11.4　Ehlers–Danlos syndrome. Skin is hyperlax and demonstrates remarkable elasticity in texture.

features and their McKusick numbers allocated at the 1986 Berlin meeting.

Most of the components of a diagnostic triad comprising extensible skin, loose joints and fragile tissue are almost always present (Figures 11.2–11.4). The skin splits on minor trauma forming gaping lacerations which heal slowly with wide papyraceous scars, often slightly pigmented and typically found over the knees and elbows. Molluscoid pseudo tumors may appear in scarred areas, sometimes forming hard, calcified subcutaneous

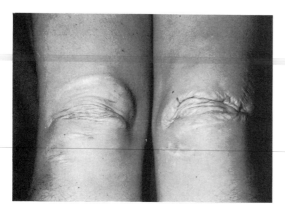

Fig. 11.3　Ehlers–Danlos syndrome. Knees may also be hyperlax, often with hyperextension. The skin heals badly with unsightly scar formation.

spheroids. Although complications are encountered in almost every system of the body, only a minority of patients, typically those with EDS type IV, experience sudden death from the rupture of large arteries[60], dissection of the aorta[61] or gastrointestinal perforation and bleeding[62]. In this account particular attention is paid to articular problems. Joint involvement is a characteristic of EDS type III in which it forms the predominant feature. It may appear to a lesser extent in types I and II. The degree of articular hyperlaxity and incidence of dislocations are closely related, the joints most frequently affected being the patellae, shoulders and digits. Congenital dislocation of the hip occurs in only a minority of patients and chronic temporomandibular joint subluxation[63] is increasingly recognized. As a result of the instability, joint effusions may occur, particularly in the knees, ankles, elbows and digits. These appear to be related to activity, often being more pronounced at the end of the day. Exceptionally hemarthrosis is seen. Muscular hypotonicity, perhaps directly associated with lax joints, also occurs.

More severe orthopedic abnormalities may be present. Spinal abnormalities of greater or lesser degree affect a proportion of patients,

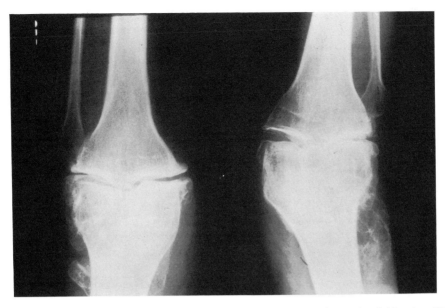

Fig. 11.5   Ehlers–Danlos syndrome. Severe osteoarthritis can occur with atopic calcification. The severity is often proportional to the degree of biomechanical abnormality.

thoracolumbar scoliosis being the most common variant. Vertebral wedging may occur at the apex of the kyphotic element of the spinal curve when a severe scoliosis is present. These features are unusual in children suggesting they may result from secondary mechanical changes. Thoracic asymmetry is common and in the foot talipes equinovarus is present at birth in 7% of patients[64], perhaps as a result of the effect of intrauterine malposition on lax ligaments. Pes planus is commonly present, related to the hyperlaxity of the feet and the loss of support from the plantar ligaments. Hallux valgus, claw toes and plantar keratomata are also all common.

The development of osteoarthritis seems to be directly related to the magnitude of joint hyperlaxity (Figure 11.5). A majority of patients with joint hyperlaxity are affected by the age of 40, the site of involvement correlating well with the hyperlaxity of individual joints. This may affect the gait. Initially the feet are placed firm and flatly on the ground with the hips hyperextended during weight bearing to counteract the genu recurvatum, enabling the pelvis to remain balanced with respect to the feet. As osteoarthritis develops, the classic gait of osteoarthritis affecting lower limb joints emerges.

Muscle cramps, common around the most lax joints, are most common during childhood. In one patient a functional proprioceptive deficit has been demonstrated[65]. Acrocyanosis is common in many patients and may mimic Raynaud's phenomenon. Chilblains are common, particularly during childhood and acro-osteolysis has been described[66].

NON-ARTICULAR COMPLICATIONS

In the heart, 'floppy mitral valves' have been described[67,68], though recently echocardiographic studies have suggested in many patients that this may not be much outside normal limits. Potentially lethal complications – dissection of the aorta and spontaneous rupture of large arteries – are mainly confined to the rare EDS type IV.

Hiatus hernia, gastric, duodenal and colonic diverticula and rectal prolapse as well as inguinal, femoral, and umbilical herniae are all more common in EDS. Gastrointestinal hemorrhage, surprisingly, is not frequently found.

Eye complications include involvement of the scleral connective tissue leading to distortion of the eyeball and consequent myopia. A divergent strabismus may occur and uncomplicated convergent squint is also common. Scleral perforation occurs except in EDS type VI. Epicanthic folds and redundant skin in the upper eyelid may produce undesirable cosmetic effects.

In pregnancy, the tissue fragility and bleeding tendency allow the frequent occurrence of antepartum and postpartum hemorrhage. It may be difficult to achieve hemostasis. Precipitant labor and premature rupture of the membranes are common. Severe perianal laceration and uterine prolapse may occur and episiotomy incisions do not heal well. Striae gravidarum, however, are rare.

Affected children, experiencing extensive bruising on minimal trauma and spontaneous dislocation of the joints, may mimic 'battered babies' and be incorrectly diagnosed as having this condition with much resultant distress for the parents.

DIAGNOSIS

The diagnosis is made on the striking clinical features, including the presence of the cardinal signs (which should always alert suspicion) and a supportive family history. Thus in about 30% of individuals, EDS appears to result from an isolated mutation without family history (Beighton personal communication, 1992). Less frequently, individuals presenting with skin abnormality may be diagnosed as having EDS on the basis of molecular genetic techniques.

'EDS' is a heterogeneous group of conditions, and there may be substantial overlap between the classical variants described earlier. Conditions that mimic the skin involvement include cutis laxis though here no organ or joint involvement is apparent. Conditions that mimic the joint involvement include benign familial hyperlaxity, though here the skin lacks the characteristic doughy elasticity found in EDS even though there may be an element of hyperextensibility. In addition, organ involvement is lacking.

TREATMENT

There is no cure and none is likely to arise in the near future in view of the heterogeneity of this condition. Treatment must be symptomatic and tailored to each individual and their relatives. The recently formed United Kingdom Ehlers–Danlos Support Group publishes a booklet providing practical advice to patients which can be used to educate their family practitioners who may be unfamiliar with this condition. The current address of the Society is 2 High Garth, Richmond, North Yorkshire DL10 4DG. Other self-help groups exist both in the USA and mainland Europe.

Involved skin should be protected from injury wherever possible. This may mean the avoidance of contact sports, particularly for children. Where laceration occurs, attending physicians should be warned of the poor healing qualities of affected skin. Sutures should be small and frequent, holding the skin together well if the typical scars are to be avoided. Hematoma formation and subsequent infection may complicate healing.

Patients should be advised that the symptoms that may affect their joints are essentially benign in nature. There is controversy among physiotherapists on optimum treatment, but on current evidence exercises to strengthen the muscle that would stabilize the worst affected joints seems the most appropriate advice, certainly for benign familial hyperlaxity. Unfortunately, patients with more extreme laxity and the muscular hypotonicity often found in EDS, seem to respond less well to these regimens. Treatment should otherwise be symptomatic with analgesics and anti-inflammatory agents, though avoidance of precipitating factors and joint fatigue is better whenever possible.

Obstetricians and other organ specialists should be alerted to the relevant complications that arise from this condition. Some may only encounter one or two affected individuals throughout the whole of their professional lives.

In general, orthopedic surgery should be avoided. Techniques to stabilize lax ligaments have proved disappointing and many surgeons intending to improve the cosmetic deformity have encountered the delayed wound healing, hematoma formation and susceptibility to infection to their cost. Skin and soft-tissue fragility, although less severe with age, may still cause problems when replacement joint surgery is considered for EDS patients with secondary osteoarthritis.

Most contentious is the extent to which such patients should be screened for aortic aneurysm and severe valvular defects. Clearly EDS type IV patients are most at risk though there may be a case for screening EDS type I patients as well. Many such patients are now offered routine chest X-ray and echocardiography on routine diagnosis. Subsequently, repeat testing perhaps every two years, to allow advance warning of aneurysm formation, may be indicated particularly in those families with a risk of sudden death from this complication. Nevertheless, corrective surgery is not without risk, patients who have most susceptibility to aneurysm presenting the most formidable technical problems to the vascular surgeon.

Genetic counselling should be made available to families once a diagnosis has been reached. Often it is the rheumatologist or the genetic counsellor who offers most local expertise in the treatment of this rare condition. Some clinical geneticists are willing to arrange for referral to rheumatologists, vascular surgeons, ophthalmologists and even dentists as

required. Parents of affected children should be warned of the danger of misdiagnosis as a 'battered baby'.

PROGNOSIS

Apart from the rare vascular accidents, particularly frequently encountered in EDS type IV and occasionally in EDS type I, longevity is normal though there may be substantial morbidity throughout life. In general, a frank approach, a well-educated patient and the continuation of as normal a lifestyle as possible, are the main objectives of treatment.

MARFAN SYNDROME

INTRODUCTION

Marfan syndrome is a hereditable generalized disease of connective tissue, predominantly involving the skeleton, ocular and cardiovascular systems. It was first described in 1896 by a Parisian professor of pediatrics[69]. The syndrome is less heterogeneous than EDS bearing a single McKusick number (15470) in the Berlin 1986 Nosology[19]. The inheritable nature of the syndrome was first clearly demonstrated in 1931[70] and the major cardiovascular complications which normally determine prognosis were first described in 1943[71]. In 1991, fibrillin was implicated as the defective gene product and a link with congenital contractual arachnodactyly was established.

PATHOLOGY

A predominantly inherited autosomal disorder of high penetrance, the incidence is thought to be approximately 1:10 000, and 30% of patients represent new mutations[35]. There is overlap with congenital contractual arachnodactyly and with dominantly inherited ectopia lentis[72,73].

In 1986, a novel component of extracellular matrix, characterized as a 350 kDa, acidic glycoprotein was identified using polyclonal and monoclonal antibody techniques[37]. Named 'fibrillin', compositional analysis revealed that it contained a high percentage of acid amino acid and cysteine residues[74]. Immediately after secretion into the extracellular matrix, fibrillin is believed to be promptly rendered insoluble by a process which involves the formation of interchain disulfide bridges. It was suggested that this might be a candidate protein in Marfan syndrome pathogenesis and genetic analysis of 10 Marfan kindreds supported this[38,75]. Concurrently, gene analysis was applied at random and gene specific polymorphic probes were applied in large collections of Marfan families, and appropriately selected for a highly penetrant dominant inheritance pattern. These studies[76,77] indicated that any protein abnormality found in the matrix gene products was a secondary effect. Subsequently, linkage analyses with random probes resulted in an exclusion map for approximately 75% of the human genome. In 1990, Kainulainem and colleagues reported the successful localization of the Marfan-associated chromosome 15Q15Q23 in five Finnish kindreds[78]. Ultimately, the Marfan gene was shown to be synonymous with the fibrillin gene on chromosome 15[43–45].

The fibrillin genes are now known to code polypeptides of unique structure which forms supramolecular aggregate 18 as 10 nm microfibrils in the connective tissue matrix. These are present in diverse tissues, including the ciliary zonule of the eye, the aorta, periosteum and perichondrium[37]. Loci for additional fibrillin may exist[43] and it would be of value to assess their possible association with other Marfan-related disorders, e.g. mitral valve prolapse syndrome and annuloaortic ectasia[79].

CLINICAL PRESENTATION

The syndrome is characterized by skeletal abnormalities (though there is wide variation

Table 11.4   Marfan syndrome diagnostic manifestations

Skeletal
  Anterior chest deformity, especially asymmetric pectus excavatum/carinatum
  Dolichostenomelia not due to scoliosis
  Arachnodactyly
  Vertebral column deformity:
    scoliosis
    thoracic lordosis or reduced thoracic kyphosis
  Tall stature, especially compared to unaffected relatives
  High, narrowly arched palate and dental crowding
  Protusio acetabulae
  Abnormal appendicular joint mobility:
    congenital flexion contractures
    hypermobility
Ocular
  *Ectopia lentis
  Flat cornea
  Elongated globe
  Retinal detachment
  Myopia
Cardiovascular
  *Dilatation of the ascending aorta
  Aortic dissection
  Aortic regurgitation
  Mitral regurgitation due to mitral valve prolapse
  Calcification of the mitral annulus
  Mitral valve prolapse
  Abdominal aortic aneurysm
  Dysrhythmia
  Endocarditis
Pulmonary
  Spontaneous pneumothorax
  Apical bleb
Skin and integument
  Striae distensae
  Inguinal hernia
  Other hernia (umbilical, diaphragmatic, incisional)
Central nervous system
  *Dural ectasia:
    lumbosacral meningocele
    dilated cisterna magna
  Learning disability (verbal-performance discrepancy)
  Hyperactivity with or without attention deficit disorder

Listed in approximate order of decreasing specificity, major manifestations indicated by*.
Berlin Nosology (1988). *Am. J. Med. Genetics*, **29**, 581–94.

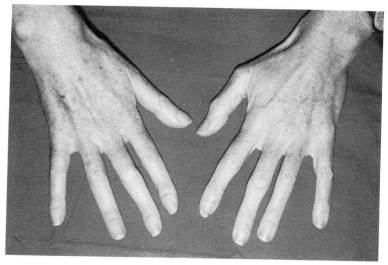

Fig. 11.6   Marfan syndrome. Fingers are long and thin (arachnodacytly).

in the precise skeletal abnormalities), ectopia lentis and aneurysms of the ascending aorta, sometimes leading to aortic dissection. A more detailed list of diagnostic manifestations, arranged in approximate order of decreasing specificity, Berlin 1986 Nosology is depicted in Table 11.4.

Skeletal aspects

The victim is said to suggest the subject of an El Greco painting. The extremities are long and the lower segment (pubis to sole) measure is in excess of the upper segment (pubis to vertex). Arachnodactyly results (Figure 11.6). The upper segment and lower segment ratio, normally 0.93, is lower than average. The change in this ratio with growth differs from normal, ending up an adult Marfan ration in the vicinity of 0.85[80]. Metacarpal index also provides an objective indication of arachnodactyly.

The length (in millimetres) of the second, third, fourth and fifth metacarpals is measured on the X-ray film of the right hand. At the exact mid-point of each shaft, the breadth is also measured and the value divided into the length. The figures for the four metacarpals are averaged. The metacarpal index is then the average ratio of length to breadth for metacarpals 2 to 5. Comparison can then be made to an appropriate histogram[81].

Hyperlaxity of the joints is common and kyphoscoliosis often occurs. The great toes may be elongated out of proportion to the others. All standard associations of joint hyperlaxity including propensity to early inflammation, flat feet, habitual dislocation of the hip and patella and genu recurvatum are found. There is a sparsity of subcutaneous fat in most cases and the epiphyses tend to close earlier than normal[82].

A high arched palate (Figure 11.7) is characteristic and pectus excavatum, spina bifida occulta and hemivertebrae may all occasionally occur in Marfan syndrome.

The eye

Ectopia lentis is almost always bilateral. The suspensory ligaments, when visualized with

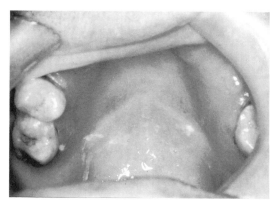

Fig. 11.7 Marfan syndrome. The palate is high and arched.

the slit lamp, are redundant, attenuated and often broken. The lens is often abnormally small and spherical[83,84]. Occasionally, there may be complete dislocation of the lens into the anterior chamber. Myopia usually results from excessive length of the eyeball. The sclerae may be impressively blue and clouding of the cornea occasionally occurs [85].

The cardiovascular system

As a result of abnormality in the base of the ascending aorta, dissecting aneurysm may occur. In addition, a 'congenital idiopathic dilatation of the pulmonary artery' is common[86] as well as occasional dissecting aneurysm of the pulmonary artery[87]. In the aorta, dilatation usually begins at the aortic ridge which, together with stretching of the aortic cuffs, usually produces profound aortic regurgitation before clear X-ray signs emerge. Aortic dilatation is usually progressive, although the patients may be free of symptoms for five or more years after the development of aortic incompetence.

Dissecting aneurysm may occur as the first aortic complication, or may be superimposed on diffuse dilatation of the ascending aorta. This causes classical features of chest pain with a risk of death, so the patient may survive

a number of years after the first dissection, even after a leak into the pericardium. Even with chronic dissecting aneurysm of the aorta, there may be little enlargement of the aorta evident on X-ray.

DIAGNOSIS

The diagnosis is made on clinical grounds in collaboration with a strong family history. With the spread of molecular biology, a diagnostic test based on the chromosome mapping of the fibrillin gene is likely to become more widely available.

Differential diagnosis is from other inherited abnormalities of connective tissue so there is likely to be pronounced overlap with dominant inherited ectopia lentis occurring in isolation and with congenital contractual arachnodactyly as well as predominantly inherited isolated mitral valve prolapse syndrome. Ultimately, these conditions may be shown to be due to closely related abnormalities of the fibrillin gene.

TREATMENT

At present there is no specific treatment for Marfan syndrome. Management should be symptomatic, based on the requirements of each individual, interpreted in relation to their family history.

The management of joint hyperlaxity has already been discussed. In general, joint laxity is much less severe in Marfan syndrome than in EDS so the muscoloskeletal problems are not so pronounced.

Management of aortic aneurysm is likely to involve early surgery with the use of valve prosthesis for incompetent aortic valves. On the whole, prognosis is better in Marfan syndrome than in EDS, the connective tissue abnormality perhaps being less severe in mechanical terms. Inevitably, some operative deaths occur (12% in one series[88]).

Obstetric complications also occur as in EDS, but perhaps not so severe. The risk of death in pregnancy is low[89]. A minimum aortic diameter of more than 40 mm, as measured by echocardiographic techniques, or the presence of any cardiac decompensation have been suggested as contraindications to pregnancy. Otherwise, antepartum hemorrhage and premature rupture of membranes may occur, but these are less severe than in EDS.

Normally, specific treatment is not indicated for ectopia lentis though surgery may be recommended when diplopia, glaucoma, retinal detachment (sometimes seen in this condition) or cataracts complicate the picture.

Ophthalmological examination and regular echocardiography would be obvious recommendations for all patients in whom the condition is diagnosed. Genetic counselling is also an important issue for families with the Marfan syndrome.

PROGNOSIS

Cardiovascular complications frequently occur and a substantial proportion of affected people die from aortic incompetence or dissection secondary to regurtive changes in the root of the aorta. The average age of death in a series of 72 patients with the syndrome was 32 years[90]. If cardiovascular complications do not intervene, the lifespan continues unaltered with only modest morbidity.

OTHER INHERITED ABNORMALITIES INVOLVING BONE, COLLAGEN AND SKIN

INTRODUCTION

Overlap between EDS and Marfan syndrome and other connective tissue disorders has already been described. Modern techniques in molecular biology are likely to identify even more genetic abnormalities, each causing their own clinical syndrome. In turn, conventional clinical classification is likely to break down. As they illustrate principals in the explosive expansion of molecular genetics and

because they occasionally present in rheumatology clinics, mention will now be made briefly of some other abnormalities of connective tissue, many of which (but not all) contribute to the observed phenotype of joint hypermobility (or joint hyperlaxity) which is a much more familiar entity in rheumatological practice.

OSTEOGENESIS IMPERFECTA

Perhaps less likely to impinge on rheumatological practice, this condition illustrates the way in which biochemical and genetic abnormalities have in general paralleled the early clinical classification, enhancing our understanding. The abnormalities center around the COL1A1 and COL1A2 genes which encode the pro-α1(I) and pro-α2(I) chains of type 1 procollagen. In turn, these genes have recently been implicated, perhaps controversially, in the pathogenesis of some variants of osteoarthritis. Table 11.5 shows a classification of the clinical variants of osteogenesis imperfecta (OI), together with our current understanding of their inheritance of biochemical and genetic abnormalities and the McKusick number, adopted in the Berlin Nosology[19]. Blue sclerae and abnormalities of the long bones occur (Figure 11.8).

The estimated incidence is 1:10 000 people in the USA and the gene prevalence although high is calculated as 5 per 100 000[91–93]. These estimates may fall short of the true prevalence and some examples of postmenopausal osteoporosis may actually be OI and masked by menopausal estrogen deficiency. Approximately 60% of OI is inherited as an autosomal dominant trait, 20% as an autosomal recessive trait and approximately 25% as a new mutation.

There have been multiple attempts at treatment of OI with hormones and drugs, mainly unsuccessful. Advocates have in turn favored mineral supplements, fluorides, calcitonin, androgenic steroids, ascorbic acid and vitamin D, on the whole without success[94,95].

Table 11.5 Clinical and genetic aspects of osteogenesis imperfecta

OI type	Clinical features	Inheritance*	Biochemical and genetic abnormalities	McKusick no
I	Normal stature, little or no deformity, blue sclerae, hearing loss in 50%, dentinogenesis imperfecta is rare and may distinguish a subset	AD	Common: 'non-functional' COL1A1 allele Rare: substitution for glycine reside in carboxy-terminal telopeptide of $\alpha 1$(IO) Substitution for glycines in the triple helix in pro-$\alpha 1$(I)	(16620)
II	Lethal in the perinatal period, minimal calvarial mineralization, beaded ribs, compressed femurs, marked long bone deformity, platyspondyly (flattened vertebrae)	AD (new)	Exon deletion in pro-$\alpha 2$(I) triple helix Common: substitutions for glycyl residues in the triple-helical domain of the $\alpha 1$(I) chain and $\alpha 2$(I) chain Rare: rearrangement in the COL1A1 and COL1A2 genes Exon deletions in triple-helical domain of COL1A1 and COL1A2	(16621)
		AR (rare)	Small deletion in $\alpha 2$(I) on the background of null allele	(25940)
III	Progressively deforming bones, usually with moderate deformity at birth. Sclerae variable in hue, often lighten with age. Dentinogenesis common, hearing loss common. Stature very short	AD	Point mutations in the COL1A1 and COL1A2 gene	(25942)
		AR (uncommon)	Frame-shift (4 bp deletion) in COL1A2 that prevents incorporation of pro-$\alpha 2$(I) chains into molecules	
IV	Normal sclerae, mild to moderate bone deformity and variable short stature, dentinogenesis is common and hearing loss occurs in some	AD	Point mutations in COL1A1 and COL1A2 genes Exon-skipping mutations in COL1A2	(16622)

AD: autosomal dominant.
AR: autosomal recessive.

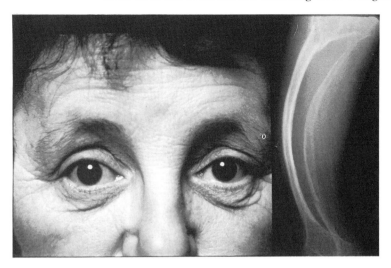

Fig. 11.8 Osteogenesis imperfecta. Characteristic features include blue sclerae and abnormalities in the shape of curved long bones.

Factors that promote bone growth, such as growth hormone and long-term, low-dose anabolic steroid, may be worthy of additional study though the appearance of osteoblasts and osteoclasts in OI is normal[96,97].

Surgery may correct deformity and facilitate weight bearing, and has been the subject of recent review[98,99]; rehabilitation and muscle strengthening exercises are important. Swimming may be particularly beneficial.

CHONDRODYSTROPHIES

Several of these are lethal at birth. Others are recognizable at birth and associated with variable survival but a normal life span. Some are not recognized at birth. Table 11.6 depicts an accepted clinical classification. All of them result from abnormalities in bone or collagen. This expanding classification avoids the confusion when, previously, all types of disproportionate short stature were called 'achondroplasia'. Recent reviews[100,101] have served to provide a more extensive clinical classification to which future specific genetic abnormalities are likely to be increasingly linked (Figures 11.9, 11.10). It seems

likely that certain phenotypes of joint hyperlaxity, particularly that associated with a wide range of movement at ball and socket joints, such as the hip and shoulder, may ultimately be linked with such abnormalities[102] as an increased number of candidate genes are explored[59].

ATHROGRYPOSIS MULTIPLEX CONGENITA

This is a heterogeneous group of disorders in which individuals are born with multiple areas of joint limitation[103]. Some types of AMC have associated anomalies. The mother is rarely affected with contractures herself, but a pregnancy carrying an affected individual can be associated with discomfort to the mother. Often there is decreased fetal movement or kicking only one area. The birth of the affected child may be complicated if it does not assume a normal attitude, breach and transverse lies are common. Affected infants often sustain bone fractures during delivery.

Some types of AMC have associated anomalies in other systems. In addition, congenital joint contractures are seen in several other specific inherited syndromes and the

Table 11.6 Chondrodystrophies

Disorders of short stature	Condition	Characteristics	Genetics
I Neonatal lethal			
1. Uniformly lethal	Achondrogenesis types I and II	Short trunk and extremities, absence of vertebral body ossification, very short underossified long bones, hyperdropic appearance	Autosomal recessive
	Thanatophoric dysplasia	Short limbs, relatively normal trunk with large head, flattened vertebral bodies, short, broad long bones	Sporadic
	Noonan–Saldino	Short limbs, narrow chest, postaxial polydactyly internal malformations	Autosomal recessive
	Majewski	Narrow chest, polysyndactyly, cleft lip or palate, short limbs, internal anomalies, short tibia	Unknown
2. Usually lethal	Chondrodysplasia punctata – rhizomelic type (rhizomelic Conradi syndrome)	Stippled epiphyses, disproportionate rhizomelic shortening of limbs, joint contractures, flat face, cataracts, skin changes	Autosomal recessive
	Infantile osteopetrosis	Dense bones, thick, dense skull, metaphyseal irregularity, hepatosplenomegaly, macrocephaly, failure to thrive	Autosomal recessive
	Infantile hypophosphatasia	Short underossified long bones, absence of ossification of skull, low serum alkaline phosphatase, urinary phosphoethanolamine	Autosomal recessive
	Neonatal lethal osteogenesis imperfecta (crumpled bone)	Short, deformed limbs, soft, large skull, blue sclerae, broad bones (crumpled) with multiple fractures	Autosomal recessive
	Homozygous achondroplasia	Short limbs, relatively normal trunk, large head, short, broad long bones, both parents with achondroplasia	Autosomal recessive
II Recognizable at birth			
1. Variable survival	Asphyxiating thoracic dysplasia (Jeune)	Long, narrow thorax, postaxial polydactyly, respiratory distress, spur-like projection of the acetabular roof	Autosomal recessive
	Diastrophic dysplasia	Multiple joint contractures, club feet, cleft palate, cauliflower ears, scoliosis, dislocated hips, club hands	Autosomal recessive
	Chondroectodermal dysplasia (Ellis–van Creveld)	Distal shortening of limbs, postaxial polydactyly, multiple frenula, dental anomalies, cardiac defects	Autosomal recessive
	Kneist syndrome	Short trunk, short limbs with prominent joints, lumbar lordosis, cleft palate, myopia, deafness, flat face	Autosomal dominant
	Spondyloepiphyseal dysplasia congenita	Short trunk, flat face, normal hands and feet, myopia, genu valgum, broad chest, delayed ossification, coxa vara	Autosomal dominant

Table 11.6 Continued.

Disorders of short stature	Condition	Characteristics	Genetics
	Chondrodysplasia punctata – asymmetric type (Conradi-Hunermann)	Stippled epiphyses, asymmetric shortening of limbs, scoliosis, ichthyosiform skin, flat face, cataracts	Autosomal dominant
2. Usually with normal lifespan	Achondroplasia	Short limbs with proximal shortening, large head, prominent forehead, trident hand, short pedicles	Autosomal dominant
	Hypochondroplasia	Short limbs, relatively normal skull, short, broad long bones, occasional mental retardation	Autosomal dominant
	Cartilage hair hypoplasia (metaphyseal chondrodysplasia – McKusick type)	Short limbs, sparse fine hair, ligamentous laxity, metaphyseal irregularities, long fibulae	Autosomal recessive
III Usually not recognized at birth	Spondyloepiphyseal dysplasia (many types)	Vertebral and epiphyseal abnormalities, all combinations and severities	Variable
	Pseudoachondroplasia	Normal newborn, normal skull, short limbs, arthritis, hyperextensibility	Autosomal dominant
	Vitamin D-resistant rickets (hypophosphatemic familial rickets)	Metaphyseal irregularities, more severe in lower limbs, bowing of legs, dental changes, hypophosphatemia, elevated alkaline phosphatasia	X-linked dominant

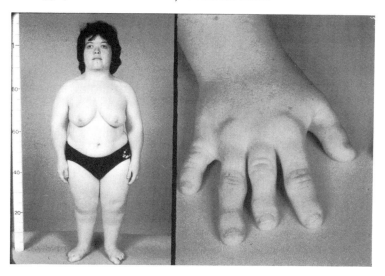

Fig. 11.9   Chondrodystrophy. Stature is often abnormal, usually short and other skeletal abnormalities may be apparent.

contractures that can occur in acquired rheumatic diseases, particularly rheumatoid arthritis and scleroderma, provide a diagnostic pitfall.

INHERITED DISORDERS OF ELASTIN

Although this description is somewhat artificial since collagen may also be abnormal, the predominant feature is felt to be an abnormality in elastin. Typically, these conditions involve the skin. Examples are cutis laxa, Menkes' kinky hair syndrome and pseudo-xanthomata elasticum. The respective McKusik numbers are 12370 and 21910 for the benign and severe forms of cutis laxis, 30940 for the X-linked Menkes' syndrome and 17785 or 26480 for the dominant and recessive forms of pseudoxanthomata elasticum respectively.

Cutis laxis currently encompasses several connective tissue disorders characterized by lax, redundant and often in elastin skin. Autosomal dominance, autosomal recessive and sex-linked variants have all been described[104–106] and an acquired form may follow the ingestion of penicillamine[107]. Unlike EDS, the skin in cutis laxis does not recoil when stretched. The autosomal dominant form is mild but the recessive variant is more severe, usually diagnosed at birth and associated with severe early cardiopulmonary complications. In neither condition are the joints hyperextensible. Cardiac murmurs have been observed in adult life and some patients develop lung abnormalities, including emphysema and cor pulmonale. Changes in the pulmonary arteries similar to those found in Menkes' syndrome[108] suggest overlap. Microscopically, there are alterations in both elastin and collagen in the dermis. Individual elastic fibers vary greatly in diameter and tend to be short and globular in outline.

Menkes' kinky hair syndrome, first described by Menkes in 1962[109] is a sex-linked disorder of copper metabolism affecting metalloenzymes essential to collagen and elastin synthesis. It provides a reminder that a more generalized metabolic abnormality in metabolism may impinge on connective tissue. The disease begins *in utero* and is apparent at birth. Hair is kinky, brittle and sparse. Hyperbilirubinemia is common and there are widespread mental abnormalities.

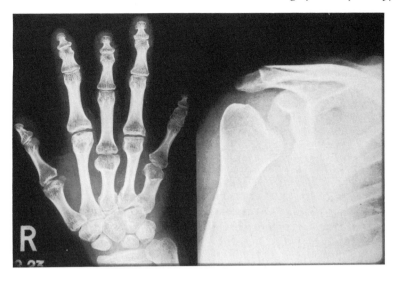

Fig. 11.10 Chondrodystrophy. Premature osteoarthritis is also common in this condition.

Skeletal demineralization occurs. Angiographic studies show characteristic corkscrew tortuosity of intracerebral, renal and intestinal vessels. There is a low serum copper, low serum ceruloplasmin and marked reduction in hepatic and brain copper content but elevated renal, skeletal muscle and placental copper content[110,111]. The common biochemical link appears to be that lysyl oxidase and its co-factor, copper, are important for the initial steps of collagen cross-linking. A putative lesion is the inability to transfer copper to cellular enzymes, resulting in neurological and connective tissue abnormalities.

Pseudoxanthomata elasticum (PXE) is a rare disorder characterized by degeneration and calcification of elastic fibers in the skin, retina and blood vessels. The estimated instance varies from 1 in 70 000 to 1 in 160 000 live births though milder cases may go unrecognized[112,113]. Classically, asymptomatic, symmetrical, yellowish-white papules appear in flexural skin folds during the third decade of life (or earlier in the recessive form). These papules have a xanthomatoid appearance mimicking cutis laxa. Mucocutaneous lesions may also occur[114] and the classical angioid streaks in the retina are radially orientated,

resembling vessels, and are the result of a break in Bruch's membrane[115]. They occur in 85% of patients but are not specific to this syndrome, being occasionally found in EDS as well. Lung lesions may be demonstrated with pleurisy on angiography. Progressive dyspnea may herald pulmonary or cardiac involvement. Genitourinary and uterine bleeding occur. The dermal elastin fibers are swollen and plump and appear to be increased in number. The centers of elastin fibers are replaced by electron-dense material, which appears to disrupt the fibers leading to degenerative calcification. Unaffected skin also contains increased amounts of this dense material, though information on the abnormality of elastin structure or synthesis is not currently available[116].

BENIGN FAMILIAL JOINT HYPERLAXITY

The pathogenesis of the phenotype, much more frequently seen in rheumatology clinics than any of the rarer disorders of connective tissue described above, remains ill understood. The range of movement observed at a joint (which varies in a Gaussian fashion throughout the population[102]) is a determinant of several features including collagen structure, the shape of the bony articulating surfaces and the neuromuscular tone. Other factors, such as skin structure, girth of the surrounding muscle and length of the limb, also serve to accentuate or limit the degree of movement. The extent to which hyperlaxity of the single joint varies between sexes, with age and with race is already well documented[52]. At present all variants are encompassed in the Berlin Nosology by a single McKusick number (14790) characterized by cardinal manifestations of generalized articular hypermobility, with or without subluxation or dislocation and absence of skin involvement. By definition, EDS type III and skeletal dysplasias with joint hypermobility are excluded though, by implication, overlap may still occur and in view of widespread clinical variations encompassed by the term 'joint hyperlaxity' this classification is likely to be an over-simplification. With time, the closer marrying of clinical and molecular genetic disciplines is likely to lead to the identification of milder abnormalities of connective tissue that produce the observed phenotype, either through alteration in collagen structure (typified by widespread laxity at many joints) or through the alteration in the shape of the bony articulating surfaces (typified by severe laxity at a small number of joints), or perhaps both. In addition, acquired factors, such as the extent to which joint laxity can be influenced by drugs used in the treatment of rheumatic disease (e.g. D-penicillamine and prednisolone), or the extent to which exercise and training can increase the range of movement at a joint and maintain this change, also require integration with genetic etiological features.

REFERENCES

1. Wordsworth, B. P. (1992) Genetic mapping in the connective tissue disorders. *Br. J. Rheumatol.*, **31**, 147–8.
2. Byers, P. H. (1989) Inherited disorders of collagen gene structure and expression. *Am. J. Med. Genet.*, **34**, 72–80.
3. Seyer, J. M. and Kang, A. H. (1989) Collagen and elastin, in *Textbook of Rheumatology*, 3rd edn, (eds W. N. Kelly, E. P. Harris, S. L. Ruddy *et al.*), W. B. Saunders Co., Philadelphia, pp. 22–41.
4. Kühn, K. and Krieg, T. (eds) (1986). *Connective tissue: Biological and Clinical Aspects*, Karger, London.
5. Robins, S. P. (1988) Functional properties of collagen and elastin, in *Biochemical Aspects of Rheumatic Diseases*, vol. 2, No. I, (eds J. Dixon and H. Bird) Baillières Clinical Rheumatology, London, pp. 1–36.
6. Kuivaniemi, H., Tromp, G. and Prockop, D. J. (1991) Mutations in collagen genes: causes of rare and some common diseases in humans. *FASEB J.*, **5**, 2052–60.
7. Byers, P. H. (1990) Brittle bones – fragile molecules: disorders of collagen gene structure and expression. *Trends in Genet.*, **6**, 293–300.
8. Pope, F. M. (1988) Genetics of inherited defects of connective tissue, in *Genetics of Rheumatic Diseases*, vol. 2, No. 3 (ed. D. M. Grennan) Baillières Clinical Rheumatology, London, pp. 673–702).
9. Sokolov, B. P., Prytkov, A. N., Tromp, G. *et al.* (1991) Exclusion of COL1A1, COL1A2 and COL3A1 genes as candidate genes for Ehlers–Danlos syndrome type I in one large family. *Hum. Genet.*, **88**(2), 125–9.
10. Oku, T., Nakayama, F., Takigawa, M. *et al.* (1990) Growth kinetics of fibroblasts from a patient with Ehlers-Danlos syndrome. *Acta Dermato-Venereologica*, **70**, 56–7.
11. Wordsworth, B. P., Ogilvie, D. J. and Sykes, B. C. (1991) Segregation analysis of the structural genes of the major fibrillar collagens provides further evidence of molecular heterogeneity in type II Ehlers–Danlos syndrome. *Br. J. Rheumatol.*, **30**, 173–7.
12. Pope, F. M. (1991) Molecular analysis of Ehlers–Danlos syndrome type II (editorial). *Br. J. Rheumatol.*, **30**, 163–6.
13. Vasan, N. S., Kuivaniemai, H., Vogel, B. E. *et al.* (1991) A mutation in the Pro-α2(I) gene (COL1A2) for type I procollagen in Ehlers–Danlos syndrome type VII: Evidence suggesting that skipping of exon 6 in RNA splicing may be a common cause of the phenotype. *Am. J. Hum. Genet.*, **48**, 305–17.
14. Nicholls, A. C., Oliver, J., Renouf, D. V. *et al.*

(1991) Ehlers–Danlos syndrome type VII: a single base change that causes exon skipping in the type I collagen α2(I) chain. *Hum. Genet.*, **87**, 193–8.

15. D'Alessio, M., Ramirez, F., Blumberg, B. D. *et al.* (1991) Characterization of a COL1A1 splicing defect in a case of Ehlers–Danlos syndrome type VII: further evidence of molecular homogeneity. *Am. J. Hum. Genet.*, **49**, 400–6.

16. Watson, R. B., Wallis, G. A., Holmes, D. F. *et al.* (1992) Ehlers–Danlos syndrome type VII B. Incomplete cleavage of abnormal type I procollagen by N-proteinase *in vitro* results in the formation of copolymers of collagen and partially cleaved pN collagen that are near circular in cross-section. *J. Biolog. Chem.*, **267**, 9093–100.

17. Chiodo, A. A., Hockey, A. and Cole, W. G. (1992) A base substitution at the splice acceptor site of intron 5 of the COL1A2 gene activates a cryptic splice site within exon 6 and generates abnormal type I procollagen in a patient with Ehlers–Danlos syndrome type VII. *J. Biolog. Chem.*, **267**, 6361–9.

18. Smith, L. T., Wertelecki, W., Milstone, L. M. *et al.* (1992) Human dermatosparaxis: a form of Ehlers–Danlos syndrome that results from failure to remove the amino-terminal propeptide of type I procollagen. *Am. J. Hum. Genet.*, **51**, 235–44.

19. Beighton, P., De Paepe, A., Finidori, G. *et al.* (1988) International nosology of heritable disorders of connective tissue, Berlin, 1986. *Am. J. Med. Genet.*, **29**, 581–94.

20. Wertelecki, W., Smith, L. T. and Byers, P. (1992) Initial observations of human dermatosparaxis: Ehlers–Danlos syndrome type V11C. *J. Paed.*, **121**, 558–64.

21. Spotila, L. D., Constantinou, C. D., Sereda, L. *et al.* (1990) Substitution of serine for glycine α2 -661 in the gene for type I procollagen (COL1A2) as a cause of postmenopausal osteoporosis. *Am. J. Hum. Genet.*, **47**, A237.

22. Nicholls, A. C., Oliver, J., Renoouf, D. *et al.* (1990) Type I collagen mutations in osteogenesis imperfecta and inherited osteoporosis. *Am. J. Hum. Genet.*, **47**.

23. Constantinou, C. D., Pack, M. A. and Prockop, D. J. (1990) A mutation of the type I procollagen gene on chromosome 17q 21.31 – q22.05 or 7q 21.3 – q22.1 that decreases the thermal stability of the protein in a woman with ankylosing spondylitis and osteopenia. *Cytogenet. Cell Genet.*, **51**, 979.

24. Shapiro, J. R., Burn, V. E., Chipman, S. D. *et al.* (1989) Osteoporosis and familial idiopathic scoliosis association with an abnormal α2(I) collagen. *Conn. Tiss. Res.*, **21**, 117–23.

25. Palotie, A., Väisänen, P., Ott, J. *et al.* (1989) Predisposition to familial osteoarthritis linked to type II collagen gene. *Lancet*, **1**, 924–7.

26. Priestley, L., Fergusson, C., Ogilvie, D. *et al.* (1991) A limited association of generalised osteoarthritis with alleles at the type II collagen locus: COL2A1. *Br. J. Rheumatol.*, **30**, 272–5.

27. Pope, F. M., Nicholls, A. C., Narcisi, P. *et al.* (1981) Some patients with cerebral aneurysms are deficient in type III collagen. *Lancet*, **i**, 973–5.

28. Kontusaari, S., Tromp, G., Kuivaniemi, H. *et al.* (1990) A mutation in the gene for type III procollagen (COL3A1) in a family with aortic aneurysms. *J. Clin. Invest.*, **86**, 1465–73.

29. Kontusaari, S., Tromp, E., Kuivaniemi, H. *et al.* (1990) Inheritance of an RNA splicing mutation (G + 1 IVS20) in the type III procollagen gene (COL3A1) in a family having aortic aneurysms and easy bruisability: phenotypic overlap between familial arterial aneurysms and Ehlers–Danlos syndrome type IV. *Am. J. Hum. Genet.*, **47**, 112–20.

30. Richards, A. J., Lloyd, J. C., Narcisis, P. *et al.* (1992) A 27-bp deletion from one allele of the type III collagen gene (COL3A1) in a large family with Ehlers–Danlos syndrome type IV. *Hum. Genet.*, **88**, 325–30.

31. Tromp, G., Kuivaniemi, H., Shikata, H. *et al.* (1989) A single base mutation that substitutes serine for glycine 790 of the α1(III) chain of type III procollagen exposes an arginine and causes Ehlers–Danlos syndrome IV. *J. Biolog. Chem.*, **264**, 1349–52.

32. Barker, D. F., Hostikka, S. L., Zhoul, J. *et al.* (1990) Identification of mutations in the COL-4A5 collagen gene in Alport syndrome. *Science*, **248**, 1224–7.

33. Eady, R. A. J. (1987) Rashes, blisters and basement membranes. *Clin. Exp. Dermatol.*, **12**, 159–70.

34. Milewicz, D. M., Pyeritz, R. E., Crawford, E. S. *et al.* (1992) Marfan syndrome: Defective synthesis, secretion and extracellular matrix formation of fibrillin by cultured dermal fibroblasts. *J. Clin. Invest.*, **89**, 79–86.

35. Ramirez, F., Lee, B. and Vitale, E. (1992)

Clinical and genetic associations in Marfan syndrome and related disorders. *Mount Sinai J. Med.*, **59**, 350–6.

36. Godfrey, M., Menashe, V., Weleber, R. G. *et al.* (1990) Cosegregation of elastin associated microfibrillar abnormalities with the Marfan phenotype in families. *Am. J. Hum. Genet.*, **46**, 652–60.

37. Sakai, L. Y., Keen, D. R. and Engvall, E. (1986) Fibrillin, a new 350-kD glycoprotein, is a component of extracellular microfibrils. *J. Cell Biol.*, **103**, 2499–509.

38. Hollister, D. W., Godfrey, M., Sakai, L. Y. *et al.* (1990) Immunohistologic abnormalities of the microfibrillar-fiber system in the Marfan syndrome. *N. Eng. J. Med.*, **323**, 152–9.

39. Francomano, C. A., Streeten, E. A., Meyers, D. A. *et al.* (1988) Marfan syndrome exclusion of genetic linkage to three major collagen genes. *Am. J. Med. Genet.*, **29**, 457–62.

40. Godfrey, M., Olson, S., Burgid, R. G. *et al.* (1990) Unilateral microfibrillar abnormalities in a case of asymmetric Marfan syndrome. *Am. J. Hum. Genet.*, **46**, 661–71.

41. Blanton, S. H., Sarfarazi, M., Elberg, H. *et al.* (1990) An exclusion map of Marfan syndrome. *J. Med. Genet.*, **27**, 73–7.

42. Kainulainen, K., Steinmann, B., Collins, F. *et al.* (1991) Marfan syndrome: No evidence for heterogeneity in different populations, and more precise mapping of the gene. *Am. J. Hum. Genet.*, **49**, 662–7.

43. Lee, B., Godfrey, M., Vitale, E. *et al.* (1991) Linkage of Marfan syndrome and a phenotypically related disorder to two different fibrillin genes. *Nature*, **353**, 330–4.

44. Maslen, C. L., Corson, G. M., Maddox, B. K. *et al.* (1991) Partial sequencing of a candidate gene for the Marfan syndrome. *Nature*, **353**, 334–7.

45. Dietz, H. C., Cutting, G. R., Pyeritz, R. E. *et al.* (1991) Marfan syndrome caused by a recurrent denovo missence mutation in the fibrillin gene. *Nature*, **353**, 337–9.

46. Tsipouras, P., Del Mastro, R., Sarfarazi, M. *et al.* (1992) Genetic linkage of the Marfan syndrome, ectopia lentis and congenital contractural arachnodactyly to the fibrillin genes on chromosomes 15 and 5. *N. Eng. J. Med.*, **326**, 905–9.

47. Peltonen, L. and Kainulainen, K. (1992) Elucidation of the gene defect in Marfan syndrome, success by the two complementary research strategies. *FEBS*, **307**, 116–21.

48. Child, A., Kainulainen, K., Pope, F. M. *et al.* (1992) Two unique fibrillin gene mutations in U.K. Marfan syndrome patients with joint hypermobility. *Br. J. Rheumatol.*, **31** (abs. suppl. No. 2), 165.

49. Miura, S., Shirakami, A., O'Hara, A. *et al.* (1990) Fibronectin receptor on polymorphonuclear leukocytes in families of Ehlers–Danlos syndrome and other hereditary connective tissue diseases. *J. Lab. Clin. Med.*, **116**, 363–8.

50. Barlati, S., Moro, L., Gardella, R. *et al.* (1991) Phenotypic correction of the defective fibronectin extracellular matrix of Ehlers–Danlos syndrome fibroblasts. *Cell Biol. Intern. Rep.*, **15**, 1183–94.

51. Colombi, M., Moro, L., Zoppi, N. *et al.* (1991) Altered fibronectin mRNA splicing in skin fibroblasts from Ehlers–Danlos syndrome patients: *In situ* hybridization analysis. *Cell Biol. Intern. Rep.*, **15**(12), 1195–206.

52. Beighton, P., Grahame, R. and Bird, H. (eds) (1989) *Hypermobility of Joints*, 2nd edn, Springer-Verlag, London.

53. Poumeau-Delille, G. and Soulié, P. (1934) Un cas d'hyperlaxite cutanée et articulaire avec cicatrices atrophiques et pseudo tumeurs molluscoides syndrome d'Ehlers–Danlos. *Bull. Soc. Med. Hôp.*, Paris, **50**, 593–5.

54. Tschernogobow, A. (1892) Cutis Laxa (Presentation at first meeting of Moscow Dermatological and Venereological Society Nov 13 1891). *Monatschrifte Pratische Dermatologische*, **14**, 76–8.

55. Ehlers, E. (1901) Cutis Laxa. Niegung zu Haemorrhagien in der Haut, Lockerung mehrerer. *Artikulationen Dermatologische Zeitschrift*, **8**, 173–5.

56. Danlos, H. A. (1908) Un cas de cutis laxa avec tumeurs par contusion chronique des coudes et des genoux (Xanthome juvenile pseudodiabétique de MM. Hallopeau et Macé de Lepinay). *Bulletin de la Societé Francaise de dermatologie et de syphiligraphie*, **19**, 70–2.

57. Beighton, P. (1970) *The Ehlers–Danlos syndrome*. William Heinemann Medical Books, London.

58. Beighton, P., Price, A., Lord, J. *et al.* (1969) Variants of the Ehlers–Danlos syndrome. Clinical, biochemical, haematological and chromosomal features of 100 patients. *Ann. Rheum. Dis.*, **28**, 228–42.

59. Iton, P., De Paepe, A., Hollister, D. W. *et al.* (1992) Molecular nosology of heritable

disorders of connective tissue. *Am. J. Med. Genet.*, **42**, 431–48.

60. McFarland, W. and Fuller, D. E. (1964) Mortality in Ehlers–Danlos syndrome due to spontaneous rupture of large arteries. *N. Eng. J. Med.*, **271**, 1309–12.

61. Beighton, P. (1968) X-linked recessive inheritance in the Ehlers–Danlos syndrome. *Br. Med. J.*, **3**, 409–11.

62. Beighton, P., Murdock, J. L,. and Votteler, T. (1969) Gastrointestinal complications of the Ehlers–Danlos syndrome. *Gut*, **10**, 1004–8.

63. Goodman, R. M. and Alison, M. L. (1969) Chronic temporomandibular joint subluxation in Ehlers–Danlos syndrome: report of case. *J. Oral Surg.*, **27**, 659–61.

64. Beighton, P. and Horan, F. (1969) Orthopaedic aspects of the Ehlers–Danlos syndrome. *J. Bone and Joint Surg.*, **51**, 444–9.

65. Bilkey, W. J., Baxter, T. L., Kottke, F. J. *et al.* (1981) Muscle formation in Ehlers–Danlos syndrome. *Arch. Physical Med. Rehab.*, **62**, 444–8.

66. Mabille, J. P., Castera, D., Chapuis, J. L. *et al.* (1972) Un cas de syndrome d'Ehlers–Danlos, avec acro-osteolyse. *Ann. Radiol.*, **15**, 781–6.

67. Cabeen, W. R., Reza, M. J., Kovick, R. B. *et al.* (1977) Mitral valve prolapse and conduction defects in Ehlers–Danlos syndrome. *Arch. Intern. Med.*, **137**, 1227–31.

68. Leier, C. V., Call, T. D., Fulkerson, P. K. *et al.* (1980) The spectrum of cardiac defects in the Ehlers–Danlos syndrome, types I and II. *Ann. Intern. Med.*, **92**, 171–8.

69. Marfan, A. B. (1896) Un cas de deformation congenitale des quatre membres plus prononcee aux extremites characterisee par l'allongement des os avec un certain degre d'amin-cissement. *Bull. Mem. Soc. Med. Hop., Paris*, **13**, 220–6.

70. Weve, H. (1931) Ueber Arachnodaktylie (Dystrophia mesodermalis congenita, typus Marfanis). *Arch. Augenheilk.*, **104**, 1.

71. Baer, R. W., Taussig, H. B. and Oppenheimer, E. H. (1943) Congenital aneurysmal dilatation of the aorta associated with arachnodactyly. *Bull. Hopkins Hosp.*, **72**, 309.

72. McKusick, V. A. (1955) The cardiovascular aspects of Marfan's syndrome: a heritable disorder of connective tissue. *Circulation*, **11**, 321–42.

73. Pyeritz, R. E. (1990) Marfan syndrome, in *Principles and Practice of Medical Genetics*, 2nd end., (eds A. E. H. Emery and D. L. Rimoin),

New York, Churchill Livingstone, pp. 1047–63.

74. Maddox, B. K., Sakai, L. Y., Keene, D. R. *et al.* (1989) Connective tissue microfibrils: isolation and characterization of three large pepsin-resistant domains of fibrillin. *J. Biolog. Chem.*, **264**, 21381–5.

75. Nakashima, Y. (1986) Reduced activity of serum beta-glucuronidase in Marfan syndrome. *Angiology*, **37**, 576–80.

76. Tsipouras, P., Borresen, A. L., Bamforth, S. *et al.* (1986) Marfan syndrome, exclusion of genetic linkage to the COL1A2 gene. *Clin. Genet.*, **30**, 420–32.

77. Dagleish, R., Hawkins, J. R. and Keston, M. (1987) Exclusion of the α2(I) and α1(III) collagen genes as the mutant loci in a Marfan syndrome family, *J. Med. Genet.*, **24**, 148–51.

78. Kainulainen, K., Pulkkinen, L., Savolainen, A. *et al.* (1990) Location on chromosome 15 of the gene defect causing Marfan syndrome. *N. Eng. J. Med.*, **323**, 935–9.

79. Glesby, M. J. and Pyeritz, R. E. (1989) Association of mitral valve prolapse and systemic abnormalities of connective tissue: a phenotypic continuum. *JAMA*, **262**, 523–8.

80. Stolz, H. R. and Stolz, L. M. (1951) *Somatic development of adolescent boys. A Study of the Growth of Boys During the Second Decade of Life.* New York, The Macmillan Co.

81. Parish, J. G., Calnan, C. D. and Lawrence, J.S. (1960) Heritable disorders of connective tissue. *Proc. Roy. Soc. Med.*, **53**, 515.

82. Van Buchem, F. S. P. (1958) Cardiovascular disease in arachnodactyly. *Acta Med. Scand.*, **161**, 197.

83. Fischl, A. A. and Ruthberg, J. (1951) Clinical implications of Marfan's syndrome. *JAMA*, **146**, 704.

84. Lloyd, R. I. (1935) Arachnodactyly. *Arch. Ophthal.*, **13**, 744.

85. Black, H. H. and Landay, L. H. (1955) Marfan's syndrome; report of five cases in one family. *Am. J. Dis. Children*, **89**, 414.

86. Castellanos, A., Jr., Ugarriza, R., de Cardenas, A. *et al.* (1957) Sindrome de Marfan. Reporte de seis casos en una misma familia. *Arch. Hos. Univ.* (Habana), **9**, 353.

87. Anderson, M. and Pratt-Thomas, H. R. (1953) Marfan's syndrome. *Am. Heart J.*, **46**, 911.

88. Donaldson, R. M., Manuel, R. W., Olsen, E. G. J. *et al.* (1980) Management of cardiovascular complications in Marfan syndrome. *Lancet*, **2**, 1178–80.

89. Pyeritz, R. E. (1981) Maternal and fetal complications in pregnancy in the Marfan syndrome. *Am. J. Med.*, **71**, 784–90.

90. Murdock, J. L., Walker, B. A., Halpern, B. L. *et al.* (1972) A life expectancy and cause of death in the Marfan syndrome. *N. Eng. J. Med.*, **286**, 804–8.

91. Wynne-Davies, R. and Gormley, J. (1981) Clinical and genetic patterns in osteogenesis imperfecta. *Clin. Orthopaed.*, **159**, 26–35.

92. Gunnear, S. (1961) *Osteogenesis Imperfecta*, Sweden, Stockholm University Books.

93. Sillence, D. O., Senn, A. and Danks, D. M. (1979) Genetic heterogeneity in osteogenesis imperfecta. *J. Med. Genet.*, **16**, 101–16.

94. Albright, J. A. (1981) Systemic treatment of osteogenesis imperfecta. *Clin. Orthopaed.*, **159**, 88–96.

95. Smith, R., Francis, M. J. O. and Houghton, G. R. (1983) *The Brittle Bone Syndrome: Osteogenesis Imperfecta*, Kent, Butterworth.

96. Sillence, D. O. and Rimoin, D. L. (1982) Morphological studies in osteogenesis imperfecta, in *AAOS Symposium on Heritable Disorders of Connective Tissue*, (eds W. J. Ackeson, P. Bornstein and M. J. Glimcher), C. V. Mosby Company, p. 259.

97. Albright, J. P., Albright, J. A. and Crelin, E. S. (1975) Osteogenesis imperfecta tarda: The morphology of rib biopsies. *Clin. Orthopaed.*, **108**, 204–13.

98. Moorefield, W. G. and Miller, G. R. (1980) Aftermath of osteogenesis imperfecta, the disease of adulthood. *J. Bone and Joint Surg.*, **62A**, 113–19.

99. Rodriquez, R. P. and Bailey, R. W. (1981) Internal fixation of the femur in patients with osteogenesis imperfecta. *Clin. Orthopaed.*, **159**, 126–33.

100. Spranger, J. W., Langer, L. A. and Wiedemann, H. R. (1974) '*Bone Dysplasias*': *An Atlas of Constitutional Disorders of Skeletal Development*, Saunders, Philadelphia, Pennsylvania.

101. Rimoin, D. L. (1975) The chondrodystrophies. *Advan. Hum. Genet.*, **5**, 1–118.

102. Bird, H. A. (1983) *Joint and Tissue Laxity. Topical Reviews in the Rheumatic Disorders*, **2**, John Wright and Sons, Bristol, pp. 133–66.

103. Hall, J. G. (1980) Arthrogryphosis, in *Klinische Genetik In der Pädiatrie, Symposium in Mainz*, (eds J. Spranger, J. Gehler and M. Tolkstorf), New York, Georg Thieme Verlag Stuttgard.

104. Beighton, P. (1972) The dominant and recessive forms of cutis laxa. *J. Med. Genet.*, **9**, 216–21.

105. Byers, P. H., Siegel, R. C., Holbrook, K. *et al.* (1980) X-linked cutis laxa; defective cross-link formation in collagen due to decreased lysyl oxidase activity. *N. Eng. J. Med.*, **202**, 61–5,.

106. Uitto, J., Ryhänen, L., Abraham, P. A. *et al.* (1982) Elastin in diseases. *J. Invest. Dermatol.*, **79**, 160s–8s.

107. Linares, A., Zarranz, J. J., Rodriguez-Alarcon, J. *et al.* (1979) Reversible cutis laxis due to maternal D-penicillamine treatment. *Lancet*, **2**, 43.

108. Meine, R., Grossman, H., Forman, W. *et al.* (1979) The radiographic findings in congenital cutis laxa. *Radiology*, **113**, 687–90.

109. Menkes, J. H., Alter, M., Steigleder, G. K. *et al.* (1962) A sex-linked recessive disorder with retardation of growth, peculiar hair and focal cerebral and cerebellar degeneration. *Pediatrics*, **29**, 764–79.

110. Willemse, J., Van Den Hamer, C. J., Prins, H. W. *et al.* (1982) Menkes' kinky hair disease. I. comparison of classical and unusual clinical and biochemical features in two patients. *Brain Devel.*, **4**, 105–14.

111. Williams, D. M. and Atkin, C. L. (1981) Tissue copper concentrations with Menkes' kinky hair disease. *Am. J. Dis. Child.*, **135**, 375–6.

112. McKusick, V. A. (1972) Pseudoxanthoma elasticum, in *Heritable Disorders of Connective Tissue*, C. V. Mosby Co., St Louis, p. 475.

113. Goodman, R. M., Smith, E. W. and Paton, D. (1963) Pseudoxanthoma elasticum: a clinical and histopathological study. *Medicine*, **42**, 297–334.

114. Goette, D. K. and Carpenter, W. M. (1981) The mucocutaneous marker of pseudoxanthoma elasticum. *Oral Surg.*, **51**, 68–72.

115. Carr, R. E. and Noble, K. G. (1980) Angioid streaks. *Ophthalmology*, **87**, 263–5.

116. Huang, S. N., Steele, H. D., Kumar, G. *et al.* (1967) Ultrastructural changes of elastic fibres pseudoxanthoma elasticum: A study of histogenesis. *Arch. Pathol.*, **83**, 108–13.

B. M. Ansell

GENETIC DISORDERS OF CONNECTIVE TISSUE

Non-inflammatory diseases of connective tissue, often heritable, have an extensive literature. The majority of these disorders are extremely rare and relatively little is known of their pathogenesis; categorization often depends on appropriate radiological examination[1].

Epiphyseal dysplasias can mimic arthritis, particularly multiple epiphyseal dysplasia and spondyloepiphyseal dysplasia. The tarda form of the latter can be inherited as an X-linked recessive, dominant or seen as a new mutation in two or three siblings[2]; it has been referred as 'pseudo juvenile rheumatoid arthritis'[3], but all acute phase reactants are normal. Serious sequelae include premature degenerative disease of joints, particularly the hips, spinal stenosis and cord injury from minor trauma because of hypoplasia of the odontoid process.

Storage disease due to the deficiency of lysosomal degradative enzymes can be mistaken for arthritis; these include mucopolysaccharidoses, particularly Scheie's syndrome due to deficiency of the enzyme alpha-1 iduronidase[4] in which the stature is well preserved, mentality is normal but there is progressive stiffening of the joints of the hands, elbows and knees without swelling and pain; presentation with carpal tunnel compression and the later development of atlantoaxial subluxation may cause clinical problems. Similarly, the Morquio–Brailsford syndrome, mucopolysaccharidosis type IV, can cause confusion, where there is normal mentality but from about the age of 3 or 4 the musculoskeletal system progressively stiffens associated with dwarfing, the hands enlarge, the knees become valgus and the gait waddling.

Among the mucolipidoses which are characterized by the intracellular accumulation of both glycosaminoglycans and sphingolipids, type III is characterized by restriction of joint mobility which does not become apparent until the second or third year of life and with mentality either normal or slightly below standard[5]. Ocular features include cloudy corneae, astigmatism, retinal and optic nerve abnormalities and visual field defects. The radiological findings are those of a dysostosis multiplex. Diagnosis is made by the characteristic inclusions found in cultured fibroblasts.

In the sphingolipidoses there is an accumulation of lipid in the cell as a result of specific enzyme deficiencies. Only three of the many different ones described have musculoskeletal signs and symptoms, notably Farber's lipogranulomatosis, Gaucher's and Fabry's disease, due respectively to deficiency of acid

Connective Tissue Diseases. Edited by Jill J. F. Belch and Robert B. Zurier. Published in 1995 by Chapman & Hall, London. ISBN 0 412 48620 2

ceramidase, acid glucocydase and α-galacto-sidase and ceramide trihexosidase.

The whole group of genetic and metabolic disorders which may involve primary bio-mechanical abnormalities of fibrous protein or connective tissue disorders will not be dis-cussed, as many have been dealt with in other chapters notably Ehlers–Danlos syndrome, Marfan syndrome, etc. (Chapter 11).

It is important to appreciate that the clinical characteristics of rheumatic disease associated with an immune deficiency syndrome are often indistinguishable from those in pre-sumed immunocompetent persons. In com-bined immunodeficiency characterized by severe defects in both cellular and humoral immunity, that associated with thymic dys-plasia and near normal immunoglobulins but defective antibody production (Nezelof's syn-drome) can be associated with severe poly-articular disease, autoimmune thyroiditis, hemolytic anemia and thrombocytopenia[6].

A quarter of boys with the combined immunodeficiency syndrome designated Wiskott–Aldrich will have an arthritis. Boys with X-linked hypogammaglobulinemia (Bruton syndrome) usually develop symp-toms from bacterial infections, including osteomyelitis and septic arthritis, from about 6 months of age. The non-X-linked hypogammaglobulinemia affecting boys and girls (common variable) tends to present later and pursue a less fulminant course. Such children develop arthritis, usually with a pauciarticular onset indistinguishable from juvenile chronic arthritis from between the age of 3 and 15 years; the frequency of this has been reported from 7–42%[7]. Such children can also develop septic arthritis and not necessarily in joints affected by the primary disorder; this has been much improved since better regimes of immunoglobulin have been employed. In addition, a dermatomyositis-like syndrome has also been recorded associ-ated with echoviral infections[8].

Genetically determined primary deficien-cies of individual components of the complement system are associated with lupus-like disorders (Chapter 2). Thus absence of Clq is the most commonly reported abnormality; such children may have symp-toms of systemic lupus erythematosus (SLE) within the first few years of life. Similarly, deficiency of Clr and often also Cls has been reported in children with lupus and these had a tendency to bacterial infections. Homo-zygous deficiency of C2 in children can be associated with anaphylactoid purpura, idiopathic glomerulonephritis, and acute syn-ovitis and other features of SLE; overall a lupus-like illness, particularly in association with heterozygous C2 deficiency, appears to be somewhat milder with less clinically sig-nificant nephritis and more florid cutaneous lesions. C3 deficiency is usually associated with severe bacterial infections, but other associations do include SLE vasculitis, glomerulonephritis and arthralgia. In syste-mic lupus in C4 deficient children, their renal course appears to be particularly severe. Further work on the familial occurrence of lupus is still required, but children with early onset disease should have their families care-fully investigated for deficiencies of selected complement components.

SYSTEMIC LUPUS ERYTHEMATOSUS

This is a multisystem disorder with similar protean manifestations to those which occur in adults. In children under 10 years of age, the sex incidence is fairly equal, but as ado-lescence approaches, females predominate. The peak incidence varies in different racial groups with Orientals, American blacks and Mexican Indians having a younger age of onset. There is also a higher incidence of familial lupus in childhood[9].

Etiological aspects are no different in child-hood from those in adult disease (Chapter 2). However, the most likely drug-induced lupus in childhood is that associated with anti-epileptic drugs[10].

The majority of children present with fever

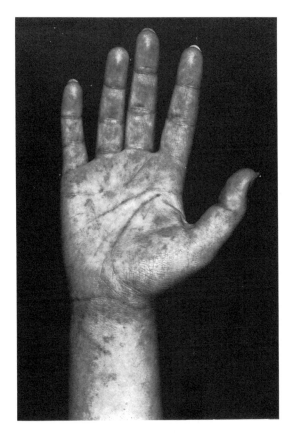

Fig. 12.1 Severe vasculitis with rash on the palm of a hand in a teenager presenting with arthralgia and a very high ESR.

and arthralgia or arthritis, sometimes apparently precipitated by a sore throat; these need differentiating from juvenile chronic arthritis which has been recorded as going on to SLE[11]. Others will present with acute hemolytic anemia or thrombocytopenic purpura and only later develop the more usual features of SLE. Some will have an insidious onset with malaise and be found to have renal or CNS involvement. Thus reviewing 30 cases aged between 3.5 and 16 years at diagnosis and followed over an 8-year period, Buoncompagni *et al.*[12] noted that renal involvement was detected in the majority of their patients on first admission. Rashes, seen in between 60% and 70% of

patients are characteristically sun sensitive, including the facial butterfly one (Plate 9), but cutaneous vasculitis, particularly of the hands and feet, is not uncommon (Figure 12.1); at times a bullous eruption precedes other features, while urticaria is not uncommon. Rash on the palate is considered particularly characteristic of the younger patient[13] as is nasal ulceration.

Very occasionally, lung presentation with pulmonary hemorrhage occurs[14]. Pleurisy is not uncommon, while interstitial infiltrates mimic pneumonitis; pulmonary function testing may document impairment even in the presence of normal X-rays. Pericarditis is the most common early cardiac manifestation being much more common than myocarditis, while Libman–Sacks endocarditis is relatively uncommon. Overall, the general clinical features in childhood do not differ greatly from that of adults, but lymphadenopathy can be very much more marked and fever more hectic and prolonged.

Although cytotoxic agents may well improve renal survival, there are long-term risks of this aggressive therapy, including decreased fertility and the potential induction of neoplasm. There is thus a need to identify children at risk for progressive renal failure. Reviewing some 71 children presenting with systemic lupus over a 13-year period, McCurdy *et al.*[15] noted 16 (22%) had progressed to chronic renal failure. Neither initial abnormalities of creatinine clearance, or 24-hour urine protein excretion, nor as an onset before puberty helped in assessing the risk of renal failure; in contrast to adults neither did male sex nor non-White race, but a renal biopsy showing diffuse glomerular nephritis was significantly associated with progression to renal failure. In biopsies both the active lesions of fibrinoid necrosis, synechiae, tubular casts and vasculitic lesions as well as the chronic lesions of glomerulosclerosis correlated with progression to renal failure. Other features of these children included persistent hypertension lasting more than 4 months, anemia, persistent abnormalities of urine analysis and early elevation of the serum creatinine level. Of the 16 children who progressed to renal failure, 2 had cadover kidney transplants and are well 5 years post-transplant, while with dialysis, 5 died from sepsis, and 4 had fulminant lupus and died within a month of commencing the dialysis. This study suggests that persistently abnormal urinary sediments calls for renal biopsy and those children showing a high activity index should be monitored carefully and considered for treatment with cyclophosphamide.

Involvement of the central nervous system is being increasingly recognized and symptoms include seizures, headaches, blurred vision, intense tremor, ocular flutter, lone chorea, behavioral problems and deterioration in school work[16], as well as bulbar symptoms and transverse myelitis[17]. High titers of anticardiolipin antibodies are frequently found in those with CNS manifestations. Neuropsychological evaluation provides an objective method for delineating changes in higher cortical function. Looking at adolescents with SLE without overt CNS involvement and comparing them to a group of children with juvenile rheumatoid arthritis (JRA), there were considerably greater neuropsychological deficiencies in the SLE group than in the JRA group, with a specific deficiency in complex solving ability as well as a marginally lower performance IQ. There was a significant inverse relationship between intellectual ability and SLE duration, with those having a longer disease showing lower measured intelligence[18].

Increased survival of young people with SLE has highlighted the morbidity of both disease and therapy. Problems include infections, particularly overwhelming ones associated with pneumococci during active disease when there is an immune complex overload with ineffective clearance of pneumococci; the possibility of prevention by specific immunization is under study[19]. The problem with atherosclerotic vascular disease has not been accurately studied, although a number of investigators have commented about this in children and young adults[20]. This has been followed by studies showing dyslipoproteinemia in active SLE and elevated very low density lipoprotein cholesterol independent of corticosteroid therapy[21].

Another important problem in children is failure to grow associated with prolonged corticosteroid therapy as well as the cushingoid appearance, both of which can give rise to serious psychological problems including failure of compliance with treatment.

Overall, the management of children with lupus is similar to that of adults; however, relatively more appear to require corticosteroids. Every effort should be made to get the child on to an alternate day corticosteroid regime as soon as possible to reduce the cushingoid state and improve the growth rate. It must be remembered in the management of joint manifestations, that the liver appears particularly vulnerable to aspirin and non-steroidal drugs in children. It is probably wise to consider an anti-platelet drug, e.g. aspirin in low dose, in any child who has anti-cardiolipin antibodies because of the risk of CNS involvement. There is still discussion on the management of renal lupus as to whether the prolonged cyclophosphamide therapy suggested for adults and for children by Lehman[22] is the best, or whether similar results can be obtained by an induction with cyclophosphamide for one or two months followed by relatively high dose azathioprine.

In the management of autoimmune thrombocytopenia in pediatric lupus, an encouraging report of the use of intravenous vincristine in two adolescents who had serious side effects on corticosteroids, and one of intravenous gammaglobulin suggest ways of perhaps managing patients who are refusing to take corticosteroids because of cushingoid features[23].

ANTI-PHOSPHOLIPID SYNDROME

Although a case of chorea in an 11-year-old child was noted to be associated with anti-phospholipid antibodies[24], overall the anti-phospholipid syndrome in childhood has not been as well recognized as in adults. In 1990 Ravelli *et al.*[25], reported on two children presenting with deep vein thromboses. Ostuni *et al.*[26], reported a 13-year-old girl with abdominal pain and vomiting with fever, hypertension, convulsions and oliguria. There was a poor response to steroids, anti-hypertensive and plasmaphoresis, but improvement after the addition of warfarin and cyclophosphamide. This represents what Asherson[27] has called the catastrophic anti-phospholipid syndrome. Inam *et al.*[28], described a 10-year-old boy fitting this description, who had recurrent loin pain, fever and weight loss and showed hematuria, a rising blood pressure and adrenal failure. Histology of the kidney showed fibrin thromboses. Two further cases, one, a 6-year-old girl, had presented with myocardial infarction and a month later chorea which remitted; two years later she had chorea again and was found to have a prolonged clotting time and a persistent lupus anti-coagulant; the other a boy of 7 years who presented with intracranial hypertension, followed by a left leg deep venous thrombosis when a high titer of anti-cardiolipin antibodies was detected; he has had recurrent thrombotic episodes[29]. A 13-year-old girl presented with chorea, who had had a diagnosis of thrombophlebitis made two years previously and for which she was on anti-coagulants at the time; she did not fulfil the criteria for lupus but she did have a positive test for anti-double stranded DNA as well as anti-cardiolipin antibodies[30]. Thus unexplained deep thrombosis in children or lone chorea, even without overt signs of SLE warrant full investigations.

NEONATAL LUPUS SYNDROMES

These present clinically as cutaneous lupus erythematosus or neonatal congenital heart block, or very occasionally both[31].

In the cutaneous form, the affected infant may present hours to days after delivery with a photosensitive rash which begins as an erythematous scaley papule expanding peripherally but leaving a depressed ecchymotic center; the lesions are multiple[32]. At this time the child will usually have a positive anti-nuclear antibody, which is only transient, and often depression of complement levels; there may be anti-Ro and anti-La or just anti-Ro antibodies. Cytopenia affecting neutrophils, thrombocytes and red cells can be present; very occasionally cytopenia is the only feature of the transient neonatal lupus syndrome. Hepatosplenomegaly may be present. The duration of this illness varies from weeks to months, but regresses spontaneously. How often such a child will ultimately develop SLE has not yet been determined, although single case reports have occurred[33].

The more serious permanent manifestation is complete congenital heart block; *in utero* this can cause sudden bradycardia resulting in congestive cardiac failure and hydrops fetalis. Histologically it is characterized by fibrosis of the conduction system and dystrophic calcification; endocardial fibroelastosis is frequent and other cardiac defects can occur. Immunoglobulin is present in the cardiac tissue[34]. Anti-Ro and anti-La antibodies are almost universally present in mothers and infants with congenital heart block, although about 50% of the mothers are asymptomatic[35]. It would appear that mothers with both anti-Ro and anti-La antibodies are at a much higher risk of giving birth to an infant with congenital heart block than mothers with only anti-Ro antibodies. All 15 ANA positive mother/baby pairs exhibiting congenital heart block had both anti-Ro and anti-La antibodies. Among those babies with cutaneous neonatal lupus erythematosus, both anti-Ro and anti-La were detected in 6, while 2 mother/baby pairs had only anti-Ro antibodies. This work suggests that both anti-Ro and anti-La antibodies are passed to those children with congenital heart block. This was supported by a mother who had originally had anti-Ro and anti-La as well as anti-U1RNP antibodies and delivered a child with congenital heart block in her second pregnancy and then had a normal child, which infant contained anti-Ro and anti-U1RNP antibodies but not anti-La. Anti-Ro and anti-La antibodies may not directly cause disease, but rather may be a marker of disease susceptibility, with other, as yet unknown, factors leading to the development of neonatal lupus. This is emphasized by reports of twins who are discordant for neonatal lupus, with heart block in only one twin. Further prospective studies are required to determine the risk factors associated with neonatal lupus. Certainly, the risk of neonatal lupus even with both anti-La and anti-Ro antibodies is not 100% and there have been reports of discordancy for both cutaneous SLE and congenital heart block. Anti-La antibodies have occasionally been seen in healthy neonates[36].

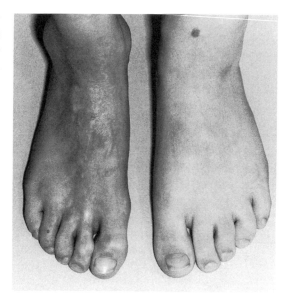

Fig. 12.2 A patch of morphea on the foot with linear scleroderma extending on to the second toe. Note the difference in size of the feet and the pigmentation and depigmentation of the skin on the affected side.

SCLERODERMA

Scleroderma in childhood is rare, but can begin at any age with boys affected almost equally with girls. There is a predominance of the localized forms, both linear and morphea. These can occur in single or multiple patches and both may occur in the same child (Figure 12.2), with linear lesions being associated with growth failure, loss of subcutaneous tissues and even bone.

Linear scleroderma in the frontoparietal region of the face and scalp is often called *en coup de Sabre*. There is atrophy not only of the skin but also the subcutaneous tissue, muscles and bone with failure of growth of that half of the face and loss of hair on the scalp and eyelids. Such patients may have intracerebral calcification and seizures. Four of 6 patients with progressive facial atrophy were evaluated for neurological defects, when 2 had seizures, 1 a left hemiplegia, and 1 learning

problems. Magnetic resonance imaging (MRI) showed increased signals in the ipsilateral white matter in all 5 patients with upper facial atrophy; cranial computed tomography showed cerebral calcification in 3[37]. The problem of the so-called Parry–Romberg syndrome of facial atrophy and its association with linear scleroderma *en coupe de sabre* is well reviewed[38]. In a further case, intractable grand mal seizures and uveitis predominantly posterior, occurred before any overt skin lesions. In this case, MRI showed involvement of orbital vessels suggestive of vasculitis, while biopsy showed diffuse chronic inflammatory cellular infiltration and lymphocytic infiltration in the lateral rectus muscle[39].

Both forms of localized scleroderma are frequently associated with anti-nuclear antibodies and occasionally rheumatoid factor. There are no clues to the etiology which may well be multifactorial. Infective agents have been suggested, thus there are case reports occurring following intercurrent infection, such as chicken pox; investigations into an infective etiology due to *Borrelia burgdoferi* have proved negative[40]. Indeed, the only suggestion of an environmental background is that of the toxic oil syndrome when children tended to have localized lesions.

With either form of localized scleroderma, children can present with stiffness in the joints associated with tendon nodules. A proportion of these have gone on to develop acrosclerosis, but anti-centromere antibodies were negative. In addition, a small proportion of children who have multiple morphea with linear scleroderma get a frank synovitis; these usually have a raised ESR and the inflammatory element appears to respond to corticosteroids which will help reduce deformity, but it has little long-term effect on the linear scleroderma[41]. The demonstration of reduction of inflammation was shown by infrared thermography[42]; however, studies on the use of thermography in monitoring linear scleroderma require further evaluation[43].

Generalized skin scleroderma has been seen with Raynaud's phenomenon and severe tenosynovitis; this seems to be particularly common in adolescence and affects girls. Initially, there is very little in the way of visceral involvement and, indeed, spontaneous regression has been seen, but there may subsequently be problems with swallowing and most recently one such patient developed an axillary vein thrombosis[44].

Systemic sclerosis is relatively uncommon in childhood, but seems to differ little from that in the adult (Chapter 3)[45]. Thus these patients develop Raynaud's phenomenon, areas of depigmentation and hyperpigmentation in the skin, spontaneous ulceration particularly in fingers and toes and, ultimately, skin tightening with contractures of joints. Difficulty in swallowing is common with typical esophogeal changes demonstrable; it has been suggested that bowel involvement may be more common in the younger age group. Pulmonary function is a particular problem, with a mild presentation being followed by progressive involvement; it has recently been suggested as the most common cause of death[46]. The myocardium can also be affected. In general, renal changes seem to be a little less common in children than in adults, but when they do occur are often rapidly progressive, particularly if hypertension develops early. The immunologic markers in systemic sclerosis in children are similar to those in the adult[47].

Fasciitis with eosinophilia can be recognized in childhood when there is apparent scleroderma affecting the limbs, but sparing the hands and feet and associated with a raised ESR and high eosinophil count. The clinical, histologic and laboratory findings are similar to those in the adult, but to date the hematologic complications have not been reported. It has been suggested[48], that corticosteroid therapy should be continued for a long time. However, while there is undoubted resolution of soft-tissue induration and the acute phase reaction following corticosteroids, a review of 10 of 17 literature cases showed residual skin lesions and fibrosis, which developed over one or more years and, indeed, affected all four of the new cases reported[49]. It has long been recognized that morphea, sometimes multiple, may occur in association with fasciitis, but it has now been noted that it can occur as a sequel.

It is generally accepted that children with overlapping features of more than one connective tissue disease (MCTD) may move into one of a number of categories. Of 26 patients with a mean follow-up of 7.5 years, 2 had died, 14 had developed sclerodermatous skin changes; only 3 had significant functional impairment and their appearance was more that of limited scleroderma (CREST syndrome)[50].

JUVENILE DERMATOMYOSITIS (JDM)

This is defined as having an onset of disease

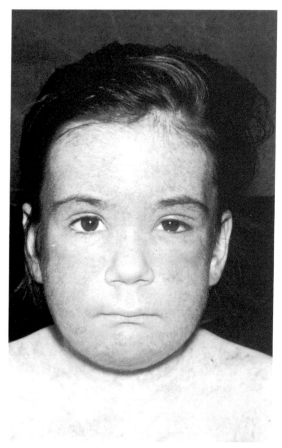

Fig. 12.3 With an exacerbation of dermato-myositis, extensive vasculitic facial rash with some loss of hair and edema, particularly around the eyes.

sign) (Figure 12.4). Rash can also be seen on the elbows and knees and down the shins. In addition, the vasculitis can cause severe ulcerations (Plate 10), which are seen particularly around the nose, armpits and groins; there can also be ulceration of the gut. Soft tissue calcinosis affecting particularly the subcutaneous tissue, and to a lesser degree but more seriously the interfascial muscle plane, eventually develops in about two-thirds of children; this can be in months from onset or may be delayed for years. It can be very severe with calcific deposits producing skin ulceration, with that in the muscle planes (Figure 12.5), further interfering with muscle function.

It should be remembered that it is not uncommon to have a normal ESR even when the disease is active, but a rise in creatinine phosphokinase and other enzymes occurs, while in the presence of an active vasculitis factor VIII von Willebrand factor antigen (VWF) is usually raised[51]. Usually the diagnosis can be made clinically; only very exceptionally is it associated with malignancy in childhood, but other problems in diagnosis include myopathies, particularly mitochondrial myopathy, when muscle biopsy is indicated[52]. An excess of the extended haplotype HLA-B8-DR3 and C4 null gene is found in idiopathic JDM. It has been suggested that prior exposure to Coxsackie virus may be important in its etiology in a susceptible population[53]. The search for a viral etiology heightened with the realization that the dermatomyositis associated with hypogammaglobulinemia is usually the result of an echoviral infection, but as yet no one organism is definitively identified. An intriguing speculation is that in a genetically predisposed host, cytokine production of lymphocytes persists in skeletal muscles as a result of the initiating factor and that the systemic features result from sharing of epitopes on connective tissue components around blood vessels in muscles and organs[53,54].

Controversies continue to exist about management. All would agree that high-dose

under the age of 16 and is characterized by an immune complex vasculitis early and subsequently a high incidence of calcinosis. It is a rare disorder and its classic presentation is that of proximal muscle weakness, which can be associated with edema masking the muscle state and a characteristic rash. There is often erythema of the face with a mauvish hue and edema around the eyes (Figure 12.3). On the hands, the characteristic rash which is considered pathognomonic consists of violacious erythematous papules or plaques over the bony prominences, particularly the meta-carpo- and interphalangeal joints (Gottron

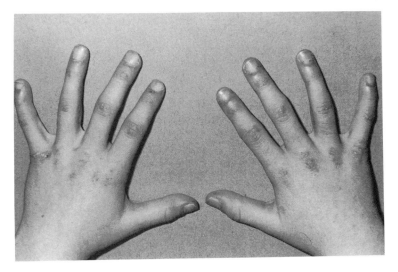

Fig. 12.4 The typical rash over the metacarpo- and proximal interphalangeal joints in dermatomyositis.

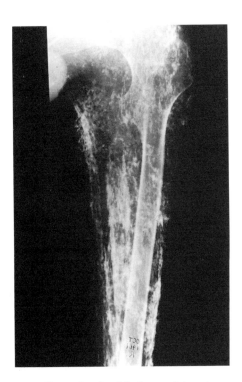

Fig. 12.5 Extensive fascial plane calcinosis associated with subcutaneous lesions some five years after the onset of dermatomyositis.

corticosteroid therapy is useful initially, but whether this should be orally, initially in divided doses because of possible malabsorption due to bowel involvement, or by intravenous methylprednisone 30 mg/kg/day has not been adequately assessed. Now one tends to start with intravenous methylprednisone given 2 or 3 times on alternate days followed by oral prednisolone and ultimately alternate day prednisolone; the possible role of deflazacort has yet to be assessed. In the past refractory cases were usually treated with methotrexate, but the preliminary results in the use of cyclosporin as a steroid sparing agent are impressive[55]. In the management of calcinosis, low-dose warfarin is not valuable and has serious side effects. In general, the important thing is to control the disease process as quickly as possible in the hope of reducing the risk of calcinosis; once it has occurred it is important to maintain control of disease activity and mobilize affected parts. Monitoring is not easy, clinical assessment can be supplemented by measurement of VWF and possibly serial *in vivo* nail fold microscopy[56]. A recently recognized sequel is the development of lipodystrophy complicated by hyperlipidemia[57,58].

Table 12.1 Vasculitic syndromes in childhood

Polyarteritis
    Macroscopic
    Microscopic
Kawasaki disease (mucocutaneous lymph node
    syndrome)
Granulomatous vasculitis
    Wegener's granulomatosis
    Churg–Strauss
Leucocytoclastic vasculitis
    Henoch–Schönlein purpura
    Hypersensitivity angiitis
Rheumatic vasculitis
    Systemic lupus erythematosus
    Juvenile chronic arthritis
    Mixed connective tissue disease
    Dermatomyositis
    Scleroderma
Giant cell arteritis

From [61].

VASCULITIC SYNDROMES

Classification of vasculitic syndromes in childhood is proving even more difficult than in adults (Table 12.1); it can also be a feature of many of the rheumatic disorders seen in childhood. Some vasculitic syndromes appear more common in children than adults; these include Kawasaki syndrome (Chapter 9), Henoch–Schönlein purpura and cutaneous polyarteritis associated with streptococcal infection (Chapter 8), and will be briefly described clinically. Manifestations and prognosis of some vasculitic disorders in childhood can be different from the adult. Thus in Takayasu's arteritis[59], a high incidence of inflammation in different systems causes fever, arthritis, skin lesions and lymphadenopathy, while the course can be aggressive and potentially lethal; in addition, alteration in growth can occur as a sequel due to impairment of blood supply.

KAWASAKI SYNDROME

While this occurs worldwide it is particularly common in Oriental stock. Criteria have been set up to assess this disorder in childhood, but incomplete disease is being increasingly recognized. Suggestive points are fewer of at least 5 days duration, 104°F or higher, with bilateral conjunctival injection, changes in the mucosa of the oral pharynx including injection of the pharynx, fissured dry lips and strawberry tongue, edema and/or erythema of the hands and feet, and ultimately desquamation usually beginning periungaly, massive cervical lymphadenopathy and polymorphous non-vesicular rashes. The incidence of cardiac problems appears to be greater with an onset under the age of 5. Other striking investigative findings include a thrombocytosis, the appearance of platelet aggregating factor and circulating immune complexes[60].

The importance of this syndrome is not only that it can cause death by coronary artery disease, but what the sequelae are likely to be. Because high-dose intravenous gamma-globulin together with aspirin may reduce cardiac sequelae, it is important to recognize the children early and treat accordingly (Chapter 14). Dillon[61] has added intravenous prostacyclin when there is evidence of myocardial ischemia or aneurysms with apparent benefit.

CUTANEOUS POLYARTERITIS

Cutaneous polyarteritis associated with streptococcal infection (Plate 11), was first described in the 1970s and most recently reviewed by Fink[62]. Our present long-term follow-up of a group of 12 such children suggests that it is not uncommon to get recurrent episodes following repeated streptococcal infection, with several having a relapsing course and two of these have now evidence of microaneurysms in the hepatic and renal arteries[63]. Thus the importance of continuing penicillin prophylaxis probably for 5–10 years following the initial episode to prevent relapses needs to be stressed.

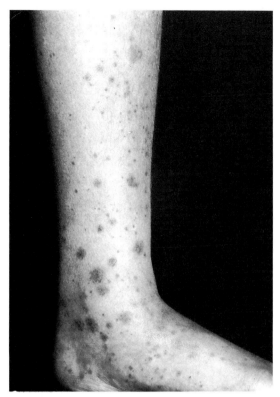

Fig. 12.6 Multiple lesions of different types and age in Henoch–Schönlein purpura.

HENOCH–SCHÖNLEIN PURPURA

Henoch–Schönlein purpura occurs particularly in young children, i.e. 2–3 years and upwards. Platelets are normal. The rash (Figure 12.6), is both macular-papular and purpuric, and tends to crop. In addition, there is frequently subcutaneous edema which may affect the face, hands, feet, scrotum and areas around the spine. There may be arthritis or arthralgia, abdominal pain with gastrointestinal hemorrhage and nephritis. These last usually come on in the first week or two of the illness. Nephritis is reputed to occur in approximately 50%, but in only 10% will it become serious and is indeed the main reason for concern in this disorder[64].

The total platelet count is normal, the ESR is often normal. Fifty per cent of children have an increase in IgA and a little less in IgM; it is characteristically in the acute phase that there are circulating IgA containing immune complexes; the etiology of the disease and these complexes is as yet uncertain (Chapter 8)[65].

BEHÇET'S SYNDROME

In childhood this is rare, it is most commonly occurring in adults (Chapter 9). In a series of 32 patients seen in northern England, a quarter had an onset in the first decade and another quarter in the second decade[66]. In the geographical areas where Behçet's syndrome is more common, figures for childhood onset disease are not easily available, but it has been suggested that the sex ratio in children might be nearer 1 to 1 in contrast to the male predominance seen in adults. From time to time, familial Behçet's syndrome is reported, while transient neonatal Behçet's disease is well recorded[67]. In general, the features in childhood are similar to those of the adult with the presence of vasculitic lesions, thus helping in diagnosis, but with an increased incidence of gastrointestinal problems and possibly also involvement of the central nervous system is thought to occur[68].

Of the characteristic clinical features, oral ulceration causes crops of extremely painful ulcers appearing on the lips, tongue, palate and also elsewhere in the gastrointestinal tract. They usually last for 3–10 days and heal without scarring, but in neonatal Behçet's syndrome extensive scarring can occur[69]. In the male there is recurrent painful ulceration of the glans penis, prepuce and scrotum, while in the female it is the vulva and vagina, where these ulcers can be penetrating; buttock vasculitic lesions can mimic Henoch–Schönlein purpura or be nodular (Figure 12.7). Erythema nodosum can be followed by skin ulceration, while at times a vesicular rash is seen. The cutaneous pustular reaction to a needle puncture has also been described in childhood. The inflammation of both the

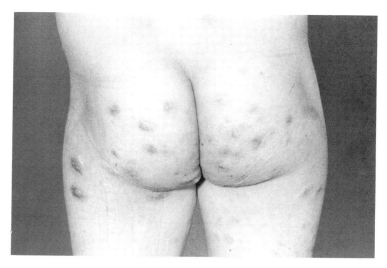

Fig. 12.7   Vasculitic lesions with nodule formation on the buttocks in a child with Behçet's syndrome; these can mimic Henoch–Schönlein purpura.

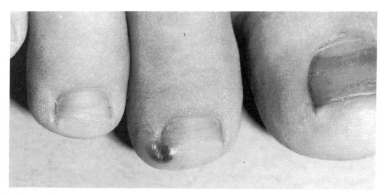

Fig. 12.8   Nail fold vasculitic lesions confirming the diagnosis of Behçet's syndrome in a child with bilateral uveitis, arthritis and a story of erythema nodosum.

anterior and posterior uveal tract is very severe, almost always bilateral and can result in blindness with hyopopyon; corneal ulceration and retrobulbar neuritis also occur. Other features include arthritis most commonly affecting knees, ankles and wrists, but it does not usually cause joint destruction. Myositis is seen occasionally[70]. Gastrointestinal manifestations appear somewhat more frequent in children and are indistinguishable from Crohn's disease or ulcerative colitis. Indeed,

the differential diagnosis may be difficult as erythema nodosum, arthritis and uveitis can be seen in both groups of diseases, although vasculitic lesions in the skin (Figure 12.8) are helpful in differentiating Behçet's syndrome. The central nervous features include meningoencephalitis, which is characterized by headache, stiff neck and drowsiness, and focal neurological abnormalities. There is no diagnostic test for Behçet's syndrome, although laboratory tests show a generalized increase in acute phase reactants; synovial histology shows only non-specific inflammation; the basic skin lesion is a vasculitis.

As in the adult it is difficult to treat. Some patients are steroid responsive, but the disease tends to run a long, relapsing course adding on features particularly ocular and CNS which can be extremely incapacitating. It does seem possible to control the severe uveitis with cyclosporin[71] (Chapter 9).

REFERENCES

1. Ansell, B. M. (1993) Disease of bone and cartilage: paediatric aspects, in *Oxford Textbook of Rheumatology*, (eds P. J. Maddison, D. A. Isenberg, P. Woo *et al.*), Oxford University Press, Oxford, pp. 1043–51.

2. Szprio-Tapia, S., Sefiani, A., Guilloud-Batsille, M. *et al.* (1988) Spondyloepiphyseal dysplasia tarda: linkage with genetic markers from the distal short arm of the X chromosome. *Hum. Genet.*, **81**, 61–3.

3. Spranger, J., Albert, C., Schilling, F. *et al.* (1983) Progressive pseudo rheumatoid arthritis – a hereditary disorder simulating juvenile rheumatoid arthritis. *Euro. J. Ped.*, **140**, 34–40.

4. Scott, H. A., Ashton, L. H., Eyre, H. J. *et al.* (1990) Chromosomal location of the human alpha 1 iduronidase gene (Iu DA) to 4p 16.3. *Am. J. Hum. Genet.*, **47**, 82–7.

5. Brik, R., Mandel, H., Aizin, A. *et al.* (1993) Mucolipidosis III presenting as a rheumatological disorder. *J. Rheumatol.*, **20**, 133–6.

6. Cassidy, J. T. and Petty, R. E. (1990) Immunodeficiencies and the rheumatic diseases, in *Textbook of Paediatric Rheumatology*, 2nd edn, Churchill Livingstone, London, pp. 467–88.

7. Petty, P. E., Cassidy, J. T. and Fuberger, D. G. (1977) Association of arthritis with hypogammaglobulinaemia. *Arth. Rheum.*, **20**, 441–2.

8. Webster, A. D. B. (1984) Echovirus disease in hypogammaglobulinaemia patients. *Clin. Rheum. Dis.*, **10**, 189–203.

9. Ward, M. M. and Studenski, S. (1990) Age associated clinical manifestations of SLE: a multicentre regression analysis. *J. Rheumatol.*, **17**, 476–81.

10. Ansell, B. M. (1993) Drug induced SLE in children (editorial). *Lupus*, **2**, 139–40.

11. Ragsdale, C. G., Petty, R. E., Cassidy, J. T. *et al.* (1980) The clinical progression of apparent juvenile rheumatoid arthritis to SLE. *J. Rheumatol.*, **7**, 50–5.

12. Buoncompagni, A., Bonbaro, G. C. and Pistoia, V. (1991) Childhood SLE: a review of 30 cases. *Clin. Exp. Rheumatol.*, **9**, 425–30.

13. Lehman, T. J., McCurdy, D. K., Bernstein, B. H. *et al.* (1989) Systemic lupus in the first decade of life. *Pediatrica*, **83**, 235–9.

14. Ramirez, R. E., Glasier, C., Kirks, D. *et al.* (1984) Pulmonary hemorrhage associated with systemic lupus erythematosus in children. *Radiology*, **153**, 409–12.

15. McCurdy, D. K., Lehman, T. J. A., Bernstein, B. *et al.* (1992) Lupus nephritis prognostic factors in children. *Pediatrics*, **89**, 240–6.

16. Yancey, C., Doughety, R. A. and Athreya, B. (1981) CNS involvement in childhood SLE. *Arth. Rheum.*, **24**, 1389–95.

17. Davies, U. M., Ansell, B. M. (1988) Central nervous system manifestations in juvenile SLE: a problem of management. *J. Rheumatol.*, **15**, 1720–1.

18. Papero, P. H., Bluestein, H. G., White, P. *et al.* (1990) Neuropsychologic defects and anti-neuronal antibodies in pediatric SLE. *Clin. Exp. Rheumatol.*, **8**, 417–24.

19. Malleson, P., Petty, R. E., Nadel, H. *et al.* (1988) Functional asplenia in childhood onset SLE. *J. Rheumatol.*, **15**, 1648–52.

20. Gladman, D. D. and Urowitz, M. D. (1987) Morbidity in systemic lupus erythematosus. *J. Rheumatol.*, Suppl 13, **14**, 223–6.

21. Ilowite, N. T., Samuel, P., Ginzler, E. *et al.* (1988) Dyslipoproteinemia in pediatric systemic lupus erythematosus. *Arth. Rheum.*, **31**, 859–63.

22. Lehman, T. J. A. (1992) Current comments in immuno-suppressive drug treatment of SLE. *J. Rheumatol.*, **19**, 20–2.

23. Lipnick, R. N., Tsokos, G. C., Bray, G. C. *et al.* (1990) Autoimmune thrombocytopenia in pediatric SLE: alternative therapeutic modalities. *Clin. Exp. Rheumatol.*, **8**, 315–19.

24. Khamashta, M. A., Gill, A., Anciones, B. *et al.* (1988) Chorea in systemic lupus erythematosus: association with cardiolipin antibodies. *Ann. Rheum. Dis.*, **47**, 681–3.

25. Ravelli, A., Caperali, R., Bianchi, E. *et al.* (1990) Anticardiolipin syndrome in childhood. A report of two cases. *Clin. Exp. Rheumatol.*, **8**, 95–8.

26. Ostuni, P. A., Lazzarin, P., Pengo, V. *et al.* (1990) Renal artery thrombosis and hypertension in a 13-year-old girl with anti-phospholipid syndrome. *Ann. Rheum. Dis.*, **49**, 184–7.

27. Asherson, R. (1992) The catastrophic antiphospholipid syndrome., *J. Rheumatol.*, **19**, 508–12.

28. Inam, S., Sidki, A., Al Marshedy, A. R. *et al.* (1991) Addison's disease, hypertension renalhepatic microthrombosis in 'primary' antiphospholipid syndrome. *Postgrad. Med. J.*, **66**, 385–7.

29. Falcini, F., Taccetti, G., Trapani, S. *et al.* (1991) Primary anti–phospholipid syndrome. A report of two paediatric cases. *J. Rheumatol.*, **18**, 1085–7.

30. Vlachoyiannopoulos, P. G., Dimou, G. and Siamopolou-Mavidrou, A. (1991) Chorea as a manifestation of the anti-phospholipid syndrome in childhood. *Clin. Exp. Rheumatol.*, **9**, 303–6.

31. Watson, R. M., Lane, A. T., Barnett, N. K. *et al.* (1984) Neo-natal lupus erythematosus. A clinical, serological and immunogenetic study with review of the literature. *Medicine*, **63**, 362–78.

32. Ansell, B. M. (1992) Neonatal lupus, in *A Colour Atlas of Paediatric Rheumatology*, (eds B. M. Ansell, S. Rudge and J. G. Schaller), Wolfe Publishing, London, pp. 103–6.

33. Fox, R. J., McCritian, C. H. and Schoch, E. P., Jr. (1979) Systemic lupus erythematosus; association with previous neo-natal lupus erythematosus. *Arch. Dermatol.*, **115**, 340.

34. Litsey, S. E., Noonan, J. A., O'Connor, W. N. *et al.* (1985) Maternal connective tissue disease and congenital heart block. Demonstration of immunoglobulin in cardiac tissue. *N. Eng. J. Med.*, **312**, 98–100.

35. Silverman, E., Mamuyla, M., Hardin, J.A. *et al.* (1991) Importance of the immune response to the Ro/La particle in the development of congenital heart block and neonatal lupus erythematosus. *J. Rheumatol.*, **18**, 120–4.

36. Silverman, E. D. (1993) Congenital heart block and neonatal lupus erythematosus: prevention is the goal. *J. Rheumatol.*, **20**, 1101–4.

37. Fry, J. A., Alvarellos, A., Fink, C. W. *et al.* (1992) Intracranial findings in progressive facial hemiatrophy. *J. Rheumatol.*, **19**, 956–8.

38. Lehman, T. J. A. (1992) The Parry–Romberg syndrome of progressive facial hemiatrophy and linear scleroderma *en coup de Sabre*. Mistaken diagnoses or overlapping conditions? *J. Rheumatol.*, **19**, 844–5.

39. David, J., Wilson, J. and Woo, P. (1991) Scleroderma 'en coup de Sabre'. *Ann. Rheum. Dis.*, **50**, 260–2.

40. Lupoli, S., Cutler, S., Stephens, C. O. *et al.* (1991) Lyme disease and localised scleroderma

– no evidence for a common etiology. *Br. J. Rheumatol.*, **30**, 154–6.

41. Ansell, B. M. (1988) Scleroderma in childhood, in *Systemic Sclerosis: Scleroderma*, (eds M. I. V. Jayson and C. M. Black), John Wiley & Sons, pp. 319–24.

42. Allen, R. C., Ansell, B. M., Clark, R. *et al.* (1987) Localised scleroderma: treatment response measured by infrared thermography. *Thermatography*, **2**, 550–3.

43. Bird, N., Shore, A., Rush, P. *et al.* (1992) Childhood linear scleroderma. A possible role of thermography for evaluation. *J. Rheumatol.*, **19**, 968–73.

44. Leak, A., Patel, K. J., Tuddenham, E. D. *et al.* (1990) Axillary vein thrombosis in adolescent onset systemic sclerosis. *Ann. Rheum. Dis.*, **49**, 557–9.

45. Lababi di, H.M.S., Nasr, F. W. and Khatib, Z. (1991) Juvenile progressive systemic sclerosis. Report of 5 cases. *J. Rheumatol.*, **18**, 885–8.

46. Garty, B-Z., Athreya, B. H., Wilmott, R. *et al.* (1991) Pulmonary functions in children with progressive systemic sclerosis. *Pediatrics*, **88**, 1161–7.

47. Blaszyk, M., Jablonska, S., Szymansker-Jagiello, W. *et al.* (1991) Immunologic markers of systemic scleroderma in children. *Ped. Dermatol.*, **8**, 13–20.

48. Grisanti, M. W., Moor, T., Osborn, T. *et al.* (1989) Eosinophilic fasciitis in children. *Sem. Arth. Rheum.*, **19**, 151–7.

49. Farrington, M. L., Haas, J. E. and Naza, S. V. (1993) Eosinophilic fasciitis in children frequently progresses to scleroderma-like cutaneous fibrosis. *J. Rheumatol.*, **20**, 128–32.

50. Allen, R. C., St. Cyr, C., Maddison, P. J. *et al.* (1986) Overlap connective tissue syndromes. *Arch. Dis. Childhood*, **61**, 284–8.

51. Bowyer, S. L., Ragsdale, C. B. and Sullivan, D. B. (1989) Factor VIII related antigen and childhood rheumatic diseases. *J. Rheumatol.*, **16**, 1093–7.

52. Ansell, B. M. (1992) Dermatomyositis, in *A Colour Atlas of Paediatric Rheumatology*, (eds B. M. Ansell, S. Rudge and J. G. Schaller), Wolfe Publishing, London, pp. 107–21.

53. Christensen, M. L., Pachmann, L. M., Schnelderman, R. *et al.* (1986) Prevalence of Coxsackie B virus antibodies in patients with juvenile dermatomyositis. *Arth. Rheum.*, **29**, 1365–70.

54. Cambridge, G. (1990) What is the role of the immune system in juvenile dermatomyositis?

in, *Paediatric Rheumatology Update*, (eds P. Woo, P. White and B. M. Ansell), Oxford University Press, Oxford, pp. 182–93.

55. Heckmatt, J., Saunders, C. and Peters, A. M. (1989) Cyclosporine in juvenile dermatomyositis. *Lancet*, **1**, 1063–6.

56. Silver R. M. and Marioq, H. R. (1989) Childhood dermatomyositis. Serial microvascular studies. *Pediatrics*, **83**, 278–83.

57. Ansell, B. M. (1991) Juvenile dermatomyositis. *Rheum. Dis. Clin. N. Am.*, **17**, 931–42.

58. Miller, L. and Schaller, J. G. (1995) *Arth. Rheum.*, (in press).

59. Marales, E., Pineda, C. and Martinex-Lavin, M. (1991) Takayasu's arteritis in children. *J. Rheumatol.*, **18**, 1081–4.

60. Rowley, A. H., Gonzalez Crussi, F., Giddy, S. S. *et al.* (1987) Incomplete Kawasaki disease with coronary artery involvement. *J. Ped.*, **110**, 409–13.

61. Dillon, M. J. (1990) Vasculitic syndromes, in *Paediatric Rheumatology Update*, (eds P. Woo, P. White and B. M. Ansell), Oxford University Press, Oxford, pp. 227–42.

62. Fink, C. W. (1988) Childhood polyarteritis, in *Vasculopathies of Childhood*, (ed R. V. Hicks), PSG Publishing Co Inc, London, pp. 273–83.

63. David, J., Ansell, B. M. and Woo, P. (1993) Streptococcal-associated polyarteritis nodosa. *Arch. Dis. Childhood*, **69**, 685–8.

64. Stewart, M., Savage, J. M., Bell, B. *et al.* (1988) Long term renal prognosis of Henoch–Schönlein purpura in an unselected childhood population. *Euro. J. Ped.*, **147**, 113–15.

65. Levinsky, R. J. and Barratt, T. M. (1979) IgA immune complexes in Henoch–Schönlein purpura. *Lancet*, **2**, 1100.

66. Chamberlain, M. A. (1977) Behçet's syndrome in 32 patients in Yorkshire. *Ann. Rheum. Dis.*, **36**, 491–9.

67. Lewis, M. A. and Priestly, B. K. (1986) Transient neo-natal Behçet's syndrome. *Arch. Dis. Childhood*, **61**, 805–6.

68. Ammann, A. J., Johnson, A., Fyfe, G. *et al.* (1985) Behçet's syndrome. *J. Ped.*, **107**, 41–3.

69. Fam, A. G., Siminovitch, K. A., Carette, S. *et al.* (1981) Neonatal Behçet's syndrome in an infant of a mother with the disease. *Ann. Rheum. Dis.*, **40**, 509–12.

70. Lang, B. A., Laxer, R. M., Thorner, P. *et al.* (1990) Pediatric onset of Behçet's syndrome with myositis. Case report and review of literature. *Arth. Rheum.*, **33**, 418–25.

71. Nussonblatt, R. B., Palestine, A. G., Chi-Cho, C. *et al.* (1985) Effectiveness of cyclosporin therapy for Behçet's disease. *Arth. Rheum.*, **28**, 671–9.

K. F. Al-Jarallah and W. W. Buchanan

Rheumatic symptoms occur frequently in systemic disorders and, indeed, may be the presenting manifestation. The present chapter reviews recent advances in not only the clinical manifestations, but also what is known of their pathophysiology.

RHEUMATIC COMPLICATIONS OF RENAL FAILURE

In the past rheumatologists were accustomed to see patients with renal osteodystrophy as a consequence of chronic renal failure. Today they are more likely to be consulted as a consequence of treatment of renal failure.

RENAL OSTEODYSTROPHY

This is a term describing a number of musculoskeletal abnormalities in chronic renal failure. These include:

1. secondary hyperparathyroidism,
2. rickets and osteomalacia,
3. osteoporosis,
4. soft tissue and vascular calcification, and
5. miscellaneous conditions.

Secondary hyperparathyroidism is caused by hyperplasia of the chief cells of the parathyroid glands due to phosphate retention and low serum calcium. The radiological features are similar to those in primary hyperparathyroidism. However, brown tumors (bone cysts) are less common, occurring in less than 2% of patients, and will probably become rarer with more extensive use of dialysis and kidney transplantation. When brown tumors occur they are usually single, unlike primary hyperparathyroidism when they are often multiple. Osteosclerosis is common in renal osteodystrophy, and is classically seen in the 'rugger jersey' spine where there is increased density of the superior and inferior portions of the vertebrae. Epiphyseal sclerosis is rare and may mimic ischemic necrosis. Osteosclerosis may be so massive as to compromise marrow function. Histology demonstrates trabecular thickening and fibrosis. Chondrocalcinosis is less common than in primary hyperparathyroidism, but periosteal new bone formation, known by the neologism, neostosis, is common occurring in 25% of patients, especially in those with periostitis[1].

The cause of osteomalacia and rickets is not entirely clear, and often histology of bone reveals no abnormality. Osteopenia is common in both children and adults and may lead to fractures. Looser's zones or Milkman fractures are rare occurring in less than 1% of patients. In children there is often irregular widening of the growth plate, and slipped femoral epiphyses are relatively common,

Connective Tissue Diseases. Edited by Jill J. F. Belch and Robert B. Zurier. Published in 1995 by Chapman & Hall, London. ISBN 0 412 48620 2

occurring in approximately 10% of patients. Certain warning signs have been described of the latter complication, including: increase in width of the growth plate, subperiosteal erosion on the medical aspect of the femoral neck and bilateral coxa vara. Soft tissue and vascular calcification is very common in renal osteodystrophy. Hydroxyapatite is frequently deposited in subcutaneous and periarticular tissues, where it may form large masses, which might cause erosion of underlying bone. Hydroxyapatite induces fibrosis, so that the lumps become encapsulated. Magnesium whitlockite material, which deposits especially in viscera, results in no tissue reaction. Deposition of hydroxyapatite in arteries may lead to vascular occlusion and gangrene.

Hyperuricemia may result in secondary gout. The radiological features are no different from primary gout. Oxalosis of bone has been described. Long standing uremia may occasionally be associated with β2-microglobulin amyloidosis leading to destructive arthropathy and spondyloarthropathy[2].

RENAL TRANSPLANTATION AND HEMODIALYSIS

A number of musculoskeletal abnormalities have recently been reported in patients undergoing treatment for chronic renal failure. It is very difficult in reviewing the literature to know whether some of these complications are the result of therapeutic intervention, or merely reflect complications of long-standing renal failure not recorded in older literature because patients did not survive long enough or because of relative lack of interest in the rheumatological complications.

The pathogenesis of avascular necrosis following renal transplantation remains a mystery. It is not entirely due to corticosteroid therapy, since it can occur in the absence of this treatment[3]. Early detection can be achieved by radionuclide scans or magnetic resonance[4]. Conservative therapy can maintain 40% of patients with hip and 70% of patients with knee avascular necrosis reasonably pain-free. Osteopenia, often developing rapidly after a transplant, occurs even with low doses of corticosteroids. Cyclosporin has not been found to decrease the severity of osteopenia and, indeed, has been considered to be a cause of musculoskeletal pain[5]. Osteonecrosis and slipped epiphyses have been reported in children following renal transplantation.

A specific type of secondary amyloidosis, β2-microglobulin amyloid, has been reported to cause a number of complications in patients undergoing long-term hemodialysis. The most common of these complications is the carpal tunnel syndrome. Arthropathy is also common and amyloid particles may be identified in joint effusions. The cell counts in such effusions are usually 3000–5000 cells/mm³. Amyloid may also be present in synovium and cartilage[6]. Baker's cysts have been reported in the knees. The shoulder joints appear to be particularly prone to involvement with amyloid, as they are in multiple myeloma[7]. A severe erosive osteoarthritis has been reported by Duncan *et al.*[8]. Destructive spondyloarthropathy due to β2-microglobulin amyloid, especially involving the cervical spine[9], may result in a myelopathy[10]. Differentiation from septic discitis can be achieved with magnetic resonance. Bone cysts, often at entheses, may lead to pathological fractures. Magnetic resonance has proven more useful in demonstrating such cysts than standard radiographs. Serum β2-microglobulin amyloid concentrations do not correlate with the extent of deposition in bones and joints, and the value of radionuclide scans remains to be evaluated. The role of aluminium and iron has been suggested in terms of localization of the amyloid deposits, as has the role of the dialysis membrane. Recent studies, however, have shown that the type of membrane has no effect[11]. β2-microglobulin amyloidosis may improve after transplantation[12].

Other complications of long-term hemodialysis include: atlantoaxial subluxation due to ligament laxity[13] as a result of increased connective tissue turnover; calcium pyrophosphate deposition disease; calcific periarthritis, staphylococcal infection of joints as a consequence of infected arteriovenous fistulae; and reflex algodystrophy after placement of an arteriovenous graft.

RHEUMATIC COMPLICATIONS OF GASTROINTESTINAL DISORDERS

The association of arthritis and inflammatory bowel disease has been recognized for over a century. Arthritis is the most common extra-intestinal complication of ulcerative colitis[14] and Crohn's disease, especially when it involves the colon. Arthritis parallels the activity of the intestinal lesion in ulcerative colitis, but in Crohn's disease it may precede the intestinal disease by years, and usually bears no relation to either the extent or severity of bowel involvement. Very rarely the arthritis may be destructive[15]. Enthesopathy and axial involvement are common in both ulcerative colitis and Crohn's disease, and the clinical picture is indistinguishable from that in primary ankylosing spondylitis. Inflammatory bowel disease complicated by peripheral arthritis is not associated with HLA-B27, but sacroiliitis and spondylitis are, but to a lesser extent than primary ankylosing spondylitis[16]. There is good evidence to believe that the incidence of both ulcerative colitis and Crohn's disease is increasing, so that the clinical rheumatologist can expect to see more patients with rheumatic complications of these diseases. Non-steroidal, anti-inflammatory analgesics may cause exacerbation of bowel symptoms in patients with these conditions[17].

There is evidence that patients with ulcerative colitis have an increased incidence of autoimmune disease. However, the only one to correlate with bowel activity is Coombs positive hemolytic anemia, which has been reported in one patient to be cured by colectomy[18]. No such association with auto-immune disease has been reported in Crohn's disease.

The problem, however, is why arthritis and spondylitis should occur in inflammatory bowel disease. The role of IgA has been studied since this is not only the most abundant immunoglobulin in humans and produced by mucosal cells of the gastrointestinal tract, but also is known to be increased in patients with ankylosing spondylitis[19]. However, recent studies by Hocini *et al.*[20] have shown that the IgA in ankylosing spondylitis is not produced in the gut but by the central immune system. In addition, ankylosing spondylitis has been reported in patients with IgA deficiency[21]. On the other hand, Shodjai-Moraodi *et al.*[22] have reported IgA antibodies to *Klebsiella* in patients with ankylosing spondylitis, although this was not confirmed by MacLean *et al.*[23]. Sulphasalazine has been shown to be effective in ankylosing spondylitis, but whether this is due to an effect on IgA producing cells in the gut or an indirect effect on gut flora is not known[24]. Moreover, sulphasalazine has also been shown to be effective in treating uveitis[25].

That abnormalities in intestinal immunity may be of importance in both the pathogenesis of ankylosing spondylitis and the rheumatic complications of inflammatory bowel disease has been strengthened by the findings of Mielants *et al.*[26], that patients with ankylosing spondylitis and other seronegative spondyloarthropathies have both acute and chronic subclinical intestinal inflammatory lesions, the latter identical to those in inflammatory bowel disease. It is of interest that Mielants *et al.*[27] found an association between the latter type of lesion and HLA-B62, which is associated with Crohn's disease. HLA-DR expression has been reported to be increased in the villi and crypt epithelial cells in the ileum in inflammatory bowel disease, suggesting that these cells may be primed for antigen presentation[28]. In this regard, it is of interest that IgA antibodies to peptidoglycans are increased in ankylosing spondylitis[29]. Earlier studies demonstrated that antisera to *Klebsiella* would lyse B27 positive lymphocytes and that fecal carriage of *Klebsiella* in ankylosing spondylitis was increased and correlated with disease activity. This latter finding has not, however, been confirmed[30]. However, antibodies to *Klebsiella* and *E. coli* have been found to be significantly increased in patients with ankylosing spondylitis, although antibodies to many other intestinal pathogens showed no difference to controls[31]. Gut permeability studies[32] have shown abnormalities consistent with chronic gut inflammation in patients with seronegative spondyloarthropathies, which unlike rheumatoid arthritis does not appear to be due to non-steroidal anti-inflammatory analgesics [33].

In coeliac disease, which is frequently associated with other autoimmune disorders especially Sjögren's syndrome, there is no evidence that these patients with IgA deficiency are any different than those with normal serum levels of IgA[34].

Intestinal bypass surgery (jejunocolostomy or jejunoileostomy) for morbid obesity is perhaps the most dramatic demonstration of an association between bowel pathology and rheumatic disease. Some 20–80% of patients subjected to this operation develop a polyarthritis some two months to three years after the procedure. The condition is considered due to bacterial overgrowth and mucosal alterations in the blind loop, but treatment with antibiotics has been singularly ineffective. Surgical reanastomosis is, however, followed by complete resolution of all rheumatic symptoms.

Approximately 10% of patients with collagenous colitis develop arthritis, including rheumatoid arthritis. This condition consists histologically of linear deposits of hyaline material and a chronic inflammatory exudate in the colonic subepithelium. The etiology remains unknown, but high concentrations of prostaglandin E_2 have been found in small intestinal aspirates and in the stools. Coexistant autoimmune disease has been noted in up to 20% of patients[35]. In this respect, the condition resembles diabetes mellitus, which is associated with autoimmune disorders, and which may be complicated by diarrhea as a result of autonomic nervous dysfunction. Perhaps the diagnosis, therefore, of collagenous colitis should be considered in patients with diabetes who develop diarrhea, but have no evidence of autonomic nervous system dysfunction.

RHEUMATIC COMPLICATIONS OF HEMATOLOGICAL DISORDERS

HEMOGLOBINOPATHIES

Among the intrinsic causes of hemolytic anemia the one rheumatologists are most likely to encounter is sickle cell disease. This is a genetic disorder where a valine is substituted at position 6 in the beta chain of globulin. Hemoglobin S may exist in the homozygous state (HbSS, sickle cell disease) or in the heterozygous state (HbAs, sickle cell trait). Polymerization of HbS causes the red cells to become rigid and sickle shaped, and undergo hemolysis. Patients with sickle cell disease are chronically anemic with hemoglobin concentrations of between 5 and 10 g/dl and reticulocyte counts of 10–30%. Inability of the rigid deformed erythrocytes to pass through capillaries leads to vascular occlusion of the microcirculation and tissue infarction. Sickle cell trait and sickle cell disease are found in those of African origin.

Osteopenia, due to compensatory overgrowth of the myeloid elements of the bone marrow, affects both axial and peripheral skeleton. The bones show widened medullary cavities, few trabeculae and cortical thinning. The skull shows thinning of the inner and outer tables and widened diploic spaces. The 'paint-brush' or 'hair on end' appearance is due to reactive new bone being laid down in the diploic space in a vertical striated pattern. As the child matures the perpendicular striae consolidate in one homogeneous mass resulting in thickening of the skull. Sickle cell disease tends to involve the frontal and parietal areas, but not the facial bones, although the mandible may be involved.

In children, dactylitis is often the initial presentation of sickle cell disease. This is due to persistence of hemopoietic marrow in peripheral skeletal sites, and is rare after the age of four when the red marrow recedes. The dactylitis is probably the result of infarction since radiolucent areas, which are often symmetrical, are replaced by osteosclerosis. The radiological appearances are similar to those seen in osteomyelitis, especially as circumferential periostitis is frequently present. The hands and feet are often swollen, painful and tender, especially in cold weather[36].

Bone infarction occurs especially in the upper humerus and upper femur. The pathogenesis of infarction may be due to increased blood viscosity with decrease in oxygen tension causing occlusion of small blood vessels by sickle-shaped erythrocytes. Alternatively, it may be due to fat embolism, as a result of infarcts in yellow marrow. In long bones infarcts may lead to concentric cylinders of bone paralleling the cortical surface: a 'bone within bone' appearance. Infarcts of other bones may result in osteosclerosis, which may resemble metastases or Paget's disease. Ischemia of the central portion of the vertebral bodies may cause H-shaped vertebrae consisting of step-like indentations of the vertebral end plates. Calcifications of infarcts may come to resemble tumors, such as enchondromata. Infarction of the femoral epiphyses may resemble Legg–Calvé–Perthes disease, but is usually easily differentiated since it occurs in Blacks and is often bilateral. Aseptic necrosis of the humeral and femoral heads may be asymptomatic even when radiologically positive[37]. The optimal therapy for osteonecrosis remains unknown but may include core decompression, limited weight bearing and

arthroplasty. In patients treated by hip arthroplasty, there is an 8% risk of surgical revision within 1 year, and a 30% risk within 4.5 years[38].

Muscle necrosis with elevations of muscle enzymes leading to fibrosis is probably due to infarction, although possibly in some cases to intramuscular injections.

Patients with sickle cell disease not infrequently develop severe mono- or pauciarticular pain, especially in the knees and elbows. Synovialysis reveals only a mild inflammation with cell counts less than 1000 cells/mm^3, and very few polymorphonuclear leucocytes. Synovial biopsy shows microvascular thrombosis and little evidence of cell infiltration. These non-inflammatory effusions are probably 'sympathetic' and due to adjacent bone infarcts. Rarely rapid destruction of joints may occur, but the cause of this remains unknown[36].

Patients with sickle cell disease may develop secondary gout, as a result of both overproduction and underexcretion of uric acid.

Patients with sickle cell disease are 100% more likely to develop bacterial infection than normal children, particularly to salmonellae and staphylococci. This is due to a deficiency in a serum opsonin, so that polymorphonuclear leucocytes are unable to phagocytose the bacteria and has been attributed to a defect in the alternative complement pathway. Bone infection is generally the result of Gram-negative organisms, while joint infection is usually due to Gram-positive bacteria[39].

Osteomyelitis is more common than septic arthritis. It usually affects diaphysis of the long bones and can be multifocal. Radiologically, osteolysis and periostitis are first evident, and may be confused with bone infarction. However, continued bone destruction, persistent fever, involucrum formation and the development of soft-tissue abscesses and sinus formation, confirm the diagnosis of osteomyelitis. The combined use of technetium and gallium scintigraphy has been found helpful in differentiating osteomyelitis from bone infarcts.

Septic arthritis usually involves the hip joint, but can be polyarticular and associated with osteomyelitis.

Involvement of the epiphyses can result in growth disturbances, and fractures can occur as a result of osteopenia, bone infarcts or osteomyelitis. Pain relief is best achieved with patient controlled analgesia. A crisis may be precipitated by intra-articular corticosteroid therapy[40].

Sickle cell trait (HbAS) is usually asymptomatic, but occasionally can be associated with osteonecrosis and salmonella osteomyelitis. Other forms of sickle cell hemoglobinopathy, e.g. HbC disease, can be associated with skull and spinal changes and osteonecrosis.

Beta-thalassemia (Cooley's or Mediterranean anemia, Thalassemia major) causes similar arthritis and skeletal abnormalities to those of HbSS sickle cell disease. The 'hair on end' appearance in the skull is even more marked than in sickle cell disease, but tends to affect the frontal and occipital bones with relative flattening of the vertex. However, unlike sickle cell disease, β-thalassemia affects the facial bones and obliteration of the air spaces in the paranasal sinuses. Maxillary involvement may cause displacement of the orbits with hyperteleorism. Overgrowth of the facial bones and malocclusion of the teeth can result in a 'chipmunk' facies with the former, and a 'rodent' facies with the latter. Beta-thalassaemia is the only hemolytic anemia to cause alteration to the facies. Changes in the long bones and vertebrae are similar but less severe than sickle cell disease. Premature closure of epiphyses is, however, more common, occurring in 10–15% of patients, and may be unilateral or bilateral. Pathological fractures are also common. Patients may develop gouty arthritis, and pseudo-gout, the latter as a consequence of hemosiderosis from repeated transfusions. Extramedullary hemopoiesis may present as paravertebral mediastinal

and retroperitoneal masses, and may cause cord compression.

The thalassemia trait (thalassemia minor) may rarely be complicated by self-limiting arthritis, and avascular necrosis of the femoral heads.

Glucose-6 phosphate dehydrogenase deficiency usually presents with acute intravascular hemolysis, often precipitated by drugs and foods. Changes may occur in bones due to marrow hyperplasia, including skull changes.

Hereditary spherocytosis usually does not manifest until adolescence. Occasional changes in long bones and in the skull may occur, with rarely the 'hair on end' appearance in the latter. Transfusion siderosis may occur in patients with severe anemia requiring frequent blood transfusions.

DISORDERS OF BLOOD COAGULATION

The most common disorders of inborn disorders of blood coagulation are hemophilia (factor VIII deficiency) and Christmas disease (factor IX deficiency). The most troublesome bleeding occurs in the joints, and commonly causes trauma[41].

An acute hemarthrosis presents with all the cardinal features of inflammation, and generally subsides in a few days or weeks. Repeated hemorrhage into joints results in deposition of hemosiderin into synovium and other joint tissues, hyperplasia of synovial lining cells, fibrosis and cartilage and bone damage. The latter is probably enzymatically rather than immunologically produced. A radiological feature of hemophiliac arthritis is the development of large bone cysts, which may either be due to intraosseous bleeding or as a result of degeneration of cartilage. Massive hemorrhage into soft tissues, such as muscle, may occur, and in bone may present as a 'pseudotumor'. The knee joint is especially involved in hemophiliac arthritis, and in addition to osteoarthritis and cystic changes in chronic disease may also demonstrate intercondylar widening on X-ray. Other radiological features of hemophiliac arthritis include enlargement of the head of the radius, flattening of the talus and 'squaring' of the inferior portion of the patella[42].

Improved therapy has certainly reduced the arthritic problem in joints, but not eliminated it. Arthrocentesis is probably best avoided in acute hemarthrosis, unless sepsis is suspected. Patients with hemophilia infected with human immunodeficiency virus are particularly prone to septic arthritis[43]. Chronic arthropathy has been described in von Willebrand's disease (factor VIII deficiency and platelet dysfunction) and secondary to anticoagulant therapy.

It is now possible with potent factor concentrates to control hemorrhage and to reduce but, as mentioned above, not eliminate destruction of joints[44].

GRAFT VERSUS HOST DISEASE (GVHD)

This is a frequent complication following bone-marrow transplantation, with up to 45% of patients developing chronic GVHD. This condition resembles a connective tissue disease in many respects, with skin thickening, keratoconjunctivitis sicca, xerostomia, pulmonary infiltrates, athralgias, myositis, Raynaud's phenomenon and polyse ositis. Treatment options include prednisolone with the addition of azathioprine and cyclosporine[45].

SARCOIDOSIS

Sarcoidosis is a disease of unknown etiology, characterized by multiple granulomatous lesions, which may affect many different organs and tissues in the body. Histologically, the sarcoid lesions consist of tubercle-like follicles composed of epithelioid cells with occasional Langhans giant cells, but fewer lymphocytes than in tubercles. The giant cells may contain calcium-rich star-shaped or conchoid inclusions (asteroid or Schaumann bodies). In contrast to tuberculosis, the lesions do not undergo caseation, although a little central necrosis may occur. These non-caseating epithelioid-cell granulomas are not diagnostic of sarcoidosis and occur in tuberculosis, brucellosis, syphilis, fungal infections and berylliosis. Diagnosis is thus based on clinical features, distribution of lesions and exclusion of the above diseases.

Sarcoid involvement of bone, joint and muscle has been well described. Acute sarcoid, Löfgren's syndrome, consists of a quaternion of acute polyarthritis, bilateral hilar lymphadenopathy, erythema nodosum and fever. Unlike chronic sarcoidosis, parenchymal lung disease does not occur, although the serum angiotensin converting enzyme may be elevated. The arthritis can involve many joints, but usually knees and ankles; in some patients tenosynovitis may be prominent. Synovial fluid is mildly inflammatory with total white cell counts up to 3000 cells/mm^3, 80% being mononuclear. Synovial biopsy shows hyperplasia of synovial lining cells without an inflammatory infiltrate[46]. When erythema nodosum is absent the polyarthritis may be mistaken for early rheumatoid arthritis, especially if there is a positive test for rheumatoid factor. In Europeans an association with HLA-B8 and DR3 haplotypes and Löfgren's syndrome has been described[46]. The HLA-B8 is in linkage disequilibrium with DR3. The course of acute sarcoid is benign and self-limited, most patients recovering in 1–6 months. Many patients with acute sarcoid are treated with oral corticosteroids but, in our opinion, is unnecessary, since both fever and arthritis respond promptly to nonsteroidal anti-inflammatory analgesics.

Joint involvement in the chronic form may rarely be associated with destructive changes and deformity. Sarcoid granulomas are frequently demonstrated in the synovium, and synovialysis has demonstrated leucocyte counts up to 6250 cells/mm^3 with predominantly mononuclear cells[47]. Tenosynovitis is also a feature of chronic sarcoidosis, and patients with extensive pulmonary

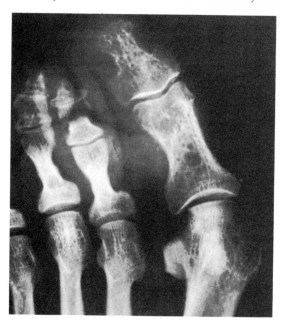

Fig. 13.1 Typical 'lattice' reticulation in the phalanges of the big toe in sarcoidosis.

involvement may develop finger clubbing and hypertrophic pulmonary osteoarthropathy. Rheumatoid factor has been reported in up to 40% of patients with chronic sarcoid arthritis, but the titers are lower than in rheumatoid arthritis. No HLA association has been reported with chronic sarcoidosis. Commonly, no abnormality is seen on radiological examination of the joints in chronic sarcoid arthritis. Soft-tissue swelling, juxta-articular osteoporosis and mild joint space narrowing may be all that is found. Eccentric erosions may occur, and in rare cases destructive arthropathy[48].

Osseous sarcoidosis is usually asymptomatic. The incidence varies widely in different reports: the true incidence is difficult to determine, although probably low. The typical appearance is of a course reticulated or lacework trabecular pattern in the bones of the hands and feet, especially the proximal and distal phalanges (Figure 13.1). Punched out round or oval cystic lesions may occur, which

may be centrally placed or eccentric; the latter leading to scalloping of bone. These cystic lesions may contain calcium. An important feature is the absence of a periosteal reaction. Osteoporosis has been recorded in chronic sarcoidosis, but whether caused by hypercalcemia and hypercalcuria has not been determined. Perhaps less commonly recognized is osteosclerosis, which may be localized or generalized[49]. Acro-osteosclerosis has been reported in chronic sarcoidosis, but occurs in a number of other conditions and also in normal subjects. Cystic foci may rarely occur in the skull, ribs, long bones and vertebral bodies. Pathological fractures have been reported and lupus pernio affecting the fingers or nose may cause destruction of underlying bone. Scintigraphy, using ^{99m}Tc pyrophosphate, may be useful in identifying the extent of osseous involvement. Sarcoid arthritis in children is rare, and may be diagnosed as juvenile rheumatoid arthritis[50].

Muscle involvement is also usually asymptomatic, although 75% of patients will have non-caseating granulomas on muscle biopsy. The types of clinical presentations are recognized: acute myositic, chronic myopathic and nodular. Sarcoid nodules in muscles may rarely be palpable, and are best identified by magnetic resonance imaging[51]. When it occurs, acute myositis may be associated with elevated creatine kinase levels and abnormal electromyographs. Chronic myopathic presentation is frequently seen with proximal symmetric muscle weakness. Neurosarcoidosis can also cause muscle symptoms[52].

The traditional diagnostic test, the Kveim test, consists of an intradermal injection of 0.2 ml of a 10% saline suspension of sarcoid tissue. A positive test consists of sarcoid granuloma formation at the site of injection. Although the test has an 80% sensitivity, it has largely become obsolete because of the unavailability of reliable Kveim antigen. Although depression of delayed-type cutaneous hypersensitivity, e.g. to tuberculin, is a characteristic, but not invariable immune feature of the disease, the relationship of sarcoidosis and tuberculosis has long been debated. It is therefore of interest that recently a murine monoclonal anti-Kveim antibody has been shown to react with epithelioid cells of sarcoid and tuberculous granuloma, thus suggesting common antigenicity[53]. Angiotensin converting enzyme is typically elevated in pulmonary sarcoidosis, but is not specific. Measurement of angiotensin converting enzyme is useful however in assessing the effects of treatment. Hypercalcemia has been reported in 25% of patients and attributed to hypersensitivity to vitamin D and increased intestinal absorption. However, recent studies have shown that sarcoid granulomas synthetize 1, 25-dihydrovitamin D, and that this might be the cause of hypercalcemia[54]. Administration of corticosteroids usually reduces hypercalcemia, as does ketoconazole, a topical antifungal.

The immunological aspects of sarcoidosis are gradually giving up their secrets, and recent advances in knowledge are admirably summarized by Mathur and Kremer[55]. It appears that the key problem is unchecked helper T-cell proliferation. Using immunohistochemical techniques and specific monoclonal antibodies, these T-cells have been shown to predominantly express α/β T-cell receptors.

RHEUMATIC COMPLICATIONS OF ENDOCRINE DISORDERS

Disorders of the endocrine system are associated with a wide variety of rheumatic conditions[56]. Although pregnancy cannot be classified as an endocrine disorder, the associated endocrine changes cause amelioration in both adult and juvenile rheumatoid arthritis in approximately 75% of patients[57,58]. Improvement usually occurs in the third trimester, but relapse is common within 3–6 months of parturition. Labor and delivery pose no serious problems in patients with rheumatoid arthritis, although cesarean section is often preferred in patients with severe hip disease. Aspirin therapy has been shown to prolong gestation and labor, and to increase both ante- and post-partum hemorrhage[57]. Why patients with rheumatoid arthritis frequently improve during pregnancy has not been explained; nor why this improvement only occurs in this disease and not in other forms of inflammatory polyarthritis, such as ankylosing spondylitis and psoriatic arthritis[57]. There is conflicting data on whether oral contraceptives[59] and nulliparity[60] are associated with a lower incidence of rheumatoid arthritis. The onset of rheumatoid arthritis is reduced during pregnancy, but increased 9 months after delivery[61]. Pregnancies occurring before the onset of rheumatoid arthritis are however, normal[62]. Men with rheumatoid arthritis have been found to have low serum testosterone levels[63], and improvement in joint inflammation has been reported following testosterone therapy[64].

PARATHYROID DISORDERS

The radiological findings in bones and joints in hyperparathyroidism have been well described by Resnick and Niwayama[65]. Radiological changes are first apparent in the hands, where subperiosteal erosions develop on the radial aspect of the middle phalanges of the index and middle fingers. Subperiosteal erosions can be seen in other bones, as can endosteal bone erosion, subchondral bone resorption, e.g. in the sacroiliac joints where it may mimic ankylosing spondylitis, brown tumors, osteopenia and bone sclerosis[65]. Inflammatory arthritis is not uncommon, and probably related to subchondral bone resorption, although crystal-induced inflammation, e.g. CPPD, may also play a role[65]. Surgical treatment is now recommended for all patients with primary hyperparathyroidism[66,67], the only exception being mild disease in the elderly. In mild disease fractures are uncommon, despite decline in bone

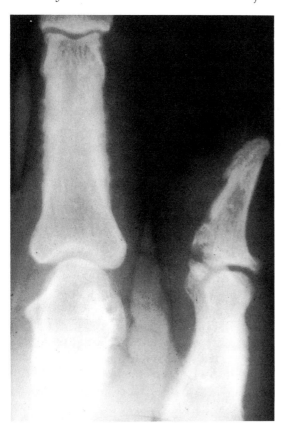

Fig. 13.2 Thyroid acropachy. Dense periostitis with feathery contour affecting both metacarpals and phalanges. The periostitis tends to be asymmetrical with a predilection for the radial aspect of the proximal phalanx of the first digit and second metacarpal.

mineral mass[67]. Osteopenia, however, improves following surgery[67].

THYROID DISORDERS

Thyrotoxicosis is associated with excessive bone turnover and hypercalcuria, leading to loss of bone mineral mass. What has recently been discovered is that physiological replacement of thyroid hormone for hypothyroidism may also lead to loss of bone mineral mass-[68,69] probably as a result of increased bone collagen breakdown[70]. However, as has been pointed out, the Scylla of osteoporosis is

less important than the Charybdis of coronary artery disease. Not surprisingly suppressive doses of thyroxine used to treat simple goiter[71] and thyroid cancer[72] have also been shown to significantly reduce bone mineral mass. However, it is of interest that Lehmke *et al.*[73] failed to show any reduction in bone mineral mass in patients treated with suppressive doses of thyroxine for thyroid neoplasm. Whether treatment with estrogens would be helpful in preventing loss of bone with thyroxine therapy remains to be demonstrated.

The association of autoimmune thyroid disease with both rheumatoid arthritis[74] and systemic lupus erythematosus[75] continues to attract attention. However, it is not known whether the association reported is related to co-existing Sjögren's syndrome or HLA-DR3 antigen.

Thyroid acropachy (Figure 13.2) and thyrotoxic myopathy in thyrotoxicosis remain to be explained. Patients with hypothyroidism may present with rheumatic complaints, including carpal tunnel compression, and muscle stiffness and pseudohypertrophy (Hoffman's syndrome)[76]. A raised serum creatine kinase concentration may lead the unwary to a diagnosis of polymyositis. The serum creatine kinase concentration usually returns to normal two months of the patient attaining the euthyroid state. How much of the serum creatine increase is due to cardiac involvement, i.e. MB isoenzyme remains to be determined. Electromyographic changes and muscle biopsies reveal no distinctive features.

Although carpal tunnel syndrome is generally considered due to mucinous deposits in the carpal tunnel causing compressing of the median nerve, it is now apparent that patients with hypothyroidism also have a generalized neuronal metabolic dysfunction causing peripheral neuropathy[77].

An arthropathy peculiar to hypothyroidism has been described. The arthritis usually develops concurrently with hypothyroidism, but occasionally antedates it, and is usually

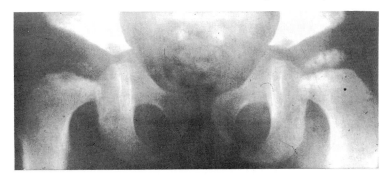

Fig. 13.3 Chondrodysplasia punctata consisting of irregular calcification of the epiphyses in a child with juvenile hypothyroidism.

bilateral affecting especially the knees. Periarticular tissues are thickened but there is ligamentous laxity. Synovial fluid is hyperviscous and generally non-inflammatory. Flexor tenosynovitis at the wrist has been attributed to hyaluronate deposition as it does not improve with thyroid therapy, but after injections of corticosteroids. The increase in hyaluronate in joint fluid and in tendon sheaths has been ascribed to increased levels of thyroid-stimulating hormone. Asymptomatic hyperuricemia occurs in men, but not in women with hypothyroidism. There is some evidence that hypothyroidism may be slightly more common in men with gout.

Retardation of skeletal maturation is the fundamental radiographic feature of juvenile hypothyroidism. This may cause slipped capital femoral ephiphysis. Ossification in the epiphyses proceeds from multiple centers rather from a simple site, the resulting appearance being known as epiphyseal dysgenesis (Figure 13.3).

this is more common in acromegalics is unknown. Compression neuropathy, especially affecting the carpal tunnel, occurs in approximately one-third of patients. Spinal cord compression with long tract signs may occur as a result of hypertrophy of the vertebral bodies and soft tissue overgrowth. A proximal myopathy may occur associated with elevation of the serum creatine kinase level and non-specific muscle fiber hypertrophy. Growth hormone promotes cartilage hypertrophy which causes widening of the articular spaces, one of the characteristic radiological features (Figure 13.4). Significant improvement in rheumatic symptoms has been reported following treatment of the disease[79]. A forgotten physical sign, the acromegalic 'rosary' has been described by Ibbertson *et al.*[80]. This consists of palpable enlargement of the costochondral junctions.

Both isolated growth hormone deficiency and multiple pituitary deficiency can result in a low bone mass[81].

PITUITARY AND ADRENAL DISEASE

Podgorski *et al.*[78] have recently described the arthritic and rheumatic complications of acromegaly. According to these authors some 75% of patients develop a peripheral arthropathy, while 50% have an axial athropathy. Synovitis may occur due to calcium pyrophosphate dihydrate (CPPD) crystals, but whether

CUSHING'S SYNDROME

The musculoskeletal complications have been well described. The most interesting recent observation is that reduced bone mineral density returns to normal with treatment[82], possibly due to preservation of trabecular architecture[83].

Small doses of oral corticosteroids, i.e. less

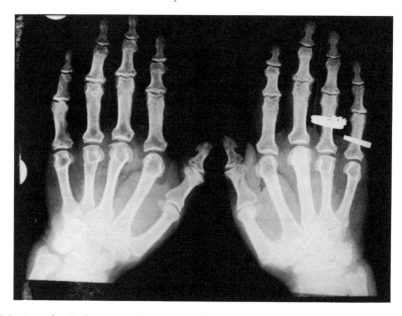

Fig. 13.4 Widening of articular spaces in acromegaly.

than 10 mg/day[84], and even normal levels of circulating cortisol[85] have been shown to have anti-inflammatory action in rheumatoid arthritis.

ADDISON'S DISEASE

Patients with adrenal insufficiency frequently complain of muscle pains, perhaps due to hypokalemia. One of the more unpleasant side effects of antiphospholipid antibodies is acute adrenal insufficiency[86]. Whether this is due to adrenal hemorrhage or thrombosis is not known. What is important is that physicians should be aware of the complication and suspect it when a patient with antiphospholipid antibodies presents with abdominal pain.

DIABETES MELLITUS

A variety of musculoskeletal abnormalities have been described in patients with diabetes mellitus. Perhaps the best known, but relatively uncommon (1 in 1000), is Charcot's arthropathy. This affects the ankle and midtarsal joints, and is always associated with a peripheral neuropathy[87]. Occasionally, other joints may be affected, and the onset often follows minor trauma[88]. Indium III labelled leucocyte scans are useful in identifying osteomyelitis in the diabetic foot[89], but magnetic resonance imaging is better[90]. Osteolysis is a common radiological finding in the diabetic foot. Arthrodesis of the ankle in Charcot's arthropathy gives poor results[91]. Joint arthroplasty for osteoarthritis in patients with diabetes melitus with no peripheral neuropathy is associated with a high infection and revision rate[92].

A thickening of the skin of the fingers occurs in a high proportion of patients with all types of diabetes mellitus. This has the clinical appearance of systemic sclerosis, but is never associated with Raynaud's syndrome or with skin hair loss or calcific deposits, and the thickening of the skin rarely extends beyond the metacarpophalangeal joints[93,94]. Patients with this cheirarthropathy, as it has been termed, cannot oppose their fingers.

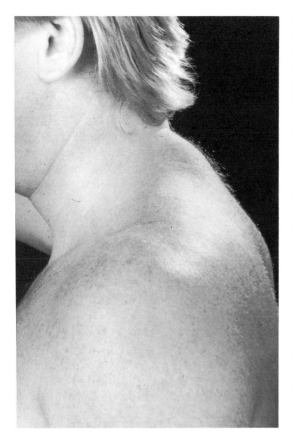

Fig. 13.5 Diabetic pseudoscleroderma (Buschke's scleroderma). This consists of a woody induration on the posterior aspect of the neck and may persist for years. (Courtesy of Dr Mark H. Arnold and the editor of *Modern Medicine of Canada* (1989).)

Nail-fold capillaries are normal in cheirarthropathy, in contrast to systemic sclerosis.

Limitation of joint mobility is a common finding in diabetes mellitus, affecting both joints in the upper and lower limbs[94]. Other common complications include Dupuytren's and Ledderhosen's contractures, flexor tenosynovitis and trigger finger, carpal tunnel syndrome and periarthritis of the shoulder [95–97]. Peyronie's disease has also been described. The relationship of these complications to retinopathy and nephropathy remains controversial[93,94,98,99] but there is some evidence that poor control[97], duration of disease[96] and cigarette smoking[100] may

play a role. These fibrosing syndromes appear to be related to abnormalities in cross-linking and increased glycosylation of collagen, increase in the hydration of connective tissues and possibly also to changes in microvasculature and peripheral nerves[98,99,101]. Decrease in glycosylation of skin collagen has been noted with improvement in diabetic control[102,103].

Diabetic psuedoscleroderma, also known as Buschke's scleredema, consists of a woody induration on the posterior part of the neck, which may persist for years (Figure 13.5). It occurs particularly in patients with long-standing diabetes mellitus.

Despite earlier doubts there now seems a clear association between diabetes mellitus, especially in older men, and diffuse idiopathic skeletal hyperostosis[104]. The exuberant ossification of spinal ligaments and enthesopathy in this disease contrasts with the finding of fewer osteophytes in osteoarthritis of the knee joints in patients with diabetes mellitus[105]. Osteoporosis has been reported in both adults and children with diabetes mellitus[106,107], which appears to be related to duration rather than severity of disease.

Multiple rheumatic complaints suggestive of systemic lupus erythematosis, systemic sclerosis and Sjögren's syndrome, have been reported in patients with diabetes mellitus who are insulin resistant due to receptor antibodies[108].

Diabetic amyotrophy causing weakness and wasting of the anterior thigh muscles has been reported in insulin-dependent elderly patients with diabetes mellitus[109,110]. The condition usually recovers after 18 months. Spontaneous muscle infarction can also occur in diabetic patients[111].

MALIGNANCY

RHEUMATIC COMPLICATIONS OF NEOPLASIA

A wide spectrum of neoplastic conditions, both hematologic and non-hematologic, may be associated with rheumatic syndromes. Perhaps the best recognized of these paraneoplastic syndromes is hypertrophic osteoarthropathy, most commonly associated with pulmonary neoplasm, but also with neoplasms in other organs, and even with lung metastases[112]. Recently, Johnson *et al.*[113] have reported a Jaccoud's-type arthropathy as the initial manifestation of carcinoma of the lung. The cause of both hypertrophic osteoarthropathy and Jaccoud's-type arthritis remains unknown.

Patients with neoplasms may also initially present with a polyarthritis, which frequently resembles rheumatoid arthritis[114,115]. However, joint involvement is often asymmetrical and the joints of the hands and wrists are frequently spared. The onset may be explosive and when fever is present the unwary may be misled into making a diagnosis of adult Still's disease. The cause is not known, histological changes in the synovium are non-specific, and synovial fluid is only mildly inflammatory. Some patients develop positive anti-nuclear factor tests and antibodies to double-stranded DNA.

Although in the past numerous authors have concluded that there is an increased incidence of polymyositis and dermatomyositis in patients with various neoplasms, Cash and Klippel[116] have recently challenged this view (also Chapter 4). Two recent papers have failed to show such an association[117,118]. Malignancies can be associated with a wide range of myopathies, and many authors in the past have not adhered to strict diagnostic criteria. There is selection bias with over-representation of hospital-based cases in most studies. At present no firm conclusion can be drawn regarding the association of neoplasm with polymyositis and dermatomyositis.

There appears, however, to be a clear association between malignancies and vasculitis[119] and this has been reviewed in Chapter 9.

Other conditions which have recently been associated with neoplasms include: reflex sympathetic dystrophy[120], Raynaud's syndrome[121] and palmar fasciitis[122]. The latter is especially associated with ovarian adenocarcinoma.

Lymphoproliferative malignancies and leukemia commonly present with rheumatological manifestations[123,124]. Leukemic synovitis may be the initial manifestation of relapse of acute leukemia. The arthritis is often migratory, but can be symmetric and rheumatoid-like and is frequently associated with bone pain and tenderness. Metaphyseal rarefaction, osteolytic lesions and periosteal reactions are useful diagnostic radiological findings. It is rare, however, to find leukemic cells in synovial fluid, even when the synovium is infiltrated[125]. Synovial fluid immunocytological analysis may be helpful in demonstrating leukemic cells[126].

MALIGNANCY IN SYSTEMIC RHEUMATIC DISEASES

There is now considerable evidence of an increased incidence of non-Hodgkin's lymphoma in rheumatoid arthritis[127]. This does not appear to be due to immunosuppressive or cytotoxic therapy[128], although Silman *et al.*[129] reported a two-fold increase in incidence in patients treated with azothioprine. Patients with rheumatoid arthritis who develop an IgA-α paraprotein have been found to subsequently develop multiple myeloma[130].

An increased incidence of non-Hodgkin's lymphoma has been reported in both primary and secondary Sjögren's syndrome (Chapter 5). It is of interest that in both rheumatoid arthritis and Sjögren's syndrome there are large numbers of CD5$^+$ B lymphocytes, which are particularly prone to clonal expansion and malignant transformation[131,132].

There continues to be controversy regarding whether there is an increased incidence of alveolar cell carcinoma of the lung in systemic sclerosis and this has been referred to in Chapter 3. Bielefeld *et al.*[133] have reported an increase in malignant blood disorders in this disease. There is no evidence of a predisposition to neoplasia in systemic lupus erythematosus, although instances of lymphoma have been recorded.

JOINT TUMORS

Malignant neoplasms of joints, such as synovial sarcoma, are extremely rare[134]. Both benign and malignant tumors of bone may, however, cause joint effusion with a low-grade inflammatory fluid. Metastatic carcinoma is usually monoarticular and most frequently involves the knee[135].

IATROGENIC MALIGNANCY

Prolonged use of oral cyclophosphamide is associated with an increased risk of hematological malignancies and reticuloendothelial tumors, and bladder tumors[136]. Although as mentioned above Silman *et al.*[129] reported a two-fold increase in lymphoma in patients with rheumatoid arthritis treated with azathioprine, no such increase has been reported by other workers[128]. An Epstein–Barr virus-associated lymphoma has been reported in a patient with rheumatoid arthritis treated with cyclosporine[137], and a case of chronic myeloid leukemia has been described in a rheumatoid patient some years after ^{198}Au synoviorthesis[138]. Rooney *et al.*[139] have recently reviewed the rheumatic complications which may arise from cancer medications. A seronegative polyarthritis has been reported following treatment of bladder cancer with intravesical BCG[140]. This human 'adjuvant' arthritis quickly disappeared when treatment was discontinued.

REFERENCES

1. Meema, H. E., Oreopoulos, D. G., Murray, T. M. (1986) Periosteal resorption and periosteal neostosis: comparison of normal subjects and renal failure patients in chronic ambulatory peritoneal dialysis using M OP-3 image analysis system and a grading method. *Skel. Radiol.*, **15**, 14–20.

2. Moriniere, P., Marie, A., Elesper, N. *et al.* (1991) Destructive spondyloarthropathy with β2-microglobulin anyloid deposits in a uremic patient before chronic hemodialysis. *Nephron.*, **59**, 654–7.

3. Mitrovic, D., Barain, T. and Kuntz, D. (1991) Osteonecrosis in a patient receiving long-term haemodialysis. *J. Rheumatol.*, **10**, 1230–1.

4. Kopecky, K. K., Braunstein, E. M., Brandt, K. D. *et al.* (1991) Apparent avascular necrosis of the hip: appearance and spontaneous resolution of magnetic resonance findings in renal allograft patients. *Radiology*, **179**, 523–7.

5. Lucas, V., Page, T., Plougastel-Lucas, M. *et al.* (1991) Musculoskeletal pain in renal transplant recipients. *N. Eng. J. Med.*, **335**, 1449–50.

6. Munoz-Gomez, J. and Sole, M. (1990) Dialysis arthropathy of amyloid origin. *J. Rheumatol.*, **17**, 723–4.

7. Athanasou, N. A., Ayers, D., Rainey, A. J. *et al.* (1991) Joint and systemic distribution of dialysis amyloid. *Q. J. Med.*, **78**, 205–14.

8. Duncan, J. S., Hurst, N. P., Sebben, R. *et al.* (1990) Premature development of erosive osteoarthritis of the hands in patients with chronic renal failure. *Ann. Rheum. Dis.*, **49**, 378–82.

9. Maruyama, H., Gejyo, F. and Arakawa, M. (1991) Clinical studies of destructive spondyloarthropathy in long-term hemodialysis patients. *Nephron.*, **61**, 37–44.

10. Chassagne, P., Dhib, M., Aitsaid, L. *et al.* (1992) Spinal cord compression revealing a destructive arthropathy of the atlantooccipital joint associated with beta-2 microglobulin amyloidosis in a haemodialysed patient. *Br. J. Rheumatol.*, **31**, 427–32.

11. Kessler, M., Netter, P., Azoulay, E. *et al.* (1992) Dialysis associated arthropathy: a multicentre survey of 171 patients receiving haemodialysis for over 10 years. *Br. J. Rheumatol.*, **31**, 157–62.

12. Campistol, J. M., Ponz, E., Munoz-Gomez, J. *et al.* (1992) Renal transplantation for dialysis amyloidosis. *Transplant Proc.*, **24**, 118–19.

13. Rillo, D., Bobini, S., Barmah, A. *et al.* (1991) Tendinous and ligamentous hyperlaxity in patients receiving long-term haemodialysis. *J. Rheumatol.*, **18**, 1227–31.

14. Scarpa, R., Del Puente, A., D'Arienzo, A. *et al.* (1992) The arthritis of ulcerative colitis:

clinical and genetic aspects. *J. Rheumatol.*, **19**, 373–7.

15. Mielants, H., Veys, E. M., Goethals, K. *et al.* (1990) Destructive lesions of small joints in seronegative spondylarthropathies: relation to gut inflammation. *Clin. Exp. Rheumatol.*, **8**, 23–7.

16. Weiner, S. R., Clarke, J., Taggart, N. A. *et al.* (1991) Rheumatic manifestations of inflammatory bowel disease. *Semin. Arth. Rheum.*, **20**, 353–66.

17. Kaufman, H. J. and Taubin, H. L. (1987) Nonsteroidal antinflammatory drugs activate quiescent inflammatory bowel disease. *Ann. Intern. Med.*, **107**, 513–16.

18. Gunaste, V., Greensten, A. J., Meyers, R. *et al.* (1989) Coombs-positive autoimmune hemolytic anemia in ulcerative colitis. *Digest. Dis. Sci.*, **34**, 1457–61.

19. Cowling, P., Ebringer, R. and Ebringer, A. (1980) Association of inflammation with raised serum IgA in ankylosing spondylitis. *Ann. Rheum. Dis.*, **39**, 545–9.

20. Hocini, H., Iscaki, S., Benlahrache, C. *et al.* (1992) Increased levels of serum IgA monomers in ankylosing spondylitis. *Ann. Rheum. Dis.*, **51**, 790–2.

21. Herrero-Beaumont, G., Armas, J. B., Elswood, J. *et al.* (1990) Selective IgA deficiency and spondyloanthropathy: a distinct disease? *Ann. Rheum. Dis.*, **49**, 636–7.

22. Shodjai-Moraodi, F., Ebringer, A. and Aboljadayel, I. (1992) IgA antibody response to *Klebsiella* in ankylosing spondylitis measured by immunoblotting. *Ann. Rheum. Dis.*, **51**, 233–7.

23. MacLean, I. L., Archer, J. R., Crawley, M. I. D. *et al.* (1992) Immune complexes in ankylosing spondylitis. *Ann. Rheum. Dis.*, **51**, 83–7.

24. Feltelius, N., Gudmunsson, S., Wennerstenl., L. *et al.* (1991) Linked immunospot (Elispot) technique to evaluate sulphasalazine effects in inflammatory arthritides. *Ann. Rheum. Dis.*, **50**, 369–71.

25. Mielants, H., Veys, E. M., Verbraeken, H. *et al.* (1990) HLA-B27 positive idiopathic acute anterior uveitis: a unique manifestation of subclinical gut inflammation. *J. Rheumatol.*, **17**, 841–2.

26. Mielants, H., Veys, E. M., Goemaere, S. *et al.* (1991) Gut inflammation in the spondyloarthropathies: clinical, radiologic, biologic and genetic features in relation to the type of

histology: a prospective study. *J. Rheumatol.*, **18**, 1542–51.

27. Mielants, H., Veys, E. M., Joos, R. *et al.* (1987) HLA-antigens in seronegative spondyloarthropathies, reactive arthritis and arthritis in ankylosing spondylitis: relation to gut inflammation. *J. Rheumatol.*, **11**, 466–71.

28. Cuvelier, C., Mielants, H., De Vos, M. *et al.* (1990) Major histocompatibility complex class 1 antigen (HLA-DR) expression by ileal epithelial cells in patients with seronegative spondylarthropathy. *Gut*, **31**, 545–9.

29. Park, H., Schumacker, H. R., Zeiger, A. R. *et al.* (1984) Antibodies to peptidoglycan in patients with spondylarthropathies: a clue to disease adiology? *Ann. Rheum. Dis.*, **43**, 725–8.

30. Van Kregten, E., Huber-Bruning, O., Vandenbroucke, J. P. *et al.* (1991) No conclusive evidence of an epidemiological relation between Klebsiella and ankylosing spondylitis. *J. Rheumatol.*, **18**, 384–8.

31. Maki-Ikola, O., Lehtinen, K., Granfors, K. *et al.* (1991) Bacterial antibodies in ankylosing spondylitis. *Clin. Exp. Immunol.*, **84**, 472–5.

32. Rooney, P. J., Jenkins, R. T. and Buchanan, W. W. (1990) A short review of the relationship between intestinal permeability and inflammatory joint disease. *Clin. Exp. Rheumatol.*, **8**, 75–83.

33. Mielants, H., Goemaere, S., De Vos, M. *et al.* (1991) Intestinal mucosal permeability in inflammatory rheumatic diseases: I. role of anti-inflammatory drugs. *J. Rheumatol.*, **18**, 389–93.

34. Collin, P., Maki, M. and Keyrilainen, O. Selective IgA deficiency and coeliae disease. *Scand. J. Gastroenterol.*, **27**, 367–71.

35. Roubenoff, R., Ratin, J., Giardiello, F. *et al.* (1989) Collagenous colitis, enteropathic arthritis, and autoimmune diseases: results of a patient survey. *J. Rheumatol.*, **16**, 1229–32.

36. Porter, D. R. and Sturrock, R. D. (1991) Rheumatological complications of sickle cell disease. *Baillieres Clin. Rheumatol.*, **5**, 221–30.

37. Milner, P. F., Kraus, A. P., Sebes, J. I. *et al.* (1991) Sickle cell disease as a cause of osteonecrosis of the femoral head. *N. Eng. J. Med.*, **325**, 1476–81.

38. Ware, H. E., Brooks, A. P., Toye, R. *et al.* (1991) Sickle cell disease and silent avascular necrosis of the hip. *J. Bone Joint Surg.*, **73B**, 947–9.

39. Epps, C. H., Bryant, D. D., Coles, M. J. *et al.* (1991) Osteomyelitis in patients who have

sickle-cell disease. *J. Bone Joint Surg.*, **73A**, 1281–94.

40. Gladman, D. D. and Bombardier, C. (1987) Sickle cell crisis following intraarticular steroid therapy for rheumatoid arthritis. *Arth. Rheum.*, **30**, 1065–8.

41. Madhok, R., York, J. and Sturrock, R. D. (1991) Haemophilic arthritis. *Ann. Rheum. Dis.*, **50**, 588–91.

42. York, J. R. (1991) Musculoskeletal disorders in the haemophilias. *Baillieres Clin. Rheumatol.*, **5**, 197–220.

43. Bleasal, J. F., York, J. R. and Richard, K. (1990) Septic arthritis in HIV infected haemophiliacs. *Br. J. Rheumatol.*, **29**, 494–6.

44. Petrini, P., Lindvaill, N., Egberg, N. *et al.* (1991) Prophylaxis with factor concentrates in preventing hemophilic arthropathy. *Am. J. Pediatr. Hematol. Oncol.*, **13**, 280–7.

45. Rennie, J. A. N. and Auchterlonie, I. A. (1991) Rheumatological manifestations of the leukaemia and graft vs host disease. *Baillieres Clin. Rheumatol.*, **5**, 231–51.

46. Kremer, J. M. (1986) Histologic findings in siblings with acute sarcoid arthritis: association with the B8, DR3 phenotype. *J. Rheumatol.*, **13**, 593–7.

47. Palmer, D. G. and Schumacher, H. R. (1984) Synovitis with non-specific histologic changes in synovium in chronic sarcoidosis. *Ann. Rheum. Dis.*, **43**, 778–82.

48. Sartoris, D. J., Resnick, D., Resnick, C. *et al.* (1990) Musculoskeletal manifestations of sarcoidosis. *Semin. Roentgenol.*, **20**, 376–86.

49. Subbarao, K. (1989) Sarcoidosis of bone, in *Radiology: Diagnosis, Imaging, Intervention*, vol. 5, (eds, J. M. Taveras, and J. T. Ferruci), Lippincott and Co. pp. 5–11.

50. Hetherington, S. (1982) Sarcoidosis in young children. *Am. J. Dis. Child.*, **136**, 13–15.

51. Kurashima, K., Shimizu, H., Ogawa, H. *et al.* (1991) MR and CT in the evaluation of sarcoid myopathy. *J. Comput. Assist. Tomogr.*, **15**, 1004–7.

52. Chapelon, C., Ziza, J. M., Piette, J. C. *et al.* (1990) Neurosarcoidosis: Signs, course and treatment 35 confirmed cases. *Medicine*, **69**, 261–76.

53. Ishioka, S., Fujihara, M., Takaishi, M. *et al.* (1990) Anti-Kveim monoclonal antibody: New monoclonal antibody reacting to epithelioid cells in sarcoid granulomas. *Chest*, **98**, 1255–8.

54. Mason, R. S., Frankel, T., Chan, Y. L. *et al.* (1984) Vitamin D conversion by sarcoid lymph node homogenate. *Ann. Intern. Med.*, **100**, 59–61.

55. Mathur, A. and Kremer, J. M. (1993) Immuno-pathology, musculoskeletal features, and treatment of sarcoidosis. *Curr. Opin. Rheumatol.*, **5**, 90–4.

56. McGuire, J. L. (1990) The endocrine system and connective tissue disorders. *Bull. Rheum. Dis.*, **39**, 1–8.

57. Buchanan, W. W., Needs, C. J., Brooks, P. M. (1992) Rheumatic diseases: the arthropathies, in *Principles and Practice of Medical Therapy in Pregnancy*, 2nd edn, (ed. M. Gleicher), Norwalk, Connecticut, Appleton, and Lange, pp. 428–9.

58. Da Silva, Jap and Spector, T. D. (1992) The role of pregnancy in the course and aetiology of rheumatoid arthritis. *Clin. Rheumatol.*, **11**, 189–94.

59. Hazes, J. M. W. and Van Zeben, D. (1991) Oral contraception and its possible protection against rheumatoid arthritis. *Ann. Rheum. Dis.*, **50**, 72–4.

60. Hazes, J. M. W. (1991) Pregnancy and its effect on the risk of developing rheumatoid arthritis. *Ann. Rheum. Dis.*, **50**, 71–2.

61. Silman, A., Kay, A., Brennan, P. (1992) Timing of pregnancy in relation to the onset of rheumatoid arthritis. *Arth. Rheum.*, **35**, 152–5.

62. Nelson, J. L., Voigt, L. F., Koepsell, T. D. *et al.* (1992) Pregnancy outcome in women with rheumatoid arthritis before disease onset. *J. Rheumatol.*, **19**, 18–21.

63. Gordon, B., Beastall, G. H., Thomson, J. A. *et al.* (1988) Prolonged hypogonadism in male patients with rheumatoid arthritis during flares in disease activity. *Br. J. Rheumatol.*, **27**, 440–4.

64. Cutolo, M., Balleari, E., Guisti, M. *et al.* (1991) Androgen replacement therapy in male patients with rheumatoid arthritis. *Arth. Rheum.*, **34**, 1–5.

65. Resnick, D. and Niwayama, G. (1988) Parathyroid disorders and renal osteodystrophy in *Diagnosis of Bone and Joint Disorders*, Vol. 4, 2nd edn, (eds D. Resnick and G. Niwayama), W. B. Saunders Co., Philadelphia, pp. 2219–85.

66. Consensus Development Conference Panel (1991) Diagnosis and management of asymptomatic primary hyperparathyroidism: consensus development conference statement. *Ann. Intern. Med.*, **114**, 593–7.

67. Mole, P. A., Walkinshaw, M. H., Gunn, A. *et al.* (1992) Bone mineral content in patients

with primary hyperparathyroidism: a comparison of conservative with surgical treatment. *Br. J. Surg.*, **79**, 263–5.

68. Baran, D. T. (1991) Thyroid hormones and bone mass (editorial). *Clin. Endocrinol. Metab.*, **72**, 1182–3.

69. Toft, A. D. (1991) Thyroxine replacement therapy. *Clin. Endocrinol.*, **34**, 103–5.

70. Harvey, R. D., McHardy, K. C., Reid, I. W. *et al.* (1991) Measurement of bone collagen degradation in hyperthyroidism and during thyroxine replacement therapy using pyridinium cross-links as specific urinary markers. *J. Clin. Endocrinol. Metab.*, **72**, 1189–94.

71. Tailman, P., Kaufman, J. M., Janssens, X. *et al.* (1990) Reduced forearm bone mineral content and biochemical evidence of increased bone turnover in women with euthyroid goitre treated with thyroid hormone. *Clin. Endocrinol.*, **33**, 107–17.

72. Diamond, T., Nery, L. and Hales, I. (1991) A therapeutic dilemma: suppressive doses of thyroxine significantly reduce bone mineral measurements in both premenopausal and postmenopausal women with thyroid carcinoma. *J. Clin. Endocrinol. Metab.*, **72**, 1184–7.

73. Lehmke, J., Bogner, U., Felsenberg, D. *et al.* (1992) Determination of bone mineral density by quantitative computed tomography and single photon absorptionmetry in subclinical hyperthyroidism: a risk of early osteopaenia in postmenopausal women. *Clin. Endocrinol.*, **36**, 511–17.

74. Leriche, N. G. H. and Bell, D. A. (1984) Hashimoto's thyroiditis and polyarthritis: a possible subset of seronegative polyarthritis. *Ann. Rheum. Dis.*, **43**, 594.

75. Vianna, J. L., Haga, H. J., Asherson, R. A. *et al.* (1991) A prospective evaluation of antithyroid antibody prevalence in 100 patients with systemic lupus erythematosus. *J. Rheumatol.*, **18**, 1193–5.

76. Klein, I., Parker, M., Shebert, R. *et al.* (1981) Hypothyroidism presenting as muscle stiffness and pseudohypertrophy Hoffman's syndrome. *Am. J. Med.*, **70**, 891.

77. Swanson, J. W., Kelly, J. D., McConahey, W. M. (1981) Neurologic aspects of thyroid dysfunction. *Mayo Clin. Proc.*, **56**, 504–12.

78. Podgorski, M., Robinson, B., Weissberger, A. *et al.* (1988) Articular manifestations of aeromy? *Aust. NZ. J. Med.*, **18**, 28–36.

79. Layton, M. W., Fudman, E. J., Barkan, A. *et al.* (1988) Acromegalic arthropathy: characteristics and response to therapy. *Arth. Rheum.*, **31**, 1022–7.

80. Ibbertson, H. K., Manning, P. J., Holdaway, I. M. *et al.* (1991) The acromegalic rosary. *Lancet*, **337**, 154–6.

81. Kaufman, J. M., Taelman, P., Vermeulen, A. *et al.* (1992) Bone mineral status in growth hormone deficient males with isolated and multiple pituitary deficiencies of childhood onset. *J. Clin. Endocrinol. Metab.*, **74**, 118–33.

82. Manning, P. J., Evans, M. C., Reid, I. R. (1992) Normal bone mineral density following cure of Cushing's syndrome. *Clin. Endocrinol.*, **36**, 229–34.

83. Aaron, J. E., Francis, R. M., Peacock, M. *et al.* (1989) Contrasting microanatomy of idiopathic and corticosteroid-induced osteoporosis. *Clin. Orthop.*, **243**, 294–305.

84. Buchanan, W. W., Stephen, L. J. and Buchanan, H. M. (1988) Are 'homeopathic' doses of oral corticosteroids effective in rheumatoid arthritis? *Clin. Exper. Rheumatol.*, **6**, 281–4.

85. Saldanha, C., Tougas, G. and Grace, E. (1986) Evidence for anti-inflammatory effect of normal circulating plasma cortisol. *Clin. Exp. Rheumatol.*, **4**, 365–6.

86. Asherson, R. A. and Hughes, G. R. V. (1991) Hypoadrenalism, Addison's disease and antiphospholipid antibodies. *J. Rheumatol.*, **18**, 1–3.

87. Giurini, J. M., Chrzan, J. S., Gibbons, G. W. *et al.* (1991) Charcot's disease in diabetic patients. *Postgrad. Med.*, **89**, 163–9.

88. Slowman-Kovacs, S. D., Braunstein, E. M. and Brandt, K. D. (1990) Rapidly progressive Charcot arthropathy following minor joint trauma in patients with diabetic neuropathy. *Arth. Rheum.*, **33**, 412–16.

89. Newman, L. G., Waller, J., Palestro, C. J. *et al.* (1991) Unsuspected oseomyelitis in diabetic foot ulcers. *JAMA*, **266**, 1246–51.

90. Wang, A., Weinstein, D., Greenfield, L. *et al.* (1990) MRI and diabetic foot infections. *Magn. Reson. Imaging.*, **8**, 805–9.

91. Stuart, M. J. and Morrey, M. D. (1990) Arthrodesis of the diabetic neuropathic ankle joint. *Clin. Orthop.*, **253**, 209–11.

92. England, S. P., Stem, S. H., Insall, J. N. *et al.* (1990) Total knee arthroplasty in diabetes mellitus. *Clin. Orthop.*, **260**, 130–4.

93. Akanji, A., Bella, A. F. and Osotimehin, B. O. (1990) Cheirarthropathy and long term

diabetic complications in Nigerians. *Ann. Rheum. Dis.*, **49**, 28–30.

94. Clarke, C. F., Piesowicz, A. T. and Spathis, G. S. (1990) Limited joint mobility in children and adolescents with insulin dependent diabetes mellitus. *Ann. Rheum. Dis.*, **49**, 236–7.

95. Buckingham, B. and Reiser, K. M. Relationship between the content of lyslrloxidase dependent cross-links in skin collagen, non-enzymatic glycosylation and long term complications in type I diabetes mellitus. *J. Clin. Invest.*, **86**, 1046–54.

96. Yosipovitch, G., Yosipovitch, Z., Karp, M. *et al.* (1990) Trigger finger in young patients with insulin dependent diabetes mellitus. *Rheumatol.*, **17**, 951–2.

97. J. Mauvikakis, M. E., Sfikakis, P. P., Kontoyannis, S. A. *et al.* (1991) Clinical and laboratory parameters in adult diabetics with and without calcific shoulder periarthritis. *Calcif. Tissue Int.*, **49**, 288–91.

98. Beacom, R., Gillespie, E. L. and Middleton, D. (1985) Limited joint mobility in insulin-dependent diabetes mellitus: relationship to retinopathy, peripheral nerve function and HLA status. *Q. J. Med.*, **56**, 337–44.

99. Mitchell, W. S., Winocour, P. H., Gush, R. J. *et al.* (1989) Skin blood flow and limited joint mobility in insulin-dependent diabetes mellitus. *Br. J. Rheumatol.*, **28**, 195–200.

100. Eadington, D. W., Patrick, A. W., Collier, A. *et al.* (1989) Limited joint mobility, Dupuytren's contracture and retinopathy in type I diabetes. Association with cigarette smoking. *Diabetic Med.*, **6**, 152–7.

101. Eaton, R. P. (1986) The collagen hydration hypothesis: a new paradigm for the secondary complications of diabetes mellitus. *J. Chronic. Dis.*, **39**, 763–6.

102. Buckingham, B. and Reiser, K. M. (1990) Relationship between the content of lyslvloxidase dependent cross-links in skin collagen, non enzymatic glycosylation and long term complications in type I diabetes mellitus. *J. Clin. Invest.*, **86**, 1046–54.

103. Lyons, T. J., Bailie, K. E., Dyer, D. G. *et al.* (1991) Decrease in skin collagen glycation with improved glycaemic control in patients with insulin dependent diabetes mellitus. *J. Clin. Invest.*, **87**, 1910–15.

104. Cassim, B., Mody, G. M. and Rubin, D. L. (1990) The prevalence of diffuse idiopathic skeletal hyperostosis in African blacks. *Br. J. Rheumatol.*, **29**, 131–2.

105. Horn, C. A., Bradley, J. D., Brandt, K. D. *et al.* (1992) Impairment of osteophyte formation in hyperglycemic patients with type II diabetes mellitus and knee osteoarthritis. *Arth. Rheum.*, **35**, 336–42.

106. Bouillon, R. (1991) Diabetic bone disease. *Calcif. Tissue Int.*, **49**, 155–60.

107. Ponder, S. W., McCormick, D. P., Fawcett, H. D. *et al.* (1992) Bone mineral density of the lumbar vertebrae in children and adolescents with insulin dependent diabetes mellitus. *J. Pediatr.* **120**, 541–5

108. Hardin, J. G. and Siegal, A. M. (1982) A connective tissue disease complicated by insulin resistance due to receptor antibodies: report of a case with high titer ribonucleoprotein antibodies. *Arth. Rheum.*, **25**, 458–63.

109. Donaghy, M. (1991) Diabetic proximal neuropathy: therapy and prognosis, (Editorial) *Q. J. Med.*, **288**, 287–8.

110. Coppack, S. W. and Watkins, P. J. (1991) The natural history of diabetic femoral neuropathy. *Q. J. Med.*, **288**, 307–13.

111. Lauro, G. R., Kissel, J. T. and Simon, S. R. (1991) Idiopathic muscle infarction in a diabetic patient. *J. Bone Joint Surg. (Am).*, **73**, 301–4.

112. Davies, R. A., Darby, M. and Richards, M. A. (1991) Hypertrophic pulmonary osteoarthropathy in pulmonary metastatic disease: a case report and review of the literature. *Clin. Radiol.*, **43**, 268–71.

113. Johnson, J. J., Leonard-Segal, A. and Nashel, D. J. J. (1989) Jaccoud's-type arthropathy: an association with malignancy. *J. Rheumatol.*, **16**, 1278–80.

114. Eggelmeyer, F. and MacFarlane, J. D. (1991) Polyarthritis as the presenting symptom of the occurrence and recurrence of laryngeal carcinoma. *Ann. Rheum. Dis.*, **51**, 556–7.

115. Lambert, C. M. and Nuki, G. (1991) Multicentric reticulohistiocytosis with arthritis and cardiac infiltration: regression following treatment for underlying malignancy. *Ann. Rheum. Dis.*, **51**, 815–17.

116. Cash, J. M. and Klippel, J. H. (1991) Rheumatic diseases and cancer. *Clin. Exp. Rheumatol.*, **9**, 109–12.

117. Lakhanpal, S., Bunch, T. W. and Melton, L. J. (1986) Polymyositis-dermatomyositis and malignant lesions: does an association exist? *Mayo Clin. Proc.*, **61**, 645–53.

118. Lyon, M. G., Bloch, D. A., Hollak, B. *et al.* (1989) Predisposing factors in polymyositis-

dermatomyositis: results of a nationwide survey. *J. Rheumatol.*, **16**, 1218–24.

119. Sanchez-Guerrero, J., Gutierrez-Urena, S., V Daller, A. *et al.* (1990) Vasculitis as a paraneoplastic syndrome: report of 11 cases and review of the literature. *J. Rheumatol.*, **17**, 1458–62.

120. Prowse, M., Higgs, C. M. B., Forrester-Wood, C. *et al.* (1989) Reflex sympathetic dystrophy associated with squamous cell carcinoma of the lung. *Ann. Rheum. Dis.*, **48**, 339–41.

121. Borenstein, A., Siedman, D. S. and Ben-Ari, G. Y. (1990) Case report: Raynaud's phenomenon as a presenting sign of metastatic melanoma. *Am. J. Med. Sci.*, **300**, 41–2.

122. Willemse, P. H. B., Mulder, N. H., Van De Tempel, H. J. *et al.* (1991) Palmar fasciitis and arthritis in a patient with an extra ovarian adenocarcinoma of the coelomic epithelium. *Ann. Rheum. Dis.*, **80**, 53–4.

123. Haase, K. L., Durk, H., Baumback, A. *et al.* (1990) Non-Hodgkin's lymphoma presenting as knee monarthritis with a popliteal cyst. *J. Rheumatol.*, **17**, 1252–4.

124. Gaudin, P., Juvin, R., Rozand, Y., *et al.* (1992) Skeletal involvement as the initial disease manifestation in Hodgkin's disease: a review of 6 cases. *J. Rheumatol.*, **19**, 146–52.

125. Fort, J. G., Fernandez, C., Jacobs, S. R. *et al.* (1992) B-cell surface marker analysis of synovial fluid cells in a patient with monoarthritis and chronic lymphocytic leukaemia. *J. Rheumatol.*, **19**, 481–4.

126. Fam, A. G., Voorneveld, C., Robinson, J. B. *et al.* (1991) Synovial fluid immunocytology in the diagnosis of leukaemic synovitis. *J. Rheumatol.*, **18**, 293–6.

127. Porter, D., Madhok, R. and Capell, H. (1991) Non-Hodgkin's lymphoma in rheumatoid arthritis. *Ann. Rheum. Dis.*, **50**, 275–6.

128. Matteson, E. L., Hickey, A. R., Maguire, L. *et al.* (1991) Occurrence of neoplasia in patients with rheumatoid arthritis enrolled in a DMARD registry. *J. Rheumatol.*, **18**, 809–14.

129. Silman, A. J., Petrie, J., Hazelman, B. L. *et al.* (1988) Lymphoproliferative cancer and malignancy in patients with rheumatoid arthritis treated with azathioprine: a 20-year follow-up study. *Ann. Rheum. Dis.*, **47**, 988–92.

130. Kelly, C., Baird, G., Foster, H. *et al.* (1991) Prognostic significance of paraproteinaemia in rheumatoid arthritis. *Ann. Rheum. Dis.*, **50**, 290–4.

131. Burastero, S. E., Casali, P., Wilder, R. L. *et al.* (1988) Monoreactive high affinity and polyreactive low affinity rheumatoid factors are produced by CD5+B cells from patients with rheumatoid arthritis. *J. Exp. Med.*, **168**, 1979–82.

132. Dauphinee, M., Tovar, Z. and Talal, N. (1988) B cells expressing DC5+ are increased in Sjögren's syndrome. *Arth. Rheum.*, **31**, 642–7.

133. Bielefeld, P. H., Besancenot, J. F., Cortet, P. *et al.* (1990) Generalized scleroderma and malignant blood disorders: accidental association? *Rev. Rhum. Mal. Osteoartic.*, **57**, 235–36.

134. Santavirta, S. (1991) Synovial sarcoma: a clinicopathological study of 31 cases. *Arch. Orthop. Trauma Surg.*, **111**, 155–9.

135. Schwarzer, A. C., Fryer, J., Preston, S. J. *et al.* (1990) Metastatic adenosquamous carcinoma presenting as an acute monoarthritis, with a review of the literature. *J. Orthop. Rheum.*, **3**, 175–85.

136. Pedersen-Bjengaard, J. (1988) Carcinoma of the urinary bladder after treatment with cyclophosphamide for non-Hodgkin's lymphoma. *N. Eng. J. Med.*, **318**, 1028–32.

137. Zijlmans, J. M. J. M., van Rijthoven, A. W. A. M., Kluin, P. M. *et al.* (1992) Epstein–Barr virus-associated lymphoma in a patient treated with rheumatoid arthritis treated with cyclosporine (Correspondence) *N. Eng. J. Med.*, **326**, 1363.

138. Lipton, J. H. and Messner, H. A. (1991) Chronic myeloid leukaemia in a woman with Still's disease treated with [198]Au synoviorthesis. *J. Rheumatol.*, **18**, 734–5.

139. Rooney, P. J., Balint, G. P., Szebenyi, B. *et al.* (1991) Rheumatic syndromes caused by antirheumatic drugs. *Bailliere's Clin. Rheumatol.*, **5**, 139–73.

140. Hughes, R. A., Allard, S. A. and Maini, R. N. (1989) Arthritis associated with adjuvant mycobacterial treatment for carcinoma of the bladder. *Ann. Rheum. Dis.*, **49**, 432–4.

RHEUMATOID ARTHRITIS

C. B. Tallman, Jr. and R. B. Zurier

Rheumatoid arthritis (RA) is a chronic inflammatory disease characterized by symmetrical polyarthritis that typically leads to articular cartilage degradation and bone erosion[1]. In addition, patients with RA exhibit characteristics of a connective tissue disease with extra-articular and systemic features; these include involvement of the pulmonary, renal, vascular and hematopoietic systems.

The diagnosis of RA is made on clinical grounds; no single test result assures the diagnosis. Several diagnostic criteria have been developed to help differentiate RA from other inflammatory musculoskeletal conditions. The most frequently used criteria are those proposed by the American Rheumatism Association (ARA) in 1958, and revised in 1987. The revised ARA criteria stipulate that 4 of 7 conditions be met before a patient may be considered to have RA. The criteria are:

1. morning stiffness lasting at least one hour,
2. arthritis of three or more joints,
3. arthritis of hand joints,
4. symmetric arthritis,
5. rheumatoid nodules,
6. serum rheumatoid factor, and
7. radiographic changes typical of RA[2].

The criteria were developed for the epidemiologic study of populations; they should not be used to diagnose individual patients, but they do provide a useful framework for the study of RA.

INCIDENCE AND PREVALENCE

RA seems to have no geographic limits. It occurs in every part of the world, and its prevalence is not influenced by climate or temperature. The incidence in different studies varies from 4.2/10 000 to 26/10 000. The prevalence of RA increases with age, peaking between the ages of 40 and 60 years; the male to female ratio is approximately 1–2:3[1]. A juvenile form of the disease also exists.

PROGNOSIS

Traditionally, most RA patients were managed conservatively, since the disease has not been considered life-threatening, and that aggressive, toxic therapy has not been thought to be warranted. However, it is becoming clear that RA is a disease that can reduce life expectancy by as much as 10–15 years[3,4]; survival rates are less than 50% at 5 years in patients with severe articular or extra-articular disease[4,5]. An elevated erythrocyte sedimentation rate, high titer rheumatoid factor, low hemoglobin level and extra-articular manifestations (except subcutaneous nodules) are associated with increased mortality[6,7]. Results of a study[7] of RA patients followed for more than 25 years indicate that if rheumatoid factor levels fall, or patients continue to be seronegative, then the overall prognosis is better. An increase in

Connective Tissue Diseases. Edited by Jill J. F. Belch and Robert B. Zurier. Published in 1995 by Chapman & Hall, London. ISBN 0 412 48620 2

disease severity as manifested by increased extra-articular features and higher incidence of joint surgery is seen in patients homozygous for the human leucocyte antigen HLA-DR4DW14.

ETIOLOGY AND PATHOGENESIS

The cause of RA is not known, but many theories have been proposed; these implicate genetic and hormonal factors, and infectious agents. The possible role of genetic factors has been studied extensively. An association between RA and class II HLA has been established, with the antigen HLA-DR4 being associated with RA in the white population[8], and a HLA-DR1 association with RA in Asian Indians[9]. HLA-DR4 is seen in 60–70% of individuals with RA as compared to 25–35% of controls. These associations are strongest for individuals with severe disease[1]. In one study, 91 of 102 patients expressed at least one of the following HLA-DR4 types: HLA-DR1, HLA-DR4DW4, or HLA-DR4DW14.

It is believed that presentation of a causative antigen to an immunogenetically susceptible host is the trigger for RA. It is therefore necessary to examine the host response before considering the antigen. Both cellular and humoral components of the immune response appear to contribute to the pathogenesis of RA. It is generally accepted that antibodies complex with antigen in the joint and activate the complement system. Indeed, reminiscent of the more traditional connective tissue diseases, an immune complex vasculitis is seen in the subsynovial blood vessels very early in the course of RA[10]. Although the very first cells to appear in the joint space are lymphocytes, most cells in synovial fluid aspirated from inflamed joints are polymorphonuclear leucocytes [PMN]. Local joint inflammation is mediated by PMN and their products. The chronic inflammatory cells, such as lymphocytes and macrophages, congregate in the synovium and produce soluble factors that cause tissue destruction and further inflammation. Microscopic examination characteristically shows proliferation of synoviocytes, villous hypertrophy, massive subintimal infiltration with lymphocytes and plasma cells, replacement of cartilage by invading chronic inflammatory cells and proliferation of subchondral connective tissue (pannus) which invades and degrades cartilage and bone[11].

It is thought that antigen-presenting cells, such as macrophages or dendritic cells in the synovium, are the first to be involved in the immune response. They ingest, process and present protein antigens to T-lymphocytes, and initiate a cellular immune response. Antigen binds to the class II major-histocompatibility complex (MHC), and the antigen-MHC complex is then recognized by helper-T-lymphocyte receptors. 'Organization' of the immune response leads to increased numbers of T-lymphocytes, which stimulate differentiation of B-lymphocytes and subsequent antibody secretion. These dramatic changes in the synovium usually occur first in perivascular areas[11].

As the inflammatory response continues, cytokines released from macrophages induce development of new blood vessels. This angiogenesis facilitates further flow of inflammatory cells into the synovium. Circulating lymphocytes attracted to the site of inflammation adhere to the endothelium of post-capillary venules. Lymphocytes then migrate out of the circulation, and aggregate near the vessel wall in the synovium[11]. Cytokines, such as interferon gamma, interleukin-1, and tumor necrosis factor increase adherence of lymphocytes to endothelial cells. Other cytokines, such as interleukin-2, stimulate T-lymphocytes which then increase proliferation of B-lymphocytes, some of which differentiate into antibody secreting cells. It is this unregulated immune/inflammatory response, with its cascade of cytokines, that leads to active synovitis in RA patients.

What is the antigen that triggers these events? Is it infectious? That other forms of chronic arthritis (such as Lyme disease (Chapter 9) and Reiter's syndrome) have been linked with an infectious cause has led investigators to continue the search for an infectious etiology of RA. Many infectious agents have been called but none have been chosen as the cause of RA[12].

Before the evidence for an infectious causation is reviewed, the mechanisms by which an infectious agent might trigger a chronic inflammatory arthritis need to be considered. These include: circulating immune complex (CIC) deposition, local antigen deposition, toxin-mediated arthritis and molecular mimicry.

CIC are found in patients with endocarditis, hepatitis B, and the arthritis associated with jejunoileal bypass surgery. CIC containing viral antigen, antibody and complement components are present in patients with hepatitis B infection when serum complement falls and joint inflammation appears[12]. Other infectious agents could stimulate a similar response, and account for a chronic arthritis.

Local antigen deposition as the inciting event for a chronic inflammatory arthritis is seen in post-chlamydial reactive arthritis in which monoclonal antibodies against a chlamydia antigen have been demonstrated by immunofluorescent staining of synovial tissue. This mechanism of injury can be reproduced experimentally in an animal model of arthritis in which a single intraperitoneal injection of an aqueous suspension of purified group A streptococcal cell wall induces a chronic destructive arthritis in rats[12].

Toxin-mediated arthritis has been described in a patient with aseptic polyarthritis in a setting of toxic shock syndrome. Arthritis associated with pseudomembranous enterocolitis has also been reported and, in some cases, c-difficile toxin has been isolated from the stool. Although the toxin was not isolated from synovial fluid, the authors assume the arthritis was toxin mediated because it resolved with treatment of the pseudomembranous enterocolitis[12].

Molecular mimicry is the fourth model to be considered. It is proposed that a normal host immune response to an infecting organism can cause an abnormal autoimmune response because of cross-reactivity between host tissue and microbial antigens. The classic example of this mechanism of tissue injury is acute rheumatic fever. Patients with acute rheumatic fever have an initial streptococcal infection and in some cases they develop cross reacting antibodies to heart tissue[12].

Epstein–Barr virus (EBV) has been considered a possible causative agent for RA for more than a decade. In one study, 80% of patients with RA had circulating antibodies against EBV. As a polyclonal activator of B-lymphocytes, EBV could stimulate production of rheumatoid factor and other immunoglobulins. Results of other studies indicate that early in the course of RA, antibody titers to EBV are not elevated compared to non-RA controls[11,12], observations which suggest that the antibodies to EBV seen in other studies develop after the early phase of RA.

Parvoviruses have also been implicated as possible etiologic agents for RA[13]. Parvoviruses are small DNA viruses that cause disease in many species. Parvovirus B19 appears to be the cause of Fifth's disease, which can be associated with a self-limiting arthritis. A report of two patients with early RA who had evidence of recent parvovirus B19 infection sparked further interest in this agent.

Other investigators have been intrigued by *Mycobacterium tuberculosis* as a cause of RA. These bacteria express heat shock proteins which are associated with arthritis in rats[11]. Arthritis can be induced in a genetically susceptible strain of Lewis rats by inoculation of heat-killed *Mycobacterium tuberculosis* in oil[12]. In some patients with RA, a relatively large number of T-lymphocytes have neither CD4 nor CD8 surface markers. It is of interest that these cells proliferate in response to mycobacteria[11,12].

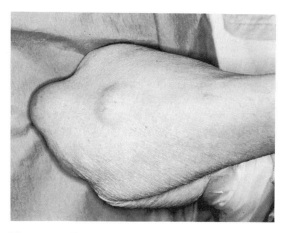

Fig. 14.1 Rheumatoid nodule on extensor surface of forearm.

ARTICULAR MANIFESTATIONS

The articular involvement in RA is a symmetrical polyarthritis which most commonly affects joints of the hands, feet, wrists and knees. The elbows, shoulders, hips and ankles are less commonly affected, but any synovial lined joint may be involved. Larger joints typically do not become inflamed until after the smaller joints have been affected. The distal interphalangeal joints are usually spared.

In order to help differentiate acute viral arthritis from RA, arthritis must be present for more than 6 weeks. Morning stiffness in joints is characteristic of an inflammatory arthritis such as RA. The course of RA is variable; a majority of patients have intermittent disease with periods of mild disease or remission. A small percentage (10–20%) of patients have one acute flare and then remain in remission. In addition, about 5% of patients experience a relentless course that leads to joint destruction and disability.

When individual joints become 'active' in RA, synovial thickening occurs, 'boggy' tissue is palpable and joint fluid accumulates. Flexion contractures often develop in part because slight flexion of joints affords patients some comfort. The proximal interphalangeal joints of the hands exhibit symmetric elliptical swelling. Persistent synovitis leads to stretching of the surrounding ligaments and this may result in subluxation. When this process occurs in the metacarpol-phalangeal joints it is often followed by the classic palmar subluxation with ulnar deviation (Figures 14.1–14.4).

The histology of the synovial lesion is well defined. Initially, clinical arthritis is associated with congestion and edema of the synovium which is most marked at the interface between synovium and articular cartilage. This is followed by migration of PMN and lymphocytes into the synovium. Lymphocytes are distributed into two distinct patterns: as diffuse infiltrates in the superficial layer of the synovium, or into small nodular aggregates. Lymphoid follicles with germinal centers often develop in longstanding lesions. The synovial tissue then thickens due to proliferation of blood vessels, fibroblasts and synovial lining cells[10].

Persistent inflammation in the synovium is usually followed by periarticular bone erosion and osteolysis. Radiographs are characteristic; periarticular soft-tissue swelling and indistinctness of the periosteum at areas of tendon insertion are seen in early lesions. Later, periarticular demineralization and uniform joint space narrowing due to cartilage degradation are seen (Figures 14.5–14.8). These radiographic changes are seen earlier and more frequently in the feet than in the hands. Thus, it is worthwhile to obtain X-rays of feet in patients with symmetrical polyarthritis of unknown cause, even when symptoms are not present in the feet.

Inflammation in the joints of the cervical spine can lead to severe pain, disability and neurological problems. Up to 70% of patients with RA will have signs or symptoms related to cervical spine involvement at some time during their illness. The entire cervical spine may be involved, but the most serious consequences occur when the atlantoaxial joint is affected. In the normal spine the distance between the posterior aspect of the odontoid

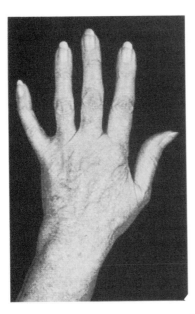

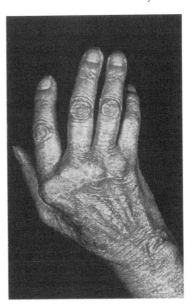

Fig. 14.2 Early RA of the hand and wrist showing swelling of the wrist with fullness over the ulnar styloid and swelling over the second and third metacarpophalangeal joints.

Fig. 14.4 Advanced RA of the hand and wrist showing spindle-shaped swelling of the proximal interphalangeal joints, dorsal swelling of the metacarpophalangeal joints, ulnar deviation of the metacarpophalangeal joints and muscle atrophy.

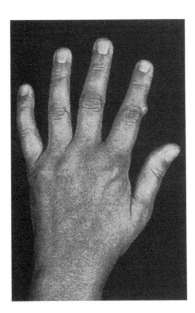

Fig. 14.3 Intermediate stage RA of the hand and wrist showing spindle-shaped swelling of the proximal interphalangeal joints and dorsal swelling of the metacarpophalangeal joints.

process and the body of the first cervical vertebra is up to 4 mm. As synovial inflammation occurs in the adjacent joints, increased pressure placed on the transverse ligament causes laxity, allowing for subluxation of the atlantoaxial joint. This can lead to paresthesias, weakness and, in rare instances, to quadriplegia or death.

EXTRA-ARTICULAR MANIFESTATIONS

PULMONARY SYSTEM

Pleuropulmonary disease is a well-recognized manifestation of RA. Infection is the major cause of death in 20–25% of RA patients[14]. Rarely, empyema is seen in the setting of a rheumatoid pleural effusion. A report of an increased incidence of bronchitis and pneumonia in patients with RA compared to patients with osteoarthritis is confounded by the fact that more RA patients than controls

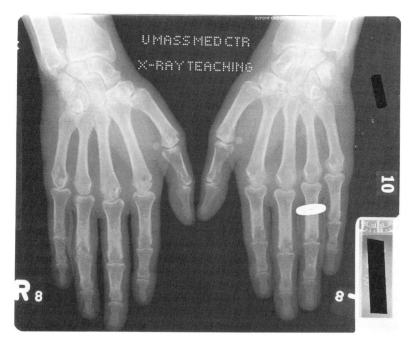

Fig. 14.5 Early RA: symmetrical joint space narrowing of the carpal joints. Narrowing of the carpometacarpal joints of the left wrist. Soft tissue swelling at the metacarpophalangeal joints of both hands.

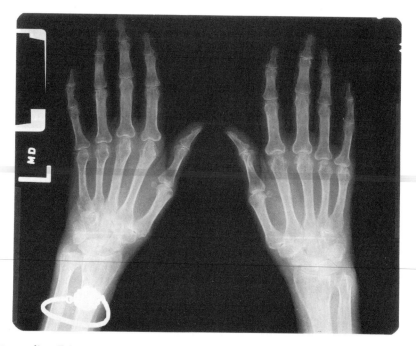

Fig. 14.6 Intermediate RA: periarticular osteopenia and narrowing of the carpal joints, carpometacarpal joints and proximal interphalangeal joints of both hands.

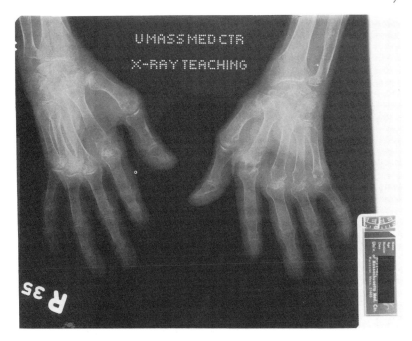

Fig. 14.7 Advanced RA: diffuse osteopenia, symmetrical joint space narrowing, and periarticular erosions. Also note ulnar deviation of the metacarpophalangeal joints.

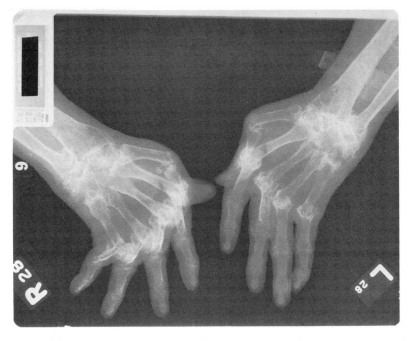

Fig. 14.8 Advanced RA: osteopenia, symmetrical joint space narrowing and erosions. Also note ulnar deviation at the metacarpophalangeal joints, and swan-neck deformities of the fourth and fifth digits of the right hand.

smoked cigarettes and the episodes of pneumonia occurred more frequently before the onset of joint disease. It is, of course, possible that a predisposition for RA also predisposes to pneumonia. On the other hand, some studies[14,15] suggest that recurrent lung infections may be a predisposing factor for development of RA by eliciting a pathologic immune response. Impaired alveolar clearance of bacteria appears to play a role in development of pulmonary infections in RA patients. Altered immunologic response to infection, bronchopleural fistula formation and immunosuppressive agents used to treat severe disease also appear to increase the risk of pulmonary infection.

Pleuritis, usually asymptomatic, is another common pulmonary manifestation of RA. In autopsy studies, pleuritis has been found in as many as 40% of patients with RA[14]. Pleuritis in association with RA occurs more frequently in males than females, and is more common in the fourth or fifth decades of life. Pleuritis may be diagnosed incidentally by chest X-ray or by presence of a pleural rub on physical examination; pleural effusion is seen in 3–5% of patients with RA. Pleurisy or pleural effusions usually occur after joint disease is established, but in about 25% of cases it may occur simultaneously or antedate arthritis. The size of the pleural effusion ranges from trace amounts of asymptomatic fluid to 1000–1500 ml of fluid that can compress adjacent lung tissue and cause respiratory distress[16].

Pleural fluid from RA patients typically is an exudate with an elevated lactate dehydrogenase concentration, very low glucose concentration, low complement levels and a leucocyte count of 100–8000/mm^3. Lymphocytes predominate, but a high concentration of PMN may be seen. Histology of biopsied pleura usually shows non-specific inflammation.

Interstitial lung disease is present in 1.6–40% of patients with RA. The higher incidence is reported in studies that use carbon monoxide diffusing capacity for diagnosis, and the lower frequency derives from studies that rely on chest X-ray for diagnosis; radiographs are relatively insensitive for detection of pulmonary fibrosis[16]. Patients with interstitial fibrosis usually present with cough, dyspnea and chest pain. Physical examination reveals nailbed clubbing and pulmonary crackles. Early radiographic features of interstitial fibrosis include bilateral soft, fluffy, cotton-like patches. After repeated episodes of inflammation, new areas of soft infiltrates evolve, often superimposed over older areas of fibrosis. A honeycomb appearance may appear as fibrosis progresses. Pulmonary function tests reveal a restrictive pattern with a reduced diffusing capacity indicative of a restrictive lesion. Pathological studies of lungs from RA patients with interstitial fibrosis show alveolar wall thickening, infiltrates of lymphocytes, fibroblasts and plasma cells, occasional lymphoid aggregates, honeycombing and, rarely, peribronchiolar fibrosis[17,18]. Methotrexate therapy in patients with RA has also been associated with the development of a pneumonitis[19] and it may be difficult to distinguish this from the interstitial lung disease of RA. High resolution computer assisted tomography (CAT scan) may be useful in making a diagnosis.

Pulmonary nodules may precede the onset of arthritis, but more typically they occur in patients with well-established and fairly severe arthritis; most of these patients are rheumatoid factor positive. Pulmonary nodules tend to occur in the periphery of the parenchyma; they are usually multiple, but solitary nodules are observed. The appearance of solitary nodules widens the diagnostic possibilities, and malignancy and infection become concerns. Pulmonary nodules typically occur in association with subcutaneous nodules[20]. Pulmonary vasculitis may lead to pulmonary hypertension and cor pulmonale.

RHEUMATOID NODULES

Subcutaneous nodules are the most common of the rheumatoid nodules. Indeed, in one study of RA patients, subcutaneous nodules were the most common extra-articular feature. The incidence of subcutaneous nodules is 20–25% in all adults with RA, and approaches 90% in severely ill RA patients. Although nodules typically are associated with severe disease, they can occur in any RA patient, including those with inactive or mild disease. Rheumatoid nodules tend to occur over sites of pressure; thus, trauma appears to play a role in their development. Also, subcutaneous nodules nearly always develop in patients who are rheumatoid factor positive. Common sites for nodules include the subcutaneous tissue over the olecranon process of the ulnar, the occiput, over the heads of the phalangeal and metacarpal bones, and overlying the ischial and femoral tuberosities[21].

The rheumatoid nodules begins as a collection of granulation tissue. In the early stages of nodule formation, elongated mononuclear cells are observed at the periphery of the nodule. As the nodule matures it takes on a characteristic structure: a necrotic core surrounded by a layer of 'palisading' mononuclear cells arranged in a radial orientation. The outer layer consists of a network of blood vessels and a perivascular infiltrate of chronic inflammatory cells[21].

HEART DISEASE

Although clinically significant heart disease is rare in patients with RA, heart involvement is observed frequently at autopsy[22]. Charcot described pericarditis in patients with RA nearly 100 years ago[22]. Myocarditis and valvular lesions (either non-specific or granulomatous) have also been described[10,22]. Pericarditis remains the most commonly reported cardiac finding in RA, a prevalence rate of 35% being reported in autopsy studies[22]. The microscopic features of pericarditis vary depending on whether inflammation is active or fibrosis is present. In the inflammatory phase of rheumatoid pericarditis, vascular granulation tissue is associated with foci of lymphocyte and plasma cell infiltrates. Fibrin deposition and areas of subacute arteritis may also be seen. Fibrotic pericarditis contains mostly dense collagenous connective tissue[22]. Although pericarditis is usually asymptomatic, it is occasionally complicated by signs and symptoms of constrictive pericarditis.

Myocardial disease can take on two forms: either granuloma formation or myocarditis. Myocardial granuloma formation is usually asymptomatic, but if the granulomas develop in the conduction system a variety of conduction defects, including bundle branch block and complete heart block, can occur[10]. In one case, granuloma were found at autopsy in both right and left coronary cusps in a patient with congestive heart failure and bradycardia.

Myocarditis occurs more commonly in patients with RA than in healthy controls, and usually occurs in association with pericarditis[22]. The pathological features of myocarditis include collections of plasma cells, histiocytes and lymphocytes. These cells tend to form foci around blood vessels, but focal myocardial fibrosis may also be seen.

Two types of valvular lesions have been described in RA: non-specific and granulomatous lesions. Most of these lesions are asymptomatic; however, cases of congestive heart failure related to valvular lesions have been reported. In a recent autopsy study[22] the association of non-specific valvular lesions with RA was questioned, as an equal number of age and sex matched control patients had these lesions.

VASCULITIS

Vascular inflammation in association with RA, termed rheumatoid vasculitis, has been described frequently since the late 1800s[23].

It can be either a necrotizing or a non-necrotizing vasculitis. It may involve blood vessels of all sizes, but it most frequently affects small arteries supplying the vasa nervorum and the digits of the hands and feet. The skin, peripheral nervous system, lungs and kidney are the organs most frequently affected by rheumatoid vasculitis. However, vessels of the heart and skeletal muscles can also be involved. Vasculitis is seen mainly in patients with long standing, seropositive, nodular, erosive RA. Cryoglobulins and depressed serum complement may also be seen in patients with rheumatoid vasculitis. In early studies[24] a higher incidence of vasculitis was observed in patients treated with corticosteroids, and it was thought that corticosteroid use might predispose to development of vasculitis. Clinically, however, vasculitis often responds to corticosteroid therapy. It is not unlikely that vasculitis is seen more often in patients treated with corticosteroids because they have severe joint and systemic disease which does not respond to more conservative treatment[25].

FELTY'S SYNDROME

Felty's syndrome, defined as RA, neutropenia and splenomegaly is a rare complication of RA which occurs in less than 1% of patients; the majority (60–70%) are female. The peak incidence is between 55 and 65 years of age. Patients with Felty's syndrome have had RA for a mean of 10–15 years before the onset of neutropenia[26]. Rarely, splenomegaly and neutropenia can predate arthritis. Patients with Felty's syndrome have a higher prevalence of other extraarticular features of RA than do hospitalized controls with RA. The spleen in patients with Felty's syndrome ranges from minimally enlarged and even non-palpable, to very large in size; the degree of neutropenia is not related to the degree of splenomegaly. Mild to moderate anemia, and mild thrombocytopenia, may be a part of Felty's syndrome. High titer rheumatoid factor is seen in 98% of cases. Antinuclear antibodies, low normal complement levels, and cryoglobulins are also seen in some patients[26].

Bacterial infections are the major cause of mortality in patients with Felty's syndrome. In two studies infections increased with a decrease in neutrophil count, a neutrophil count less than $1000/mm^3$ being most associated with infections. However, in a third study no increase in infections was observed even in patients with markedly reduced neutrophil counts. Results of other studies indicate that even patients with a normal leucocyte count are at increased risk of infection because of impaired neutrophil function[26].

EYE

Ocular manifestions of RA include keratoconjunctivitis sicca (KCS), scleritis, episcleritis and corneal melting[27]. KCS, a manifestation of Sjögren's syndrome (SS), is characterized by dry and gritty eyes. Reduction in tear formation in SS patients is accompanied by physical and chemical changes in tears. The tear film becomes less stable, and greater exposure of the cornea to the environment leads to corneal erosion[27,28] (also Chapter 5).

Episcleritis is inflammation of the superficial layers of the sclera, fascia bulbi or tenons capsule. Attacks of episcleritis are self-limited and typically resolve within 10 days. Attacks usually recur but do not cause serious damage[27].

Scleritis is a serious problem and if left untreated may lead to blindness. It occurs in 0.6% of patients with RA, most frequently in patients with other extra-articular manifestations, especially vasculitis. If scleritis is not treated, the inflammation can spread to the episclera, choroid, ciliary body or retina. Secondary complications, such as choroidoretinitis, retinal detachment, keratitis, glaucoma, cataracts or perforation, may follow[27]. Extreme thinning or melting of the cornea may lead to ulceration or perforation of the cornea; this may be a complication of scleritis or may occur without involvement of other ocular structures[27]. Corneal melting associated with conjunctival vasculitis in a patient with otherwise inactive RA has been described.

TREATMENT

Patient education should be initiated with any therapy for RA; patients should be educated about the likely course and prognosis of their disease; they should also be taught what they can do when their disease becomes active. The role of exercise and rest should also be discussed with the patient; the amount of rest that should be prescribed remains controversial. A study in 1963[29] showed that during periods of exacerbation of synovitis, complete immobilization was more beneficial than bedrest with intermittent exercise. However, a 1971 study[30] showed that in hospitalized patients, activity as tolerated was better than complete bedrest. Results of a 1983 study[31] suggested that patients with active disease do better with rest, and patients with less active disease do better with mild activity.

Range of motion (ROM), strengthening and aerobic exercises have all been advocated for RA patients. ROM exercises relieve stiffness and increase flexibility; strengthening exercises facilitate activities of daily living. Decreased aerobic capacity in RA patients is secondary not only to disease, but also to inactivity[32]. Isometric exercises and water exercises strengthen muscles with minimal stress across damaged joints[33].

The standard therapeutic approach for treatment of RA has been the 'pyramid' approach. In this regimen all patients are treated with education, rest, exercise and salicylates or other non-steroidal antiinflammatory drugs (NSAID). As disease progresses, the 'disease modifying anti-rheumatic drugs' (DMARD) are introduced. Under the pyramid system, hydroxychloroquine or oral or parenteral gold are the first DMARDs to be introduced. Parental gold is reported to have favorable effects on the course of RA[34], but other studies[35] have failed to confirm a beneficial effect from therapy with this agent. The second line DMARDs traditionally have been: methotrexate, azathioprine and D-penicillamine. Treatment with each of these agents results in varying degrees of success[36–41].

Methotrexate is now often the first DMARD used in many patients with RA, due to ease of administration, efficacy and relatively manageable adverse effects. Long-term (8 years) studies indicate that about half of patients remain on the drug at 5 years[42,43]. A good deal of sentiment is building in the rheumatology community for 'inverting the pyramid'. A greater awareness of the severity of the disease, its potential threat to life, and a better understanding of how to use the more toxic drugs, has prompted rheumatologists to treat RA patients more aggressively earlier in the course of disease[44]. Indeed, several authors[44–48] have suggested the use of combinations of DMARDs as early treatment of RA; many combinations have been studied. Several studies show clinical benefit[49–51], whereas others show increased toxicity[52] without much benefit. DMARD combination therapy in treatment of RA remains an uncertain enterprise, and must be considered experimental until long-term controlled studies are done.

Corticosteroids have been used to treat RA since 1949 when Dr Philip Hench and his colleagues[53] showed that corticosteroids rapidly reduce articular inflammation in RA. However, it soon became apparent that corticosteroids had many adverse effects[54], and the precise role of corticosteroids in the treatment of RA has remained controversial. As use of corticosteroids became more widespread, it was noted that patients treated with high doses for prolonged periods of time were more likely to develop adverse effects from the corticosteroids. Since the 1960s, efforts have been made to find a low dose that would be symptomatically beneficial without major side effects[55,56]. At this time the search for the optimal place for oral corticosteroids in therapy of RA continues. One strategy is to use low doses (<10 mg/day of prednisone) as a short-term bridge between beginning a DMARD and the onset of symptomatic relief from the DMARD. The work of Wilder and his colleagues[57] suggests that very low doses of prednisone 1–3 mg) given twice daily to mimic the normal diurnal rhythm may be useful.

Corticosteroids are also administered by intra-articular injection. Clinical experience and investigation since 1950 show a temporary beneficial effect from corticosteroids injected into inflamed joints[58]. This beneficial effect may last weeks to months if combined with joint rest. This technique of corticosteroid administration is very useful if one or two joints have active inflammation from RA. The beneficial effect is only temporary, but a repeat injection may be done at a later date.

Although we do not now usually include rheumatoid arthritis in discussion of connective tissue diseases, it is clear that the pathological changes of RA may be indistinguishable from those of the other visceral connective tissue diseases, particularly systemic lupus erythematosus, vasculitis, progressive systemic sclerosis and polymyositis. Klemperer, who coined the term 'collagen vascular disease'[59] and Pagel and Treip[60] who spoke of 'viscerocytaneous collagenosis' recognized that the tissue changes of the more traditional connective tissue diseases could be found in RA.

ACKNOWLEDGEMENTS

The work was supported in part by NIH Grant AR38501. The manuscript was prepared by Mrs Carol Mader.

REFERENCES

1. Spector, T. (1990) Rheumatoid arthritis. *Rheum. Dis. Clin. N. Am.*, **16**(3), 513–37.

2. Arnett, F. C., Edworthy, S. M., Bloch, D. A. *et al.* (1988) The American Rheumatism Association 1987 Revised Criteria for the Classification of Rheumatoid Arthritis. *Arth. Rheum.*, **31**(3), 315–24.

3. Pincus, T. and Callahan, L. F. (1989) Reassessment of twelve traditional paradigms concerning the diagnosis, prevalence, morbidity and mortality of rheumatoid arthritis. *Scand. J. Rheumatol.*, Suppl. **79**, 67–95.

4. Winchester, R. (1992) Genetic determination of susceptibility and severity in rheumatoid arthritis. *Ann. Intern. Med.*, **117**(10), 869–71.

5. Rasker, J. J. and Cosh, J. A. (1989) Course and prognosis of early rheumatoid arthritis. *Scand. J. Rheumatol.*, Suppl. **79**, 45–56.

6. Erhardt, C. C., Mumford, P. A., Venables, P. J. W. *et al.* (1989) Factors predicting a poor life prognosis in rheumatoid arthritis: an eight year prospective study. *Ann. Rheum. Dis.*, **48**, 7–13.

7. Reilly, P. A., Cosh, J. A., Maddison, P. J. *et al.* (1990) Mortality and survival in rheumatoid arthritis: a 25 year prospective study of 100 patients. *Ann. Rheum. Dis.*, **49**, 363–9.

8. Statsny, P. (1978) Association of the B-cell autoantigen DRw4 with rheumatoid arthritis. *N. Eng. J. Med.*, **298**, 869–87.

9. Woodrow, J. C., Nichol, F. E. and Zaphiropoulos, G. (1981) DR antigens and rheumatoid arthritis: a study of two populations. *Br. Med. J.* **283**, 1287–8.

10. Gardner, D. L. (1992) *Pathological Basis of Connective Tissue Diseases*, Lea and Febiger, Philadelphia, London.

11. Harris, E. D. (1990) Rheumatoid arthritis: pathophysiology and implications for therapy. *N. Eng. J. Med.*, **332**, 1277–89.

12. Inman, R. D. (1991) Infectious etiology of rheumatoid arthritis. *Rheum. Dis. Clin. N. Am.*, **17**(4), 859–70.

14. Abeles, M., Weinstein, A. and Zurier, R. B. (1980) Infections Complicating Rheumatic Diseases, in *Infections in the Abnormal Host*, (ed. M. H. Grieco), York Medical Books, USA, pp. 666–92.

15. Mathiew, J. P., Stack, B. H. R., Dick, D. C. *et al.* (1978) Pulmonary infections and rheumatoid arthritis. *Br. J. Dis. Chest*, **72**, 57–61.

16. Popp, W., Rauscher, H., Ritschka, L. *et al.* (1992) Prediction of interstitial lung involvement in rheumatoid arthritis. *Chest*, **102**(2), 391–4.

17. Gordon, D. A., Stein, J. L. and Broder, I. (1973)

The extra-articular features of rheumatoid arthritis. *Am. J. Med.*, **54**, 445–52.

18. Roschmann, R. A. and Rothenberg, R. J. (1987) Pulmonary fibrosis in rheumatoid arthritis: a review of clinical features and therapy. *Semin. Arth. Rheum.*, **16**(3), 174–85.

19. Carroll, G. J., Thomas, R., Phatouros, C. C. *et al.* (1994) Incidence, prevalence and possible risk factors for pneumonitis in patients with RA receiving MTX. *J. Rheumatol.*, **21**(1), 51–4.

20. Rubin, E. H., Gordon, M. and Thelmo, W. L. (1967) Nodular pleuropulmonary rheumatoid disease. *Am. J. Med.*, **42**, 567–81.

21. Ziff, M. (1990) The rheumatoid nodule, *Arth. Rheum.*, **33**(6), 761–7.

22. Bonfiglio, T. and Atwater, E. C. (1969) Heart disease in patients with seropositive rheumatoid arthritis. *Arch. Int. Med.*, **124**, 714–9.

23. Bywaters, E. G. L. (1957) Peripheral vascular obstruction in rheumatoid arthritis and its relationship to other vascular lesions. *Ann. Rheumat. Dis.*, **16**, 84–103.

24. Kemper, J. W., Baggenstoss, A. H. and Slocumb, C. H. (1957) The relationship of therapy with cortisone to the incidence of vascular lesions in rheumatoid arthritis. *Ann. Int. Med.*, **46**, 831–51.

25. Theofilopoulos, A. N., Burtonboy, G., LoSpalluto, J. L. *et al.* (1974) IgM rheumatoid factor and low molecular weight IgM: an association with vasculitis. *Arth. Rheum.*, **17**(3), 272–84.

26. Rosenstein, E. D. and Kramer, N. (1991) Felty's and pseudo-Felty's syndromes. *Semin. Arth. Rheum.*, **21**(3), 129–42.

27. Hazleman, B. L. and Watson, P. G. (1977) Ocular complications of rheumatoid arthritis. *Clin. Rheum. Dis.*, **3**(3), 501–26.

28. Friedlaender, M. H. (1992) Ocular manifestations of Sjögren's syndrome: keratoconjunctivitis *Sicca*. *Rheum. Dis. Clin. N. Am.*, **18**(3), 591.

29. Partridge, R. E. H. and Duthie, J. J. R. (1963) Controlled trial of the effect of complete immobilization of the joints in rheumatoid arthritis. *Ann. Rheum. Dis.*, **22**, 91–9.

30. Mills, J. A., Pinals, R. S., Ropes, M. W. *et al.* (1971) Value of bed rest in patients with rheumatoid arthritis. *N. Eng. J. Med.*, **284**(9), 453–8.

31. Alexander, G. J. M., Hortas, C., Bacon, P. A. *et al.* (1983) Bedrest, activity and the inflammation of rheumatoid arthritis. *B. Med. J.*, **22**, 134–40.

32. Beals, C. A., Lampman, R. M., Banwell, B. F. *et al.* (1985) Measure of exercise tolerance in patients with rheumatoid arthritis and osteoarthritis. *J. Rheumatol.*, **12**, 458–61.

33. Semble, E. L., Loeser, R. F. and Wise, C. M. (1990) Therapeutic exercise for rheumatoid arthritis and osteoarthritis. *Semin. Arth. Rheum.*, **20**(1), 32–40.

34. Capell, H. A. *et al.* (1986) A three year follow-up of patients allocated to placebo, or oral or injectable gold therapy for rheumatoid arthritis. *Ann. Rheum. Dis.*, **45**, 705–11.

35. Epstein, W. V., Henke, C. J., Yelin, E. H. *et al.* (1991) Effect of parenterally administered gold therapy on the course of adult rheumatoid arthritis. *Ann. Intern. Med.*, **114**(6), 437–44.

36. Bunch, T. W., O'Duffy, J. D., Thompkins, R. B. *et al.* (1984) Controlled trial of hydroxychloroquine and D-penicillamine singly and in combination in the treatment of rheumatoid arthritis. *Arth. Rheum.*, **27**, 267–76.

37. The Australian Multicenter Clinical Trial Group (1992) Sulfasalazine in early rheumatoid arthritis. *J. Rheumatol.*, **19**, 1672–7.

38. Taggart, A. J., Hill, J., Astbury, C. *et al.* (1987) Sulphasalazine alone or in combination with D-penicillamine in rheumatoid arthritis. *Br. J. Rheumatol.*, **26**, 32–6.

39. Wilkins, R. F., Urowitz, M. B., Stablein, D. M. *et al.* (1992) Comparison of azathioprine, methotrexate and the combination of both in the treatment of rheumatoid arthritis. *Arth. Rheum.*, **35**, 849–56.

40. Weinblatt, M. E., Polisson, R., Blatner, S. D. *et al.* (1993) The effects of drug therapy on radiographic progression of rheumatoid arthritis. *Arth. Rheum.*, **36**, 613–19.

41. Arnold, M. H., O'Callaghan, J., McCredie, M. *et al.* (1990) Comparative controlled trial of low-dose weekly methotrexate versus azathioprine in rheumatoid arthritis: 3-year prospective study. *Br. J. Rheumatol.*, **29**, 120–5.

42. Weinblatt, M. E., Weissman, B. N., Holdworth, D. E. *et al.* (1992) Long-term prospective study of methotrexate in the treatment of rheumatoid arthritis. *Arth. Rheum.*, **35**(2), 129–37.

43. Kremer, J. M. and Phelps, C. T. (1992) Long-term prospective study of the use of methotrexate in the treatment of rheumatoid arthritis. *Arth. Rheum.*, **35**(2), 138–45.

44. McCarty, D. J. (1990) Suppress rheumatoid inflammation early and leave the pyramid to the Egyptians (Editorial), *J. Rheumatol.*, **117**, 1115–8.

45. Brooks, P. M. and Schwarzer, A. C. (1991) Combination chemotherapy in rheumatoid arthritis. *Ann. Rheum. Dis.*, **50**, 507–9.

46. Paulus, H. E. (1990) The use of combinations of disease-modifying antirheumatic agents in rheumatoid arthritis. *Arth. Rheum.*, **33**(1), 113–20.

47. McGuire, J. L. and Ridgway, W. M. (1993) Aggressive drug therapy for rheumatoid arthritis. *Hosp. Prac.*, Sept., 33–40.

48. Croghan, J. E. and White, P. H. (1992) Challenging the pyramid: earlier, more aggressive treatment of RA. *Drug Therapy*, Nov., 17–31.

49. Kantor, S. M., Willin, B. A., Grier, C. G. *et al.* (1990) Combination of auranofin and methotrexate as initial DMARD therapy in RA. *Arth. Rheum.*, **33**, S60.

50. Brawer, A. E. (1988) Combined use of oral methotrexate and intramuscular gold in rheumatoid arthritis. *Arth. Rheum.*, **31**, R10.

51. Farr, M., Kitas, G. and Bacon, P. A. (1988) Sulphasalazine in rheumatoid arthritis: combination therapy with D-penicillamine or sodium aurothiomalate. *Clin. Rheumatol.*, **7**, 242–8.

52. Gibson, T., Emery, P., Armstrong, R. D. *et al.* (1987) Combined D-penicillamine and chloroquine treatment of rheumatoid arthritis – a comparative study. *Br. J. Rheumatol.*, **26**, 279–84.

53. Hench, P. S., Kendall, E. C., Slocumb, C. H. *et al.* (1949) The effect of a hormone of the adrenal cortex (17-hydroxy-11-dehydrocorticosterone; compound E) and of pituitary adrenocorticotropic hormone on rheumatoid arthritis: preliminary report, *Proc. Staff. Meet. Mayo Clin.*, **24**, 181–97.

54. Bollet, A. J., Black, R. and Bunim, J. J. (1955) Major undesirable side-effects resulting from prednisolone and prednisone. *JAMA*, **158**, 459–63.

55. DeAndrade, J. R., McCormick, J. N. and Hill, G. S. (1964) Small doses of prednisolone in the management of rheumatoid arthritis. *Ann. Rheum. Dis.*, **23**, 158–62.

56. Harris, E. D., Emkey, R. D., Nichols, J. E. *et al.* (1983) Low dose prednisone therapy in rheumatoid arthritis: a double blind study. *J. Rheumatol.*, **10**(5), 713–21.

57. Boumpas, D. T., Chrousos, G. P., Wilder, R. L. *et al.* (1993) Glucocorticoid therapy for immune-mediated diseases: basic and clinical correlates. *Ann. Intern. Med.*, **119**(12), 1198–208.

58. Hollander, J. L. (1985) Arthrocentesis technique and intrasynovial therapy, in *Arthritis and Allied Conditions*, (ed. D. J. Mcarty), Lea & Febier, Philadelphia, pp. 541–53.

59. Klemperer, P., Pollack, A. D. and Baehr, G. (1942) Diffuse collagen disease; acute disseminated lupus erythematosus and diffuse scleroderma. *J. Am. Med. Assoc.*, **119**, 331–2,

60. Pagel, W. and Treip, C. S. (1955) Viscerocutaneous collagenosis. A study of the intermediate forms of dermatomyositis, scleroderma and disseminated lupus erythematosus. *J. Clin. Pathol.*, **8**, 1–18.

E. H. S. Choy and G. S. Panayi

INTRODUCTION

Rheumatic diseases continue to be a major burden to health care systems worldwide. Patients' lives are blighted by pain, loss of mobility and function that result in substantial physical and psychological morbidity. Furthermore, a number of rheumatic diseases, such as rheumatoid arthritis (RA), systemic lupus erythematosus (SLE), scleroderma and vasculitis have an increased mortality. Current therapies of rheumatic diseases are associated with toxic side effects and have failed to affect the long-term outcome significantly. The mechanism of action of many current conventional treatments remains unknown as their entry into rheumatological practice was by serendipity rather than through rational drug research. The goal of rheumatological research is to elucidate pathogenic mechanisms from which rational, specific and non-toxic treatments can be developed. Ideally, such treatments should involve a short course of therapy but produce prolonged disease remission. The obvious advantages will be convenience and lack of toxicity. Alternatively, maintenance treatment, which is non-toxic but effective, may be acceptable but will be inconvenient and expensive. In this chapter we shall review recent advances in the treatment of rheumatic disease with biologics and their potential to lead to long-term disease remission.

PATHOGENESIS OF AUTOIMMUNE DISEASES

Although aspects of pathogenesis have already been covered by Chapter 1, it is worthwhile emphasizing some of these because of their importance with respect to future therapies. Chronic inflammatory diseases are characterized by continuous activation of cellular and humoral immune responses. The crucial event in the initiation of the immune response is the presentation of antigenic peptides by antigen presenting cells in the context of major histocompatibility complex (MHC) molecules to T-cells equipped with the appropriate T-cell receptor (TCR). The engagement of this trimolecular complex (MHC/antigen/TCR), in the presence of other co-stimulatory signals, results in T-cell activation and initiation of the immune and inflammatory cascades, including activation of the humoral immune response with B-cell proliferation and maturation into plasma cells and the production of antibody.

T-cell activation is a complex process with much of the detailed mechanisms remaining unknown. Antigen or autoantigens are first taken up by professional antigen presenting cells, such as Langerhan's cells of the skin, macrophages or B-cells. Antigens are processed and broken up enzymatically either in the cytoplasm (endogenous pathway) or endoplasmic reticulum (exogenous pathway)

Connective Tissue Diseases. Edited by Jill J. F. Belch and Robert B. Zurier. Published in 1995 by Chapman & Hall, London.
ISBN 0 412 48620 2

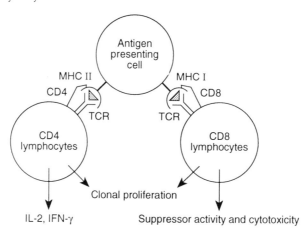

Fig. 15.1 The activation of CD4 and CD8 T-cells by antigenic peptides presented in the context of major histocompatibility complex (MHC) class I and class II molecules respectively via the T-cell receptor (TCR). IL-2: interleukin-2; IFN-γ: interferon-γ.

into small peptide fragments[1,2]. These peptides are brought into association with either MHC class I molecules and β2 microglobulin or class II molecules, respectively. In the case of MHC class I molecules, this process is controlled by the transport associated protein(TAP) I and II[3]. The association of antigenic peptide with the MHC molecules stabilize the complex which is then transported to and inserted into the plasma membrane. The detailed structure of MHC molecules has been elucidated by X-ray crystallography[4,5]. Both the MHC class I and class II molecules have certain structural similarities. Each is composed of two α helices and a β pleated sheet which form a peptide binding groove in which is located the antigenic peptide. Certain regions of the MHC molecules are particularly important because they are essential for binding antigenic peptides. One region of MHC class I and II molecules are highly polymorphic while others are non-polymorphic (Figure 15.1). The antigenic peptide binding in the groove of the MHC class I molecule is about 9 amino acids in length while in the case of MHC class II it is 11–14 amino acids or longer. To date, the only known function of the MHC class I and II molecules is to present antigenic peptides to

CD8 and CD4$^+$ T-cells equipped with the appropriate TCR. This restriction is due to the fact that CD4 binds specifically to a non-polymorphic region of the MHC class II molecule while, conversely, CD8 binds specifically to MHC class I molecule. Engagement of the TCR with the MHC/antigen complex leads to co-aggregation of a number of molecules on the surface of the T-cell which include CD3, TCR and CD4 or CD8[6]. The cytoplasmic tails of the CD3-TCR and CD4-CD8 molecules contain binding domains for tyrosine phosphokinase (p59^{fyn} and p56^{lck} respectively)[7]. Juxtapositioning of these tyrosine phosphokinases leads to tyrosine phosphorylation and initiation of a number of cellular events, including activation of protein kinase C, which eventually result in clonal proliferation and production of various cytokines such as interleukin-2 (IL-2), interferon-γ (IFN-γ) and cytokine receptors such as the IL-2 receptor (IL-2R). There is convincing evidence to suggest that optimal T-cell activation requires the presence of other co-stimulatory signals (Table 15.1). Engagement of the trimolecular complex in the absence of these co-stimulatory signals may lead to the induction of immunological tolerance rather than activation. Immunological tolerance has

Table 15.1 Co-stimulatory molecules on T-cells and their respective ligands on antigen presenting cells

T-cells	Antigen presenting cells
CD4	Non-polymorphic region β chain of major histocompatibility complex class II molecule
CD2	Leukocyte function antigen 3
Leukocyte function antigen 1	Intercellular adhesion molecule 1
Very late activation antigen 4	Vascular cellular adhesion molecule 1
CD28	B7

Table 15.2 Molecules involve in leukocyte-endothelial cell interaction

Phase of leukocyte migration	Leukocyte	Endothelial cell
Rolling	Sialyl-Lewis X acid	E-selectin
Strong adhesion	CD2 LFA-1 VLA-4	LFA-3 ICAM-1 VCAM-1
Migration	Unknown	Unknown

LFA: leukocyte function antigen.
ICAM-1: intercellular adhesion molecule 1.
VLA-4: very late activation antigen 4.
VCAM-1: vascular adhesion molecule 1.

been studied intensively because of its therapeutic implications for many autoimmune diseases and transplantation. The ability to 'reprogramme' the immune response and hence the chance of a cure is an exciting prospect[8]. There is plenty of evidence both *in vitro* and *in vivo* that tolerance can be induced by antibodies directed against T-cell surface molecules such as CD4 and LFA-1[9] or by manipulation of the antigen[10].

Cytokines, which are proteins secreted by many different cell types, have diverse biological functions. They convey signals between different cells, paracrine stimulation, or to the same cell, autocrine stimulation, leading to amplification or downregulation of the inflammatory response. A vast number of cytokines have now been discovered (also Chapter 1). Some have argued that certain cytokines, such as tumor necrosis factor-α (TNF-α), by virtue of its ability to induce production of other cytokines, is the main control cytokine[11]. However, the 'central' role of TNF-α in RA, for example, remains a controversial issue. As discussed above, T-cells upon activation secrete IL-2 as well as expressing IL-2R on their surface. IL-2 amplifies the T-cell response further by activating other IL-2R bearing T-cells. Activated T-cells

also secrete other cytokines such as IL-3, IL-4, IL-5 and IL-6. These cytokines are essential for the development of the humoral response. B-cells require cytokines in order proliferate, to undergo isotype switching and to mature to plasma cells secreting antibodies. IFN-γ activates monocytes, which secrete a number of pro-inflammatory cytokines, such as IL-1 and TNF-α. Both IL-1 and TNF-α induce production of cytokines, such as IL-6, which act on hepatocytes resulting in production of acute phase proteins, such as serum amyloid A protein. IL-1 and TNF-α also stimulate the release of metalloproteinases, such as collagenase, which are responsible for tissue damage. IL-1, IFN-γ and TNF-α can act synergistically in upregulating the expression of adhesion molecules on endothelial cells, including E-selectin (formerly, endothelial leucocyte adhesion molecule 1 or ELAM-1), intercellular adhesion molecule 1 (ICAM-1) and vascular adhesion molecule 1 (VCAM-1)[12,13]. These adhesion molecules mediate accumulation of leucocytes into inflammatory lesions by enhancing leukocyte adhesion and migration. Initially, the leukocyte rolls along the endothelial surface; this phase is controlled by E-selectin and sialyl-Lewis acid residues on the surface of endothelial cells and

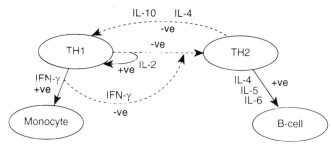

Fig. 15.2 Lymphokines secreted by TH1 and TH2 subsets are autocrine growth factors and inhibit the development of the other type of TH type response. IL: interleukin; IFN-γ: interferon-γ; solid lines and +ve: induction; dotted lines and −ve: inhibition.

leukocytes respectively. The interaction between these molecules is rather weak but leads to a stronger adhesion mediated by ICAM-1 and leucocyte function antigen 1 (LFA-1) as well as leucocyte function antigen 3 (LFA-3) and CD2. After this interaction, between VCAM-1 and very late activation antigen 4 (VLA-4) finally leads to migration of leukocytes through the blood vessel. A summary of the molecules and their respective ligands in different phases of leukocyte migration is shown in Table 15.2 and illustrated graphically in Chapter 1.

Interestingly, most of these molecules have also been shown to be of importance in providing co-stimulatory signals during T-cell activation[14]. ICAM-1 and VCAM-1 are also present on the surface of antigen presenting cells and are the ligands for LFA-1 and VLA-4, respectively, found on T-cells. Hence, they act not only as mediators of T-cell migration but also as co-stimulatory signals during T-cell activation. Although the exact role of these molecules during T-cell activation remains unknown, their absence may induce anergy rather than T-cell activation.

So far, we have emphasized the role of cytokines in the amplification of the immune response but it is clear that they also have a role in the negative feedback control of inflammation. T-helper cells are defined as T-cells which are able to provide 'help' to B-cells to produce antibodies. Murine T-helper cells can be further divided into two

types, TH1 and TH2, depending on the pattern of cytokines which they secrete. TH1 cells produce mainly IL-2 and IFN-γ, while TH2 cells produce IL-4, IL-5 and IL-10 (Figure 15.2). The former are thought to lead to a predominantly cellular immune response while the latter leads to a humoral immune response[15]. Although the TH1 and TH2 subsets have not been conclusively demonstrated in human lymphocytes, it is clear that there are TH1 and TH2 type responses such as that seen in leprosy and parasitic infections[16]. Various treatments can change the type of response. IL-2 enhances TH1 type responses but inhibits TH2 cells while IL-4 has opposite effects[17]. Indeed, certain form of immunological tolerance may be caused by the switching from a TH1 to a TH2 response.

THERAPEUTIC TARGETS AND TREATMENT GOALS

In this complex network of inflammatory cells and mediators, there are ample opportunities to manipulate the immune response. Possible targets include cytokines, adhesion molecules and cells. Many of these will be discussed in more detail in the latter part of this chapter. Ideally, new treatments should be non-toxic, effective in a large number of patients and lead to a permanent cure. Short of this perfect solution, a treatment that leads to prolonged disease remission will still be economical and convenient. Table 15.3 shows a list of possible

Table 15.3   Possible therapeutic targets including lymphocyte surface markers, cytokines, adhesion molecules and MHC molecule

Lymphocyte	Cytokines	Adhesion molecules	Others
CD4	Tumor necrosis factor α	Intercellular adhesion molecule 1 (CD54)	MHC II
CD5	IL-1	E-selectin	
CD7		Vascular adhesion molecule 1	
CDw52			
CD8			
Leukocyte function antigen 1			
Very late activation antigen 4			
IL-2 receptor			
T-cell receptor			

MHC II: major histocompatibility complex class II molecule.

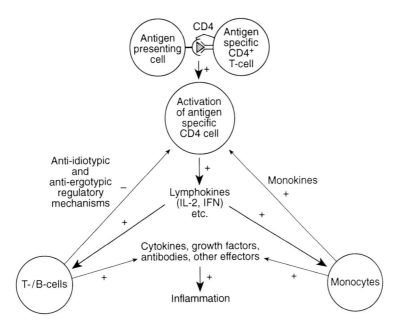

Fig. 15.3   Pathogenic pyramid of CD4$^+$ T-cell driven autoimmune disease. IL: interleukin; IFN: interferon-γ.

targets, their specificity and their potential for 'cure' or prolonged disease remission.

It is obvious from the discussion on the pathogenesis of inflammation that intervention at the top of the inflammatory cascade (Figure 15.3) is more likely to be effective and specific. Plainly, the perfect solution in many inflammatory diseases is to remove the pathogenic antigen but, unfortunately, for the majority of autoimmune diseases, the autoantigens are unknown. The only hope of a 'cure' in this case must rely on 'reprogramming' the immune response so as to develop 'immunological tolerance' to the autoantigen.

Table 15.4 Major pro- and anti-inflammatory cytokines and their modes of action

Pro-inflammatory cytokines	Mode of action	Anti-inflammatory cytokines	Mode of action
IL-1	Induce production of cytokines	IL-1 receptor antagonist	Inhibits IL-1
Tumour necrosis factor-α	Induce production of cytokines	*Transforming growth factor β	Inhibits T-cells and monocytes
IL-2	Activate IL-2R⁺ T-cells	IL-10	Inhibits T-cell activation
Interferon-γ	Activate monocytes	IL-13	Inhibits monokine secretion
IL-4	Promote antibody production		
IL-5	Promote antibody production		
IL-6	Acute phase response		
IL-8	Leukocyte chemotactic factor		

IL: interleukin.
* Transforming growth factor β is also a pro-inflammatory cytokine.

Short of targeting the antigen or auto-antigen, therapies directed against the TCR or MHC molecules should be very specific treatments. Lymphocytes and other inflammatory cells are also possible targets but they are more non-specific. The cytokine network is an obvious target for intervention. As discussed above there is a fine balance between pro-inflammatory cytokines, such as IL-2, IL-1 and TNF-α and anti-inflammatory cytokines, such as transforming growth factor β (TGF-β) and IL-10. Table 15.4 shows a list of pro- and anti-inflammatory cytokines and their modes of action. Therapy using anti-inflammatory cytokines or anti-cytokines can alter this fine balance. However, it is unlikely that targeting cytokines alone will lead to a permanent cure. Nevertheless, anti-cytokine therapy may lead to significant disease improvement for a long period of time so that treatments given at regular intervals may then be sufficient to control disease activity.

TOOLS IN BIOLOGICAL TREATMENT

Having identified possible therapeutic targets, what can we use to target them? In the case of cytokines, nature has already provided us with ready made agents such as anti-inflammatory cytokines, like TGF-β, IL-10, or natural occurring cytokine antagonists, like soluble cytokines receptors. Examples of these will be discussed in more detail later. Although at the moment these agents are either given as intravenous or subcutaneous injections, it may be possible to implant fibroblasts in which genes of cytokine antagonists or anti-inflammatory cytokines have been inserted. Constitutional secretion of anti-inflammatory cytokines or cytokine antagonists by these fibroblasts at the site of inflammation will avoid the need to give parenteral treatment. Another way of utilising nature's providence is to manipulate the immune response of the patient by T-cell vaccination or oral tolerance. These methods enhance suppressive elements in the immune response and their use in autoimmune diseases will be discussed later.

We have already discussed the important role of the trimolecular complex during T-cell activation. In the center of the complex is the antigenic peptide. *In vitro* experiments have shown that it is possible to generate peptides

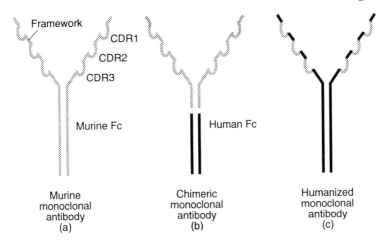

Fig. 15.4 Structural difference of murine, chimeric and humanized monoclonal antibody. Stippled lines indicate murine protein while human proteins are indicated by dark lines. CDR: complementarity determining region.

which bind to either the MHC or TCR but which do not result in T-cell activation (Figure 15.4). Interfering with the interactions of the trimolecular complex is therefore a possible strategy which is attractive because it would be highly specific for the disease in question.

Gammaglobulin given in large doses is also effective in some inflammatory conditions (Chapters 8 and 9). Although their exact mechanism of action remains unknown, there are a number of interesting possibilities. First, they may competitively inhibit binding of pathogenic autoantibodies to Fc receptor on the surface of mononuclear cells. Secondly, the presence of anti-idiotypic antibodies in the polyclonal gammaglobulin may reduce the pathogenicity of autoantibodies by binding to their F(ab)$_2$. Thirdly, since monocytes and T-cells carry FCγR on their surface, gammaglobulin may inhibit their function through binding to these receptors and generate negative signals.

In order to pursue a treatment that is specific, many have turned to monoclonal antibodies (mAb). This is an attractive option because mAb are highly specific and the action of the antibody may be changed by altering the immunoglobulin heavy chain subtypes. The advent of hybridoma technology and molecular biology allow the generation of large amounts of mAb which can be used in therapy[18]. Initially, many of these antibodies were murine in origin but when they were used in therapeutic trials, almost all patients developed a human anti-mouse antibody response[19]. Consequently, there was a risk of anaphylaxis and reduced efficacy on re-treatment. Chimeric antibody is a construct of antibody in which the murine Fc has been replaced by human Fc fragment. In the case of humanized antibody[20], only the murine complementarity determining region of the F(ab)$_2$ has been left, the framework regions having been replaced by human sequences (Figure 15.5). It is hoped that such antibodies will be less antigenic. Indeed, they have now been used in the treatment of autoimmune diseases and transplant rejection[21]. However, as will become clear later, although both chimeric and humanized antibodies are less antigenic than their murine counterparts, many patients still develop an anti-antibody response upon retreatment but it seems that anaphylactic reactions are rare

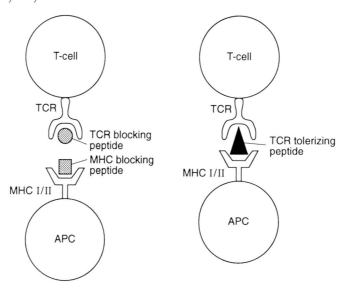

Fig. 15.5 Mechanisms of action of different types of peptide in blocking major histocompatibility complex class II (MHC II) and major histocompatibility complex class I (MHC I) molecules and the T-cell receptor (TCR). APC: antigen presenting cell.

even after repeated treatment and with little or no loss of efficacy.

Most antibodies and cytokines bind to their cell surface antigens and cytokine receptors with high specificity and avidity. It is, therefore, possible to use antibodies and cytokines as a 'guidance system' to deliver drugs or toxins. Based on this principle, immunotoxins have been developed. These are constructs of biological toxins conjugated to antibodies or cytokines. Examples of immunotoxins include CD5+, IL-2-DAB$_{486}$ and anti-Tac (IL-2R) conjugated to yittrium. All these bind specifically to their respective ligands and once bound to the cell surface, the toxins conjugated to the antibodies or cytokines lead to killing of the cell. All these have been used in the treatment of autoimmune diseases and T-cell leukemias. In the case of CD5+, murine anti-CD5 mAb was conjugated to ricin A chain. Once CD5+ binds to CD5, the ricin binds to cell surface glycoprotein and glycolipid and is then endocytosed killing the cell by inhibiting protein synthesis. IL-2-DAB$_{486}$ is a conjugate of IL-2 to truncated diphtheria toxin. IL-2 binds to IL-2R with

high affinity and the diphtheria toxin binds to an epidermal growth factor-like receptor on the cell surface which, after endocytosis, kills its target by suppressing protein synthesis. The disadvantage of using a large protein toxin, such as ricin and diphtheria toxin, is the induction of host antibody directed against the toxin. One alternative is to use radio-labelled antibodies such as ^{90}Y-anti-Tac which is anti-IL-2R mAb labelled with yttrium-90. It has been used in the treatment of lymphoid malignancy with very promising results[22] and its use in RA is evaluated.

One of the most exciting therapeutic prospects in recent years has been the generation of anti-sense oligonucleotides as immuno-modulators. Short fragments of specific oligonucleotide can be generated targeting mRNA of cytokines, cell surface molecules, specific proteins or enzymes. Such binding will inhibit translation of mRNA products and hence protein synthesis. This again should allow highly specific targeting and minimize possible side effects. Although it has not been used in clinical trials, this strategy is being actively pursued.

CLINICAL EXPERIENCE OF TREATMENT WITH BIOLOGICS

MAJOR HISTOCOMPATIBILITY COMPLEX AND THE T-CELL RECEPTOR AS THERAPEUTIC TARGETS

Many autoimmune diseases are associated with the MHC. One of the best examples is RA in which susceptibility and severity of disease are both associated with HLA-DR4 and HLA-DR1. Gregersen *et al.* showed that the amino acid sequence in the third hypervariable region of the β-chain is conserved among disease associated HLA-DR molecules[23]. They hypothesized that the disease-specific antigen or autoantigen is bound in the HLA groove thus initiating and maintaining the cellular immune response. *In vitro* experiments have shown that specific peptides can be generated which competitively bind to the MHC groove but which do not generate an immune response[24]. However, a high concentration of the inhibitory peptide is required to block immune activation and, in chronic diseases, maintaining such a high concentration of inhibitory peptide may be difficult[25]. Recently, Sloan-Lancaster *et al.* have shown that a minor alteration in the amino acid sequence of the antigenic peptide may not only inhibit T-cell activation but may induce a state of tolerance to the original peptide[10]. This offers the possibility of using peptide therapy in autoimmune disease in order to achieve long-term remission after a short course of treatment.

T-cell vaccination

This therapy is based on the observation in animal models of autoimmune disease which are induced by the injection of an antigen can be transferred by antigen-specific, disease-causing T-cell lines or T-cell clones. A good example of this is the induction of experimental allergic encephalomyelitis (EAE) by myelin basic protein or adjuvant arthritis by mycobacterial protein extract in Freund's complete adjuvant. Lymphocytes from the lymph nodes of the affected animal are rich in disease specific T-cells. These cells can be further expanded *in vitro* with the pathogenic antigen. When these cells are injected into another susceptible animal and in the complete absence of immunization with the initiating antigen, a similar autoimmune disease can be induced as effectively as the original antigen. This confirms the important pathogenic role of T-cells in autoimmune disease. Interestingly, if the lymphocytes are pre-treated with mitomycin C or irradiated before immunization, the animal becomes resistant to further disease induction either by antigen injection or by transfer of antigen activated lymphocytes[26]. This method of inducing disease suppression is termed T-cell vaccination because of its resemblance to the use of attenuated bacteria or virus as vaccines. It is based on the hypothesis that the recipient will generate an immune response directed against idiotypic structures on the injected T-cells[27]. The disease-causing T-cells are attenuated either by irradiation, high barometric pressure or mitomycin C and treatment with gluteraldehyde before use as a vaccine. Only a small dose of T-cells (1000–100 000 cells) need be used. Although this method of treatment is effective in a number of animal models of autoimmune diseases, the exact mechanism of action remains unknown. T-cell vaccination has been used by three independent groups in the treatment of RA[28–30]. All groups adopted similar strategies. In RA, the antigen is unknown but the highest concentration of disease specific T-cells is likely to be found in the rheumatoid joint. Lymphocytes were obtained from the synovial fluid, expanded *in vitro* by IL-2 and anti-CD3 mAb treated with gluteraldehyde and injected subcutaneously into the patients as a vaccine in three separate doses. Overall, the clinical response from the treatment has been disappointing so far: van Laar *et al.* treated 13 RA patients in an open study and found that, although a number of patients might have responded, none obtained complete disease remission[29] and Kingsley *et al.* performed a double blind placebo controlled trial in six patients, with half the patients receiving active vaccine[30]. One patient from the active vaccine group responded. Although the results seem disappointing at first glance, there are a number of important observations to be made. First, from a disease like leprosy, we know that the frequency of antigen specific T-cells is approximately 1 in 500 or lower. Hence, synovial fluid mononuclear cells may only contain a small population of antigen-specific T-cells and this will result in a very low dose of 'active' vaccine being given to the patient. Secondly, the method of T-cell expansion with IL-2 and anti-CD3 mAb tends to expand activated T-cells non-specifically, unlike antigen stimulated expansion, and this is likely to reduce further the effectiveness of the vaccine. This hypothesis is in part supported by the observation by van Laar *et al.* that only a few patients developed a cellular immune responses towards the vaccine[29]. A similar observation was made by Kingsley *et al.* in that only one out of the three patients developed an anti-vaccine response[30]. Interestingly, this occurred in the patient who improved clinically. Thirdly, Lohse *et al.* have shown that in addition to the anti-vaccine response, another possible mode of action of T-cell vaccination is the generation of an anti-ergotypic response which is antigen specific and is mediated by T-cells which include both CD4$^+$ and CD8$^+$ subsets[31]. These T-cells are counter-regulatory and suppress activation of antigen specific T-cells. Anti-ergotypic responses may be a naturally occurring mechanism downregulating the immune response and augmenting this may be a useful way to control inflammation. Further efforts with T-cell vaccination should continue with the hope that an anti-ergotypic response is elicited.

T-cell receptor peptide therapy

The disadvantage of T-cell vaccination is that the method is time consuming, treatment has to be tailored for each individual patient and the patient must have a large synovial effusion in order to generate the vaccine. However, one way of overcoming this obstacle is to use T-cell receptor peptides. In experimental autoimmune conditions such as EAE, the pathogenic T-cells utilize a restricted Vβ gene repertoire and, consequently, a peptide can be synthesized corresponding to a specific region of the TCR receptor. This peptide can then be used as a vaccine to induce the formation of T-cells reacting against the TCR of the pathogenic T-cells so as to downregulate them. This approach has been effective for the treatment of EAE, an animal model of multiple sclerosis[32]. Consequently, a similar approach has been attempted in patients with multiple sclerosis (MS) although it is not widely accepted that there is a restricted TCR usage in the disease. However, in the cerebral spinal fluid of patients with MS there is an increased expression of Vβ5.2 and Vβ6.1 T-cells[33]. Two peptides generated from these Vβ proteins have been used to vaccinate 11 patients with MS[34]. A delayed type hypersensitivity reaction to the peptides was demonstrated in the treated patients and the anti-TCR T-cells which were elicited were shown to be CD4$^+$. The long-term efficacy of this treatment is still awaited. In rheumatic diseases, whether T-cell Vβ gene usage is restricted remains a controversial issue. There is some evidence that in RA there is a preferential expression of Vβ1, Vβ14 and Vβ16 among the IL-2R$^+$ T-cells[35] but the findings are variable and a general consensus has not developed. Hence, such therapy does not seem likely for the rheumatic diseases at present.

Oral tolerance

Tolerance can be generated by feeding an animal with an antigen prior to systemic immunization[36]. This phenomenon may be due to unique properties of the mucosal immune system which are yet to be fully understood. This method of tolerance induction has been shown to be effective in the treatment of animal models of autoimmune disease, such as EAE, by feeding animals with myelin basic protein[37] and, in collagen type II arthritis, collagen[38]. This strategy has been employed in MS by Weiner *et al.*[39] in a controlled study in which placebo or bovine myelin was fed to 30 patients with relapsing-remitting MS. Patients were assessed by measuring the number of subsequent attacks and the level of disability. Early results suggested that there was some clinical benefit and, in addition, there was a reduction in the number of circulating myelin basic protein reactive T-cells in the active treatment group. Results of a clinical trial to assess the effectiveness of oral feeding of chicken type II collagen in patients with RA indicate a modest but encouraging improvement in joint inflammation[40]. It is of interest that titers of antibody to type II collagen were not altered by administration of collagen. Weiner *et al.* have proposed that oral feeding induces CD8+ T-cells which home to the site of the lesion in MS patients, where they release TGF-β which then suppresses immune-mediated inflammation[41]. Hence, if it were possible to induce such cells in patients with RA by feeding with type II collagen, the cells would home to the joint and exert anti-inflammatory effects regardless of the exact status of collagen type II immunity. More recent work has suggested that very small amounts of antigen can be used to induce systemic tolerance if given through the nasal or pulmonary mucosa[42]. This finding may be of some considerable practical importance if the amount of autoantigen available is limited.

T-LYMPHOCYTES

The pivotal role of T-cells in the initiation and maintenance of chronic inflammation has been emphasized previously. Targeting T-lymphocytes with biologics is therefore an obvious therapeutic option. In the past, the use of lymphocyte depleting therapy in the form of lymphocytopheresis, thoracic duct drainage and total lymphoid irradiation have all been shown to be beneficial[43]. However, these procedures are laborious to perform, have unacceptable side effects and are not suitable for routine clinical use. A number of drugs have been shown to act specifically on T-lymphocytes, such as cyclosporin A, FK506 and rapamycin. Cyclosporin A and rapamycin bind to immunophilins while FK506 binds to FK-binding protein in the cytoplasm of T-lymphocytes and inhibit transcription of the IL-2 gene and hence suppress the production of IL-2[44]. Cyclosporin A has already established itself as an important drug for transplantation and a number of autoimmune diseases. Its main mechanism of action is inhibiting IL-2 production by suppressing transcription of NF-kB. To date only cyclosporin A has been used in the treatment of RA with some beneficial effect[45]. Unfortunately, it is a non-specific immunosuppressant and has significant renal and other side effects so that its eventual place in the treatment of RA may be circumscribed.

Protein kinase C is essential for T-cell activation. Inhibitors of protein kinase C can lead to suppression of T-cell *in vitro*. Recently, several new protein kinase C inhibitors have been developed which seem to be specific for the T-cell enzyme[46]; they have been successfully used for the treatment of adjuvant arthritis in rats. They may soon be used in clinical trials in patients with RA.

Anti-CD7 monoclonal antibody

CD7 is an early marker of T-cells and is expressed on pluripotential hemopoietic cells in the thymus and bone marrow. A subset of peripheral blood T-cells also expresses CD7. Its function is unknown. Both murine and chimeric anti-CD7 mAb have been used in the treatment of refractory RA[47,48]. No significant clinical improvement was seen despite significant decreases in the number of peripheral blood and synovial CD7$^+$ lymphocytes. Recently, Lazarowits *et al.* have demonstrated that CD7$^+$ cells may not be important in inflammatory diseases[49]. Although the majority of peripheral blood lymphocytes are CD7^{bright}, synovial fluid lymphocytes are mainly CD7^{dim}. T-cells which are CD7^{dim} appear to be a stable population which may have different functions from those which are CD7^{bright}. Hence, the lack of response to anti-CD7 may reflect the fact that CD7^{bright} T-cells are not found in the rheumatoid joint. It is of interest to note that CD7^{bright} T-cells are found in human renal allografts: a situation in which anti-CD7 mAb has been shown to be successful in preventing graft rejection[21].

CD5 plus

CD5 is expressed on most thymocytes, all mature T-cells and a subset of mature B-cells. CD5$^+$ B-cells polyreactive antibodies, mostly IgM, which recognize a variety of self- and foreign antigens and have been implicated in the pathogenesis of autoimmune diseases such as RA[50]. CD5$^+$ is an immunoconjugate composed of the murine anti-CD5 mAb conjugated to the ricin A chain. The latter is toxic to cells. It has been used in the treatment of both refractory as well as early RA[51]. CD5$^+$ was administered as daily intravenous infusions for 5 days. Disease improvement was assessed by the Paulus criteria. Fifty-four patients with longstanding refractory RA and 24 with early RA (mean disease duration 1.8 years) were recruited. After treatment, 40% and 70% respectively of the refractory and early RA patients showed a 50% improvement in disease activity criteria. After 1 month of therapy, 22 out of 67 patients had >50% and 31 out of 67 had >20% reduction in erythrocyte sedimentation rate (ESR), C reactive protein (CRP) or rheumatoid factor (RF) values. More patients in the early arthritis

group improved after treatment. There was a marked reduction in the number of circulating CD5$^+$ CD3$^+$ T-cells which involved both CD4$^+$ and CD8$^+$ T-cell subsets. Recovery of lymphocyte number was not affected by concurrent treatment with methotrexate or azathioprine. Seventy-five out of 76 patients developed a human anti-mouse antibody response by day 15. The median half-life of CD5$^+$ was 3.5 hours. Side effects included nausea, vomiting, fever, chills, weakness, fatigue, headache, flushing, fluid retention, skin rash and one case of myositis. Most of these reactions were mild and resolved spontaneously, and only 6 patients had to be withdrawn from the study because of side effects. Anaphylaxis occurred in 3 patients but symptoms resolved with adrenaline. Two patients suffered from pulmonary edema. Other side effects included exacerbation of anemia, leukocytosis, mild to moderate rise of liver enzymes (in patients receiving concurrent immunosuppression), hypoalbuminemia and hypertriglyceridemia. The cause of these complications is unknown. The exact role of CD5$^+$ in RA remains to be elucidated. A multi-center placebo controlled study has been undertaken but the results have not yet been published.

Campath-1H

Campath-1H is a humanized anti-CDw52 mAb. The CDw52 molecule is a glycoprotein present on the surface of thymocytes, T-cells, monocytes, B-cells and a proportion of granulocytes and eosinophils. Although the function of CDw52 is unknown, it is an exceptionally good target for complement mediated cell lysis. Hence, Campath-1H, with a human IgG1 Fc engrafted, is extremely lytic. In a patient with systemic vasculitis refractory to therapy with steroid and conventional immunosuppressants, treatment with Campath-1H led to disease improvement although the patient relapsed later. When he was retreated with Campath-1H followed by anti-

CD4 mAb, there was a sustained improvement in disease activity lasting up to 8 months[52]. In an open labelled phase II study, 9 patients with refractory RA patients were treated with daily infusions of Campath-1H for 5 days[53]. Significant clinical improvement was seen after treatment with approximately 50% reduction in Ritchie index and joint score; the disease relapse could be retreated. There was no significant change in ESR and CRP. Campath-1H induced a rapid drop in the circulating lymphocyte number whose severity and duration was related to the dose. In addition to lymphopenia, there was also a monocytopenia lasting 3 months. Disease improvement did not correlate with either lymphopenia or monocytopenia. Side effects were common and included pyrexia (up to 40°C), nausea, rigor, skin rash and hypotension. These features are consistent with the 'cytokine release syndrome' seen after immunotherapy with IL-2 and anti-CD3 mAb[54]. Other side effects included oral ulceration, renal impairment and infective complications. In this study, Campath-1H did not induce a significant anti-globulin response after a single treatment course although 3 out of 4 patients after re-treatment did so. This was a mixed anti-isotype and anti-idiotype response. In order to simplify treatment, Campath-1H has been given as subcutaneously[55] but lymphopenia and monocytopenia were still noted, side effects were similar to those after intravenous infusions but were less severe and disease improvement seemed to be less effective.

Anti-IL-2 receptor monoclonal antibody

Anti-IL-2R mAb was used in an open study of 3 patients with RA. Two patients had significant disease improvement[56]. No immunological data was presented in this report.

IL-2-DAB$_{486}$

IL-2-DAB$_{486}$ is a fusion toxin of human IL-2 conjugated to the toxic membrane translocating domains of diphtheria toxin. It targets all IL-2R$^+$ cells which include activated T-lymphocytes, B-lymphocytes, monocytes, lymphomas and leukemias. IL-2-DAB$_{486}$ binds to the human IL-2R with high affinity. The diphtheria toxin is internalized and results in killing of the cells. IL-2-DAB$_{486}$ has been used in the treatment of RA, lymphomas, leukemias and diabetes mellitus. In a preliminary dose ranging study (from 150–300 ku/kg/day) in 19 patients with refractory and active RA, it was given as an intravenous infusion daily for 5–7 days[57]. Clinical improvement was seen by 7 days and persisted for 4–30 weeks beyond the treatment period. Side effects included fever, lower extremity edema and transient elevation of hepatic transaminases. Subsequently, a double blind placebo-controlled trial was carried out in 45 patients with severe refractory RA in which patients were randomized to receive either 150 ku/kg/day of IL-2-DAB$_{486}$ or placebo daily for 5 days. Clinical improvement was assessed by the Paulus criteria. No improvement was seen in the placebo treated group while in the treated group 4 out of 18 patients had >50% and 2 out of 18 had >20% clinical improvement. There was a significant reduction in the number of peripheral blood IL-2R$^+$ lymphocytes. Interestingly, most patients developed antibody response to IL-2-DAB$_{486}$ but these were all directed against the diphtheria toxin and did not interfere with the activity of IL-2-DAB$_{486}$. A larger study using a further genetically engineered modification of IL-2-DAB$_{486}$: IL-2-DAB$_{389}$ to enhance its potency and reduce its toxicity is currently underway to assess its efficacy in RA.

Anti-CD4 monoclonal antibody

Anti-CD4 monoclonal antibodies have been used extensively for the treatment of experimental autoimmune diseases. It is clear from the earlier discussion on the pathogenesis of autoimmune diseases that CD4$^+$ T-cells are central to the initiation and control of the inflammatory response. Therefore, CD4 lymphocytes are an attractive target for immune modulation especially after Benjamin *et al.* demonstrated that concurrent administration of antigen with anti-CD4 mAb was able to induce tolerance to the antigen[58]. This was later shown also to be the case in streptococcal cell wall arthritis and in adjuvant arthritis[59], if anti-CD4 mAb was given at the same time as injection of the relevant arthritis inducing antigen. Furthermore, re-challenging the animal with antigen 6 weeks later failed to induce disease. Anti-CD4 mAb therapy has been used in animal model of transplantation, type I diabetes mellitus and systemic lupus erythematosus. In the non-obese diabetic mouse which spontaneously develops diabetes, anti-CD4 mAb given at the time of appearance of diabetes can abort further worsening of disease by the induction of tolerance. Thus, tolerance may also be induced therapeutically not just prophylactically. If tolerance could be induced in established human autoimmune disease by the infusion of anti-CD4 mAb, there is the tempting possibility that long-term remission after a single treatment course could be achieved.

In human trials both murine and chimeric anti-CD4 monoclonal antibodies have been used in several conditions including RA, relapsing polychondritis and systemic lupus erythematosus. Relapsing polychondritis, an autoimmune disease directed against human cartilage, is rare but can occasionally be lethal. Fortunately, most patients respond to treatment with steroids. Two groups have reported cases of severe refractory relapsing polychondritis responding to treatment with anti-CD4 mAb. Murine anti-CD4 mAb MT-151 was given to a patient with severe life-threatening relapsing polychondritis[60] because of tracheal involvement requiring ventilatory support. However, the disease remained very active despite treatment with steroid and immunosuppressant. After treatment with 7 daily doses of MT-151 there was a

drastic reduction in disease activity with improved respiratory function. Encouraged by this initial report, we subsequently used the chimeric anti-CD4 mAb, cM-T412, in a patient with relapsing polychrondritis refractory to conventional treatments including steroid and methotrexate[61]. Disease activity improved after 3 doses of 50 mg of cM-T412 given intravenously fortnightly. Sustained improvement was seen and lasted at least 3 years. Unlike the murine antibody, CD4 lymphopenia was more prolonged lasting at least 1 week but after 3 fortnightly doses, lymphopenia lasted some 3 months. Lymphocyte proliferation to tuberculin PPD was reduced after treatment but recovered.

Anti-CD4 mAb has been used successfully in the treatment of murine models of systemic lupus erythematosus[62]. Because of these reports, Hiepe *et al.* used the murine anti-CD4 mAb MAX.16H5 in 3 patients with severe intractable lupus nephritis[63]. After 7 daily treatments with anti-CD4 mAb there was a reduction in the overall disease activity and, in particular, a decrease in the quantity of proteinuria and an increase in serum albumin. The titer of anti-dDNA antibodies dropped after treatment from 1:64 to 1:8.

Most of the work relating to the clinical efficacy of anti-CD4 monoclonal antibodies have been carried out in RA. Murine anti-CD4 monoclonal antibodies have been used by three groups in open clinical studies in refractory RA patients[64–66]. Detailed comparison between these trials is impossible since different anti-CD4 monoclonal antibodies, antibody doses and treatment regimens were used. Overall, treatment was well tolerated. The commonest side effects were fever, chill and rigor but these were self-limiting and were attributed to cytokine release during treatment[67]. These were only troublesome during the first dose since symptoms improved or disappeared on subsequent treatment. Clinical response was variable but most patients improved by 50%. A few patients have been reported in these studies with very prolonged disease remission lasting at least 6 months. Unlike other murine antibodies, such as anti-ICAM-1 mAb[68], only 70% of the patients developed human antibody to the murine antibody (HAMA). This supports the notion that anti-CD4 mAb may be able to induce tolerance to itself. CD4 lymphopenia developed soon after treatment and lasted 24 hours. Prolonged CD4 lymphopenia was uncommon, the only report being in a patient who had had a previous splenectomy[69]. The mechanism of action of murine anti-CD4 mAb was unclear since clinical response did not correlate with the degree of CD4 lymphopenia. Radio-labelled murine antibody showed that antibody concentrated mainly in the liver (30%), spleen (7.5%) and bone marrow (50%) and only 2.5% of the radiolabelled antibody was found in the inflamed joints[70].

Chimeric anti-CD4 mAb, cM-T412, has been used in a number of clinical trials in refractory RA. Studies thus far have shown that, despite the more prolonged half-life of chimeric antibody, single or weekly doses of cM-T412 have failed to produce any clinical improvement despite extended CD4 lymphopenia[71]. This confirms the experience with murine antibody that peripheral CD4 lymphopenia does not predict clinical response. Daily treatment with cM-T412 was effective in most of the patients[72,73]. Some patients have prolonged disease remission after a single course of treatment (daily cM-T412 for 5–7 days). In others, improvement occurred but relapsed 4–6 weeks after the last treatment. We have made a most interesting observation in a study using daily 50 mg doses of cM-T412 for 5 days: the amount of antibody reaching the synovial joint varies a great deal among patients. Thus, when paired synovial fluid and peripheral blood samples obtained before and after treatment on day 1 and 5 were examined, there was a clear discrepancy between changes in the peripheral blood and synovial fluid[74]. After a single dose of cM-T412 there was a drastic reduction in the number of circulating CD4 lymphocytes in the peripheral blood, the majority of which were coated with the anti-CD4 antibody, while in the synovial fluid the CD4 T-cells changes were minimal after a single dose and only after 5 daily infusions was there a reduction in the number of synovial fluid CD4$^+$ lymphocytes of which a significant percentage were coated with anti-CD4 mAb. Interestingly, CD4 reduction and cM-T412 coating in the synovial fluid was variable. Most importantly, the percentage of synovial fluid CD4 lymphocytes coated with anti-CD4 mAb after 5 daily infusions correlated with the degree of clinical improvement seen after treatment. This suggests that synovial concentration of cM-T412 may be surrogate marker for effective dosing and that efficacy is directly related to the inhibition of events taking place within the joint. One event within the joint of critical importance would be inhibition of T-cells responding to the rheumatoid antigen. Indeed, we have produced *in vitro* evidence to suggest that one mechanism of action by which anti-CD4 mAb may be acting is the induction of antigen specific apoptosis[75]. In these experiments, we showed that if lymphocytes are pre-incubated with cross-linked anti-CD4 mAb, subsequent challenge with cognate antigen does not lead to stimulation and proliferation but to death by apoptosis. Hence, elimination of antigen specific lymphocytes in the joint by apoptosis may explain the long-term disease remission seen in some patients treated with anti-CD4 mAb, but only when it is given in a sufficient dose to enter the joint to coat almost all the synovial CD4$^+$ T-lymphocytes. Thus, the most important question concerning therapy with anti-CD4 mAb is deciding the ideal dose and the treatment regimen to maximize antibody entering the synovial joint in order to induce long-term remission. This raises an important point concerning biological treatment. Antibodies, though highly specific in their target, will bind to many targets which may not be relevant to the pathogenesis of the disease. This is illustrated in the case of anti-CD4 mAb in RA. When antibody is given intravenously, it binds to CD4 molecules on lymphocytes, monocytes and cells of the reticulo-endothelial system. Most of these do not have significant contribution to the inflammatory process in the rheumatoid joint. Only after sufficient antibody has entered the joint, will it be able to ameliorate inflammation by binding to $CD4^+$ lymphocytes to inhibit their function. The majority of the $CD4^+$ lymphocytes at the site of inflammation are recruited non-specifically so that although downregulating their function may reduce inflammation it is unlikely to lead to long-term remission. Only when a high proportion of all the lymphocytes in the joint are coated with anti-CD4 mAb is there a significant chance of eliminating the pathogenic lymphocytes.

The most consistent feature after treatment with anti-CD4 mAb is CD4 lymphopenia. The duration of CD4 lymphopenia is longer with chimeric antibody than murine antibody. Higher dosage also leads to more prolonged depletion. Concomitant treatment with methotrexate undoubtedly leads to severe and prolonged CD4 lymphopenia; this type of combination therapy is therefore to be avoided. The mechanism of CD4 lymphopenia remains unknown but is probably multifactorial: antibody dependent cell-mediated cytotoxicity, antibody mediated clearance by the reticuloendothelial system and complement-mediated lysis which is unlikely since cM-T412 is poor in inducing complement mediated lysis. One of the main worries concerning the prolonged CD4 lymphopenia is the possibility of severe life-threatening infections. Although there is one report only of pneumocytsis pneumonia with death occurring in an elderly patient who was taking steroid and methotrexate concurrently with cM-T412, the cM-T412 was thought not to have been implicated in the cause of death[76]. Hence, to date the fear of infectious complications is more apparent rather than real.

GAMMAGLOBULIN

Although the mechanism of action of gammaglobulin remains unknown, its therapeutic efficacy in certain autoimmune diseases is now well established. Indeed, it is currently the treatment of choice in Kawasaki's disease, a childhood illness characterized by acute systemic vasculitis[77] leading to death through coronary arteritis. High-dose intravenous immunoglobulin (single dose of 2 gm/kg) used early during the disease has dramatically reduced the incidence of coronary abnormalities and mortality.

Gammaglobulin has also been used in systemic juvenile chronic arthritis (Still's disease) with encouraging initial results[78]. When gammaglobulin was given during the acute systemic illness, there was clinical improvement in most of the patients. Childhood dermatomyositis may also respond to high-dose gammaglobulin[79]. In a pilot study, 5 children with steroid resistant juvenile dermatomyositis were treated with high-dose gammaglubulin. All patients improved in muscle strength and the skin rash. As further evidence of efficacy, prednisolone was either discontinued or the dosage reduced in patients after treatment. A larger study involving 20 patients, was conducted by Cherin *et al.* in adult patients with refractory inflammatory myositis[80]. Fourteen patients had polymyositis and 6 had dermatomyositis. The dosage ranged from 0.4–1 gm/kg daily given for 2–5 days each month. Most patients showed clinical and biochemical improvement in disease activity with improvement in muscle strength and decrease in serum creatine kinase. High-dose gammaglobulin has also been used in RA[81]. In an open study, 9 patients with refractory RA were treated with high-dose of gammaglobulin (400 mg/kg) monthly for 6 months. Clinical improvement was seen in most patients although no patient had disease remission. There was no change in the ESR or C reactive protein. Since gammaglobulin has also been shown to be useful in idiopathic thrombocytopenic purpura, two reports have suggested that severe thrombocytopenia due to systemic lupus erythematosus may also respond to high-dose gammaglobulin[82]. Antineutrophil cytoplasmic antibody related vasculitis and Wegener's granulomatosis may also respond to gammaglobulin according to Richter *et al.* who reported 9 such patients[83]. The long-term efficacy of treatment is not yet available.

CYTOKINES AND ANTI-CYTOKINES

As already discussed cytokines have very important regulatory roles in the inflammatory process; it is not surprising, therefore, that several anti-inflammatory cytokines and cytokine antagonists have been used in the treatment of rheumatic diseases.

Interferon gamma

IFN-γ, is an important T-cell cytokine which is secreted by TH1 type T-cells. It is an autocrine growth factor for TH1 cells and inhibits growth of TH2 cells. IFN-γ has many important biological functions including: upregulation of endothelial cells adhesion molecules often in synergy with IL-1 and TNF-α, activation of monocytes to express HLA-DR molecules as well as secretion of various monokines such as IL-1 and TNF-α, has anti-viral properties by inhibiting the replication of herpes simplex type I virus[84], acting synergistically with TNF-α. It has anti-cancer properties possibly by augmenting the immune response[85], inhibits angiogenesis and endothelial cell proliferation[86] and inhibits the development of streptococcal cell wall arthritis in rats[87].

Recombinant IFN-γ has been used in several double-blind placebo controlled trials in RA[88–91]. Direct comparison of these trials is difficult because of the use of different IFN-γ dosages and treatment regimens. It is given as subcutaneous injections in divided doses each day. In general, patients treated with IFN-γ showed significant clinical improvement although placebo treated patients often improved slightly as well although the number of responding patients was greater in the active treatment group. A negative study was reported by Cannon *et al.*[90] but this may have been due to the small number of patients (105 patients) involved in the study and hence the possibility of a type I error cannot be excluded. However, two large studies[88,89] subsequently demonstrated that IFN-γ was superior to placebo in patients with RA. Unfortunately, these studies were mainly short term and the end points were set at 3 or 4 months. Besides clinical improvement, there was also a significant but small decrease in ESR. Interestingly, a decrease in circulating B-cells was noted after treatment although there was no significant change in serum RF titer or immunoglobulin level. The mechanism for this is unknown and it did not correlate with clinical improvement. In the only long-term study there was a high drop out rate (44 out of 70 patients) although some patients had sustained disease improvement[92]. The large number of patients required in order to demonstrate a statistically significant benefit raises the question as to whether the small degree of benefit is clinically and therapeutically useful. The side effects of IFN-γ were fever, chill, myalgia, headache and night sweats, but the treatment was generally well tolerated.

IFN-γ has been used in a single case of systemic lupus erythematosus[93,94] and in an open pilot study in 9 patients with systemic juvenile RA, 7 patients improved[95]. Its exact role in this and other conditions will need to be assessed by further controlled studies.

Interleukin-1 receptor antagonist

IL-1 is a monokine which has pro-inflammatory properties. It is present in two forms: IL-1α and IL-1β, which bind to type I and type II IL-1 receptors (IL-1R) although IL-1α binds better to type I IL-1R while IL-1β binds to type

II IL-1R. Mature monocytes and macrophages have been shown to secrete a IL-1 antagonist interleukin-1 receptor antagonist (IL-1ra). Structurally it is very similar to IL-1α and it competes with IL-1α for the type I IL-1R but itself has no agonist activity. The level of IL-1ra has been shown to be elevated in inflammatory sites such as the rheumatoid joint. *In vitro* it inhibits the action of IL-1 and *in vivo* reduces inflammation in animal models of sepsis, graft vs host disease and arthritis. However, a high excess (10–500 fold) of IL-1ra is required to inhibit 50% of the biological activity of IL-1.

Recombinant IL-1ra was used in an open label phase I study in patients with refractory RA[6]. Fifteen patients were treated with two courses of IL-1ra administered 4 weeks apart. Each course involved IL-1ra being given as subcutaneous injections daily for 7 days. After one course of treatment there was a 50% reduction in the number of tender and swollen joints. There was no change in circulating lymphocyte subsets and lymphocyte proliferation to mitogens and antigens. The only side effect was irritation at the injection site.

Anti-TNF-α monoclonal antibody

TNF-α is thought to have a pivotal role in the pathogenesis of RA[11]. There is no doubt that it is a very potent pro-inflammatory cytokine inducing the secretion of other cytokines including IL-1 and IL-6. Interestingly, transgenic mice, which produce TNF-α in excess, developed a spontaneous inflammatory arthritis[97]. *In vivo* anti-TNF mAb was effective in abrogating the development of collagen type II arthritis in DBA/l mice[98]. Elliott *et al.*[99] used chimeric anti-TNF mAb in 10 patients with refractory RA in an open phase I/II study. Antibody (50 mg/kg) was given as intravenous infusions in two or four doses. The treatment was well tolerated. Significant clinical improvement was seen after treatment in all patients. There was a concomitant decrease in the acute phase reactants including ESR, CRP and in RF. This confirms that TNF-α is a potent inducer of the acute phase response. However, the ability of anti-TNF-α mAb to inhibit the acute phase response may render many acute phase reactants such as ESR and CRP unsuitable for assessment of disease activity in anti-TNF-α mAb treated RA patients. Data on the pharmacokinetics of the chimeric anti-TNF mAb and of the human anti-chimeric antibody response are not yet available.

ADHESION MOLECULES

Anti-ICAM-1 monoclonal antibody

Control of leucocyte migration into inflammatory sites has obvious therapeutic potential. In addition, some adhesion molecules, such as LFA-1, ICAM-1 and VCAM-1, have very important co-stimulatory roles during T-cell activation (Chapter 1).

Antibody directed against LFA-1 given at the time of T-cell activation may produce an anergic signal[9]. This has led to the use of mAb directed against adhesion molecules in autoimmune diseases. Murine anti-CD54 mAb (anti-ICAM-1) was used by Kavanaugh and his colleagues in 15 refractory RA patients[100]. Antibody was given as daily intravenous infusions for 5 consecutive days.. Nine out of 13 patients had >50% disease improvement after treatment but most of the patients relapsed 3 months after treatment. All the patients developed human anti-mouse antibody by day 15. Transient lymphocytosis was noted in all the patients suggesting that anti-CD54 mAb was blocking migration of lymphocytes from peripheral blood into inflammatory sites. This was supported further by the observation that cutaneous response to antigen (tuberculin PPD) was diminished during treatment but returned to normal after treatment. Interestingly, there was no change in circulating neutrophil, monocyte numbers or B-cell numbers. Increases occurred in both

CD4$^+$ and CD8$^+$ lymphocytes and in the naive (CD45RA$^+$) and memory (CD45RO$^+$) subsets. Proliferation of peripheral blood mononuclear cells to anti-CD3 mAb was decreased after treatment. This may be due to inhibition of interaction between T-cells and antigen presenting cells since ICAM-1 is present on antigen presenting cells and interacts with LFA-1 on the surface of T-cells to provide co-stimulatory signals. Serum concentration of anti-CD54 mAb dropped rapidly after treatment. No circulating anti-CD54 mAb was found 1 week after treatment.

CONCLUSION

Research invested into the basic science of the immune response and pathogenic mechanisms in autoimmune diseases have allowed us to generate treatment hypotheses which have been tested both *in vitro* and *in vivo*. With the help of the biotechnology industry, we now have the right tools with which to try to interfere and possibly reprogramme the immune response. Biologics are obviously very different from conventional pharmacological agents and much hard work needs to be done in order to define the correct way of using them. Biologics not only provide us with the opportunity to assess their efficacy as treatments but also as probes by which to gain a greater insight into the immunopathogenetic basis of rheumatic diseases. The ultimate goal in the treatment of autoimmune disease must surely be to translate any successes gained by the use of biologics into the development of simple compounds active orally as this will reduce the cost of the treatment and, hence, make the treatment more widely available unless, of course, treatment with a biologic induces specific tolerance and permanent disease remission.

REFERENCES

1. Braciale, T. J. (1992) Antigen processing for presentation by MHC class I molecules. *Curr. Opin. Immunol.*, **4**, 59–62.

2. Unanue, E. R. (1992) Cellular studies on antigen presentation by class II MHC molecules. *Curr. Opin. Immunol.*, **4**, 63–9.

3. Monaco, J. J. (1992) Major histocompatibility complex-linked transport proteins and antigen processing. *Immunol. Res.*, **11**, 125–32.

4. Auffray, C. and Strominger, J. (1985) Molecular genetics of the human major histocompatibility complex. *Adv. Hum. Gen.*, **15**, 197–247.

5. Brown, J. H., Jardetzky, T., Saper, M. A. *et al.* (1988) A hypothetical model of the foreign antigen binding site of class II histocompatibility molecules. *Nature*, **332**, 845–50.

6. Rudd, C. E. (1990) CD4, CD8 and the TCR-CD3 complex: a novel class of protein-tyrosine kinase receptor. *Immunol. Today*, **11**, 400–6.

7. Mustelin, T. and Altman, A. (1989) Do CD4 and CD8 control T-cell activation via a specific tyrosine protein kinase? *Immunol. Today*, **10**, 189–92.

8. Waldmann, H. and Cobbold, S. P. (1991) Is tolerance therapy a plausible possibility? *Br. J. Rheumatol.*, **30**(suppl 1), 75.

9. Benjamin, R. J. Qin, S. X., Wise, M. P. *et al.* (1988) Mechanisms of monoclonal antibody-facilitated tolerance induction: a possible role for the CD4 (L3T4) and CD11a (LFA-1) molecules in self-non-self discrimination. *Eur. J. Immunol.*, **18**, 1079–88.

10. Sloan-Lancaster, J., Evavold, B. D. and Allen, P. M. (1993) Induction of T-cell anergy by altered T-cell-receptor ligand on live antigen-presenting cells. *Nature*, **363**, 156–9.

11. Brennan, F. M., Maini, R. N. and Feldmann, M. (1991) TNF alpha – a pivotal role in rheumatoid arthritis? *Br. J. Rheumatol.*, **31**, 293–8.

12. Oppenheimer-Marks, N., Davis, L. S., Bogue, D. T. *et al.* (1991) Differential utilization of ICAM-1 and VCAM-1 during the adhesion and transendothelial migration of human T lymphocytes. *J. Immunol.*, **147**, 2913–1921.

13. Shimizu, Y., Newman, W., Gopal, T. V. *et al.* (1991) Four molecular pathways of T cell adhesion to endothelial cells: roles of LFA-1, VCAM-1, and ELAM-1 and changes in pathway hierarchy under different activation conditions. *J. Cell Biol.*, **113**, 1203–12.

14. Makgoba, M. W., Sanders, M. E. and Shaw, S. (1989) The CD2/LFA-3 and LFA-1/ICAM-1 pathways: relevance to T cell recognition. *Immunol. Today*, **10**, 417–22.

15. Romagnani, S. (1991) Human TH1 and TH2 subsets: doubt no more. *Immunol. Today*, **12**, 256–7.

16. Romagnani, S. (1992) Induction of TH1 and TH2 responses: a key role for the 'natural' immune response? *Immunol. Today*, **13**, 379–81.

17. Maggi, E., Parronchi, P., Manetti, R. *et al.* (1992) Reciprocal regulatory effects of IFN gamma and IL-4 on the *in vitro* development of human Th1 and Th2 clones. *J. Immunol.*, **148**, 2142–7.

18. Kohler, G. and Milstein, C. (1975) Continuous cultures of fused cells secreting antibody of predefined specificity. *Nature*, **256**, 495–7.

19. Isaacs, J. D. (1990) The antiglobulin response to therapeutic antibodies. *Semin. Immunol.*, **2**, 449–56.

20. Winter, G. and Milstein, C. (1991) Man-made antibodies. *Nature*, **349**, 293–9.

21. Lazarovits, A. I., Rochon, J., Banks, L. *et al.* (1993) Human mouse chimeric CD7 monoclonal antibody (SDZCHH380) for the prophylaxis of kidney transplant rejection. *J. Immunol.*, **150**, 5163–74.

22. Waldmann, T. A., Pastan, I. H., Gansow, O. A. *et al.* (1992) The multichain interleukin-2 receptor: a target for immunotherapy. *Ann. Intern. Med.*, **116**, 148–60.

23. Gregersen, P. K., Silver, J. and Winchester, R. J. (1987) The shared epitope hypothesis. An approach to understanding the molecular genetics of susceptibility to rheumatoid arthritis. *Arth. Rheum.*, **30**, 1205–13.

24. Metzler, B., Pairchild, P. J. and Wraith, D. C. (1993) MHC binding peptides as therapeutic agents. *Clin. Exp. Rheumatol.*, **11** (Suppl. 8), S45–6.

25. Adorini, L. (1991) Peptide interactions with MHC class II molecules. *Br. J. Rheumatol.*, **30**, 10–13.

26. Cohen, P. L., Naparstek, Y., Ben-Nun, A. *et al.* (1983) Lines of T lymphocytes induce or vaccinate against autoimmune arthritis. *Science*, **219**, 56–8.

27. Lider, O., Reshef, T., Beraud, E. *et al.* (1988) Anti-idiotypic network induced by T cell vaccination against experimental autoimmune encephalomyelitis. *Science*, **239**, 181–93.

28. Lohse, A. W., Bakker, N. P., Hermann, E. *et al.* (1993) Induction of an anti-vaccine response by T cell vaccination in non-human primates and humans. *J. Autoimm.*, **6**, 121–30.

29. van Laar, J. M., Miltenburg, A. M. M.,

Verdonk, M. J. *et al.* (1991) T cell vaccination in rheumatoid arthritis. *Br. J. Rheumatol.*, **30**, 28–9.

30. Kingsley, G., Verwilghen, J., Chikanza, I. *et al.* (1992) T cell vaccination (TCV) in rheumatoid arthritis: a controlled double-blinded pilot study. *Arth. Rheum.*, **35**, S44.

31. Lohse, A. W., Mor, F., Karin, N. *et al.* (1989) Control of experimental autoimmune encephalomyelitis by T cells responding to activated T cells. *Science*, **244**, 820–2.

32. Offner, H., Hashim, G. A. and Vandenbark, A. A. (1991) T cell receptor peptide therapy triggers autoregulation of experimental encephalomyelitis. *Science*, **251**, 430–2.

33. Chou, Y. K., Bourdette, D. N., Offner, H. *et al.* (1992) Frequency of T cells specific for myelin basic protein and myelin proteolipid protein in blood and cerebrospinal fluid in multiple sclerosis. *J. Neuroimmunol.*, **38**, 105–13.

34. Vandenbark, A. A., Bourdette, D. N., Whitham, R. *et al.* (1993) T-cell receptor peptide therapy in EAE and MS. *Clin. Exp. Immunol.*, **11**(Suppl. 8), S51–3.

35. Howell, M. D., Diveley. J. P., Lundeen, K. A. *et al.* (1991) Limited T-cell receptor β-chain heterogeneity among interluekin 2 receptor-positive synovial T cells suggests a role for superantigen in rheumatoid arthritis. *Proc. Natl. Acad. Sci. USA*, **88**, 10921–5.

36. Melamed, D. and Friedman, A. (1993) Direct evidence for anergy in T lymphocytes tolerized by oral administration of ovalbumin. *Eur. J. Immunol.*, **23**, 935–42.

37. Higgins, P. J. and Weiner, H. L. (1988) Suppression of experimental autoimmune encephalomyelitis by oral administration of myelin basic protein and its fragments. *J. Immunol.*, **140**, 440–5.

38. Staines, N A. (1991) Oral tolerance and collagen arthritis. *Br. J Rheumatol.*, **30**, 40–3.

39. Weiner, H. L., Mackin, G. A., Matsui, M. *et al.* (1993) Double-blind pilot trial of oral tolerization with myelin antigens in multiple sclerosis. *Science*, **259**, 1321–4.

40. Trentham, D. E., Dgnesius-Trentham, R. A., Orav, E. J. *et al.* (1993) Effects of oral administration of type II collagen on rheumatoid arthritis. *Science*, **261**, 1727–30.

41. Khoury, S. J., Hancock, W. W. and Weiner, H. L. (1992) Oral tolerance to myelin basic protein and natural recovery from experimental autoimmune encephalomyelitis are

associated with downregulation of inflammatory cytokines and differential upregulation of transforming growth factor beta, interleukin 4, and prostaglandin E expression in the brain. *J. Exp. Med.*, **176**, 1355–64.

42. Dick, A. D., Cheng, Y. F., McKinnon, A. *et al.* (1993) Nasal administration of retinal antigens suppresses the inflammatory response in experimental allergic uveoretinitis. A preliminary report of intranasal induction of tolerance with retinal antigens. *Br. J. Ophthalmol.*, **77**, 171–5.

43. Norment, A. M., Salter, R. D., Parham, P. *et al.* (1988) Cell-cell adhesion mediated by CD8 and MHC class I molecules. *Nature*, **336**, 79–81.

44. Schreiber, S. L. and Crabtree, G. R. (1992) The mechanism of action of cyclosporin A and FK506. *Immunol. Today*, **13**, 136–42.

45. Wells, G. and Tugwell, P. (1993) Cyclosporin A in rheumatoid arthritis: overview of efficacy. *Br. J. Rheumatol.*, **32**(Suppl. 1), 51–6.

46. Hallam, T. J. (1993) Functional significance of protein kinase C in human T-cell activation: a new therapeutic class? *Clin. Exp. Immunol.*, **11**(Suppl. 8), S131–4 (Abstract).

47. Kirkham, B. W., Pitzalis, C., Kingsley, G. H. *et al.* (1991) Monoclonal antibody treatment in rheumatoid arthritis: Clinical and immunological effects of a CD7 monoclonal antibody. *Br. J. Rheumatol.*, **30**, 459–63.

48. Kirkham, B. W., Thien, F., Pelton, B. K. *et al.* (1992) Chimeric CD7 monoclonal antibody therapy in rheumatoid arthritis. *J. Rheumatol.*, **19**, 1348–52.

49. Lazarovits, A. I., White, M. J. and Karsh, J. (1992) CD7-T cells in rheumatoid arthritis. *Arth. Rheum.*, **35**, 615–24.

50. Casali, P. and Notkins, A. L. (1989) CD5⁺ B lymphocytes, polyreactive antibodies and the human B-cell repertoire. *Immunol. Today*, **10**, 364–8.

51. Strand, V., Lipsky, P. E., Cannon, G. W. *et al.* (1993) Effects of administration of an anti-CD5 plus immunoconjugate in rheumatoid arthritis. Results of two phase II studies. The CD5 Plus Rheumatoid Arthritis Investigators Group. *Arth. Rheum.*, **36**, 620–30.

52. Mathieson, P. W., Cobbold, S. P., Hale, G. *et al.* (1990) Monoclonal-antibody therapy in systemic vasculitis. *N. Eng. J. Med.*, **323**, 250–4.

53. Marrack, P., Endres, R., Shimonkevitz, R. *et al.* (1983) The major histocompatibility complex-restricted antigen receptor on T cells. II. Role of the L3T4 product. *J. Exp. Med.*, **158**, 1077–91.

54. Alegre, M. L., Vandenabeele, P., Depierreux, M. *et al.* (1991) Cytokine release syndrome induced by the 145-2C11 anti-CD3 monoclonal antibody in mice: prevention by high doses of methylprednisolone. *J. Immunol.*, **146**, 1184–91.

55. Johnston, J. M., Hays, A. E., Heitman, C. K. *et al.* (1992) Treatment of rheumatoid arthritis (RA) patients by subcutaneous injection of Campath-1H. *Arth. Rheum.*, **35**, S105.

56. Kyle, V., Coughlan, R. J., Tighe, H. *et al.* (1989) Beneficial effect of monoclonal antibody to interleukin 2 receptor on activated T cells in rheumatoid arthritis. *Ann. Rheum. Dis.*, **48**, 428–9.

57. Woodworth, T. G. (1993) Early clinical studies of IL-2 fusion toxin in patients with severe rheumatoid arthritis and recent onset insulin-dependent diabetes mellitus. *Clin. Exp. Rheumatol.*, **11**(Suppl. 8), S177–80.

58. Benjamin, R. J. and Waldmann, H. (1986) Induction of tolerance by monoclonal antibody therapy. *Nature*, **320**, 449–51.

59. Van den Broek, M. F., Van de Langerijt, L. G., Van Bruggen, M. C. *et al.* (1992) Treatment of rats with monoclonal anti-CD4 induces long-term resistance to streptococcal cell wall-induced arthritis. *Eur. J. Immunol.*, **22**, 57–61.

60. van der Lubbe, P. A., Miltenburg, A. M. and Breedveld, F. C. (1991) Anti-CD4 monoclonal antibody for relapsing polychondritis. *Lancet*, **337**, 1349.

61. Choy, E. H., Chikanza, I. C., Kingsley, G. H. *et al.* (1991) Chimaeric anti-CD-4 monoclonal antibody for relapsing polychondritis (letter). *Lancet*, **338**, 450.

62. Wofsy, D. and Seaman, W. E. (1985) Successful treatment of autoimmunity in NZB/NZW mice with monoclonal antibody to L3T4. *J. Exp. Med.*, **161**, 378–91.

63. Hiepe, F., Volk, H., Apostoloff, E. *et al.* (1991) Treatment of severe systemic lupus erythematosus with anti-CD4 monoclonal antibody. *Lancet*, **338**, 1529–30.

64. Horneff, G., Burmester, G. R., Emmrich, F. *et al.* (1991) Treatment of rheumatoid arthritis with an anti-CD4 monoclonal antibody. *Arth. Rheum.*, **34**, 129–40.

65. Reiter, C., Kakavand, B., Rieber, E. P. *et al.* (1991) Treatment of rheumatoid arthritis with monoclonal CD4 antibody M-T151. Clinical

results and immunopharmacologic effects in an open study, including repeated administration. *Arth. Rheum.*, **34**, 525–36.

66. Wendling, D., Racadot, E., Morel-Fourrier, B. *et al.* (1992) Treatment of rheumatoid arthritis with anti-CD4 monoclonal antibody. Open study of 25 patients with the B-F25 clone. *Clin. Rheumatol.*, **11**, 542–7.

67. Horneff, G., Krause, A., Emmrich, F. *et al.* (1991) Elevated levels of circulating tumor necrosis factor-alpha, interferon-gamma, and interleukin-2 in systemic reactions induced by anti-CD4 therapy in patients with rheumatoid arthritis letter. *Eur. Cytokine Netw.*, **3**, 266–7.

68. Horneff, G., Winkler, T., Kalden, J. R. *et al.* (1991) Human anti-mouse antibody response induced by anti-CD4 monoclonal antibody therapy in patients with rheumatoid arthritis. *Clin. Immunol. Immunopathol.*, **59**, 89–103.

69. Horneff, G., Emmrich, F., Reiter, C. *et al.* (1992) Persistent depletion of CD4$^+$ T cells and inversion of the CD4/CD8 T cell ratio induced by anti-CD4 therapy. *J. Rheumatol.*, **19**, 1845–50.

70. Becker, W., Horneff, G., Emmrich, F. *et al.* (1992) Kinetics of 99mTc-labelled antibodies against CD4 (T-helper) lymphocytes in man. *Nuklearmedizin*, **31**, 84–90.

71. Choy, E. H. S., Chikanza, I. C., Kingsley, G. H. *et al.* (1992) Treatment of rheumatoid arthritis with single dose or weekly pulses of chimaeric anti-CD4 monoclonal antibody. *Scand. J. Immunol.*, **36**, 291–8.

72. van der Lubbe, P. A. Reiter, C., Riethmuller, G. *et al.* (1991) Treatment of rheumatoid arthritis with chimaeric CD4 monoclonal antibody. *Arth. Rheum.*, **34**(Suppl), S89.

73. Moreland, L. W., Bucy, R. P., Tilden, A. *et al.* (1993) Use of a chimeric monoclonal anti-CD4 antibody in patients with refractory rheumatoid arthritis. *Arth. Rheum.*, **36**, 307–18.

74. Choy, E. H. S., Pitzalis, C., Kingsley, G. H. *et al.* (1993) Daily treatment with chimaeric anti-CD4 monoclonal antibody (mab): clinical and immunological response in peripheral blood and synovial fluid. *Br. J. Rheumatol.*, **32**, 55.

75. Kingsley, G. H., Choy, E. H. S., Adjaye, J. *et al.* (1993) Induction of apoptosis is one mechanism of action of anti-CD4 monoclonal antibody. *J. Immunol.*, **150**, S5424 (Abstract).

76. Moreland, L. W., Parks, W., Pratt, R. *et al.* (1992) Clinical status of rheumatoid arthritis patients 18 months after treatment with chimaeric anti-CD4 antibody. *Arth. Rheum.*, **35**, S44.

77. Leung, D. Y. (1991) New developments in Kawasaki disease. *Curr. Opin. Rheumatol.*, **3**, 46–55.

78. Fink, C. W. (1990) Medical treatment of juvenile arthritis. *Clin. Orthop. Relat. Res.*, **259**, 60–9.

79. Lang, B. A., Laxer, R. M., Murphy, G. *et al.* (1991) Treatment of dermatomyositis with intravenous gammaglobulin. *Am. J. Med.*, **91**, 169–72.

80. Cherin, P., Herson, S., Wechsler, B. *et al.* (1991) Efficacy of intravenous gammaglobulin therapy in chronic refractory polymyositis and dermatomyositis: an open study with 20 adult patients. *Am. J. Med.*, **91**, 162–8.

81. Muscat, C., Agea, E., Bini, P. *et al.* (1992) Long-term treatment of rheumatoid arthritis (RA) with intravenous gammaglobulin (IVGG). *Clin. Rheumatol.*, **11**, 161.

82. ter Borg, E. J. and Kallenberg, C. G. (1992) Treatment of severe thrombocytopenia in systemic lupus erythematosus with intravenous gammaglobulin. *Ann. Rheum. Dis.*, **51**, 1149–51.

83. Richter, C., Schnabel, A., Csernok, E. *et al.* (1992) Treatment of Wegener's granulomatosis with intravenous immunoglobulin. *Clin. Rheumatol.*, **11**, 161.

84. Balish, M. J., Abrams, M. E., Pumfery, A. M. *et al.* (1992) Enhanced inhibition of herpes simplex virus type 1 growth in human corneal fibroblasts by combinations of interferon-alpha and -gamma. *J. Infect. Dis.*, **166**, 1401–3.

85. Kruit, W. H., Goey, S. H., Monson, J. R. *et al.* (1991) Clinical experience with the combined use of recombinant interleukin-2 (IL2) and interferon alfa-2a (IFN alpha) in metastatic melanoma. *Br. J. Haematol.*, **79**(Suppl. 1), 84–6.

86. Sidky, Y. A. and Borden, E. C. (1987) Inhibition of angiogenesis by interferons: effects on tumor- and lymphocyte-induced vascular responses. *Cancer Res.*, **47**, 5155–61.

87. Allen, J. B., Bansal, G. P., Feldman, G. M. *et al.* (1991) Suppression of bacterial cell wall-induced polyarthritis by recombinant gamma interferon. *Eur. Cytokine Netw.*, **3**, 98–106.

88. Veys, E. M., Mielants, H., Verbruggen, G. *et al.* (1988) Interferon gamma in rheumatoid arthritis – a double blind study comparing human recombinant interferon gamma with placebo. *J. Rheumatol.*, **15**, 570–4.

89. Anonymous (1992) Double blind controlled

phase III multicenter clinical trial with interferon gamma in rheumatoid arthritis. German Lymphokine Study Group. *Rheumatol. Int.,* **12**, 175–85.

90. Cannon, G. W., Pincus, S. H., Emkey, R. D. *et al.* (1989) Double-blind trial of recombinant gamma-interferon versus placebo in the treatment of rheumatoid arthritis. *Arth. Rheum.,* **32**, 964–73.

91. Machold, K. P., Neumann, K. and Smolen, J. S. (1992) Recombinant human interferon gamma in the treatment of rheumatoid arthritis: double blind placebo controlled study. *Ann. Rheum. Dis.,* **51**, 1039–43.

92. Cannon, G. W., Emkey, R. D., Denes, A. *et al.* (1990) Prospective two-year followup of recombinant interferon-gamma in rheumatoid arthritis. *J. Rheumatol.,* **17**, 304–10.

93. Wandl, U. B., Nagel Hiemke, M., May, D. *et al.* (1992) Lupus-like autoimmune disease induced by interferon therapy for myeloproliferative disorders. *Clin. Immunol. Immunopathol.,* **65**, 70–4.

94. Wandl, U. B., Nagel-Hiemke, M., May, D. *et al.* (1992) Lupus-like autoimmune disease induced by interferon therapy for myeloproliferative disorders. *Clin. Immunol. Immunop.,* **65**, 70–4.

95. Pernice, W., Schuchmann, L., Dippell, J. *et al.* (1989) Therapy for systemic juvenile rheumatoid arthritis with gamma-interferon: a pilot study of nine patients. *Arth. Rheum.,* **32**, 643–6.

96. Thompson, R. C. (1993) IL-1 receptor antagonist in arthritis and arthritis models. *Clin. Exp. Immunol.,* **11**(Suppl. 8), S169.

97. Keffer, J., Probert, L., Cazlaris, H. *et al.* (1991) Transgenic mice expressing human tumour necrosis factor: a predictive genetic model of arthritis. *EMBO J.,* **10**, 4025–31.

98. Williams, R. O., Feldmann, M., Maini, R. N. (1992) Anti-tumor necrosis factor ameliorates joint disease in murine collagen-induced arthritis. *Proc. Natl. Acad. Sci. USA,* **89**, 9784–8.

99. Elliott, M. J., Maini, R. N., Feldmann, M. *et al.* (1993) Treatment of rheumatoid arthritis with chimaeric monoclonal antibodies to TNF-α. Safety, clinical efficacy and control of the acute phase response. *Clin. Rheumatol.,* **12**, 34.

100. Kavanaugh, A. F., Nichols, L. A. and Lipsky, P. E. (1992) Treatment of refractory rheumatoid arthritis with an anti-CD54 (intracellular adhesion molecule-1, ICAM-1) monoclonal antibody. *Arth. Rheum.,* **35**, S43.

INDEX

Page numbers appearing in **bold** refer to figures and page numbers appearing in *italics* refer to tables.

Note: Systemic lupus erythematosus is referred to as SLE in sub-headings.

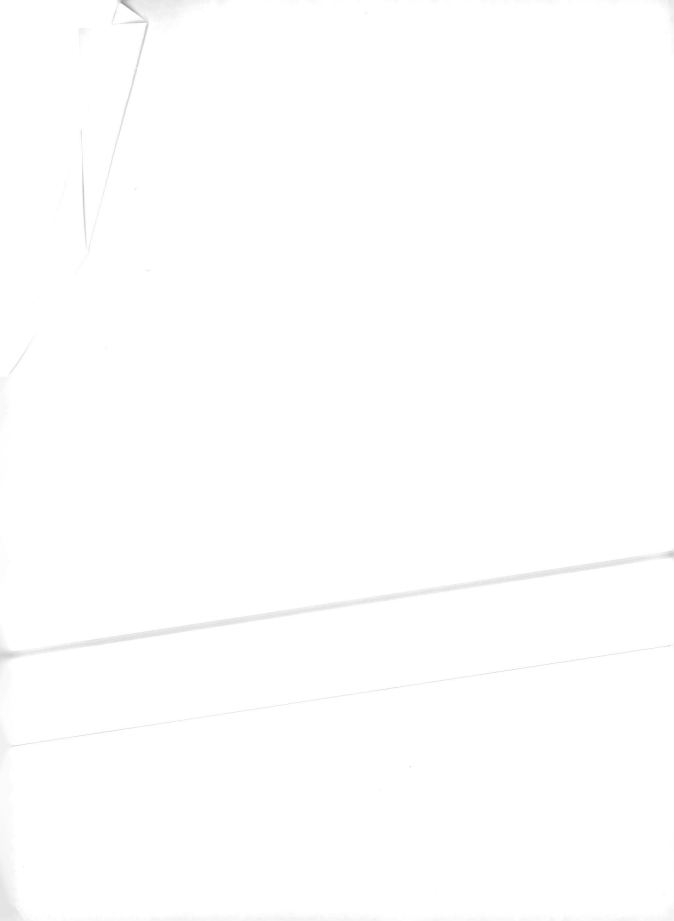